HUMAN LIFE ITS PHILOSOPHY AND LAWS

AN EXPOSITION OF THE PRINCIPLES AND PRACTICES OF ORTHOPATHY

Contents: Health and Its Conditions and Requirements; The Laws of Life; Living Matter Cures Itself; Is Disease Fried or Foe; Early Orthopathic Ideas of Disease; Acute Disease a Curative Process; Self-Limited Disease; The Rational of Inflammation and Fever; Physiological Compensation; Acute Disease not a Radical Cure; Unity of Disease and Symptoms; Causes of Disease; Germs; Perversions; Feeding; Fasting; Sunshine and Sun-Baths; Physical Exercise; Hygiene of Health; Care of Wounds; Place of Art; Passing of the Plagues; Suppression of Disease and its Results; The Declusion of Cure.

Herbert M. Shelton

ISBN 1-56459-714-8

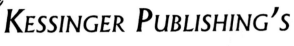
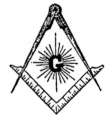

Warning—Disclaimer

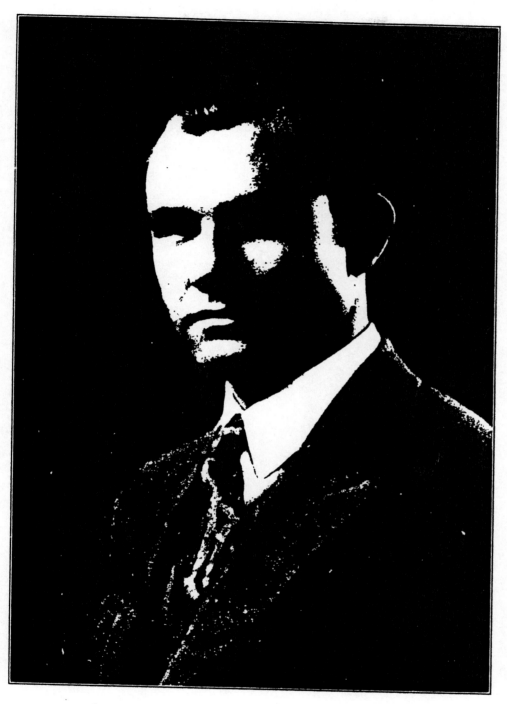

Yours for Health Truth

Herbert M. Shelton

TABLE OF CONTENTS

DEDICATION

To all men everywhere, in all countries, all ages and all professions and all schools of medicine, who have either directly or indirectly contributed to our konwledge of Orthopathy and Orthobionomics, and especially to:

ISAAC JENNINGS
RUSSELL T. TRALL
SYLVESTER GRAHAM
JOEL SHEW
GEORGE H. TAYLOR
ROBERT WALTER
EDWARD H. DEWEY

EMMET DENSMORE
CHARLES E. PAGE
FLORENCE NIGHTENGALE
FELIX L. OSWALD
O. S. FOWLER
JAMES C. JACKSON
JOHN H. TILDEN

This book is respectfully dedicated by

THE AUTHOR.

PREFACE

THE human mind is very largely a product of its environment. It absorbs its food from its surroundings and digests and assimilates this, rejecting some portions of it and organizing the remainder into its own substance. It is for this reason that so few people ever get beyond the age in which they live, and why the vast majority never advance beyond the community in which they reside.

We are prone to regard life as static and to look upon those conditions under which we grow up as the natural and eternal order of things. It is for this reason that we resist change and are often found foes of progress and enlightenment. To the ancients slavery seemed to be the natural order of things and within the lifetime of many now living there were advocates of slavery as a divine institution. The subjection of women was, and yet is, in many quarters, regarded as the natural order of existence. Kings were once thought to be natural institutions and the advocates of the divine rights of kings are not all dead yet. The physician, no less than the layman, is a creature of his education and environment and may be depended on, in the majority of instances, to rely upon the traditions and procedures he has been taught to employ and to be antagonistic to change or innovation or what he may regard as heresy. When education and training have caused a thought to crystalize into habit, its eradication is exceedingly difficult.

Every advance that the human race has made has had to meet and overcome the old order, and because the old order was part and parcel of the makeup of the minds of the period, advance could come only through a mental revolution. People had to be taught to see things differently. They had to learn that progress does not mean the destruction of the universe. They had to acquire a new view of things.

Progress in living reform is no exception to this law of mental evolution. Before men and women can be persuaded to reform their modes of living, they must acquire a new perspective of life. They have to acquire a new understanding of health, a revolutionary new conception of the essential nature of disease, a new attitude towards the body and the laws which govern it, a new view of the causes of disease and of the conditions and requirements of recovery. Living reform must not be looked upon as a cure, which, having accomplished its work of restoring health, can be laid aside like a medicine bottle or a pill box, until one becomes sick again. Living reform requires the individual understanding of the why and wherefore of reform and can never depend on the obedience, by the patient, of his doctor or teacher.

Perhaps nowhere else is a revolution in our thinking more necessary than in our manner of viewing health and disease. Yet, so prone are men and women to regard their own ingrained prejudices as established first principles, that, it is difficult to attack and expose old error without offending those who hold to these. For, men usually regard an attack upon their inherited beliefs and prepossessions as an attack upon their persons. The lapse of time invests old ideas with authority and sanctity and history reveals that but few ever escape from the tyranny of these. This accounts for the persistence of many ancient, coarse and grotesque speculation in what we are pleased to call the *Modern Science of Medicine.*

To primitive man disease was an entity—an unseen evil spirit which attacked him to maim and destroy. He feared it. He surrounded suffering and pain with a psychology of fear, dread apprehension and awe. He did not understand it so he attempted to combat and destroy it. Man knew nothing of the protecting influence of discomfort and pain and, even yet, there are few who are capable of understanding the language of their sensations. They still either ignore them until a formidable and recognizable pathological state has been developed or else they seek to combat or suppress them. For, we still regard disease in the same light with which the "cave-man" viewed it.

Each disease state and each location of an affection came to be looked upon as a specific disease—a "special creation." Due to the persistance of the ancient notion that each form of disease is a "special creation" and to the idea that disease is an entity, an idea that exists, incarnate, in the germ theory, little progress has been made in the field of medicine.

The principles of *Continuity* and *Unity* which underlie all of modern science and which permeate all of its literature, have never found an acceptance in the field of medicine, and particularly in the field of disease, its causation and development.

Another fact—namely, that so-called disease represents a peculiar type of behavior of an organ or a system of correlated organs of the body has yet to find recognition in what is called *Medical Science*. That the symptoms of disease depend on the same vital powers as the signs of health is a fundamental fact of Orthopathy, but un-recognized by medical men. Back of all of these peculiar types of behavior lie the *causes* or *occasions* for this type of behavior and these should be of chief interest to us in preventing or "curing" disease.

Some medical men do recognize asthma, for instance, as merely a peculiar type of behavior of the respiratory apparatus, back of which lie its causes. But they do not recognize that vomiting or diarrhea, or fits and convulsions or inflammation or fever or coughing and sneezing are all mere types of behavior. They completely ignore the fact that the living organism is capable of many and varied and complex responses and reactions to excitation and stimulation and that it behaves in a certain way with reference to a given *cause* or *occasion* for action in obedience to fixed and definite laws of action inherent in living matter. We are watching the behavior of the living being, and not of the dead thing, when we observe the symptoms of disease and the so-called "actions of remedies."

But we must not stop with the recognition that disease action is vital or organic behavior. Vital action is determinate and end-serving. When vomiting serves to eject a poison; when diarrhea eliminates a mass of putrescence; when coughing and sneezing clear the air passages of irritants and obstructions; when inflammation serves to heal a flesh wound, knit a broken bone, or remove a foreign body or an infection from the flesh; and when fever serves to increase cellular activities and heighten the body's toxin-destroying powers, these are all definitely beneficial actions—that is, beneficial to the organism. None of them are so simple as we may at first suppose. Fever, for instance, is not merely a rise in temperature. The rise in temperature is the end-result of a complicated series of antecedent phenomena, all of which work, automatically, towards the end in view—the rise in temperature. The fever then results, automatically, in other actions equally as camplicated. The entire series of phenomena is beneficial and protective, and represent an "organic" unit.

It is upon the above briefly skeletonized theory of the essential nature of disease that Orthopathy is based, and this is the central theme of this book. For writing this book, I deserve either to be crucified as a savior, or hung as a dangerous man. For, this is either the most important book of the kind ever written and brings to its readers the most important message they could possibly receive, or, else, it is the most dangerous book ever published and will be the means of great injury to many.

The philosophy of life, health, disease and cure herein unfolded is either true or false. If true no other book can equal this one in importance—if false, no other book can equal it in potential evil.

The book is not perfect. But I believe the principles herein unfolded are sound and know from experience that they work in practice. I am, at the same time, well aware that many of the details of application yet remain to be fully worked out.

It has taken over two thousand years of human labor and effort to write this book and it required four years for me to put it together. All of us who have labored on the book have worked with an earnestness and a zeal born of white-hot convictions and an honest desire to understand and present the truth on the subjects herein considered. We have only one desire in presenting the book to you—your own good.

THE AUTHOR.

INTRODUCTION

"Nature ever shows the true and perfect way,
Therefore learn betimes ne'er from her path to stray!"

NO man, conscious of his moral integrity, intellectual ability and studied efforts to present what he conceives to be the truth upon any subject will ever apologize for speech or book, hence I offer no apology for having written this book. I deal with a subject which I consider to be one of the highest, if not the highest studies to which the human mind can turn—life, health, disease and correct living. That my subject is unpopular does not frighten nor deter me. Indeed, this is an added incentive to clearly present the matter.

At the outset permit me to disclaim literary merit and originality for most of what is contained in this book. I have spent years in careful and extended research in the field I am here trying to present and, although, much of what I have learned from my studies of the works of others is given in the form of quotations from these works, it is not possible to put it all into this form. I have followed their words very closely in some instances. I do claim originality, although, perhaps not priority, for some of the matter in these pages. But my work has been for the most part, that of sifting, selecting and testing what those who have gone before have left us as a heritage. Several years of experience in caring for the sick and in the use of many and varied means of treating them, followed by more years of experience with the purely hygienic system have proven, to my satisfaction, the truth of what I write in this book.

There is a theory that the Over Lord of the universe selects His instruments by which He releases certain truths from an unfathomable source at stated times, and that these truths are released when the public mind is ready for them. It may be so, I do not know; but I do know that a flood of light broke over the world about a hundred years ago and that it came almost simultaneously from a number of independent sources. The astounding harmony that exists in the teachings promulgated by these various sources and the readiness with which many thousands of people accepted them, would seem to lend credibility to the above mentioned theory. No one mind is capable of grasping all there is to know of truth. Enthusiasm may have blinded some of these men so that they failed to recognize errors that are patent to those who follow, and may have caused some of them to stray, often, from the path of truth, but each man who has identified himself with this movement and who has hesitated to tread the way of digression has done something to advance the truth a little farther towards complete enlightenment.

In its very nature enthusiasm is ardent and streaming. It either moderates as time passes, and dissolves into memory, or, else it cools and hardens into an unshakable conviction, the foundation of which must rest as well in facts as in reason and experience. Enthusiasm gives rise to extremes, and evangelism and these serve their purpose. We have need of the extremest, the dogmatist and the evangelist to arouse the lethargic public to an awareness of a new idea, and during this incubation period it is unavoidable that many errors will be committed. A wise selectionism and differentiationism belongs to experience and a liberal view. Once a new idea is accepted, "the gyroscope of time establishes equilibrium." The Hygienic or Orthopathic movement is now over a hundred years old and has proved itself worthy of a higher place than is accorded it in the minds of the leaders of the world's thought.

At this point a definition of Orthopathy is in order that we may the better understand what we are studying. The following definitions are taken from Jennings, who coined the term Orthopathy to express his conception that *"Nature is always upright—moving in the right direction,"* in disease as in health.

"*Orthopathy:*—From two Greek words,*Orthos,* upright, erect, true, and *pathos,* affection,—right affection. The vital economy always maintains an upright position. The tendency of all her movements, in the lowest depths of disease, as well as in the most vigorous natural action, is as true to the pole star of perfect health, as is the needle to the poles."

To the other systems then in vogue he applied the term *Heteropathy.* It is equally applicable to all systems of today other than the Orthopathic. Defining this last term he says:

"*Heteropathy:*—From two Greek words, *eteros,* another, different, and *Pathos,* affection, changed condition or disease, differing kind from the natural unchanged state; wrong or subservive action. Opposed to orthopathy."—*Philosophy of Human Life.*

The term Orthopathy was coined to express a new conception of the essential nature of disease, a conception that is the very antithesis of the ancient and still prevailing Heteropathic conception. The Orthopathic conception of health and disease leads to pure hygiene, while the Heteropathic tradition places its chief reliance on *therapeutics.* The one is a natural system the other an artificial structure. Therapeutics changes from day to day, hygiene remains always the same. Its principles are eternal.

Dr. Isaac Jennings of Oberlin, Ohio, deserves first mention in any account, however brief, of the development of this movement. In 1822, after twenty years spent in the practice of regular medicine, he gave up the pills, plasters, powders and potions of the saddle bag and launched out into a new and untrodden field. Many experiences during his twenty years of practice had caused him to rely less and less upon the curative agents of the Faculty and more and more upon regimen and the powers of life. In the year 1822 some of his experiences knocked the last remaining props from under his practice and caused him to abandon drugs entirely and rely wholly upon hygiene. But he did not feel that it would be professionally safe to tell his patients of his intentions. Therefore, for the next twenty years, he satisfied their faith in the power of potions to restore health by giving them bread pills, colored water and starch powders.

"Dr. Isaac Jennings, the greatest pathologist (or, at least pathgnomist) of our century, was sadly misunderstood, chiefly, I believe, because he called his plan the 'Let alone plan.' Prevention plan, or Unmedicinal Cure, would have been a better word." Thus spoke Dr. Felix Oswald, *Physical Education,* p. 200, a Prince of Hygienists, of Dr. Jennings. Of Jennings, N. Bedortha, declared in a lecture on *Medical Reform,* which appeared in *The Water-Cure Journal,* of August, 1853:

"We have one more of the wonders of medical reform which we will mention. This had its origin in the State of Connecticut, the land of wooden nutmegs and other yankee notions. A pupil of the celebrated Prof. Ives, of New Haven, a man of science and good practical common sense and judgment, having commenced a course of medical practice under very favorable auspices, and while in the tide of prosperity, and enjoying a good share of popular favor, was seized with the very unpopular idea, that he was doing his patients more harm than good by the system of drug medication he had been taught to practice. Under this conviction he began to practice some duplicity upon his patients, and instead of giving them medicines, he gave those who were not seriously ill bread pills and cold water drops under the name of medicine. These he found worked admirably, and emboldened by his success, he ventured still further, and after a time he treated the most serious and complicated diseases with his bread pills and pure water. For fifteen or twenty years he continued his experiments, becoming more and more confirmed in his novel practice, until his mind became fully settled in its convictions, when he burst the bubble he had been so long inflating and came out before his medical brethren and before the world a sworn enemy to all drug medication.

"Surprise and chagrin seized his medical friends, but the effect upon the community in which he practiced was various. Some denounced him as an imposter, unworthy of confidence or patronage, and ready to stone him for deceiving them; while others, who were the more elevated portion, though confounded by the ruse practiced upon them, took the doctor by the hand and said, 'if you can cure our diseases without the use of medicine, then you are the doctor for us.' Thus encouraged, he went forward with his reform till he had perfected a theory of disease and of medical practice entirely diverse from any which had preceded him. Disease in his theory is a unit, and the manifestations of disease in the forms of fever, coughs, colds, etc., are kindly efforts of nature entirely true to the laws of life and health, which cannot be aided by any system of drug medication whatever, relying solely upon the *vis med. naturae*, placing the patient in what he supposes is the best possible condition by rest, pure air, and proper diet. This man is Isaac Jennings, of Cleveland, Ohio. He still lives to advocate his theory with much zeal. He has written two books in defense of his system, which he styles Orthopathy. He has never succeeded to any great extent in getting his practice into popular favor, although he has some warm friends who have adopted his views."

In his justly famous lecture on "*The True Healing Art, or Hygienic vs. Drug Medication*," delivered in the Smithsonian Institute, Washington, D. C., in February, 1862, Dr. Trall said of Jennings:

"Who has not heard of Dr. Jennings, now of Oberlin, Ohio? Some years ago he practiced medicine in Derby, Conn. Being a close observer and a very conscientious man, and, withal, something of a philanthropist, he became a 'reformer,' and what all true reformers must be in the world's estimation a 'radical' and 'Ultraist,' a 'one-idealist,' a 'fanatic,' etc. He became fully convinced that the system of drug medication was all wrong; that drugs instead of curing persons, or aiding nature to cure them, really hindered the cure, or changed the primary malady to a drug disease as bad or worse; and to put the matter to the proof, he practiced for several years without giving a particle of medicine of any kind. But his patient's did not know it. The people did not mistrust that they were *humbugged* out of their diseases; cheated into health; deceived into saving the greater part of their doctor's bills, all of their opothecary's bills, and the better part of their constitutions. Under Dr. Jennings' administration, diseases seemed to have lost all their malignancy and danger, and to have assumed a singularly mild and manageable form, type, and diathesis. He gave harmless placebos—colored water, sugar pellets, and starch powders—to keep up confidence and furnish the mind with some charm of mysteriousness to rest its faith upon, and then he directed such attention to hygienic conditions as would enable nature to work the cure in the best possible manner and in the shortest possible time.

"His success was remarkable. His fame extended far and wide. The praises of his wonderful skill were heard in all the regions roundabout. In a few years, having conclusively demonstrated the principle involved, he disclosed to his medical brethren the secret of his extraordinary success. And do you think that they were all swift to adopt the no medicine plan of Dr. Jennings? Not quite—no, not one of them. Dr. Jennings has not at this day a single disciple, perhaps in all Connecticut. The Connecticut doctors all thought, doubtless, with Dr. Flint, of New York, 'This no-medicine plan may do in public hospitals, but it will never answer in private families. It may do for Dr. Jennings or for the people, but will never answer for us.' "

This reference to Professor Austin Flint, M. D., then of the New York Medical College, really related to a statement made by Dr. Flint, only a few weeks previously, in a *clinical* lecture to his class of medical students that in treating pneumonia in the hospitals he did not give any medicine at all and lost no patients. In speaking of private families, the professor said, "There it would not do to refuse to prescribe medicine." At that time the deaths from pneumonia in private families in New York were thirty to forty a week.

In his *Exact Science of Health*, pp. 238-9, (1903) Dr. Robert Walter, then an old man and a graduate of Dr. Trall's school, declared of Jennings:

"A leading thought of our system was imbibed from the writings of Dr. Isaac Jennings, of Oberlin, Ohio. Dr. Jennings was a regular practitioner of the old school who located at Oberlin in its early days. He had a remarkable experience; was twenty years a regular practitioner; twenty years a practitioner with bread pills and colored water, and twenty years he practiced with no medicine or any other treatment than simple nursing, and claimed to enjoy wonderful success in the later years. In these years he sought to establish a system that he called Orthopathy. His leading thought was, 'Disease is right action'; when the patient is very low his vitality is being recuperated, and when he is active, he is expending it in doing work, but in either case nature is doing the right thing."

Again he says, *Life's Great Law*, p. 178:

"Dr. Isaac Jennings, of Oberlin, Ohio, had a wonderful success fifty years ago in the treatment of fevers, choleras, etc., by the use of bread pills and colored water—a success which there is reason to believe has never been equaled in purely medical practice."

Jennings says he was well satisfied with the early part of his practice, but before long began to suspect there was something wrong. A number of cases conspired to shake his faith. He also found, as did Trall, that the older physicians gave less medicine than the younger ones, and "were much more wary in their interference with disease, or attempts to break it up." Older physicians with whom he often consulted and whose opinions he respected, cautioned him against a free use of medicine and told him that many cases would get well quicker without than with medicine.

A case which came under his observation in the summer of 1815 served greatly to give bent to his new investigations. A family was suffering with a fever. He was in attendance. While on one of these calls the head of the house called him back, as he was preparing to leave and asked him to tell him what ailed him as he had not been well for a few days. He presented the "characteristic symptoms of the prevailing fever fully developed." The doctor began to re-open his saddle bags, in order to supply him with medicine. The man objected, saying that should he grow worse he would send for him. Jennings says:

"A number of days elapsed without my seeing or hearing anything of Mr. P., when on passing near his house, I saw him in a lot nearby at work. Jumping from my horse, I went to him to ascertain what had become of his fever. To my surprise, I found that he had recovered entirely from his indisposition, and that too without the use of any medicine or means of any kind to arrest the disease.

"All that he had done was to keep quiet, refrain from eating while his appetite was lacking, and drinking freely of water as long as his febrile thirst called for it.

"Up to that time I had attended a large number of cases of fever in that district that season, and in no instance had one recovered in so short a time, or with so mild a set of symptoms as had Mr. P.; and yet, I had spared no pains in giving those whom I had treated the best possible chance—according to my sense of what was best in the cases—for recovering rapidly, safely and thoroughly, entirely eradicated of disease. I had watched the progress of disease by night and by day; had been prompt in meeting the symptoms with the kind and degree of remedial force that the respective cases seemed to call for, and apparently too, with signal success;—for I seldom made a prescription without seeing, or fancying I saw, good results; and my patients and their friends were satisfied, yea, more than satisfied with my practice. I obtained and enjoyed their warmest approbation, and their strongest confidence; and the enjoyment was heightened by a conviction that they were merited for I could but indulge the belief that I had used due and exemplary diligence in qualifying myself for the important post which I then occupied.

"This case was, indeed, a severe rebuke to professional greatness, but I felt unwilling to lose the benefit which the lesson was calculated to teach.

"From this time my large saddle-bags were thrown out of employment, and it was not long before a small pair that had taken the place of the large ones, shared the same fate, and a pocket or two made to carry all the medicine I judged to be necessary in my practice."

Bread-pills, sugar pills, starch powders and colored water soon took the place of the medicines and he embarked upon what he calls his bread-pill practice.

"At the time I launched forth into the 'do-nothing' mode of treating diseases," he says, "vigorous practical medicine was the vogue of the day. Popular teachers and leading medical men discarded the doctrine of 'cure by expectation,' which had been brought considerably into notice and practice in the preceeding century, by *Van Helmont*, *Stahl*, and others, as based upon a fanciful and visionary theory, and tending only to the use of inert and frivolous remedies, and on the contrary, recommended bold and energetic practice; and in this common sentiment I had participated largely, while a student of medicine, and in the first years of my medical life. It was no light affair therefore, to face square about on a subject which involved human lives, and attempt to stem the long established, broad, deep and powerful professional current, aware too, as I was, that such a course would be likely to alienate me from the warm affection and sympathy of those with whom I had taken sweet counsel, and whose favor was as dear to me as the apple of my eye."—*Introduction to Philosophy of Human Life.*

His lancet, also, was sheathed, and no more blood did he spill for the sick. His debut in medicine was "made under the flag of *Cullen*," he was now sailing under a new flag the *no-medicine practice*. "After having thoroughly tested the 'no-medicine' practice in disguise," and having reached a point where he "was able to give a reason for the course" he "was pursuing," he "made a full disclosure of his "pathological views, and general plan of treating disease" to confidential friends and, later, to the whole world.

Jennings wrote three books as follows, "Medical Reform," 1847, "Philosophy of Human Life," 1852, "Tree of Life, or Human Degeneracy, its Nature and Remedy, as based on the Elevating Principle of Orthopathy," 1867. This last was published just 45 years after he had forever broken away from drugs and treatments. However, he was not a crusader. A busy practice kept his nose to the grinding stone. A few physicians took up his work, but they were unable to follow the master all the way. When Dr. Jennings died, Orthopathy ceased to be heard of, although the influence of his work is still felt. It had a great influence upon Dr. R. T. Trall who will be discussed later. With Jennings, began the Hygienic movement.

In 1799 there was born in Austria a man who was destined to make medical history. This man, Vincent Priessnitz, a Presasant, opened the world's first "water cure" institution at Greaffenberg in the Silesian mountains in 1826. He had had but little education, but according to his biographers, was a natural genius in the "healing art." His institution grew, its fame spread throughout the world, others took up his methods and "water cure" institutions sprang up everywhere. By 1853 there was not less than seventy-five such establishments in the United States.

The "water cure," often called, also the "cold water cure," was the parent of modern hydrotherapy. It was, and is, only a palliative method with little or no virtue to commend it to the hygienist. However, the water cure broadened out, and long before Priessnitz's death, it gave much attention to hygiene, particularly to diet, exercise and out door life. Several names are linked with the early days of the "water cure" in Europe chief among which are, Rausse, Hahn, and Metcalf. Priessnitz died in 1851.

The medical profession has adopted hydrotherapy but claims Winternitz as its father. Winternitz studied water-cure under Kneipp who in turn had studied under Priessnitz.

The next great apostle of Hygiene, a man who exerted a great and profound influence upon his contemporaries, and whose influence is not yet dead, despite the efforts of many to supplant him with German Water-Cure pioneers, was Sylvester Graham. Graham was born in 1794 and was the 17th child of his father. He was descended from a family of some distinction and in the reign of George I, one branch of the family was promoted to the title of Duke of Montrose. It was in 1718 that the Rev. John Graham, after being graduated at Oxford, arrived in Boston, Mass. Sylvester Graham was his last child. He was of a "nervous mental temperament," a very weak and delicate child whose life was despaired of. At the age of 16, he developed symptoms of tuberculosis of the lungs. After various attempts at a career, all of which were wrecked by ill health, he entered Amherst College in 1823 to prepare himself for the ministry. It was here that he proved himself to be a talented orator, as well as being gifted with writing poetry and drawing portraits. While in college he studied anatomy and physiology.

Before the fame of Peissnitz had reached America and before the name of Jennings had gone abroad, Graham came forward as a champion of Hygiene and living reform.

Graham was too sincere to remain in the ministry. He was a truly religious man, and it seems was desirous of doing something of real and lasting good for his fellow-men. In 1830 he was engaged by the Pennsylvania Temperance Society to present the cause of Temperance. Two years later, 1832, he became conspicuous as the advocate of the principles set forth in his "Lectures on the Science of Human Life." These principles were first put forth as a preventive of cholera, and thousands followed his advice with beneficial results. He says:

"But the most signal demonstration of the truth of the principles which I am contending for, was afforded in the city of New York during the prevalence of cholera in the summer of 1832. The opinion had been imported from Europe, and generally received in our country, that a generous diet embracing a large proportion of flesh-meat, flesh-soups, etc., with a little good wine, and a strict abstinence from most fruits and vegetables, were the very best means to escape an attack of that terrible disease. Nearly four months before the cholera appeared in New York, I gave a public lecture on the subject in that city, in which I contended that an entire abstinence from flesh meat and flesh-soups, and from all alcoholic and narcotic liquors and substances, and from any kind of purely stimulating substances, and the observance of a correct general regime in regard to sleeping, bathing, clothing, exercise, the indulgence of the natural passions, appetites, etc., would constitute the surest means by which anyone could rationally hope to be preserved from an attack of that disease. I repeated this lecture after the cholera had commenced its ravages in the city. Notwithstanding the powerful opposition to the opinions which I advanced, a very considerable number of citizens strictly adhered to my advice. And it is an important fact that of all who followed my prescribed regime uniformly and consistently, not one fell victim to that fearful disease, and very few had the slightest symptoms of an attack."

Medical men in Graham's day were no different in their intolerant attitude towards the ideas of others than they are now. They opposed and misrepresented him, as they do all who present the same principles today. In a foot-note Graham adds:

"During the prevalence of cholera in New York in 1832, it was most extensively, clamourously, and continually asserted, that the 'Grahamites' were dying by scores with the epidemic, and this opinion has gone abroad through the country, and is perhaps generally believed. Yet I solemnly declare that I made the most diligent search in every part of the city where any such case was reported, and called on every physician who I heard had made any such assertion, and in the newspapers of the city, publically called for the specification and proof of such cases, yet I could not find a single instance in which an individual who had adopted and consistently observed the regime I had prescribed had died of cholera or any other disease, and but two or three instances in which there had even been a slight attack, and in each of these there had been decided imprudence."

J. Bradford, Sax, of West Aurora, New York, in his "The Organic Laws" (1851), confirms Graham's statements in these words:

"During the prevalence of cholera in New York, in 1832, not a single 'Grahamite,' and they were quite numerous, died of the epidemic. Only two or three were slightly attacked, and they had been decidedly imprudent."

As an evidence of the lay and medical ignorance against which Graham had to battle in his fight for living reform, I offer the following resolution, by the Board of Health of Washington, on August 16, 1832:

"The Board of Health, after mature deliberation, have Resolved, and they do now Declare, that the following articles are, in their opinion, highly prejudicial to health at the present season. Believing them, therefore, in the light of nuisances they hereby direct that the sale of them, or their introduction within the limits of this city be prohibited from and after the 22nd instant, for the space of ninety days:

"Cabbage, green-corn, cucumbers, peas, beans, parsnips, carrots, egg plants, cimblings or squashes, pumpkins, turinps, watermelons, cantaloupes, muskmelons, apples, pears, peaches, plums, damsons, cherries, apricots, pineapples, oranges, lemons, limes, cocoanuts, ice-creams, fish, crabs, oysters, clams, lobster and crawfish.

"The following articles the Board have not considered it necessary to prohibit the sale of, but even these they would admonish the community to be moderate in using:

"Potatoes, beets, tomatoes and onions."

Against such ignorance, Graham had an easy battle. There was no one to oppose him—that is no one worthy to fight. His lectures were well received every where and the Grahamites multiplied rapidly. The *Graham Magazine* and other magazines of a similar nature grew and spread the message far and wide. Hotels and eating houses were opened to feed the Graham diet. Many men of prominence and influence in that day, joined the ever growing ranks of the Grahamites, and the mighty movement for Living Reform, Medical Reform and Hygiene went forward by leaps and bounds. Some idea of the influence Graham exerted, especially upon the reform schools of that day, is gained from the remark made by Dr. Trall, that Graham knew more of the human body than any other man that had ever lived.

His "*Lectures on the Science of Life,*" was first published in 1837. It was a veritable encyclopedia and ran through many editions.

His premature death in 1851 was due largely to the fact that he worked himself to exhaustion in the cause he was advancing, and partly to the fact that in his extremity he forgot his principles and permitted the doctors to give him stimulants.

The great evangelist and crusader in the cause of Hygeiotherapy, as he called it, was Russel Thacker Trall, M.D. Dr. Trall was born in Conn., in 1812, and after graduating from a regular or Allopathic school of medicine, he practiced in the regular way for twelve years. He was one of those rare genuises who help to make every year of the world's history an epoch of progress.

It is evident from a remark made in after years by one of the professors under whom he studied, that Trall's was an independent and thinking mind, even while in medical college. The old professor said to one of the readers of Trall's Journal (The Water-Cure Journal), "I NEVER EXPECTED TRALL TO AMOUNT TO MUCH."

Shortly after Graham began his lectures and writings, this bold and fearless champion of the hygienic system, who was destined to eclipse all his predecessors and contemporaries, and who had grown tired of writing prescriptions in Latin almost before he had begun the practice, joined the ranks of the Hygienists. To the untiring efforts and indomitable spirit of this man, hygienists of today owe much more than most of them realize. He worked vigorously as a writer, lecturer, and teacher. One of his pupils declared him to be "the master mind among them, (the Hygienists) in America, at least."

Shortly after the first reports of the success of the "water-cure" reached America, he, along with several other American physicians, sailed to Europe to investigate and study this new method. However, influenced more by the works of Jennings and Graham than by that of Preissnitz, Dr. Trall built up a system which he called Hygieo-therapy. Something of the influence which Graham exerted upon him may be gained from the fact that, he stated that Graham knew more about the human body than any other man who had ever lived. Graham founded no healing system and developed no "cures." His system was purely hygienic. Dr. Dodds records the following:

"In the history of this world-wide reform the fact must ever remain, that while Hydropathy paved the way for the introduction of Hygeiotherapy, it was Trall who reduced the new methods to a science. ·He combined in one great system the use of *all* the hygienic agents; though many of his best thoughts on dietetics, etc., were derived from Dr. Sylvester Graham, who was his intimate friend, and perhaps equally talented. Trall once said of Graham that he came as near discovering the truth of Hygeiotherapy as any one could, not to do it."—*Drugless Medicine*, p. 117.

Again she says of him:

"The mind of Trall was strictly analytical; he examined his premises carefully, and conclusions were logically drawn. The doctrines that he advanced, whether in *Life Illustrated*, the *Water Cure Journal*, or in his books, were not only interesting and instructive, but sensational. No such brilliant thinking on these subjects had before been done. The consequence was, that his writings though revolutionary and schismatic were carefully studied, and often severally criticized. Trall was then in the zenith of his intellectual powers. His thoughts were clean cut, his arguments forcible; and woe to the adversary who challenged him to debate. He always came out victor. The

truth as he portrayed it was so self-evident, that his readers wondered why these things had not occurred to them before. By his admirers he was loved and venerated in the highest degree; by his adversaries he was hated, and often misrepresented. But in the work to which he gave his life he was without a peer; and the principles that he has left behind him will remain as a perpetual legacy to mankind. Through his writings alone, the name of Trall will long be a household word in this and other lands. There are thousands yet unborn, who will live to do him honor, to render that tardy justice, which, though it come late, is due to the brave and fearless pioneer of a great reform."
—*Drugless Medicine*, pp. 114-15.

He began an investigation of the premises of medicine and their relation to Nature, and finding them, as he said, "self-evident absurdities," set himself to the task of discovering the premises that must underlie any true system of caring for the well and sick.

He was both an iconoclast and a builder. Without a doubt he was one of the most prodigious workers who ever lived; and it is largely due to his untiring labors that the Nature Cure movement made the progress it did in those early days of its history. He was a missionary, crusader, scholar, thinker, writer, lecturer, professor, editor, and a physician all wrapped up in one bundle.

Dr. Dodds says of him:

"Like many other distinguished men, Trall was not a born financier. Possibly it was just as well that he was not. It has been truly said, that to plan and execute even one great and good enterprise is more than has fallen to the lot of most men. Dr Trall undertook a work so extensive that it could scarcely be compassed by a single mind. First, he must shake the public confidence in an institution venerable with age, its history reaching far back into the shadows of the past. Next, he must place in its stead a new system, in every way unlike the old, and with scarcely a friend to defend it. The principles underlying it must also be clearly expounded, and speedily put into practice. How much of this work he actually did is next thing to marvelous; and his failures, if such they were, might rather be termed successes, judged by the immense progress that has been made in hygiene since his death. He left the work clearly defined, so clearly indeed, that those who followed had but to pick up the broken threads of the warp, splice them, and weave on; filling in woof, and completing the wonderful web whose patterns he was permitted only to design."—*Drugless Medicine*, p. 115.

Speaking of the many works undertaken by Trall, Dr. Dodds says:

"He even essayed to do more; he desired to found a college in which the principles of hygeiotherapy should be taught. And but for the lack of financial aid, not to say active sympathy which would have secured it, the college might have been successful, and alive today. It was founded in 1852; though the charter was not obtained until 1857. For twenty years and more, from the different states in the Union, from the Canadas and even from abroad, there came to him men and women to learn those great principles which he was expounding in his books, and also teaching year after year to his medical classes. In the meantime, financial disaster overtook him, leaving him completely bankrupt; and his death, hastened no doubt, by his reverses, occurred in 1877, putting an end to the college as well as to his other work."—*Drugless Medicine*, p. 116.

The New York Hydropathic and Physiologist School, the name of which was later changed to The New York College of Hygeo-Therapy, was founded by Dr. Trall and first opened its doors Oct. 1, 1853. In 1857, it was chartered under the laws of the State of New York, with the right to confer the degree *Doctor of Medicine*. This seems to be the only degree it ever conferred upon its graduates. Both sexes were admitted to the college, a very daring thing for a medical school to do in those days.

It was not until during the War for Southern Independence that Medicine, teaching and clerical work was opened to women. Trall was ever in the forefront of progress and reform.

This school, located at 15 Laight St., near St. John's Park, New York City, was well equipped with apparatus and laboratory and a large library. Students received practical work in Trall's Hydropathic and Hygienic Institute, "a commodious establishment," located at the same address and which was "the oldest and most extensive water-cure in the United States." Students visited the hospitals of the city on Saturday afternoons. Clinics were held on Fridays. In 1854 the college announced:

"The course of instruction in this Institution embraces not only all the positive facts and ascertained principles of Medical Science taught in other schools, and the theory and practice peculiar to the Hydropathic system, but contemplates also, a critical examination of all past and existing systems, with a recognition of whatever truths they embody, and an exposition and recognition of the falsities they contain. It embraces indeed, a much wider range of subjects than are taught, or even introduced, into any other Medical School."

The school taught its students the following subjects: Anatomy, Physiology, Chemistry, Organic Chemistry, Pathology, Psychology, Hygiene, Dietetics, Calesthenics, Theory and Practice of the "Healing Art," diagnosis, Therapeutics, Jurisprudence, nature cure, water cure, and other subjects. Students were given work in Dissection, and the school taught subjects supplementing High School Education. Its methods of teaching represented a radical departure from the methods then in vogue and were more in keeping with the more advanced principles of the newer educational methods of today.

Among its list of Faculty members are the following names:

Dr. R. T. Trall, Institutes of Medicine, Materia Medica, Female diseases; G. H. Taylor, M.D., Chemistry, Surgery, Obstetrics; James Hambleton, M.D., Anatomy, Physiology, Hygiene; J. E. Snodgrass, M.D., Medical Jurisprudence; H. F. Briggs, M.D., Philosophy of voice and speech; Asa Christie, M.D., Medical and Special Gymnastics; L. N. Fowler, Phrenology and Mental Science; Miss A. S. Cogwell, Chemistry and Physiology; Joel Shew, M.D., taught regularly for the first term of the school, after this he lectured occasionally.

Graduates of this college held commissions in the Medical Corps of the Federal Armies during the War for Southern Independence and have a very good record. Of this Trall declared while the war was still on:

"I have visted the camp and hospitals of our armies in this vicinity, and I learned —just what I knew before. One of the surgeons told me yesterday that his regiment was the most healthy one in the department. *He gives no medicine*, and his associate almost none. They have had several cases of *typhoid fever*, many cases of *pneumonia*, and some hundreds of cases of dysentery to treat, and have lost none.

"I will not mention their names here, for prudential reasons. It might compromise their position. But when this war is ended—on or before the Fourt of July I hope —the names will be given to the world, and these facts will be certified. Suffice it to say now that they are of my school and my faith."—*True Healing Art.*

In 1861 the College presented a petition to the legislature of New York asking this body to endow the college and the hospital connected therewith. Among the reasons set forth as entitling the college to an endowment were:

"The general design and object of this school are preeminently beneficent, and calculated to promote the welfare of mankind more directly and effectually, perhaps, than any educational institution in the world (not of a religious character) in diffusing abroad a knowledge of the laws of life and the conditions of health, so as to prevent or lessen sickness in the community, and to teach a safe, sure, and economical method of curing all curable persons; and in thus accomplishing the purposes of this School, the people are necessarily indoctrinated into the principles, and led into the practices, which correct injurious personal habits, reform morbid appetences, establish hygienic rules, improve social usages, and lay the foundation for permanent temperance, health, virtue and happiness.

"The special purpose of this school is to qualify, male and *female* practitioners of the Healing Art in accordance with the principles of the *Hydropathic*, or more properly, the *Hygienic or Hygeio-Therapeutic System*, which we believe to be the *true medical system;* and also, in the language of its charter, 'to educate and send into the fields of Human Progress competent Health-Reform Teachers and Lecturers.' Much has been already accomplished in the furtherance of these purposes. Already the graduates of this school number nearly *two hundred*, nearly one half of whom are females; and the majority of them are now gaining an independent livelihood for themselves, while they are more successfully treating the maladies of their patients by the employment of simple hygienic agencies alone, than is done, or can be done, by the physicians of any other school or system.

"Health is pre-eminently the great want of the age. A precise, intimate, and practical knowledge of its conditions, and of the circumstances which induce disease, as well as of the way to remove diseases without incurring other evils as great, or worse, is the great need of the people. We believe the physical salvation of the race depends on it. *In no medical school on earth except this are these things taught*, nor are they pretended to be taught in any other. On these points, we speak advisedly.

"*The Hygeio-Therapeutic College* has inaugurated a new era in medical science. Its advent is an epoch in the Healing Art. It was the first medical school in the world—and so far the only one—to adopt hygienic or normal agencies, as *light, air, temperature, water, food, sleep, clothing, exercise and rest, bathing, electricity, or magnetism, mental influences, etc.*, exclusively in the treatment of diseases, rejecting wholly and totally, as not only unnecessary, but injurious, each and all of the *poisons* known to the *materia medicas* of other medical schools, under the name of 'drug medicines.'

"It has not only introduced a new *materia medica* and a new practice, but also a new theory and philosophy of medical science, at variance with and in opposition to all of the fundamental doctrines or dogmas on which medical systems have heretofore been built. In a word, it claims to have ignored the falsities of the old systems, and to have based its philosophy and its practice on the *unerring and demonstrable laws of nature;* while its practitioners claim to be successful in the treatment of all forms of disease, to an extent unheard of before in the world's history, and unknown to any other medical school."

"Hygeio-Therapy (erroneously called 'Hydropathy,' or 'water-cure'), "he declared, "restores the sick to health, by the means which preserve health in well persons." "Diseases should not be 'cured.' So long as causes exist, the disease should continue. But the causes of disease should be removed and the patient cured." "Truly remedial agents are materials and influences which have *normal* relations to the vital organs, and not drugs, or poisons, whose relations are *abnormal* and *anti-vital.*"—*The Hygienic System.*

In a lecture to one of his classes he once made the following remarks which show unmistakably that he was working for a disease-free and doctor-independent world:

"I cannot forbear a word in allusion to the prospects before us in a business point of view The system which we advocate naturally and necessarily destroys the professional business and emoluments of its practitioners. If we cannot practice the Healing Art with a higher motive than to get a profitable trade out of the ignorance and falsities and infirmities of society, it would be well for us, and better for the world, if we should seek some other vocation. We cannot practice our system without educating the people in its principles. No sooner do they comprehend them, than they find themselves capable of managing themselves, except in rare and extraordinary cases, without our assistance. Not only this but our patrons learn from our teachings, examples, and prescriptions, how to live so as to avoid, to a great extent, sickness of any kind. When you become physicians, you will be continually teaching the people how to do without you. You must, therefore, continually extend your field of practice by making new converts, or your occupation will soon be gone. And whenever the world becomes so intelligent as to adopt our system in all of its parts, to the exclusion of all others, they will be their own doctors. They will not need us; indeed, there will then be no practitioners of medicine in demand, or in existence, except *male* surgeons and *female* midwives."—*The Hygienic System.*

The "Civil" War came very near wrecking the college and it did not long survive the war. As a matter of fact, the War set our movement back at least a hundred years. We can truthfully claim that we are now where we were in 1853. Our movement only began to revive about thirty years ago, since which time, we have been making great gains.

Dr. Robert Walter, one of Trall's illustrious students says:

"In speaking of my predecessors I ought not to neglect the teachings of Drs. Russell T. Trall, and James C. Jackson, to whom I am indebted for valuable truth. Dr. Trall was an acute thinker and had many valuable ideas, but because of an unfortunate mental constitution, aggravated by his extreme notions of diet, he was extremely narrow, and his practice was an utter failure. A man of few words, he was equally a man of limited resources; the very elements which made him a successful popular writer made him also utterly impracticable. Jackson, on the contrary, was resourceful, eloquent, voluble, but eminently practical, even though his theories were quite indefinite. The one rock on which these men foundered was vegetarianism; their antipathy to the use of drugs as medicines was their typical virtue. If the so-called hygienic school of practice would really accord to nature the opportunity, as well as the power of cure, and cease their fads and fancies, it would be more successful. If these men could have imbibed a little of Samuel Hahnemann, it would have helped them wonderfully."—*Exact Science of Health*, p. 239.

Between the obvious dislike of Trall and Jackson by Dr. Walter on the one hand, and the equally obvious over enthusiasm of Dr. Dodds for Dr. Trall, on the other, the truth probably lies. I am personally inclined to the opinion that Dr. Dodds is nearer the truth. I also think that Dr. Walter's criticism of these men was wrongly directed. To say that Dr. Trall was narrow or that "his practice was an utter failure" is only to reveal an ingrained prejudice that was probably born of jealousy. No narrow minded man is ever found in the fore-front of all the reform movements of his day, as Trall was. No "utter failure" ever achieves the success this man did. He was not practical in a business way. This much is certain. But his success in practice must have been far greater than that of the medical men of that day or this. It could not have been otherwise and the testimony shows this to have been so.

Vegetarianism and lack of Hahnemannian fallacies were not the things that vitiated the practices of these men. It was the "water-cure" which they incorporated with the Hygienic practice that prevented their practice from being what it might have been. It was the "water-cure," homeopathy and electrotherapy that did the same thing for the practice of Dr. Walter.

Among Trall's many works are the *Hydropathic Encyclopedia*, 2 vols., 1851; *The Hygienic Handbook, Sexual Physiology; Digestion and Dyspepsia; Diseases of the Throat and Lungs; The Alcoholic Controversy; True Temperance Platform; Water-Cure for the Million*, 1860; *Scientific Basis of Vegetarianism; Diphtheria: Its Nature, History Causes and Prevention; Uterine Diseases and Displacements*, 1854; *Hydropathic Cook-Book; Illustrated Family Gymnasium; Popular Physiology; Hydropathy for the People; Theory of Population; Home Treatment for Sexual Abuses; Woman's Hygienic Hand Book; Tobacco Using*, 1872; *The Hygienic System*, 1872; etc. While his justly celebrated lecture on *The True Healing Art*, delivered in the Smithsonian Institute, in February, 1863, was published and enjoyed a wide circulation. All of Trall's books ran through many editions before they finally passed into the "out-of-print" list.

Trall was also editor of the *Water-Cure Journal*, published by the Fowler and Wells Publishing Company, which later became known as the *Hydropathic Review*. In 1853 this Journal enjoyed a monthly circulation of over 50,000 copies.

It was a Journal of Living Reform. It advocated Woman's Suffrage, the Single Standard of Conduct for the Sexes, teaching of physiology and sex hygiene to the young, and joined Mrs. Amelia Bloomer, who often contributed to its pages, in her fight for bloomers for women instead of skirts. *Life Illustrated*, published by the same publishers and also edited by Trall, was an equally valient fighter for progress, freedom and right living.

In the December, 1913, *Stuffed Club*, Dr. J. H. Tilden wrote of him:

"He wrote many books and sowed the seed of medical liberty that has had more or less influence ever since."

Dr. Trall fought for medical liberty as never man fought. He battled against fallacies and frauds with the might of a Goliath. He went about as a roaring lion in his endeavor to get some medical man to meet him on the public platform for a discussion of the differences between his school and the medical schools. He defied them, and they feared him. He hurled his challenge into their very teeth, and taunted them with the charge that they knew that if they ever dared get on the platform with him, there would not be another drug doctor in all the land with the rising of tomorrow's sun. They dared not meet him.

He hurled his challenge at the Allopaths, Homeopaths, Eclectics, Physio-Medicalists, Reformed Botanic School, and to all others, but they dared not measure lances with him. They realized too well the truth of his remark during the course of his memorable lecture in the Smithsonian Institute:

"The Drug Medical System cannot bear examination. To explain it would be to destroy it, and to defend it even is to damage it. Its only safety consist in non-agitation, and all its asks is to be 'let alone'."

Dr. Trall also conducted a sanitarium and private practice. With workers like this, with sincere and earnest men, with tireless and determined men, the Nature Cure movement had to go forward. It required a War to stop it, but even a war will not stop it again.

Susanna Way Dodds, M.D., who was one of Dr. Trall's most brilliant students, and who left her monumental work, *Drugless Medicine,* (1915), together with her sister-in-law, Mary Dodds, M.D., and Alexander Milton Ross, M.D., etc., etc., of Toronto, Ontario, Canada, founded the Hygienic College of Physicians and Surgeons in St. Louis, Mo., in 1887. The college was first opened on October of that year and conducted classes for five or six years thereafter. It offered a three-year course, but at the expiration of this the course was increased to four years. Students enrolling were required to have "high school entrance standing." On its staff were: Dr. Luteys, a Homeopath, who taugh chemistry; Dr. Stickney, an Allopathist, who taught anatomy and surgery; Dr. S. W. Dodds, a Hygeiotherapist, who taught the theory and practice of the Hydro-Hygienic system; Dr. Mary Dodds, who taught Obstetrics; Dr. Sanborn, who taught microscopic anatomy and biology, and two other physicians of the "regular" or allopathic school. Besides being taught the hydro-hygienic theories and practices the students were taught enough of allopathic theories and materia medica to enable them to pass the state Board examinations. The College was well liked by many regular medical men who had lost their faith in the stupidities of the drugging schools.

A former student of this school, George Nebden Corsan, Sr., of Echo Valley, Islington, Ontario, Canada, who cared for the cadavers assigned to this school, informs me that, although he thinks it was against the law to have "syphilitic" subjects for anatomical work, he is sure that all "syphilitic" subjects that could be secured were sent to this school, which "received an extraordinary number in comparison with the number of students."

Because the Hospitals in St. Louis were crowded with medical students, the college was unable to secure a day at the hospital for its own work and its students were forced to do their hospital work on the same afternoon, Wednesday, that the American Medical College and the Eclectic Medical School received their hospital lectures. The first two years of the existence of the College there were twenty-one women students and a smaller number of men students in attendance. The Hospital lectures were given by one Dr. Bogart, a "regular," and Mr. Hebden says he "would bring up all the revolting syphilitic cases when the young women students were present." This may well show the animosity that existed in "regular" circles against the school.

Dr. Dodds also founded the Hydro-Hygienic Institute, a sanitarium devoted to the methods and theories of Trall, in St. Louis.

Since the closing of this school the Macfadden College of Physcultopathy, (Chicago), the Lindlarh College of Natural Therapeutics (Chicago), and the American School of Naturopathy, (New York), have been about the only schools that have kept alive the work. The first two of these are now defunct while the other one cannot be called an Orthopathic school. Indeed neither of them ever merited the name.

Among the others who demand recognition for the work they have done in the Hygienic movement are:

Joel Shew, M.D., author of several books on the water-cure.

G. H. Taylor, M.D., head of the Lowell Water-Cure establishment, and author of *Pelvic and Hernial Therapeutic*, 1885; *Health by Exercise*, 1857, etc.

James C. Jackson, M.D., head of Glen Haven Water Cure, Courtland Co., N. Y., and author of a number of valuable books.

S. O. Gleason, M. D., author of a number of books on living and sex reform.

A. Kalm, M.D., a Priessnitzian from Germany, who opened the New York Hydropathic Medical College on 60th St., in New York City, in 1856. The "Civil" War forced the closing of this school

F. W. Meyer, M.D., West Feliciana, La.

Dio Lewis, M. D., author of a number of works on Hygienic Reform.

L. N. Holbrook. M.D., author of books and editor and publisher of a magazine devoted to living reform.

Profs. O. S. and L. N. Fowler, who not only wrote and lectured extensively upon the reforms for which the Hygienic movement stood, but as members of the Fowler and Wells Publishing Co., were the chief publishers, in America and England of Hygienic and water-cure books and magazines.

Charles E. Page, M.D., of Boston, author of *The Natural Cure*, 1883; *How to Feed the Baby*, 1882.

Emmet Densmore, M.D., author of *How Nature Cures*, 1891; and a work on the Natural Cure of Consumption.

Felix L. Oswald, M.D., author of *Nature's Household Remedies*, 1890; *Physical Education*, 1882; *Vaccination and Crime*, 1901, *The Poison Habit*, 1887; *Fasting, Hydrotherapy and Exercise*, 1901, and other books.

Robert Walter, M.D., founder of the famous Walter's Sanitarium, Walter's Park, Pa., and author of *Vital Science*, 1899; and *The Exact Science of Health*, 1903.

Edward Hooker Dewey, M.D., erroneously called the *Father of the Fasting Cure*, author of *The No-Breakfast Plan and Fasting Cure*, 1900. *The True Science of Living*, 1894; *The Radical Cure of Chronic Alcoholism*, 1899; *New Erea for Woman*, 1896, etc.

Wm. A. Olcott, M.D., author of many works and co-worker with Graham in the spread of vegetarianism.

In Europe the chief contributions have been made by Arnold Rikli, Rausse, Kuhne, Lahman, Ragnor Berg, Andrew and George Combe, and a few others. Except for our knowledge of the value of the organic salts, and Rikli's contributions to our knowledge of the sunlight, Europe has really contributed but little to *Orthopathy*. The Water-Cure, so widely mixed with the Hygienic movement, in its early years came from Europe, but as a plague, not as an advancement.

Among living contributors to our knowledge, J. H. Tilden, M.D., of Denver, Colo., founder of the Tilden Health School, *A Stuffed Club*, later changed to *Philosophy of Health*, *Dr. Tilden's Health Review and Critique*, and author of numerous books, stands at the head.

During the years that have passed since Orthopathy was born many earnest and sincere students have attacked its problems and added to our knowledge of Nature Cure. But it has been found hard to shake off old dogmas and superstitions and few of these students, capable and honest though they were, were able to divorce themselves from many theories and practices that are really foreign to true nature cure. They adhered to the idea that nature must be aided, and so as various of these developed their *aids to Nature*, there arose a counterfeit system called, today, *Naturopathy*.

Morris Fishbein, paid propagandist of the medical trust, declares that Osteopathy is the back door to medicine while Chiropractic is the cellar entrance. After noticing the hodgepodge of methods and conglomeration of theories that make up what is called Naturopathy, he declares: "Obviously here is a medical cesspool." An Osteopath once declared that Chiropractice is the first six weeks of Osteopathy. The conflict between the rival camps of cure-mongers is amusing. There is no doubt that Naturopathy is a medical cesspool constituted of every form of therapeutic system and method that departs from allopathy, but at that, it is not more of a cesspool than is Allopathy and is still less ruinous to its victims. *It does not cure more, it kills less.*

As I said long ago Naturopathy may be defined as an incoherent aggregation of disrelated, antagonistic and mutually exclusive theories, hypotheses, principles, methods, systems, practices, machines, apparatuses and drugs. In short, it is a strange mixture of all non-allopathic methods of treating the sick; without a single coordinating principle running throughout. It does not differ in its principles of application from the allopathic system but is a treatment of symptoms by many methods, many systems, *a case of where one fails try another.*

"Naturopathy is 'systematized drugless healing,' " says Dr. Benedict Lust. "Osteopaths are in the strict sense of the term Drugless Physicians. Drugless physicians are Naturopaths. They cure by Natural methods."

His statement that drugless physicians are naturopaths, that they cure by natural methods, his frequent use of the expression "all natural drugless or natural systems" together with the statement that naturopathy is systematized drugless therapy, reveal, as nothing else could, that naturopathy is considered by its leading advocates to be merely a hodgepodge of drugless methods and systems. The loose and indiscriminate way in which they apply the term natural to any and all drugless methods, reveals the confusion that exists in their minds. Any non-allopathic method, regardless of its true relation to vitality, is called natural and no one dares challenge the idea. It is one of the chief purposes of this book to point out the true natural method. The terms drugless and natural are not synonomous.

Naturopathy traces its lineage to Germany to Preissnitz, Kuhne, Kneipp, Bilz and others. It is doubtful if any of these men would recognize it as their off-spring or acknowledge it as their heir. These men, as I shall show had many false ideas, but they did make an effort to escape from the confusion of the bizarre methods and theories that exist in what is called naturopathy.

Naturopathy is only an abortive escape from Allopathy. It has a bastard heritage of curative theories and almost as many curative agents as its illegitimate sire. It does not know any difference between the terms natural and drugless and its treatments are wholly symptomatic and suppressive in character. Its advocates think they can gather together an arm full of "branches" some of pine, some of hickory, oak, spruce, and mosquit and tie them together with string and make a tree. They do not know that branches grow out from a trunk and never develop independently of it. They are all nourished from the same sap (principles) and not from all manners of incompatible saps.

The Age-long controversy between the various schools of healing has been fought around the question: *What is the proper way to aid nature?* No one seems ever to have thought of the primary question: *Does nature require aid?*.

Louis Kuhne wrote:

"The natural method as hitherto applied, which far excels other systems, is the foundation of the new art of healing without drugs or operations. I have found it necessary, however, to follow more the great discoverers and founders of the system—Preissnitz, Schroth, Rausse and Theodor Hahn—rather than its later representatives. The latter, in their excessive zeal for individualization run the risk of degenerating into artificiality and deviating from the clear and simple paths of nature."

Speaking of his own restoration to health he wrote:

"This has only been rendered possible, however, through my thinking out, after long reflection, a new manner of taking the sitz-bath. This has proved so effective, that I can with certainty affirm that every disease, whatever name it may bear, is positively curable. I say every disease, not every patient."

Again: "The Natural method commands a wealth of forms in which water may be applied; packs, enemas, douches, shower-baths, half-baths, whole-baths, sitz-baths and steam baths of various descriptions. These many remedies, however, prove in part superfluous when once insight into the true nature of disease has been gained. The new art of healing simplifies the application of water as much as possible."

Lastly, he said:

"Our aim, therefore, must be to bring about the expulsion of the matter still lying quiescent in the body. For this purpose I have introduced the friction hip and sitz-baths which I shall afterwards describe, by the aid of which the system is excited to expel the morbid matter from the body."

Kuhne, it is here seen, observed the ever increasing number and complexity of the "aids to nature," and attempted to simplify the matter. What he failed to do, however, was to settle the primary question: Does nature require aids? Therefore, what he actually succeeded in accomplishing was simply to add to the number and complexity of the "aids."

A few years later Adolph Just writes:

"I saw so much quarreling and controversy among the individual champions of the nature cure method. One or another process was represented as false or even injurious.

"Were the opponents right or wrong? Could it be possible that the nature cure method was even harming me? Or were all my sacrifices again in vain? If I got no help from the nature cure, where then was I to place my faith? Was I simply to resign myself to my fate? The dissentions among the nature cure people were at least suspicious."

Observing, the failure of his predecessors and contemporaries to reach an understanding he was led to an effort to found a system upon natural instincts. He made many serious blunders in this effort, however. Following in the footsteps, not of instinct, but of his predecessors, who, he said: "sought rather to cleanse the sick body of its foreign matter, and that, indeed, with but one natural remedy—with water," he set about to invent a "natural bath" which formed the chief part of his system. Of this he says:

"The Nature-Cure method was in the beginning only a water-cure method, and only water-cure institutions were at first established.

"Therefore it was my first endeavor to obtain from nature herself directions for the right use of water applications."

Mr. Just did not stop to ask the primary question:

Are water applications of any kind needed? These he assumed were needed, because his predecessors and contemporaries had used and were using them. Starting with this assumption which could not do otherwise than bias his mind, he turned to a study of "land animals" and found that they not only do not take "full baths" but "they are actually afraid of them." The "voice of nature" having been hushed by the water-cure philosophy and practice he was unable to see in this fact that bathing was unnatural. Finding that, deer and wild boars often lie down in small muddy swamps or pools, usually dirty pools, (a thing they do to escape the flies or the heat) he invented his "natural (?) bath."

Like Kuhne, he expected his bath to take the place of all other forms of water application. Not having solved the primary question, however, instead of his bath supplanting the older forms it was merely added to them. Thus every effort to simplify error only increased its complexity and confusion.

Mr. Just declares "the nature-cure method was, in the beginning, only a water-cure method." This statement is true only in so far as it relates to Germany and Austria and the movement started by Priessnitz. Neither Jennings nor Graham founded a water-cure method while Jennings distinctly condemned their methods, although endorsing many of their theories. His words were:

"The great Hydropathic experiment is also most effectively sustaining the claims of Orthopathy, and nullifying those of Heretopathy. Hydropathic physicians as a body, discard medicine as the *rule* in practice as much as Orthopathists do; and when they come to steer clear of the old Heteropathic bug-bear notion of disease, and depend less on water as a *curative* means, their practice will be admirable.

"The Hydropathic organ of intelligence, 'The Water Cure Journal,' has a very extensive circulation, has obtained a stronghold on the public mind, and, all things considered, takes a very commendable stand on the subjects of medical and dietetic reforms, and is exerting a wide-spread and salutary influence in these directions. The name, if applied to individual cases of disease, is a misnomer, but viewing the work in its adaptation to effect a thorough eradication of the whole evil of human physical disorders, to its deepest foundation, the name is entirely appropriate. As this work is now in the field under a good organization and extensive patronage; it seems to me that economy would dictate that all the friends of health reform possessing a general similarity of views with those promulgated through this periodical, on its main topics, should throw the whole weight of their influence into this medium of communication with the public mind, do what they can to augment its circulation, and improve its matter."—*Philosophy of Human Life,* pp. 251-2-3.

In 1854 Dr. Jennings, in connection with Dr. G. W. Strong, a hydropath, opened the Orthopathic Water Cure Institute in Forest Dale, Cleveland, Ohio.

From the beginning the Hygienic movement was forced to battle its way against ignorance, superstition, age long traditions and organized medicine. Despite this fact it made rapid headway at the start. This was due to several factors, chief of which are, (1) Its advocates were sincere and fought a clean vigorous fight. Its books and journals were written and issued for the sole purpose of spreading knowledge. They were not merely written to sell, nor were they sensationalized. Sober thinkers wrote and spoke in those days; (2) Medicine made no pretense of being scientific, and so great were the damages produced by its heroic dosage that the people feared drugs as much as the doctors; (3) Puritanism taught the doctrine of personal responsibility; (4) medicine was not as well organized and had not captured the state and national government. It had not gained control of the schools and was not dictating what people could and could not be taught; (5) The press was more open and liberal and was not dominated by the medical societies; (6) People were still imbued with the spirit of liberty which had descended from the period of the revolution.

The Civil War impoverished the movement, wrecked its schools and institutions and so impoverished the people that there was no sale for books on health, and hygiene. The movement practically stood still for many years and did not begin to revive until about thirty years ago. Its progress has been very slow since this time, however, due to several causes chief of which are:

(1) Its advocates are few and can offer but a feeble fight; (2) Medicine pretends to be scientific and both the profession and the laity have been hypnotized into believing this; (3) Evolution and Socialism deny personal responsibility and destroy confidence in the fixed laws of nature; (4) Medicine is the most powerfully organized profession in the world. It has captured the schools, government, army and navy and all commercial and industrial organizations. It dictates what can and cannot be taught in the schools; (5) The press is closed, intolerant, antagonistic and does not hesitate to lie in the interest of medicine and to the detriment of the Hygienic movement; (6) The spirit of liberty is dead. Mussolini is the embodiment of the present world ideal; (7) A greater obstacle than all of these has been the rise of a whole array of miracle-mongering cults that have held out to a people that is rapidly losing confidence in drugs, serums and surgery, the vain hope of escaping the results of their misdeeds through drugless methods of palliation. These systems, beginning with Osteopathy and coming on up through Christian Science, New Thought, Chiropractic, Naprapathy, Naturopathy, Sanipractic, Spondylotherapy, Psycho-analysis, Lindlar's Natural Therapeutics, Physio-therapy, The Electronic Reactions of Abrams, the Bio-dynamic, chromatic diagnosis and treatment, of White and a much larger list of minor systems and methods, have done more to divert the attention of the people, who were seeking an escape from medicine, away from hygiene than has regular medicine itself. These methods have corrupted a large number who would otherwise have been good Orthopaths. Its progress has been hindered more by its barnacles than by organized medical opposition. None of these cults which have attached themselves to the hygienic reform have long survived, but they have all diverted attention from its true principles. (8) The publications that have pretended to be devoted to the hygienic movement have been devoted primarily to money grabbing. They have not been edited by men who had a knowledge of hygiene or who were interested in hygiene. The pages of these magazines have been devoted to the interests of the advertisers. The text-matter

has been sensationalized. It is written to amuse or to sell goods and not to instruct. For the most part, sober men and men who know their work have been excluded from their pages. The same is true of the great majority of books that have been written. Few of the books are worth the paper they are written on. Most of them are misleading. They represent a conglomeration of all drugless fallacies extant; (9) There have been no leaders. Those who could have led were insincere. Those who were sincere found no one who was willing to be led. The rank and file adopted first one fad, then another as these rode the wave of popularity.

It is encouraging to know that at the present time, the bankruptcy of drugless Heteropathy is beginning to be recognized and the Orthopathic movement is taking on renewed life. The signs of the times indicate that ere long Orthopathy will supplant the Heteropathic practices. One by one the barnacles are losing their attachments. The bankruptcy of drugless "healing" is growing more and more apparent every day.

"The dawn is at hand, though daylight spreads devilishly slow," once remarked Dr. Felix Oswald. His untimely death by accident cut short the career of one of America's greatest hygienists and the nature cure movement thereby lost one of her boldest and most useful champions. The dawn is still just at hand because the clouds of therapeutics have so long obscured the sun of true nature cure. But the better day is coming. There are rifts in the clouds and the light is breaking through. The number of physiological practitioners—that is, practitioners who employ hygienic instead of unhygienic methods—is increasing. And, what is a more hopeful sign, the people are beginning to wake up to the fact that they have been hoodwinked, by the machine operators and apparatus peddlers. Machine made health is beginning to fall into disrepute.

"As from roots wide-spreading, deep and sturdy, springs the oak in pillared strength," so from the most basal principles of organic existence spring the practices of Orthopathy, or true nature cure—the Hygienic system. Other systems, not content with laws and principles that are as fixed and eternal as existence itself, continue the world-old quest for some strange occult and hitherto inoperable law which will set aside all kown laws and enable them, through the use of some serum, drug, machine or apparatus, to cure disease and thus do away with the natural condition of obedience to the law of being.

These systems remind us strongly of the amusing story told of a young man who, one pleasant summer evening many years ago, was on a small sailing vessel going north on the Chesapeake Bay. The captain, becoming weary called on his young passenger to take his place at the helm, while he retired to the cabin for a bit of rest. He directed the young man to steer by the north star. After a time the young man also became drowsy and fell asleep. The flapping of the sails in the wind soon awakened hint, and, finding the ship quite out its course, he hastened to the cabin shouting: "Captain, Captain: come up and give me another star to steer by; I have passed the one you gave me." These therapeutic systems have all lost their way. They have passed the pole-star and are wandering aimlessly and hopelessly about on a sea of confusion.

When the cowardly and perplexed Pilate, amid the clash of conflicting creeds and cults, dispairingly asked the question, "What is Truth?" little did he know that it was to resound throughout the ages to come. He lived in a day when the creeds of his fathers were tumbling; he was stationed in a land where the mighty conflict between the Roman and Hebrew creeds, Greek philosophy and the revolutionary new doctrines of Jesus and his disciples had locked horns for a "free for all." They all possessed THE TRUTH, or at least, all claimed to posses it. Each was charged by the others with hyprocrisy and of being in cahoots with His Satanic Majesty, Emperor Diabolis, the First.

Pilate, being of a thoughtful mind and a broadly tolerant disposition, was much perplexed. He saw that error is so interwoven and interlaced with everything human that great research and discrimination are required to distinguish the true from the false. He knew that all of the warring creeds did not have truth, but knew not where to turn. Thus his dispairing cry; "What is Truth?"

No doubt many had asked that question before; millions have echoed it since. With every step in the advancement of human progress there has been a clash of creeds, a conflict of opinions and the despairing cry of many: "What is truth?"

Always the great leaders of human thought have been met with the same spirit of bigotry and intolerance that demanded the crucification of Jesus in the same breath with which it asked for the release of a murderer. The great gods or authorities of things as-they-unfortunately-are and all their thoughtless followers think, by such suppression, to hinder the onward march of progress and the ultimate triumph of truth. The impotency of such efforts would render them ridiculous, only that their very insignificance substitutes pity for ridicule.

"Yet it moves," said Galileo to the intolerant bigots who persecuted him and who vainly imagined that by imprisoning him they could suppress the truths and great principles which he so boldly proclaimed in the face of despotic power. Who, in reading of his trial, does not sense a great admiration for his boldness in declaring the laws which govern the Heavenly Orbs? Who remembers the bigots, who persecuted him, except to execrate them? Some one has made the indomitable Pisan say: "I was reviled by wise men; but the facts were not overthrown thereby." This simply means that intolerance of truth, because it chances to conflict with some long cherished belief or superstition; or that strong prejudices against everything of a revolutionary character, or that tends to change the existing order of things, cannot prevent the forward march of the eternal verities.

"All great truths begin as blasphemies," says G. B. Shaw. All great truths have been beset by the greedy pack and every effort has been made to tear them to shreds. They have conflicted with what has previously passed for knowledge; or they have threatened the entrenched interests of the bell-wethers of orthodoxy. The fight against every new truth has always commenced at the top. The "authorities" are afraid of new truths; it is they who try to suppress them. The herd only follows along in the foot-steps of their bell-wethers.

It is a strange state of affairs when those who dwell in the intellectual empyrean are unable to expose the fallacies that lie on the surface of the philosophies of "sciosophists," and must resort to the thumb-screw and the rack as a reply. The desire of those who sit in high places, to suppress all who differ with them arises out of their own weakness; a weakness they dare not confess aloud. The medieval practice of suppressing divergent opinion, would, if successful, shut us up in little water-tight compartments and hold us there that we might descend to the intellectual level of the hottentot, and the wheels of progress rust from inaction.

Those whom training has made contented slaves to tradition, and whose native originality and ingenuity have been crushed out of them by the mechanizing routine of the modern training system, will find in this book much which will be new and strange and perhaps distasteful to them. The modern straight jacket method of education prevents the normal development of the mind and fails to draw out originality. Rather it forces the mind into pre-determined moulds, evokes mere echoes and tends to fasten the thoughts and habits of an older generation indelibly upon the plastic minds of the young. It is a stereotyping process. A healthful sign is seen, however, in the widespread revolt of modern youth against the jails for thought that our standardized and over-institutionalized training system presents.

It is to those with intelligence enough and courage enough to revolt against the "stored-up wisdom of the experts who know all about a thing and know it all wrong," and against the traditional beliefs, customs and standards, which, although they may have been good enough for people in the past, are now stubbornly in the way, that this book is addressed. To those who have substituted the new critical mindedness for the all too common gullibility which enables so many men and women to swallow without question or protest the steady stream of false and misleading propaganda of those whose economic interests incline them to do anything and all they can to maintain themselves in power and to maintain the *status quo* to which they are accustomed; and to those who do not permit their salaries and their dividends to dictate what they shall think and say and how they shall feel and act; to those who are free, or are seeking freedom and truth, I appeal for a fair hearing and a critical examination and trial.

Full well do I know that I might as well speak to the tides and currents of the ocean, and expect them to stop at my command, as to waste words with some on the matters contained in these pages. But such are free. Let them obey their own inclinations. Let them follow their own desires. I wish to control the actions of no man by any other influence save that of reason, and truth. Were men and women as ready and willing to investigate, comprehend, appreciate and acknowledge as they are to doubt, disbelieve, condemn there would exist far greater truth and harmony in the affairs of earth than at present.

In the words of Dr. Felix Oswald:

"The progress of Medical Reform has reached a stage which to all who can read the signs of the times is a sufficient pressage of its victory. Its exponents have obtained a hearing. The transition period of the present age still struggles with the mists of the past, and thousands wander aimlessly from doubt to doubt; but they have at least ceased to follow the *ignus fatuus* of the long night. A spirit of free inquiry is abroad; the morning dawns, and light has ever been the ally of Truth. Scrutiny, even with the most hostile intent, has, indeed, never prevented the growth of a doctrine rooted in fact. For the laws of Nature, if read aright, reveal and confirm each other, and by just as much as perverse criticism succeeds in attracting the attention of honest inquirers, it will defeat its own purpose by leading to the discovery of additional evidence in behalf of Truth. 'If the right theory should ever be discovered,' says Emerson,' we shall know it by this token, that it will solve many riddles.'

"The mere announcement of a new truth has thus more than once led to its general recognition. It was in vain to legislate against the spread of the Copernican theory; the heavens refused to ratify the veto of the Inquisition. Newton's principals and the doctrines of Evolution could dispense with the favor of critics. They prevailed by 'solving many riddles,' nature, Logic and Experience, conspired to insure their triumph; in their theorems friend and foe found the solution of mysteries which other keys failed to unlock. The gospel of Natural Hygiene, too, can appeal to the evidence of that crucial test."—*Nature's Household Remedies*, pp. 1 and 2.

We have faith in the progressive power of truth. We do not believe that anything else than truth is worth the united efforts of man. He who labors to discover the *laws of nature* and who makes these the basis of his art and science should not be asked to harmonize with the reckless and selfish demogogue who is either too shallow pated to discern the distinctions between truth and error, or else to dishonest to choose the former and reject the latter. Both dissent and opposition should be raised against all who would teach error and suppress and villify truth and right. Opposition here is the highest virtue. What is called science has proved itself both wrong and arrogant too often in the past, for the conscientious seeker after truth to turn aside from his investigations, because of the scoffing and taunts of "science." The reigning clique of "eminent scientists" and recognized authorities do not have and have never had a monopoly on the facts and principles of nature and we need have no fear in withdrawing our faith from the hocum that now hallows the system

It is a humiliating fact that men and women in general, everywhere, when they see a "great" name believe in it. They are always more ready to bow to the authority of a great name, than to yield to the evidence of truth. It does not matter how incontestible your evidence and how irrefragable your reasoning; if you have not gained a mental and moral sovereignity of the minds of men, your evidence and your reasoning are weighed and measured by the obscurity of your name, and are sneered at in proportion as they lack the authority of great names. In this state of affairs, integrity, research, science, Philosophy, fact, truth, are no shield against the ridicule, abuse and misrepresentations of those who sit in high places and those who worship at the shrine of authority.

If, by any means, you may gain a conquest over men's minds, you may sit down upon this intellectual throne and wield the sceptre of intellectual despotism and few will concern themselves to question whether your word is sustained by truth or not. Your word is law and men will submit to it with zealous alacrity, as if each were emulous to be nearest to the chariot-wheels of such a despot, in his triumphal march through the world of thought. If anyone arises to dispute the crown with such an one he is simply told: "We have not educated you; you teach not our doctrines," and this often silences him. For, how can a man know anything if the authorities or their echoes have not educated him? Must not every man drink at the fountain of knowledge the authorities have established or remain forever in ignorance as dark as that which hovered over Egypt?

If those convention bound, tradition blinded hibernators in antiquity find in this book many things that are new and strange and greatly displeasing to them I only ask that they lay aside their prejudices and pre-conceptions for a while and give its pages a candid and thoughtful consideration. Let them test its principles and practices and withold their ready made condemnation until they have qualified themselves by investigation of our subject to properly appraise the value of that which is contained herein.

"So limited is the human capacity, that the most exalted genius, and the deepest powers of investigation, have not been able to raise their possessors above the errors and prejudices of their age, on subjects which have not been made the peculiar object of their reflection."

The great and learned in other fields of human endeavor have been, for the most part, unable to rise above the popular medical fallacies, prejudices and traditions of their time. For this reason the movement for living reform must progress slowly and meet with much unintelligent opposition as it goes along. Opposition is naturally expected from those whose livelihood is derived from exploiting the sick and suffering, but from those who derive no benefits from the sufferings of others, we have a right to expect an intelligent and open-minded hearing.

Theology and medicine are the two greatest fields of graft in human activities. The priests and medicine men of all ages have known that they are fakers and pretenders; they have known that they were playing the public as suckers and getting away with it. These two spheres of graft really had a common origin, and did not become separated into distinct professions until an advanced stage of civilization had been reached. Indeed they show every sign of attempting to again merge into one great system of hokum and exploitation. Christian science, Doweism, the Emanuel movement, divine healing cults and kindred movements are all based primarily upon doctrines of healing. Psychology, psychotherapy, practical metaphysics, metaphysical healing and Coueism are all curious mixtures of medicine and theology. They are all employed as means of exploitation. They are in many ways more remunerative than the purely medical systems and also less immediately harmful. The best that can be said of them is that *they do not cure more, they only kill less.*

The schools of medicine—Allopathy, homeopathy, Eclecticism, bio-chemistry, Osteopathy, Chiropractic, Physio-therapy, Naturopathy, Neuropathy, Naprapathy, Sanipractic, etc.—while, all of them are systems of humbugging and exploiting the sick and suffering, are more immediately destructive than the theological methods. They range in harmfulness all the way from chiropractic and naprapathy at one end of the scale to physio-therapy and allopathy at the opposite end. Naprapathy is probably the least harmful.

The professional healer, be he Allopath, Homeopath, Eclectic, Bio-chemist, Osteopath, Chiropractor, Christian Scientist, or a member of some other cult insists upon the need for treatment, for if this were ended the *healer* would be out of a job. Hence their bitterness against all Orthopaths and against each other. They are equally as bitter against their competitors as against those who would abolish the whole motley crew.

The Allopaths, arrogantly assuming that they alone are the guardians of public health and that to them only has been entrusted all skill and knowledge in heaven and in earth pertaining to health, disease and treatment, have waged and continue to wage a bitter war of extermination upon all competing cults. All cults pretend that they are scientific, but the Allopathic cult is the loudest and most arrogant in this boast. It is scientific and all other cults are quackery and charlatanism. It is frankly acknowledged by the truly big men in this cult that what they are pleased to term *modern medical science* is not scientific and that its progress is all in the future, but these admissions do not deter this cult from pursuing its ruthless course.

"Today Medicine is a science in the making, and its progress all in the future." Dr. Alexis Carrel of the Rockefeller Institute, (Scientific Monthly, July 1925.)

He also makes the common allopathic claim to having "conquered infectious diseases" through the Pasteur reveaiations, but "doubts whether this victory has so far brought much happiness to the world."

Medicine is a business, a profession, a means of securing money. Its votaries are men and women. They are actuated by the same motives, desires, ambitions nad vanities as the members of any other profession. They are surrounded by the same social and economic conditions and forces as carpenters, brick-layers and book-keepers and pursue their calling for the same purpose and with the same feelings as do these classes. Doctors are not super-men and super-women, elevated above the great mass of mankind and freed from the immoral and selfish interests and forces against which we all struggle and to which many of us frequently succumb. No *healer* and no school of *healing* should be regarded as any more than he or it is—a tradesman and a trade exploiting the sick for profit.

Why one cult should be woven into the warp and woof of our government, exalted, by law, to the position of diety, and permitted to use the advantages thus gained, to crush out all other cults and all anti-medical movements, is difficult to understand. Why in choosing the cult to thus enthrone, was the most destructive and deadly of all the cults selected? This cult has been permitted to use public funds to carry on its propaganda and to employ the police power to force its schemes and methods upon the indifferent or even antagonistic public. It has gradually worked its way into the public schools, the army and navy and has gained complete control of these. State medicine is the result. All of this has been done, of course, under the pretense of protecting the public health. But their real motives are both apparent and transparent. The Allopathic cult has no more interest in the public health than any of the other cults and none of them are bent on preserving public health since this would spoil their incomes. Physicians do not secure their fees from the well but from the sick. They are interested in selling their wares not in destroying the market for such wares. Put a member of any of the *healing* trades in a healthy community where no one calls for his services and he will not remain there long. He will move to a community where he can find employment. He would no more remain in a disease-free community than a carpenter would remain in a community where there is no building. He is interested in the sick, not in the well.

The Allopathic cult is said now to dominate no less than forty departments of our government and it is straining with might and main to gain controll over all others. Power, more power and still more power over the health and lives of the nation is its insistent and increasing demand, while the vast political power it wields, and the vast amount of wealth at its disposal make this cult the most dangerous enemy of the public health of all the cults. Its treaments are the most destructive and its confessed aims the most dangerous.

The situation is rapidly becoming intolerable to the thinking man and woman. My good friend, Mrs Annie Riley Hale, truly says in her remarkable book *These Cults*, P 257.

"The time has come when a majority of the lay world has pierced this pious disguise of the medical hierarchy; have learned also that much of its boasted 'science' is about as scientific as the voodoo practices of an African witch doctor. It is this disillusioned and aroused laity which is serving notice on State medicine where it may get off. Not the drugless cults, not rival practitioners, but plain, every-day laymen and taxpayers are saying to the learned medical profession: If you know so much more than the drugless schools and are so superior to the 'quack', prove it to the world by getting back into your offices in your own legitimate field of private practice, and do what you force the drugless men to do, earn your livelihood by the patronage of those who believe in you enough to consult you of their own free will and to pay for the service out of their own pockets. But henceforth take your hands out of the public funds, contributed by all the people, and stop using that to boost your practice and spread your peculiar doctrines."

Heteropaths start and wonder
At the Orthopathic thunder;
While it shakes their sandy footing,
    From the mountain to the shore.

And the doctors in their raging,
Seem to think the war that's waging,
Will be all their thoughts engaging,
    Making trouble ever more.

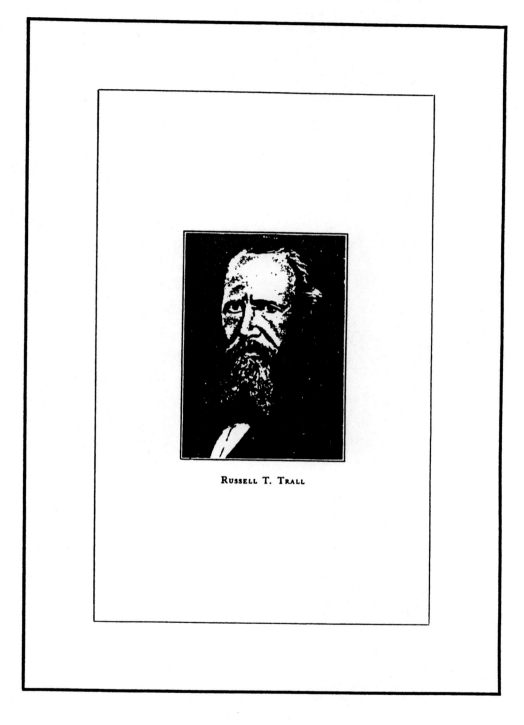

RUSSELL T. TRALL

HEALTH—ITS CONDITIONS AND REQUIREMENTS

Chapter I

"Nor rank, nor crown, nor power, nor wealth
Weigh 'gainst the worth of Radiant Health!"

FOR ages the study of disease has progressed. One by one the various symptoms and symptom-complexes that are presented by the diseased human body have been studied with painstaking care an praisworthy minuteness, both upon living and dead bodies. Pathology has reached a degree of perfection unknown to most of the collateral sciences that form what is called the science of medicine. Knowledge of pathology increased by leaps and bounds after the invention of the microsocope until today pathology is the one most important study of the medical student. Physiology, anatomy, histology, biology, etc., are all made subservient to pathology. The study of disease has held the student fascinated for ages.

Health has received scant attention. Strange as it may appear, health has been considered of so little importance as to be unworthy of investigation. No schools ever existed for teaching health. Medical schools existed to train the student in a knowledge of disease and *cures*. Even today no school exists that has as its purpose the teaching of the conditions and requirements of health. The conditions of a healthy life are but little understood by the various healing professions and and still less so by the general public. Health is not in the technically professional line of the physician. This chapter shall be devoted to a presentation of health, its conditions and requirements.

At the outset it may be broadly stated that the conditions and requirements of health are the conditions and requirements of life. In its broader sense, life, the state of being alive, is a condition in which animals and plants exist with capacity for exercising their functions. Perfect life is that condition in which those functons are exercised perfectly. Death is the cessation of life. Between these two extremes of perfect life, on the one hand, and death on the other, are found all those various degrees of health and disease which exist today. From this stand point both health and disease are states or conditions of being or life.

Briefly stated, health consists in the correct condition and action of all the vital powers and properties of the living body, and this necessitates the proper development and vigorous function of all the organs and tissues of the body and a close adherence to the laws and requirements of life. It is the normal or natural state of all organic existence and always obtains where the laws and proper conditions of life are observed.

Health is spontaneous. This is to say, it is the legitimate and inevitable result of the normal operation of the organs and functions of the living body. Every organ in the body is constituted to commence its normal and healthy action from the first and perform it spontaneously throughout life. They are constituted for health and unless deranged or prevented by violated law will from the beginning of life perform their functions with all the regularity of the sun in a natural and vigorous manner, because they cannot do otherwise.

Each individual organ of the body has its own appropriate work to perform. It must perform this function so long at it has power to work. If it has a sufficient amount of power it will work perfectly. If its supply of power is inadequate it must do the best it can. The liver, for instance, must secrete bile—good bile—if it has the necessary power, and the best it can under the circumstances, if power is low. It is so constituted that while it possesses power to act at all, it must act in a given direction and in no other The same is true of all other organs and tissues of the body.

We see, then, that the essential element of health is the healthy condition and function of the organs of the body. Full health of the body consists not in the full development and vigorous activity of some of its parts, but in the full development and vigorous activity of all of them. These organs and their functions are preserved in their highest integrity by a strict conformity to the laws of life and are impaired and destroyed by every violation of these. "Life and health are proportionate to each other," said Prof. Fowler. "Viewed in any and all aspects, *Health is Life.*"

3

Observe the painstaking labor nature has put forth to construct the body and all its organs and tissues with a degree of perfection unknown to the human work shop. The organs are perfectly constructed for the work they are to perform and their functions are no less perfect. Indeed, this structural perfection was expressly devised to secure a corresponding perfection of function. The flow of health from such organs is as natural as the return of the river's water to its ocean home.

Prof. Fowler used to illustrate the spontaneousness of function by the story of the little boy who inadvertently whistled in school and who upon being scolded by his teacher replied that he didn't whistle, "it whistled itself." The Prof. after reciting this story would say of the organs of the body: "It breathes itself, sees itself, moves itself, sleeps itself, digests itself, thinks and feels itself, everthing itself;" and breathes, sees, feels thinks, digests, moves and does everything exactly right so long as the proper conditions are fulfilled. Indeed, as the Professor often pointed out, the organs of the body perform their functions normally with less difficulty than they do abnormally.

It is not difficult to breathe or to breathe right or enough or to breathe wholesome air, but it is difficult to refrain from breathing or to breathe too little or to breathe a noxious atmosphere. It is not hard to eat or to eat enough. It is not hard to eat healthful foods. These things are easily accomplished and what is here true of breathing and eating is equally true of every function in the body. Every organ is constituted to commence its normal and healthy action from the first and peform it spontaneously throughout life and they are so constituted that they can function normally much easier and with much less waste than they can function abnormally.

Their powers are astonishing. They are often capable of continuing their healthy function in spite of being habitually abused and outraged, and, even after they have been thus broken down, they still endure the abuse and go on year after year till one wonders that they yet live. It requires great and long continued abuse of the body to impair its healthy function sufficient to produce that state of impaired health known as disease. Few realize how much abuse they are in the habit of daily heaping upon their bodies. Yet in spite of this abuse many live on to eighty or a hundred and enjoy what now passes for good health.

Alcohol, tobacco and other drugs that poison and gradually undermine the constitution are used by millions. Many drink, often to drunkenness, for years, without destroying their health, although they do greatly impair it.

Nature seems to have done her best to bestow vigorous and uninterrupted health upon all living things. She has constituted them for health and supplied them with a wonderful amount of physical stamina and energy. There would seem to be no more need for ever beccomming sick—for ever being in any other state than that of good health—than for refusing to breathe or see or eat. Life is made for health and under natural conditions health is as inevitable as the rise and fall of the tides. Living matter cannot be otherwise than healthy, if the conditions of health are present. It is easier to have good health than to have poor health.

The universal tendency of all oragnic existence—animal or vegetable—is towards health. Every organ and tissue in the living body is striving ceaselessly to maintain itself in as ideal a state as possible. To this there is no known exception. Life strives always toward perfection. *"It is as natural to be healthy as it is to be born."*

In general terms it may be said that one's health depends upon the body as it was inherited and upon what one has done or is doing with his or her inheritance. Many are born with inherited structural weaknesses which cannot be entirely overcome. There is such a close harmony and interdependence existing between all parts of the body—one part with every other part and every other part with the one—that if one part is disordered or impaired the whole body suffers more or less.

The student should keep ever in mind that the human body is not like a doll made up of separate parts and materials with no vital connection. No part of the body can be affected independent of the other parts. The human body is a unit. Each organ has its particular function to perform, yet no organ can perform its function independently of the others, and no organ can sustain itself by its own function alone. The Alimentary canal digests food for the whole system, the lungs supply oxygen and throw off carbon dioxide for the entire body, the skin and kidneys execrete waste and toxins for the whole system, the heart and vascular system carry blood for the whole vital economy. Such is the dependence of each organ upon the whole system and of the whole system upon each organ that the function of no one organ can be impaired, without involving the whole system in the consequences. The body is a unit, a community of interdependent organs, every part of which is vitally essential to wholeness and the highest degree of health and vigor.

So great is the dependence of the whole body upon some of its parts, such for instance, as the brain, lungs, heart, etc., that if they are destroyed or if their functions cease death results instantly. Sound health and vigorous function of the body, therefore, depend upon the proper development and harmonious operation of all its parts and not merely upon the vigorous action of one or two organs. The body is an unit, not a mere aggregate, and functions best as a whole rather than by parts.

Present day specialism in medicine treats each part of the body as though it were an independent isonomy with no special community value attached to it. Organs are removed on the theory that this can be done without any special injury resulting to the rest of the body. However, there are no useless organs and, while some may be removed with less serious consequences than others, perfect health is never possible after one of the body's organs are removed. The disastrous consequences that invariably followed the removal of tonsils and ductless glands should have shown medical men the error of their ways. Instead, it only led to the creation of another field for specialism and now there exists a brand of specialists who regard the human body as a few ductless glands and a few unimportant appendages.

Natural extinction carries off—not those whose constitutions are merely impaired, or those which are merely degenerate in structure, for multitudes of these do actually survive and produce others with similar defects—but those only, whose impaired constitutions, or whose defective structures, are absolutely incompatible with prolonged existence. However, a penalty is visited upon each individual organism, commensurate with the degree of its departure from the normal. This is true whether the departure is inherited or acquired.

The loss or degeneration in an individual or breed of any one of the positive features of its species results in an increased liability to disease, shortened life, decreased fertility and a higher death rate in the young. The maintenance of the normal reciporcal balance of all the organs and parts of the species constitutes full physiological perfection, and when any part or parts are impaired or wanting this balance is impaired. The evil resulting therefrom is over and above the mere deficiency in parts as shown by the lessened fertility and constitutional vigor in the individual.

How far much of the constitutional weakness that exists today can be overcome by proper selection of wives and husbands remains to be discovered. Just now those who busy themselves with human genetics are not concerned with this problem except indirectly. In fact, they seem not to have recognized its importance.

What is called natural selection is, at best, only a struggle against degeneration. It should be known that the adverse conditions which occasion natural selection, do more than kill off the weakest. They also cause a degeneration, both of those which have barely escaped extinction and of the stronger and more vigorous. For instance, if what Darwin called the "directly injurious action of climate" kills off the less hardy, less fit, it will also produce degeneration in the more vigorous and most fit. This fact Darwin saw, saying: "in going Northward, or in ascending a mountain, we far oftener meet with stunted forms, due to the directly injurious action of climate, than we do in proceeding southward, or descending a mountain."

It should be obvious then that health and vigor depend not alone upon the perfection of the organism but upon the congeniality of the conditions under which life exists. Briefly, if the seed, egg or ovum of plant or animal is to develop into the being that exists potentially in it, certain conditions are essential. These are moist heat, air, water, food, and protection from violence. When the young bird emerges from the shell, it still must have warmth, air, food and protection from violence plus light. The young plant just coming up through the soil requires the same. Given these they develop into full grown birds and plants.

This same is true of human beings. They require light, air, water, food and freedom from violence. They like the bird also require exercise and rest, sleep and cleanliness. Given these as required the baby develops into a wholesome well formed man or woman; provided other elements are not introduced to retard, subvert and pervert development. Health is potential in life and under natural conditions is, barring accidents, as inevitable as the rise and fall of the tides. Living matter cannot be otherwise than healthy if the conditions of health are present. But it lies in man's power to place himself under conditions other than those of health and these impair his health.

The tendency toward health is universal and as unceasing as time itself. This tendency is an inherent property of living matter or protoplasm. It is a necessity of existence. It is inseparable from life.

If the laws of life are complied with—if the conditions of healthy life are present —there is no power known to man which can prevent him from manifesting superb health. If these conditions are not present, the body must manifest as much health as the conditions present will permit. If health is already impaired, and the laws and conditions of healthy life are complied with there is nothing that will prevent the living organism from returning to normal health, unless the destruction of vital parts or exhaustion of vital power have progressed beyond the body's power of repair and recuperation. Its healthward movements, will be as inevitable and spontaneous as the rise of a depressed cork to the water's surface after the weight that holds it down is removed.

Health is potential in life. Its realization depends wholly upon an observance of those simple laws and conditions upon which life depends. The requirements of life are few and simple and if these are complied with and all hindering influences removed, health, by virtue of this inherent effort of the living organism to preserve its functional and structural integrity, will always be the result. It may be either the result of a fortuitous concourse of favorable circumstances or of an intelligently ordered life. Intelligent direction is preferable.

"As from roots wide-spread, deep and sturdy, springs the oak in pillared strength," so from the most basal principles of organic existence springs that condition of the living organism denominated health. Dr. Emmet Densmore well sums the matter up in the following words:—

"Health is the undeviating expression of animal (indeed all organic) life, always concomitant where the conditions natural to the animal are undisturbed."

A fact unknown to physicians and laymen alike is that all the functions of the body are performed with as much promptness, regularity and efficiency, as under exsting circumstances, is compatible with the safety and highest welfare of the body. In "disease" and in "health," that is, so long as life contiues, every organ and tissue of the body is at its post, ready and disposed to perform its particular function, to the full extent of its ability. They do good work when they have the power to do so, and when lacking in power to produce a perfect work, must do the best they can. They can never take on wrong action. When the laws of gravitation become confused and cause water to reverse itself and run up hill of its own self, then will we expect to see the vital laws permit the organs of the body to take on wrong action.

Impaired health, or disease, is simply a lessened degree of the action of the organs of the body, taken as a whole, than is performed by these same organs in the highest state of health, together with such impairments of structures, and secretions as flow naturally from such depressed action.

The present health standard is a false one. Indeed, it represents just the condition of things described above. A true health standard would be the highest possible degree of healthy action in a perfect organism. Anything short of this is impaired health— disease. In this view, the highest action in the most perfect human organism of which we now know is a condition of disease. That is, mankind is sick, is far short of perfection, and those whom we call healthy are just a little less sick than those whom we call sick or, to put it more naturally, those whom we call sick are only a little less healthy than those we call well.

6

Health is the natural condition of life. Perfect health is an ideal state. The condition of the body is not fixed—static. It fluctuates continuously. Health may be represented by a waving line, the waves of which rise up to good health or dip down to poor health as the conditions of life change. The health standard of civilized man is a decidedly low one, when contrasted with that of the wild animals in a state of nature, or even when contrasted with that of so called primitive man where he exists far away from the haunts and contamination of civilization. There are many reasons for believing that the health standard of modern man is far below that enjoyed by primitive man.

Long life, well developed muscles, a powerful bony frame-work, great strength, vigorous health, and sound teeth which, without the "aid" of tooth brush and dentrifice, lasted throughout life, are, qualtiies that seem to have belonged to all primitive people. Many of the so-called primitives of today possess good, sound teeth which last throughout life. Cushman tells us that "mental and nervous diseases were unknown among the ancient Choctaws; and idiocy and deformity were seldom seen." Catlin tells us the same thing of the Indians in both North and South America which he visited.

All authorities agree that measles, smallpox, scarlet fever, mumps, and whooping cough were unknown to the Indians until after the white man had changed their mode of living. The infant death rate was almost negligible.

Among civilized peoples deformities and defects of many kinds are everywhere met with. Strength, beauty and symmetry are absent in both sexes. Civilized man is rapidly becomming a race of bald heads, false teeth, glass eyes, and wooden legs. Every resource of the tailor and cosmetitian are resorted to to give an appearance of health, strength, symmetry and beauty. Both sexes seem to be content with imitation. Men and women in civilized countries may almost be said to be caricatures of man. Even our so-called beautiful women are like masterpieces in oil—they look better from a distance. They will not bear close inspection.

Women are rapidly losing their abilities to bear and nurse children. Pregnancy is a disease and parturition a surgical operation. Her brother fares no better. The shameful revelations of the examinations of the draft revealed, in part, the pitiably low standard of health maintained by the male element of civilized life.

What does all this deformity and misshapen ugliness and defective organs and faltering functions mean? They mean that mankind has degenerated far below his natural health standard. The health of both "savages" and wild animals is far higher than that of civilized man. Take a thousand codfish or antelope or lions or eagles and they are all sound and healthy. They are beautifully and symmetrically developed and present a uniform type. They not only do not suffer from the many and varied forms of disease from which man suffers, but there is no deformity among them. Health is the rule; disease the exception. Among the animals there is no "weaker sex."

So long as the average man is able to get out of bed in the morning, and, with the aid of various condiments, sauces and dressings, whip up a jaded appetite to enable him to eat three square meals a day, which is two squares too many, and, by the use of a cold bath, coffee, tobacco, alcohol and other stimulants, force himself through his days work, he considers himself to be in good health. His friends are satisfied with his "healthy" appearance. If, however, he should sicken and die suddenly, they exclaim: "how sudden! He was a picture of perfect health."

A picture, indeed! A picture and but little more. They call him healthy. And he is by their standard. How low the standard!

It is a sad commentary upon the intelligence of mankind that such a health standard is considered normal and that a mode of life that results in such a low state of health continues to be tolerated and even defended by the so-called brightest minds of the dominant school of medicine.

Consider a moment the beauty and perfection of nature and the constant tendency towards the normal in both plant and animal kingdoms, and reconcile with these facts, if you can, the theory that disease is more or less unavoidable. Yet place along side of this the strange anomaly that the human body, the masterpiece of creation, is more than any other animal in nature subject to disease.

More than half the race perishes in infancy, childhood and youth—by its eighteenth year. The remainder are victims of pains and sufferings more or less constantly. Of those who arrive at maturity, the greater part get little more than a glimpse of life and die prematurely. If we examine, closely, those who appear to be strong and healthy we find them defective in some one or more respects, or suffering from some secret uneasiness which detracts from their present comfort and gives rise to anxious thoughts and apprehensions for the future. The whole world of mankind is sick. Even those who are said to be healthy, if they are not suffering in some way today will be tomorrow. Health, it has been said, can be represented by a wave rather than by a line. It might be added that today at least, the wave, while it often goes rather low, seldom or never rises very high. Such is a faithful outline of the habitual condition of mankind. Indeed, we have underdrawn rather than overdrawn the picture.

There is no reason to mince words. Mankind, constituted for perfect health, falls far short of it. Every ache and pain, every defect, however slight or large, is evidence of this lack. Bald heads, glass eyes, wooden legs, false teeth, pimples, blotches, obesity, emaciation, weakness, lack of endurance, "susceptibility to disease" fear, worry, irritability, restlessness, war, crime, sensuality, the stimulant habit; these and many more things all evidence man's fall from his primtive standard of perfection. These represent a health standard that is far below that enjoyed by the lowest of the animals of the forest and field.

Every doctor's office, every hospital, santiarium, asylum, jail house, every house of prostitution, every grog shop and coffee house, every Christian science church, every drug store and drug and serum manufacturing plant, every health magazine and every book dealing with health, all singly and combined prove that mankind is laboring under a health standard that borders perpetually on death.

The very national salutations of the various nations all of which are substantially: "How are you" are constant witnesses to man's usual poor health. And those who pretend to possess good health are usually only bluffing.

The average life span of today is about one-third what it should be and this short period is usually filled with aches and pains, weaknesses and diseases without number. This is so universally so that mankind have acquired the habit of accepting the average of a diseased humanity as representing the normal man or woman. "Normal" standards for body weight, blood pressure, rate of heart beat, acidity of the urine, etc., are all mere averages of what a bunch of abnormal and overstimulated men and women present in these things. They do not represent an approach to the ideal. Normality cannot be found by averaging up abnormality. This places the health standard far too low.

Much is said today about the increasing life-span. However, this increase is only apparent and not real. Relatively fewer people are reaching old age today than ever before. The average length of life has increased, but not its actual length. Infant mortality has been greatly decreased. More infants grow up and reach maturity now than in the past.

The California State Journal of Medicine for Nov. 1922, states: *"Never in the history of the world was there more sickness than there is today."* It is estimated that in the United States alone approximately 148,650 persons die annually of influenza and pneumonia; 49,585 of other respiratory diseases; 15,100 of liver disorders; 10,915 of bronchitis; 10,400 of stomach disorders; 10,185 of intestinal disorders; 4,000 of anemia and many thousands more of numerous other disorders. It is claimed that relatively fewer people today reach 100, 80, 60 or even 50 years than formerly. Vital statistics reveal that every year 366,000 persons die in this country before the age of 30; 449,000 before the age of 40; 543,000 before the age of 50; 655,000 before the age of 60; 786,00 before the age of 70; and 919,000 before the age of 80. So few pass the age of 80 that it is hardly worth considering. Yet 80 years is far short of the age man would naturally be expected to attain if judged solely by the animal standard. Animals live on an average, from five to seven times the length of time they require

8

to reach complete physical maturity. Judged by this standard the least that should be expected of man is 120 years. He does not average half this.

Prof. Irving Fisher, of Yale, made the following statements in an address, a few years ago, before the Twentieth Century Club:—

"The truth is, we are witnessing a race between two tendencies—a reduction of acute or infectious diseases such as typhoid and an increase in chronic or degenerative diseases, such as hardening of the arteries and Bright's disease.

"Such process bids fair soon to change our net gain in the average life span into a net loss unless we attack the degenerative problem very soon. This situation is especially alarming for us in the United States because the tendency towards degeneracy seems to be more in evidence here than elsewhere.

"The number of persons now dying from diseases of the blood vessels (arteriosclerosis) is nearly four times as great as a decade ago. The mortality from these constitutional diseases in three decades has increased eighty-six per cent in Massachusetts and ninety-four per cent in fifteen American cities."

In this country 132,000 people die annually from tuberculosis; 120,400 of heart disease; 90,000 of cancer; and 77,500 of kidney disease. One man out of every ten dies of cancer. One woman out of every seven dies of cancer of the womb. It is estimated that 25,000,000 of the present population of civilized nations will die of cancer. 75,000 people died of cancer in the United States in 1913; 110,000 in 1923, an increase in ten years of nearly 47%. In 1900, the death rate in twenty-three cities, aggregating 20,839,737 people was 62.9; in 1923 it was over 108.5 per 100,000, an increase of over 72% in a little more than two decades. 25% of this increase occurred from 1900 to 1913, and 47% from 1913 to 1923, making the increase in the last 10 years over the preceeding 13 years, 88%.

Cancer, consumption, heart and circulatory diseases, Bright's disease, diabetes, nervous and mental diseases and other chronic and degenerative diseases are rapidly increasing. There are today in Great Britain, one insane person to very two hundred people as contrasted with one in every six hundred and fifty in 1870.

This state of affairs is a sad commentary upon our boasted civilization. These are the very diseases that are practically unknown among those so-called savage peoples whom we affect to despise as our inferiors. These diseases are wholly unknown among wild animals in their natural state.

That the modern health standard is a very low one is shown by the fact that, as a rule, from three to ten times as many soldiers "fall victims of disease" in all wars as are wounded and killed and that four times as many "die of disease" as from the casualties of war.

A mode of living and a system of treatment which, together, are more deadly than war should cause thoughtful people to pause and give careful consideration to the problems of health and disease. No one would be bold enough to claim that a mode of living and a plan of treatment which are productive of such disastrous results are in harmony with natural law or the requirements of a healthy life.

The final conclusion must be that man is going along under a very low health standard—one that represents universal impairment of body and mind. And yet there is nothing more certain than that health—*good health*—is his natural or normal state. Nothing is more true than that good health is the only legitimate result of the unimpaired operation of any and all of the organs and functions of the human body. Good health is man's birth-right. That he does not possess it is no fault of his structures and functions; and no fault of the laws governing his being, nor is it the fault of the natural forces and conditions around him. The true causes of man's impaired health are to be found in his failure to comply with the laws and requirements of life. All his evils arise from a misuse of his natural powers, and not from the right and proper use of any of them.

If man is sick it is not because he was made so. The Creator cast him in a nobler mold. In shape and form and power, he stands at the apex, of creation, a glowing tribute to the infinite Designer. He is constituted for health and happiness and the Divine intention is stamped on each and every organ and is declared by every function performed by them. Adolph Just well says:—

"Man originally came from the hand of the Creator absolutely healthy and good, without any blemish in body and soul. The handiwork of the All-Mighty, All-wise Creator could not, indeed have been from the start, an imperfect and defective, a diseased and sinful, a miserable and unhappy being." "Out of the primeval spring of eternal love the whole universe was created: God has created the world out of love, and out of love he maintains it. From the infinite love of God, from his omnipotence and omniscience, only the good, the beautiful and noble could evolve, as long as man did not step between disturbing it, while pains, diseases, anguish, misery, bad and worse could not originally emanate out of eternal kindness."

THE LAWS OF LIFE
Chapter II

NO one accustomed to observing the exact order and harmony that prevail in the world about him will question that his own body is constituted upon precise and fixed principles and that the vital machinery is controlled by express law. Physicians of all schools profess to believe in the existence of a law which governs the vital organism, and most of these profess to believe that in a perfect state of the body, this law is fully adequate to the government of all the vital forces and their actions. But in a disordered or impaired state of the body, Physicians of all schools hold that the economy of life is incompetent alone, to exercise the entire supervision and direction of all the internal affairs of the organism. It needs and must have counsel and aid from the human mind; backed by agents and forces other than those inherent in the organism.

The *law of animal life* is an inherent principle or tendency in the animal organs, by means of which they perform certain specific functions or acts, and this law, principle or tendency is immutable, always in force, and always acting in one direction with as much positiveness and unerving certainty as that water will run down hill, or heavy bodies tend towards the center of the earth.

The general law of the vital economy is a unit In all its operations, whether in perfect or impaired health, its tendency is one and indivisible: *the highest and best interest of the whole organism.* Nor can this unity be broken so long as life continues.

For the purpose of showing, more clearly, the nature and tendency of the law of life, and its adaptation to the purposes of life and health, it will be necessary to examine it under a number of separate divisions. These divisions reflect a grand system of order that is ultimately based on the same principles and which give rise to a grand harmony which can but excite the wonder and admiration of every man or woman who studies them. Before entering into this, however, it is deemed advisable to say a few words about what is meant by the terms, laws of nature, laws of life, etc., which we shall have frequent occasion to use throughout this book.

We are in the habit of saying the Universe is governed by law and, while we shall use this convenient expression throughout this work, we desire it understood that we do not use the word law in any legislative or coercive sense. The laws of nature are not legislative enactments. Natural events do not take place in obedience to natural laws. Natural laws, as we call them, govern nothing. They are "uniformities of nature which are classified in universal formulas describing all possible happenings of nature. Thus the law of gravitation does not govern the motion of falling bodies and the coursing planets, meteors and suns. The law, so-called, is a descriptive formula which states in the tersest way possible the mode of action which things of a definite quality will take under certain conditions." Natural laws are formulas which describe uniformities or regularities of nature. The uniformities of nature are not mere haphazzard coincidences but intrinsically necessary conditions. They are based on the nature of things and constitute an intrinsic and necessary part of the world-order, or, rather, of the universal order. The uniformities of nature are eternal. They are uncreated and uncreatable.

Well does Graham say:—

"But when we speak of laws and properties of matter, what do we mean? We talk of the law of gravity; and so far as size, weight, distance velocity, etc., of attracting bodies are concerned, we can reason with mathematical accuracy and precision; but with all this extent and accuracy of knowledge in regard to the fixed order of the phenomena of gravity, what do we know of the essence of that power which we call the attraction of gravitation? Absolutely nothing. The chemist also speaks of the molecular affinities of matter, and the laws which govern the conbinations of his experimental elements; yet he is totally ignorant of that power or property which he calls affinity, and the fixed order of whose phenomena he calls law.***** We use the word law then, in regard to matter, as an abstract term, to signify a fixed order of phenomena that are produced by a power of which we are entirely ignorant.**** While, therefore, we cannot, from our knowledge of things, affirm what the essence of life is, we know as certainly as we know anything concerning matter, that it could not spring from any of the properties or powers of inorganic matter, and that its relation to the organization of matter is of necessity in the nature of things, and has ever been since the first establishment of the vital economy in connection with organized matter, THAT OF A CAUSE AND NOT OF AN EFFECT."—*Science of Human Life*, p. 201.

We however, do not require to know the essential nature of life in order intelligently to obey its laws any more than the chemist must know the essential nature of matter, or the electrician must know what electricity is in order to work with these intelligently. Whatever hypothesis a chemist may hold in regard to the essential nature of matter he must still observe the same laws in his work as a chemist as his fellow chemist who perhaps holds to an essentially different hypothesis of what matter is. Just so, in giving us power, light and heat all electricians, whatever their ideas concerning the nature and essense of electricity, must observe the same laws.

Just as our ideas about the essential nature of matter and electricity do not change them one iota, just so, our ideas about the essential nature of life do not change the phenomena and laws of life. Life will not change it's "fixed order" to suit our changing conceptions of its essential nature. It continues to "saw wood" at the same old stand and in the same old way.

All the various conditions and requirements of life herein set forth, that is, air, water, food, light, warmth, exercise, rest, sleep and freedom from poison and violence, structural and functional integrity of the organism, etc., are not life nor the causes of life. These are but the necessary conditions of life without which life would cease. But these conditions cannot produce life. The responses of the living organism or of the fertile seed or egg to these conditions are the results of the operations of a force inherent in and peculiar to the living being. This force, called by various names, strives always to preserve and maintain the organism in as near perfect condition as possible. The reaction of the living thing to any adverse condition or circumstance is always calculated to defend and preserve its integrity. In fact, so strong and universal is this effort at self-preservation that it has been called the first law of nature. The instinct of self-preservation is inherent (1) in the smallest microscopic unit of organic existence, (2) in cells associated as a community, (3) in cells organized into distinct organs, and (4) as organized into organisms. Every particle of living matter is under the control of life or vital force and is endowed with the instinct of self-preservation.

Self-preservation is the primary or controlling expression of life and, normally, is subordinate to no other law except, at times, to the instinct of race preservation, in which case the individual often sacrifices itself for the protection of the young or of the flock. However, in such cases, there is no true sacrifice, but rather, the individual is killed while trying to defend itself and young or herd from danger.

Dr. Robert Walter formulated this law as follows, and denominated it:

LIFE S GREAT LAW: "*Every particle of living matter in the organized body is endowed with an instinct of self-preservation, sustained by a force inherent in the organism, usually called vital force or life, the success of whose work is directly proportioned to the amount of the force, and inversely to the degree of its activity.*"

A law is a "constant mode of action of a force;" that is, it describes how the force works. The life force in its operations works, as do all other forces, according to well defined *laws* or *uniformities*. Laws have no validity except as expressions of the forces back of them. Primarily, life seeks to preserve itself or rather the organization it has built for itself. All the functions of life have reference to this effort at self-preservation either of the individual or the race. This is as much true of the single cell as of the complex organism.

In the organic as in the inorganic realm, there exist also, secondary laws or "the observed order" of facts which grow out of the primary law which produces them. Dalton's laws of chemistry and Kepler's laws of the heavenly bodies form secondary laws to the primary laws of chemical affinity and gravitation respectively. So in life we have certain laws secondary to "*Life's Great Law*" called the *Laws of Vital Relation*. First among these we have:—

THE LAW OF ACTION: *"Whenever action occurs in the living organism, as the result of extraneous influences, the action must be ascribed to the living thing which has the power of action, and not to the dead whose leading characteristic is inertia."*

There is a vast difference between living and dead protoplasm. Chemically, they may be the same, physically they may present identical appearances, but they answer to different tests. The living protoplasm or the living organism possesses the power of action; dead protoplasm, in common with all other lifeless matter, does not. Lifeless matter may be moved, but it cannot move itself. Living matter can move itself and other matter as well. The action of living matter under various conditions and when subjected to various stimuli does not represent the action of these conditions or stimuli upon the living organism, but, rather, the response of the living thing to the conditions or stimuli. The response is from within, the power to respond is inherent. When the power of response is lacking as in dead protoplasm there is no response to changed conditions or to the application of various stimuli. In the relations between lifeless and living matter, the living matter is active, the lifeless matter passive. If the power is low the response is correspondingly low. The work of vital force is "DIRECTLY PROPORTIONED TO THE AMOUNT OF THE FORCE."

We may illustrate the above law by the common practice of taking purgative or laxative drugs to force bowel action. The expression is common that certain drugs "act on the bowels" or on the liver or on the kidneys or act on some other organ. Apparently this is the case, but actually the reverse of this is true. The taking of a dose of epsom salts is soon followed by a movement of the bowels. Dr. Trall's question, "which acted and which was acted upon," is a very pertinent one. The only action of which any drug is capable is chemical action and no one will maintain that the bowel action in this case is chemical. No one will dispute that it is bowel action. From first to last the living organism is the actor, the salts are acted upon.

Why do the bowels act; why the hurry following the ingestion of the salts? The answer is: Self-preservation. The chemical union of salts or any other drug with any of the fluids and tissues of the body is destructive to them, impairing their structure and function and even resulting in death. They act as irritants and are irritating in direct proportion to their destructiveness. The bowels act to cast them off, to eliminate them. They but perform their God-ordained function of elimination in order to self-preservation, in hurrying the dose of salts from the body.

This bowel action is vital action, as much vital action as the beating of the heart or the act of hearing, and the power of the action is inherent in the bowels, not in the salts or other drug. Vital action is accomplished by vital power and this leads us naturally to the:—

LAW OF POWER: *"The power employed, and consequently expended, in any vital or medicinal action is vital power that is, power from within and not from without."*

It is the living thing that acts, it is the life power that produces the action. A dose of salts or calomel will produce no movement in the bowels of a dead man. The body of a man who is nearly dead will not respond to medicines. Why? Because the power of response is absent. It is living power, not drug power that is back of the action. Vital force is the cause of the action, the threatened danger to the organism, due to the presence of the drug is but the occasion for the action.

Dr. Trall well illustrates this law as follows:—

"It is urged that, as escharotics or caustics applied to the skin occasion rapid decomposition of the structures, the drugs must, in these cases, act on the system; for, it is asked, would the living system destroy itself? Is that remedial action which results in death? I answer: Remedial action is not necessarily successful in always accomplishing its purposes. It is defensive action. It aims to rid itself of the enemy; to remove the abnormal and offending material. It may wear itself out in the struggle. It may die in the attempt. It *must* oppose and war upon whatever is injurious, whatever is incompatible with its functions, so long as they are present, otherwise it could not be vital. And this is precisely the distinction between living and dead matter; the dead is passive and quiescent everywhere; the living will not tolerate the presence of the dead.

"That caustic does not act on the skin any more than ipecac acts on the stomach, or caster-oil on the bowels, is demonstrated in this way. Apply a blistering plaster to the skin of a healthy, vigorous, young person. It 'draws' readily and the skin is soon vesicated. Apply it then to a feeble, pale, anemic, or dropsical invalid. It 'draws' with difficulty or not at all. Before it will vesicate, the skin must be rubbed with some pungent or irritant, as hot vinegar or red pepper. Then apply the blister to the skin of a dead person. It will produce no effect whatever. What is the explanation of these facts?

"If the blister acted on the skin, the effect would be greater instead of less in the cases of feeble persons, for the reason that there is less vital resistance. But the contrary happens to be the fact. The *effect* of the blister is precisely according to the vigor, integrity, and resisting power of the living and acting machinery; and this I regard as proof positive that it is the living system, and not the dead drug, which acts. And the principle herein indicated explains how it is, and why it is that healthy vigorous persons, when equally exposed to the causes of disease, have more acute and violent maladies. Disease being remedial action, and their vital machinery being in vigorous condition, the defensive action, the disturbance, the disease, will manifest proportionally more violent symptoms."—*The Hygienic System.*

Dr. Walter used Herschel's rules for determining the real cause of an effect, to show that this explanation is correct. These rules are:—

First—Invarible connection between cause and effects.

Second—Invarible absence of effect with absence of cause.

Third—Increased or diminished intensity of effect with increased or diminished intensity of cause.

Now, let us apply these rules to our law and see how it works. Our law says that vital force is the cause of the action, while the living organism is the actor. Already, we have used a dose of salts to illustrate the *Law of Action,* and we shall use it to illustrate the present. No amount of salts can "move" the bowels of a dead man. The giving of salts to the dead produces no effect. Yet, if salts were the cause of the movement we should get a movement. Bowels do not move, whatever the occasion or condition, where life is lacking. Dead bowels cannot be made to act. The more vigorous a person is, the more vitality he possesses, the more vigorous will be the response to the salts, on the part of the bowels, while, if the person is very low, the response may be hardly perceptible. In the relations between living and lifeless matter, the living matter is active, the dead matter is passive. The action of living matter is in proportion to the need for action and to the amount of *power of action* that is present.

If salts act on the bowels, to move them, they should always do so regardless of the condition of the bowels. But if the bowels act on the salts, to expel them, it is obvious that there will be no bowel action following the ingestion of a dose, if the power of movement is lacking. Where the power of movement is present, the movement must be in proportion to the power possessed and to the need for action. The salts cannot give power to the bowels for they possess no power to give. But they do occasion the expenditure of the power already possessed by the bowels. The same thing is true of other substances and agencies which apparently strengthen us. They occasion the expenditure of power already possessed but do not add power. Power is felt only in its expenditure, never when it is passive. One, therefore, feels stronger while he is growing weaker, and feels weaker when he is actually growing stronger through recuperation of power. The man who has had a drink of alcohol is led to believe that he is strengthened by it, while, in reality, the alcohol has only occasioned the expenditure of the power he possesses.

In this way strychnine may "strengthen" the heart until it exhausts this wonderful organ. A cold plunge or a short hot bath produces a general feeling of strength and well being by occasioning the expenditure of power which they do not and cannot give.

14

The thing which seems to give strength is the thing which is taking it away, the thing which appears to be curing the patient is the thing that is hastening his death, the very agents which seem to be "supporting" and "sustaining" life are the very things that are undermining the foundations of life.

Following the period of apparent increase in vigor (stimulation) there comes a period during which there is a feeling of lessened vigor (depression). There are two effects following the use of every force or agent.

THE LAW OF DISTRIBUTION: *In proportion to the importance and needs of the various organs and tissues of the body is the power of the body, whether much or little, apportioned out among them.*

The laws of life are as fixed and uniform as the law of gravitation, or any other uniformity of nature. They are immutable, always tending toward the perfection, in every particular, of the organism, whether the power which they sway is sufficient for the accomplishment of this end or is greatly inadequate therefor. The distribution of this power is under control of immutable law which wisely and minutely appropriates it where most needed and supplies every organ with as much as it can use so long as there is sufficient power to distribute.

Art cannot, by any possibility expedite the recuperation or generation of power or increase its quantity at any given time in good health or impaired health.

Art can by no possibility secure a more efficient and advantageous distribution and use of the vital powers than would be made by the vital laws if these are left to the undisturbed administration of organic affairs

Every organ of the body has its particular and specific functions to perform, and with an adequate supply of power, will do its work promptly and well. But with an inadequate supply of power it falters in its functions and fails to accomplish its work in a thorough, workmanlike manner, yet it always does the best it can with the power at its disposal. Its calls for power will be urgent and in proportion to its needs. The *Law of Distribution* will be as vigilant and discriminationg in its appropriation of power when all or a number of organs are calling loudly for it, as when all parts are adequately supplied.

THE LAW OF DUAL EFFECT: *The secondary effect upon the living organism of any act habit indulgence or agent is the exact opposite and equal of the primary effect.*

Perhaps no better illustration of this law can be given than that of the phenomena of Anaesthesia. About eighty years ago it was a common practice in parts of this country for persons to inhale the fumes of ether for its exhilirating effects. This practice often formed the chief means of entertainment at country parties. During these ether frolics the stage of excitement was often followed by unconsciousness and loss of sensation. It was this later effect that probably first suggested its use as an anaesthetic, it being first employed as such by Dr. Crawford Long of Georgia.

Complete anaesthesia is divided into three stages:— (1) induction, (2) maintenance, (3) recovery.

The stage of induction is divided into two periods:—(1) the period of cerebral and muscular excitement, (2) the period of relaxation.

The stage of recovery is divided into two periods:—(1) the return of the reflexes, (2) the return of consciousness.

The stage of *induction* extends from the beginning of the administration of the anaesthetic to the point of *general muscular relaxation.* It is evidenced, during the first period, that of *excitement*—called "exaltation of function"— by an unusually rapid pulse, irregular sighing respirations, anxious expression, fidgety movements of hands and feet, constant clearing of the throat, licking of the lips and other movements and struggles. There is universal excitement and commotion in the organic domain. Recovery takes place in inverse order to induction. The following description of the phenomena of anaesthesia from the *International Encyclopedia of Surgery*, Vol, 1, p. 406, is illuminating:—

"A description of the symptoms occasioned by the inhalation of the vapor of ether or of chloroform will convey a sufficiently accurate idea of the manner in which artificial anaesthesia ordinarily supervenes. The first effect*** is a local excitement cf the nervous apparatus of the respiratory passages. The senses of taste and smell**** are powerfully excited. The activity of the salivary glands is aroused, the acts of deglutition are stimulated.**** The initial effect is disturbance of function; the subsequent effect is paralysis of function. Disturbance usually assumes the form of exaltation.*** There is a humming sound in the ears and subjective impressions of light flash in varied forms across the visual field. The pulsations of the heart can be felt, and the vermicular movements of the intestines can sometimes be perceived. The arteries throb, the brain seethes, waves of heat flush the surface of the body, perspiration appears on the face, and may become general, the pulse rises, respiration is accelerated, the pupils contract, the eyes close, reflex irritability is exalted, and in its general appearance the patient resembles a person in the early stages of alcoholic intoxication. To this period of excitement succeeds the state of diminishing function; cutaneous sensibility grows less, the temperature falls, the pulse recedes, the blood-pressure diminishes, the respiratory movements become deep and full, voluntary movements cease, consciousness gradually fails, reflex movements are abolished, and the patient becomes utterly insensible."

The above description well illustrates not only the law of dual effects but, those of action and power and shows, as well, how strongly the living organism battles in self-defense. When the vapor of ether or chloroform is inhaled its poisonous character is instantly recognized by the organic sensibilities of the parts upon which it comes in immediate contact, and the alarm is promptly spread throughout the whole organic domain. Every organ of the body is more or less powerfully and extensively effected and there is a general effort of the vital powers to resist the poisonous effects of the anaesthetic and to expel it from the system. The integrity of the vital domain is in jeopardy and it puts up a strong fight in self-defense. Under such conditions, the extent to which the physiological operations of the system deviate from their normal course, must always be proportionate to the force of the poisonous or injurious influence, and the physiological power of the disturbed economy. This violent reaction against the drug is referred to in the above quotation as "exaltation" of function, a "period of excitement."

Truely there is reason for excitement and for vigorous action. The whole organism is endangered and true to its instinct of self-preservation it puts up a fight. Every organ, every tissue, every living cell in the body enters the fight for every particle of living matter is endowed with the instinct of self-preservation. The increased action is still vital action and the power employed and consequently expended is vital power. It will be shown later that healthy sleep differs from the state of coma and apparent death induced by drugs, in that, the organism aroused from sleep feels refreshed and renovated and is ready for action, while the organism aroused from coma is languid and exhausted and utterly unfitted for action. The reason should be obvious. Sleep is a renovating, recuperating process, its first and temporary effect being weakness and reduced function, its second and lasting effect being strength and increased function. Anaesthesia is a poisoning process, the first and temporary effect of which is increased function, its second and lasting effect diminished or abolished function. The inactivity of sleep, not the increased activity of stimulation, is the great representative process of recuperation and health. The primary effect of stimulation, increased activity and an increased feeling of well being, produces weakness and exhaustion, as its secondary and lasting effect. This is true regardless of whether the stimulant is chemical, electrical, mechanical, or mental. *The degree of weakness that follows is commensurate with the degree of stimulation that preceeded.*

Alcohol which apparently strengthens and which for a very brief moment increases function results in diminished function and weakness. Alcohol like ether and chloroform does not add power to the system. It only occasions the expenditure of power already possessed. It is properly classed as a caustic irritant and the exalted function which first follows its use is not due to any power it communicates to the body and mind but to the vital resistance and consequent expenditure of vital power its irritating effects occasion. Its secondary effect is due to the exhaustion of the vital powers and its destructive effects upon the tissues of the body.

A cold plunge or a short hot bath acts as a stimulant. There is an increased feeling of well being, an increase of physiological function. It is always and necessarily followed by an equal amount of mental and physiological depression. Prolonged cold baths act much the same as chloroform or ether. The temporary exhiliration of function is soon followed by a decrease in function. The heart action is reduced, the circulation and respiration slowed down and nervous activity decreased. Muscular activity is decreased even to the point of stopping such activity. Prolonged application of cold to the chief trunk of a nerve will greatly diminish or entirely abolish its activity. The feeling of warmth that comes with the reaction from the first shock of the cold gives way to a feeling of chilliness and cold. The apparent increase of strength gives way to a feeling of weakness and lassitude, and if the cold is continued, numbness and abolition of function follow. Anaesthesia can be produced by prolonged cold. It is a vital depressant and the feeling of increased strength with the increase of activity which comes primarily upon its application is one of vital resistance. The organism resists the cold as truly as it does alcohol or ether. Cold does not supply functional power but it does occasion its expenditure.

Moderate heat applied to the surface of the body occasions the dilation of the arteries, capillaries, veins and lymph vessels. This temporarily increases skin activity. If this is prolonged or repeated often the result is a weakening of the skin and a lessening of its reactive power—debility and exhaustion. This is always the result of prolonged or repeated stimulation whatever the agent used to produce the stimulation. More will be said upon this point in the chapter on stimulation.

All medical authors agree that if the use of a tonic is long continued, the effect is debility. A tonic medicine first strengthens, and then debilitates. Such results are accounted for by the law of dual effect. Alcohol permanently weakens because it temporarily strengthens. Opium permanently produces sleeplessness, nervousness and pain, because it temporarily relieves these conditions. A cup of coffee will relieve a headache but in so doing it permanently fastens the headache habit upon the patient. It will relieve mental depression, but when the user is deprived of his coffee he becomes doubly depressed. Tobacco steadies the nerves only to unsteady them. Tonics strengthen only to debilitate. Purging produces constipation, diuretics produce inactivity of the kidneys, cholagogues result in torpidity of the liver. If the habitual user of any drug will cease its use for a few days he will experience in their fullness all its secondary effects. If he then returns to his use of the drug he will be delighted to find that these secondary effects are "cured" by it. The disease is "cured" by its cause—coffee cures the headache which it produced; whiskey restores the (feeling of) strength it has wasted; tobacco, the steadiness of nerve it has destroyed.

Give opium to cure a man of pain! Who has pains equal to those of the opium addict? The nomenclature of medicine needs revision. Opium and other anodynes and antispasmotics should be classed as odynes and spasmotics. The whole class of tonics should be classed as atonics. Stimulants should be called depressants. These substances should be classed according to their *secondary* and *lasting* effects and not according to their *primary* and *temporary* effects.

There is no such thing as a strengthening medicine. The manner in which so-called tonics act in *strengthening* the body or any part of it resembles the methods of marching of the Corporal who used to command his squad to, "*Advance five paces backwards!*" They strengthen us after the principle of *progress* illustrated by the frog in the well—*two* feet out in the morning and four feet back at night. They take away the strength they appear to give. They cause the sleeplessness they appear to cure. These substances and destructive agencies enslave their victims, because of their poisonous nature, which first arouses vital activity, giving an appearance and feeling of strength, at the very time and by the same means that the patient is being exhausted. Utter destruction would promptly follow their use were it not for the *Law of Vital Accommodation*, which we shall discuss a little later.

The energy of medication by poisons, is the energy of defense. Only that which arouses the organic energies to desperation brings about prompt action. The action wastes vital power and results in weakness.

This law of dual effect admits of no exceptions. It applies to all departments and all the actions of life. Labor or exercise arouses vital activity thus giving an appearance of increased vigor. This is their first effect. But their secondary effects are tiredness, fatigue, decreased vigor and exhaustion. How often do we hear the invalid advised that he must keep up, because if he goes to bed he will lose strength. This is the first effect. The secondary effect is a gain in strength. Travel or excitement makes the invalid feel stronger and better as a first effect. But the secondary effect is languor, weakness, exhaustion. Rest and sleep, on the contrary, produce as their first effects, weakness and languor, but no one doubts its recuperative value. Rest and sleep, are the only means whereby recuperation and re-invigoration can be secured. But these are its *secondary* and *lasting* effects. The invalid must be weak that he may grow strong.

The same is true of eating. Those foods that are most stimulating, such as tea, coffee, cocoa, chocolate, spices, meat, etc., invariably weaken, as their secondary effect, in proportion to the strength they appear to give.

This law is equally applicable to the sex function, but, as this will be described in a later chaper, no attempt will be made at this place to show its application.

THE LAW OF LIMITATION:—*Whenever and wherever the expenditure of vital power has advanced so far that a fatal exhaustion is eminent, a check is put upon the unnecessary expenditure of power and the organism rebels against the further use of even an accustomed stimulant.*

This is a very poor formulation of this law which I have attempted to make. However, it will serve, together with the following explanation to convey the meaning to the reader.

It often happens that a physician employs a certain stimulant in the treatment of a very depleted patient. This seems to "work like a charm." The patient responds readily. But it becomes necessary to give the stimulant in increasingly larger doses, and finally the body ceases to respond to it and rebels against its use. In the days when brandy was the medical man's stand-by, after this had been given for some time in low states of disease, it would pall upon the senses and be loathed by the patient.

If the patient is not too low, after one drug has ceased to produce the "desired" effects, it is usually possible to produce these by changing drugs. But when the patient is very low, near death, no drug will produce such effects. When over stimulation has wasted the energies of life almost to the fatal point the law of limitation interposes a hand and prevents their further use. The desire for tobacco, alcohol, opium or other irritant ceases. There is a loathing for the accustomed drug. It is this law also that withdraws power from the voluntary muscles and from the digestive organs in acute and frequently in chronic disease.

In future chapters other examples of this will be given and it will be shown that this *Law of Limitation* is frequently enforced against one organ or group of organs, in order that the whole may be saved. It is a conservative principle which says to stimulants "thus far shalt thou go an no farther."

In their pure and perfect state, the least violence done to the nerves by stimulants, excitants and disturbing agents, is felt and announced by them in full. But when they have been impaired by the habitual use of these things, a moderate excitation or flagellation with an agent such as that which impaired them, just sufficient to *exalt* the sensibilities to a comfortable state is relished, while an excess of the accustomed excitation is insipid or unpalatable. But in the degree as the sensibility and excitability of the nerves are depressed and impaired, in that proportion will it require force of excitation to raise them temporarily from their depression and despondency.

So long as power is present to respond to the lash of stimulation these agents are "delighted" in by the impaired nerves. But when the necessary force is no longer present and none is available to be dragooned to the relief of the unfortunate victim of his habits, until the nerves have had an opportunity of replenishing their storehouses, then the true character of the act of stimulation is revealed in all its naked deformity and is abominated by the thoroughly depressed sensibilities.

Inveterate tobacco users sometimes get so low that the tobacco is rejected until the flagging energies are partially recuperated. Inordinate users of alcohol or tea or coffee are liable to the same changes. Women whose very lives seem to be bound up in coffee, and who think they cannot live without it, will some times have periods during which they loath it. At such times they are regarded as "very sick," and they are, but they are sick because of the great depletion of their energies.

THE LAW OF SPECIAL ECONOMY:—*The vital organism, under favorable conditions, stores up all excess of vital funds, above the current expenditures, as a reserve fund, to be employed in a time of special need.*

Power in reserve is the surest guarantee against disease. The body seeks always to maintain a certain reserve of power and we can get this power out only by supplying emergencies such as this reserve is stored up to meet. Thus irritants, miscalled stimulants, produce an emergency that call out the body's reserve power in an effort to overcome these.

If no stimulants are employed the body will always have on hand a reserve of power to meet other emergencies of life.

During rest and sleep the body stores up power. During favorable weather it stores up power. During activity power is expended in doing work. During unfavorable weather power is exepending in defending the body against the excessive cold or excessive heat, etc.

The growth and development of the body takes place by "spurts." Periods of rapid growth alternate with periods of slow growth. The body seems to take a rest and accumulate power for the period of rapid growth. In periods of rapid growth there are new developments to be made, or incomplete ones to be finished and these things cannot be accomplished without an outlay of energy above the ordinary expenditure. In preparation for such a work there always precedes a period of comparative rest, as just prior to the onset of and in preparation for puberty at which time the forces of development go forward with a rush.

Some who have been ailing through more or less of the period of childhood are "carried by the force of development, which in a cyclonic fashion sweeps everything before it into health—and that, too, often in spite of wrong life, and a medical treatment that might prove fatal if administered at any other time in life.

"These health storms, typhoons, revolutions, often sweeps invalids into health, starting up with no apparent cause, and carrying many victims of ill-health into physical states approximating good health?"—*Impaired Health*, Vol. I, p. 153, by J. H. Tilden, M.D.

It is as though the Miller, in preparation for a busy season, shuts his sluce gates and lets the water accumulate above the mill-dam until he has a head of power sufficient to meet the demands of the season.

We may make use of this same principle when the actions of the body falter due to lack of power. If the action of the mill falters from a decrease of water-power the gates are closed for the purpose of accumulating power. Activities are ceased and no power is expended. In cases of impaired health the closing of all the waste-gates through which vital power is needlessly expended permits the accumulation of power.

THE LAW OF VITAL ACCOMMODATION—*Natures Balance wheel*—"*The response of the vital organism to external stimuli is an instinctive one, based upon a self-preservative instinct which adapts itself to whatever influence it cannot destroy or control.*"

The man who habitually indulges in stimulation would exhaust and destroy himself with but few indulgencies if the organism had no means of curbing its reactions against the stimulation and thereby lessening the expenditure of vital power. The first effect of stimulation is exaltation of function; if it is long continued, or often repeated, exhaustion with an almost total abolition of function results. The repeated use of stimulants would soon result in death. But their repeated use soon brings about a condition in which the organism ceases to respond so readily and violently to the stimulant. If the former amount of stimulation is to be received from the stimulant a larger amount of the stimulant must be used.

The first smoke or the first chew of tobacco usually occasions a very powerful reaction against it on the part of the organism. The young man or woman is made very sick; there is headache, nausea, vomiting, loss of appetite, weakness, etc. So long as the physiological powers and instincts are undepraved and unimpaired they instantly perceive the poisonous character of the tobacco and give the alarm to the whole system. A vigorous effort is made to destroy and eliminate it and the user is forced to throw away his tobacco. But if he continues to repeat the performance the reaction against it grows less and less with each repetition until, finally, he is able to use many times the original amount without producing such results. His system learns to tolerate it and adapts itself to its use as far as possible. The system soon becomes depraved and its power impaired by the use of the tobacco, its poisonous character is no longer detected and no alarm is given, rather a craving for the substance is developed. However, the habitual use of any substance that is injurious in itself cannot in any way render it harmless or beneficial and the habitual presence of any such substance is injurious to life, even, though, no energetic effort is made to resist its action.

What is here said of tobacco is true of other poisonous substances. Ordinarily the user of drugs such as tobacco, opium, alcohol, cocaine, etc., becomes so accustomed to their use that he is able to take at one time enough of his favorite drug to kill several non-users outright, and yet, it only produces in him an apparent normal condition of comfort and strength. There was the ancient King who, in order to protect himself against poisoning by his foes, accustomed his body to various poisons by gradual increase in the amount taken, until, when a time finally arrived when he desired to take his own life, by poisoning, he failed in the attempt. The first effort of the living organism, in response to adverse and inimical influences, is to overcome and destroy these. Failing in this it attempts to accommodate itself to such conditions and influences. For, what it cannot overcome, it must learn to endure or perish.

Men live in almost every conceivable climate and under almost every conceivable condition, are subject to all kinds of influences and indulge in many and often very opposite habits. If given time the body is able to adapt itself to these varying conditions. Only sudden and violent changes become immediately destructive of life. We cannot quickly transfer the esquamaux to the tropics nor the Hottentot to Greenland. We can suddenly force upon the non-user the amount of alcohol, arsenic or opium used by the habitue, only at the expense of life itself.

Habits, gradually built and long established, cannot usually be suddenly broken. There is no immediate danger to life as a result of the sudden breaking off of a habit, long practiced, but it is often followed by one or more crises more or less severe as the organism seeks to accommodate itself to the changed conditions. Because a habit does not seem to be immediately destructive is no evidence that it is not destructive or that it is beneficial. Its secondary effects alone can furnish us with the clue to its influence. A cup of coffee produces an immediate feeling of well being while no such feeling accompanies the taking of a glass of orange juice. But when the secondary effects of these two substances are viewed, no room for doubt is left as to which of these is really beneficial and which is injurious.

When the French revolutionists destroyed the Bastile, they found a man who had been confined for eighteen years in one of the cells, and his only bed a hatchel, or plank pierced with nails, the points of which protruded on the side on which he was forced to lie without protection from the points of the nails.

The man's sufferings had been almost beyond endurance for the first two weeks of his incarceration, yet when he was removed by his friends, and supplied with a soft bed, he begged to be restored to his bed of nails for he could now rest no where else. But the same kind *law of accommodation* which had made his *hatchel* endurable, would soon have accommodated him to a soft bed. This law cushions the bottoms of the feet of bare-foot boys, girls and adults, and guards the hands of the manual laborer by a similar cushion.

In the mouth, throat, stomach, intestine and bowel, a similar hardening and thickening takes place to guard the at first sensitive linings of these organs against the constant irritation to which they are ignorantly subjected by those who use, tobacco, antiseptic dentrifices, mouth washes and gargles, alcohol, coffee, tea, salt, pepper, mustard, horse-radish, spices, cathartics, mineral waters, etc. But this is an expensive business— this business of keeping the system accustomed to the action of *irritants* so that the sensibilities shall not be kept under torture by these. Such protection does not render them harmless.

That hard (mineral) waters do contain substances that are unfriendly to life is obvious from their effects upon the hands that are much washed in such waters. The skin of the hands is firmer and more resistant to such influences than is the delicate membrane which lines the digestive tract and the lining of the internal surfaces of the arteries and veins. Yet these latter must come in contact with such substances if they are taken into the body.

When such waters are first taken the irritation they set up occasions a diarrhea. But as their use is continued thickening and hardening of the lining of the digestive tract occurs to protect these and the diarrheas cease. A similar hardening and thickening must take place in the arteries and veins. Hardening of the arteries is due to irritation caused by toxins and irritants of all kinds.

Other, and perhaps less important, laws no doubt exist, but they have not yet been formulated. One of these which may rightly be denominated the *Law of Selective Elimination* remains to be formulated. It is known that *all injurious substances, which by any means, gain admittance within the domain of vitality, are counteracted, neutralized and expelled in such a manner and through such channels as will produce the least amount of wear and tear to the system.* This law accounts for the fact that some drugs apparently act on the bowels, some on the liver, some on the kidneys, etc. These are the organs which are *selected* to act on the drugs.

The *Law of Stimulation* remains to be formulated. Also the *Law of Repose*. These I shall attempt to formulate in the chapters on *Rest* and *Stimulation*.

LIVING MATTER CURES ITSELF

CHAPTER III

THE power of cure is inherent in living matter. Beginning with the tiniest microscopic cell or germ and extending to the most highly complex organism of which we know, the power of healing or cure is seen in operation. This power shall be discussed at length in this chapter.

Samuel O. L. Potter, A.M., M. D., in his compend of *Materia Medica and Therapeutics,* in classifying therapeutics, gives first:—

"Natural Therapeutics, including the operations of the *Vis Medicatrix Naturae,*—The modes and processes of healing which occur independently of art, for the spontaneous decline and cure of disease. There is no fact in science more fully established than that the living organism is in itself adequate to the cure of all its curable disorders."

Here is a great truth, one that is capable of shedding a flood of light upon the many vexed problems of the various cults. But this great light is so obscured by the false theories and hypotheses of the cults that their members are walking around in darkness as thick as that which hovered over Egypt.

"*The living organism is adequate to the cure of all its curable disorders*" by "*modes and processes of healing that occur independently of Art, for the spontaneous decline and cure of disease.*" Yea! More! The diligent student of medical history cannot but be aware of the stupendous fact that the living organism often cures its disorders in spite of methods of treatment that are not only not beneficial but are, more often than otherwise, positively harmful and destructive. More about this in another chapter. At present I wish to present briefly the powers by which the living organism heals and cures itself. These are:

I. THE CAPACITY OF REDINTEGRATION FOLLOWING THE DISINTEGRATION OF TISSUES. Of this power, no evidence is needed, for it is well known by physiologists, and even, by the unlearned in science. It is the process of repair which is continually making good the eternal wear and tear of the tissues consequent upon the operations of life. Regeneration of tissue is a continuous physiological process in health and disease and operates to restore tissues that have been destroyed, although here its sphere is more limited. Were it not for this process of repair and replenishment the bodies of all animals would begin to gradually wear and waste away from the moment of birth and in the course of a few days would perish or wear out. Animals would not live through the period of infancy.

Carrell and Burrows discovered that cells which showed signs of what is called old age require only to be placed in a new culture media to become young again and to multiply and grow. Dr. Woodruff kept groups of cells alive for 8,500 generations without loss of cellular vitality.

Parts of the stomach, the kidney, the lungs, the liver and other organs have been rebuilt by being fed with blood. Lung tissue added to the piece of lung, kidney tissue to the kidney, liver tissue to the liver, etc. Almost all parts of the body have been subjected to experiments of this kind and have proven themselves capable of growth and repair under such conditions. Each part of the body renews and repairs itself, by its own intrinsic power to absorb nutritive material from the surrounding medium and assimilate, organize and transform it into material identical with its own substance and endow it with vital properties.

Part of a newly-born rabbit was placed in cold-storage and allowed to remain there for a year. It was then placed on a slide, given food and warmth and it began to grow as soon as the proper temperature was reached. A piece of bone of a young pig began growing quickly, but a piece of bone from an old pig was slow in beginning its growth. Experiments have shown that parts taken from very young life begin to grow soon, those from middle life require more time to start growing while those from old life require much more time. The practice of grafting plants and trees is familiar to all, in fact, it is so common that everyone considers it a matter of course. In recent years grafting of animal parts has been successfully accomplished. For instance, pieces of skin have been put in cold storage to prevent decay, and after they have been there several months, have been taken out and fed warm blood and they began to grow. New pores and layers were built in perfect order, and all the intricate apparatus involved in perspiration was constructed. Fresh pieces of skin placed on the denuded flesh where the skin was torn or burned away grew and united with the surrounding skin.

Pieces of bone have been taken from freshly killed animals and fed with fresh blood with the result that they selected from the blood the elements necessary to the building of new bone and rejected the rest. Pieces of new bone have been grafted into the bones of those who from some cause have had part of their bone destroyed. The bone grew and united with the surrounding bone

The power to regenerate impaired, degenerated, atrophied parts depends not alone upon the abilities of depleted and "aged" cells to revive and grow young again, but also upon the power of the organism to replace dead and dying cells with new ones. This power has its limits. Tissues that are destroyed and have had their places filled by other tissues of a lower grade cannot regenerate, at least, not fully. Thus in cirrhosis of the liver, where the functioning cells have been replaced by connective tissue the system has no means of dissolving the connective tissue and filling the space occupied by it with liver cells. Experiments upon all the tissues of the body, both of young middle aged and old animals have shown this power of regeneration to belong to all of them. Cells of young animals begin to regenerate most quickly and those of aged ones least quickly. The exercise of this power of regeneration, however, depends upon the existence of certain definite conditions which need not be discussed here.

2. THE POWER OF HEALING WHICH IS EVIDENCED EITHER BY WHAT IS TERMED "HEALING BY FIRST INTENTION," OR "HEALING BY SECOND INTENTION," UPON THE OCCURRENCE OF ANY WOUND OR ABRASION.

Whether the continuity of the tissues has been broken either by bursting of an abscess or by a clean cut, the process of repair is always the same. The wound is filled with new connective tissue, its surface is covered by the proliferation of the surrounding epithelium, the nervous and circulatory channels are re-established and the wound healed. Clean cuts, on healthy individuals heal with a minimum amount of connective tissue so that the results are scarcely apparent to the naked eye. This is called "healing by first intention" or "primary union."

"Healing by second intention" does not differ in any great respect from "healing by first intention." There is, however, an obvious formation of connective tissue and the formation of a superficial scar. The same formation of granulation tissue (embryonic connective tissue) coagulation, fibrin formation and proliferation of capillaries and connective tissue takes place in both forms of healing. Both are accompanied by more or less of inflammation resulting in the destruction of some tissue. Bone and nerve tissue are the best regenerators, although there is more or less regeneration in other tissues.

3 THE POWER TO IMMEDIATELY REPRODUCE A LOST PART. A power displayed to the fullest extent by the lower orders of animals, and, measurably, by even the highest. Darwin referred to this power as the "Reparative power which is common, in a higher or lower degree, to all organic beings, and which was formerly designated by physiologists as the *nisus formativus.*" He said, also, this "power is greater in animals, the lower they are in the scale of organisms." The reason for this lessened reproductive power, in the higher animals, is, that such animals are more complex, the conditions of growth are correspondingly more complex and less easily supplied and, therefore, lost members are less likely to be supplied, when required.

Experiments upon protozoa show that if the cell is divided into two parts, the part containing the nucleus soon again becomes a complete cell with all the properties and powers which it originally possessed. If even a small part of the nucleus remains in the cut-off piece of cytoplasm, reconstruction may take place.

It is the contention of the present writer that the power of healing and cure is inherent in living protoplasm and that it does not inhere in anything else. Living matter cures itself where cure is possible. Where cure is not possible no outside "aids"

23

will or can effect it. All cure is self-cure. It is spontaneous and independent of art. Indeed, with the exception of a few surgical cases, art is a hindering agent or force, impeding or preventing cure or healing and both increasing and prolonging the suffering. This last statement will be made clear in future pages of this book.

The glass snake, which scientists insist is a lizard and whose family name is *squamata lacertilla anguidae ophisaurus ventralis*, if caught by the tail, will snap it off and hurry on in its effort to escape from its enemy. It then, without trouble or pain, grows a new tail that serves just as well as the original one. The slow-worm, the sphenodon and many other lizards can do likewise. Many fingers, the tips of which have been cut off in accidents, grow new tips including even the nails. A finger nail or a toe nail which has been seriously damaged is slowly thrown off as a new nail forms underneath.

Oscar Hertwig in his "The Biological Problem of Today" says:

"Although in many higher animals and plants one sees that cells with the capacity for reproduction are limited to special areas, still, the capacity for regeneration often is very great. In a wonderful fashion animals will reproduce lost parts, sometimes of most complicated structure; just as a crystal, from which a corner has been chipped, will perfect itself again when brought into a solution of its own salt. A Hydra, from which the oral disc and tenacles have been cut off, a Nais deprived of its head or of its tail, a snail of which a tentacle with its terminal eye has been amputated, will reproduce the lost parts, sometimes in a very short time. The cells lying at the wounded spot begin to bud, producing a layer or lump, the cells of which resemble embryonic cells. From this embryonic mass of cells the lost organs and tissues arise—in Hydra, the oral disc with its tentacles; in Nais, the anterior end with its sense-organs and special groups of muscles; in the snail the tentacle with its compound eye built up of elements as different as retinal rods, pigment cells, nerve cells, lens, and so forth.

"Even among vertebrates, in which the capacity for regeneration is the least, as in the restoration of the wounded parts small defects occur, lizards can reproduce a lost tail, tritons an amputated limb. From a bud of embryonic tissue there are elaborated in the one case whole vertebrae with their muscles and tendons, and part of the spinal cord with its ganglia and nerves in the other case, the numerous differently shaped skeletal pieces of the hand or foot, with their appropriate muscles and nerves. The regeneration, morevoer, is in strict conformity with the character of the species concerned."

Again he says:

"Heteromorphoses are well known in plant physiology. When one cuts a slip from a willow, one may make the cut at the bottom of the slip and the cut at the top in any part of the willow-twig, yet still the lower end of the slip always produces rootlets, which are organs not normal to that part of the twig, while shoots will rise from the upper end. Moreover, either end of the slip may be made the root portion." He presents many other examples of a similar character.

Cut off a leaf from a begonia plant, place it in a suitable soil and water it; it puts out roots and shoots and in due time a full grown begonia plant results. Cut off a minute part of the leaf, as small as can be seen, and care for this properly and a full grown plant, just like one grown from the seed, will result. Something like a hundred plants may be produced from the fragments of a single leaf.

If Planaria are cut into small pieces and the pieces placed where they can absorb nourishment, each of them will grow into a whole worm. If they cannot get nourishment, they cannot grow; each piece, therefore, completely rearranges its materials and becomes a perfect but very minute worm. The piece that happens to contain the pharnyx finding this too large for his present size, will dissolve it and make a new one that fits its new size. Many other worms when cut grow new heads or tails.

The tubularia is a kind of sea anemone which grows on a stalk with two rows of tentacles surrounding the head and mouth. If the head with its tentacles is cut off, the first sign of regeneration consists of two rings of lines, one above another, running down the sides of the stem from the cut. These are gradually stripped off keeping one end attached and thus forming new tentacles. The head then forms in their midst. But if, before this, you cut off part of the stem, leaving only one of the two rows of

24

lines,, the creature, as if in disgust, sometimes erases the one row left and then divides it in the middle thus forming two lines, one end of each, thus forming two very small tentacles, and then grows these to their proper length and size.

The following quotations are selected from "Animals and Plants Under Domestication," by Chas. Darwin:

"It is notorious that some of the lower animals, when cut into many pieces, reproduce so many perfect individuals. Lyonnet cut a Nais, or fresh water worm, into nearly fifty pieces, and these all reproduced perfect animals. It is probable that segmentation could be carried much further in some of the protozoa, and with some, of the lowest plants, each cell will reproduce the parent form."

"Now, when the left leg, for instance, of a salamander, is cut off, a light crust forms over the wound, and beneath this crust, the uninjured cells, or unities of bone, muscles, nerves, etc., are supposed to unite with the diffused gemmules of those cells which in the perfect leg come next in order; and these as they become lightly developed, unite with others, and so until a papilla of soft cellular tissue, the 'budding leg,' is formed; and in time a perfect leg. Thus, that portion of the leg which has been cut off neither more nor less, would be reproduced. If the tail or leg of a young animal had been cut off, a young tail or leg would have been reproduced, as actually occurs with the amputated tail of the tadpole."

"Spallanzani, by cutting off the legs and tail of a salamander, got in the course of three months, six crops of these members; so that 687 perfect bones were produced, by one animal, during one season. At whatever point the limb was cut off, the deficient part, and no more, was exactly reproduced. Even with man as we have seen in the twelfth chapter, when treating of polydactylism, the entire limb, while in an embryonic state, and supernumary digits, are occasionally, though imperfectly reproduced after amputation. When a diseased bone has been removed, a new one sometimes gradually assumes the regular form, and all the attachments of muscles, ligaments, etc., become as complete as before."

"This power of regrowth does not, however, always act perfectly; the reproduced tail of a lizard differs in the forms of the scales from the normal tail."

Kellogg tells us that "the long 'domesticated' Mulberry silkworm larva possesses the capacity of regenerating any of its legs, if the mutilation has not removed the whole appendage."

Craw-fish are able to grow new parts if a limb or tentacle is destroyed. Experiments have shown that almost every part of a craw-fish may be reproduced.

The regeneration of a nerve fiber is an interesting and instructive process. I present the following brief description after Howell (Text-book of Physiology), of course, stripping it of all theories and hypotheses of how it is accomplished.

When a nerve trunk is cut or killed at any point by crushing, heating or by any means, all the fibers from the point of injury to the periphery undergo degeneration. The definite changes included in this degeneration are observed only in a living nerve. A dead nerve or the nerve of a dead animal does not undergo these changes. The time required for the degenerative change to begin differs for the different kind of fibers found in the animal organism. In the dog they begin in four days. In the frog from thirty to a hundred and forty days depending on the season of the year. It has been found that if the frog is maintained at a high temperature (30 degrees C) degeneration will proceed as rapidly as in the mammal. In a cold temperature more time is required. In the dog it goes on so rapidly that the process appears to occur simultaneously throughout the whole of the peripheral stump. In the frog and rabbit it is observed to begin at the point of injury and progress peripherally.

The nerve fibers break up into ellipsodal segments of myelin, each of which contains a portion of the axis cylinder. These segments in turn break up into smaller pieces which finally are absorbed. The central stump, the fibers of which are still connected with the nerve cells, undergoes a similar degeneration for a short distance immediately contiguous to the wound.

In the peripheral portion of the nerve regeneration begins almost simultaneously with the beginning of degeneration. The nuclei of the neurilemmal sheath begin to multiply and form around them a layer of protoplasm so that as the fragments of the

25

old fibers disappear their places are filled by numerous nuclei and their surrounding cytoplasm. This eventually forms a continuous strand of multi-nucleated protoplasm. This fiber bears no structural resemblance to the normal nerve fiber and is described as "embryonic fiber."

In the adult animal regeneration ceases at this point unless an anatomical connection is made with the central stump. However, such a connection is almost always accomplished unless special means are taken to prevent it. The two ends of the severed nerve find each other in a remarkable way and several ingenuous theories have been invented to account for this. After the two portions of the nerve have grown together the "embryonic fibers" of the peripheral end are gradually transformed into normal nerve fibers with myelin sheath and axis cylinder.

The earlier physiologists thought that if the severed ends of a nerve were brought together by suture they might unite by "*first intention*" without degeneration of the peripheral end. It is now known that this degeneration is inevitable once the living continuity of the fibers has been interrupted by any means. Any functional union that occurs is a slow process involving the degeneration and subsequent regeneration of the peripheral fibers. As if in disgust, nature tears down the old fibers and builds them anew.

Another interesting phenomenon that is but added evidence of what has gone before is reported by Prof. C. M. Child, of Chicago University. He chopped some small flat worms up into small pieces and each piece grew into a brand new worm. The new worm was a young worm although the piece from which it grew was from an old worm.

In his *Human Psysiology*, (1836), Robley Dunglison, M.D., in the chapter on "*Life*" (Vol. 2., p. 531), wrote:

"Again, the similarity of the actions of the instinctive principle, in the animal and vegetable, is exhibited by the reparatory power which both possess when injuries are inflicted upon them. If a branch be forcibly torn from a tree, the bark gradually accumulates around the wound, and cicatrization is at length accomplished. The great utility of many of our garden vegetables,—such as spinach, parsley, cress, etc.,—depends upon the possession of a power to reapir injuries, so that new shoots speedily take the place of the leaves that have been removed. Similar to this is the reparative process, instituted by the lobster that has lost its claw, in the water-newt lost an extremity, or, the eye; in the serpent deprived of its tail, and in the snail that has lost its head. These parts are reproduced as the leaves are in the spinach or the parsley.

"Few animals, however, possess the property of restoring lost parts; whilst all are capable of repairing their own wounds when not excessive, and of exerting a sanitive power, when laboring under disease. If a limb be torn from the body, provided the animal does not die from hemorrhage, a reparatory effort is established, and if the severity of the injury does not induce too much irritation in the system, the wound will gradually fill up, and the skin form over it. To a lesser extent we see this power exerted in the healing of ordinary wounds, and in cementing broken bones; and although it may answer the purposes of the surgeon to have it supposed, that he is possessed of healing salves, etc., he is well aware, that the great art in these cases, is to keep the part entirely at rest, whilst his salves are applied simply for the purpose of keeping the wound moist; the edges in due apposition, where such is necessary, and extraneous bodies from having access to it—his trust being altogether placed in the sanative influence of the instinctive power situated in the injured part, and in every part of the frame.

"It is to this power, that we ascribe all the properties ascribed to the famous sympathetic powder of Sir Kenelm Digby,—which was supposed to have the wonderful property of healing wounds, when merely applied to the bloody clothes of the wounded person, or to the weapon that had inflicted the mischief;—a powder, which at one time enjoyed the most astounding reputation. The wound was, however always carefully defended from irritation by extraneous substances; and it has been suggested, that the result furnished the first hint, which led surgeons to the improved practice of healing wounds by what is technically called the *First intention*. It is to this instinctive principle, so clearly evidenced in surgical or external affections, but, at times, not less actively exerted in cases of internal mischief, that the term *Vis Medicatrix Naturae* has been assigned; and whatever may be the objections to the views entertained regarding its manifestations in disease, that such a power exists can no more be denied than that organized bodies are possessed of the vital principle. We have too many instances of recovery from injuries, NOT ONLY WITHOUT THE AID OF A PRACTITIONER, BUT EVEN IN SPITE OF IT, to doubt for a moment, that there is, within every living body a principle, whose operations are manifestly directed to the health and preservation of the frame, and of every part of such frame." (Caps mine. Author.)

I believe any reasoning mind will concede, after reviewing medical history, that not only do external injuries often recover in spite of the practitioner but that the gravest internal diseases just as often recover in spite of his murderous methods. Dunglison seemed to think that the inherent curative power possessed by the living organism was actively engaged in defending the body against internal mischief, only at times. This is not the case. This reparative and defensive power, which is nothing more nor less than the ordinary powers of healthy life, never rests day or night asleep or awake, so long as life lasts, and even, after somatic death has occurred, many cells in the body continue, for some time, to repair and defend themselves. This reparative power is inseparable from life and is exercised only by life. It never begins but once—when life begins—and never ends until death. It does not depend upon any special conditions or treatments. The snail only asks for the ordinary or natural conditions of snail life in order to grow a new head. He requires no drugs, serums, salves, antiseptics, vaccines, antitoxins, electrical currents, x-rays, radium, nor any drugless treatment. The celery or parsley stalk needs only the ordinary or natural conditions of plant life in order to grow a new shoot or leaf to take the place of the destroyed one. The same is true of the crab that has lost its claw. Given these conditions, even though not in their perfection, and life is capable of accomplishing all the reparative work possible. What life cannot do, cannot be done by treatment.

Advocates of the idea that cure is accomplished by anything that will effect the mind strongly enough will please note that no mental influence aids the decapitated snail to grow a new head, nor does the asparagus plant receive any help from this source, in growing a new shoot. Crabs do not employ mental influences in growing new claws, nor do trees in healing a wound where a limb has been torn away. Man cannot grow a new head like the snail, nor a new limb like the crab, and treatment cannot grow these for him. Man can heal a wound or a broken bone, but treatment, beyond bringing the edges of the wound together or setting the bone, cannot aid him in healing these. A wet cloth applied over a wound will accomplish all that Dunglison claimed for salves and ointments and even this is not necessary. Cleanliness and rest are all that wounds require and many heal without either of these, although, not so rapidly.

There is not the slighest evidence that the living organism can make any use whatever of any influences or agents in the cure of disease or repair of injury that it does not and cannot use in maintaining health. There is, however, a world of evidence that the living organism can get along without all these therapeutic agents and influences and equally as much evidence that it does often get along in spite of them. There is, also, a world of evidence, that many, if not all, methods and systems of therapeutics are harmful and as a consequence, retard healing and cure. The voice of history and the laws and powers of life cry aloud in praise of hygiene, and in denouncing therapeutics.

Thus far, we have considered four phases of the living organism's power of self-repair. A few words here about the oneness of this power may not be amiss. Animals begin life as a single microscopic cell and by processes of cell proliferation and differentiation are organized into complex organisms with many dissimilar organs with their varied powers and functions The organism is apparently self-evolving dependent only upon certain natural conditions. Each of the three phases of the power of self-repair we have considered are accomplished by the same processes and are subject to the same natural conditions as are involved in the development of the animal from ovumhood to adulthood. Regarding this Darwin wrote:—

27

"Between the powers, which repair a trifling injury in any part, and the power which previously was occupied, in its maintenance, by the continued mutation of its particles, there cannot be any difference and we may follow Mr. Paget in believing them to be the self-same power. As at each stage of growth, an amputated part is replaced by one in the same state of development, we must likewise follow Mr. Paget in admitting, that the powers of development, from the embryo are identical with those exercised for the restoration from injuries."

This power of repair of re-integration goes beyond the individual. In close inter-breeding of animals many characters are suppressed or "stopped down." As an example, I may mention that there is in many cases of close in breeding the loss of one or more vertebrae in the spinal column. In cases of cross-breeding or in "spontaneous" reversions these suppressed characters are restored. Darwin wrote:

"No doubt the power of reparation, though not always quite perfect, is an admirable provision, ready for various emergencies EVEN FOR THOSE WHICH OCCUR ONLY AT LONG INTERVALS OF TIME." (Caps mine. Author).

Again: "That there is a tendency, in the young of each, successive generation, to produce the long-lost characters, and that this tendency, from some unknown cause, sometimes prevails."

Lastly: "This subject has been here noticed, because we may infer, that when any part or organ is either greatly increased in size, or wholly suppressed, the co-ordinating power of the organization will continually tend to bring all the parts again into harmony with each other."

This shows that, with each species, there is a certain ratio of development of its several characters, which cannot normally be varied from, and which could not be varied from very greatly under any conditions without resulting in such disproportionate development and loss of physiological coordination, and all their attendant evils, as are seen in the results of close-interbreeding. If Darwin had adhered to the principle he states above, in his treatment of the facts of breeding and variation, he could never have propounded a theory of the deriviation of one species from another. He himself produced ample evidence to show that the more a form diverged from the primitive normal form the less its chances of survival and the more need it had for "repair." On the other hand, cross-breeding and "reversion," by restoring one or more of the suppressed characters, increase the ability to survive.

If this power of repair, after being kept down for hundreds or even thousands of generations by adverse conditions—Darwin's "unknown cause"—is able, when the adverse conditions are removed, to "sometimes prevail" and "BRING ALL THE PARTS AGAIN INTO HARMONY WITH EACH OTHER," how much more successful should we expect it to be in repairing ordinary injuries when the organism is placed under proper conditions?

5. THE POWER OF THE LIVING ORGANISM TO REJECT AND ELIMINATE ALL WASTE, USELESS AND INJURIOUS SUBSTANCES. The first three powers which we have just considered all depend upon the power peculiar to living things to appropriate dissimilar material from their environment, transform it into matter like themselves, and incorporate it into their own structure. The power to reject and refuse waste, useless and injurious substances and to eliminate these is as fundamental as the power of appropriation and transformation or assimilation. *Each of these two powers are equally essential to the continuance of the living state and the living organism equally serves its own end in either set of actions.*

The complex animal body is adequately equipped with organs and structures, the function of which is to excrete and eliminate from it all waste matter, toxins, etc., chief among these are the lungs, skin, kidneys, bowels, liver and the mucous surfaces of the hollow organs of the body. No special notice will be given these organs at this place. I do desire, however, to direct attention to one phase of the work of keeping the body clean that is frequently overlooked. I refer to the work performed in the nose and throat in filtering the air we breathe and in removing from the air passages dust, etc., that get into these.

These passages are lined with fine hairlike projections called cilia. These are very close together and continually wave to and fro like the stalks of grain in a wheat field. However, the stroke made in one direction is sharp and decisive, the recovery is slower and more gentle, reminding one of the stroke of a whip or an oar or of the movements of the hands in swimming. These cilia are overlaid with a thin film of moisture or mucous which is kept moving by their strokes. Any small particles of dust, germs, etc., which adhere to the surface of these passages are carried along with the moving film. In the bronchial tubes the movement is from below upward toward the throat so that dust that might otherwise accumulate in the lungs and result seriously is continually cleared away. It is carried to and gathered temporarily about the root of the tongue where it is usually swallowed but sometimes coughed up and spit out. One physiologist compares us to vacuum cleaners "freeing the air of part of the suspended material and depositing it in their own stomachs." But it is not allowed to remain in the stomach. It passes out with the food and after traversing the entire length of the digestive tract, is expelled from the bowels.

There remains some doubt about the direction of the ciliary currents in the nose. It is disputed whether the movement is toward the nostrils or toward the pharnyx. Movements in each direction may be present, depending on the part of the nasal passage one views. It is sufficicnet for us, however, that it occurs and keeps the nasal passages clean.

The nose and trachea filter the air we breathe, warm it and moisten it and thus fit it for entrance into the lungs. The atmosphere is nowhere pure enough and usually not warm and moist enough for man's breathing until it has passed through this process. The air which enters the lungs is as different from that which enters the nostrils as distilled water is different from that which entered the still.

The man with weak or diseased lungs finds it painful to breathe through his mouth but experiences no such difficulty in breathing through his nose. The mouth does not prepare the air for the lungs as does the nose. Some dust does escape the action of the cilia and gets into the lower portions of the air passages where no cilia exist, where it may accumulate and stain the lungs. This is seen in the lungs of coal miners, inhabitants of smoky cities and workers in other dusty places. Further mention of this will be made in the chapters on what is disease.

Cilia surrounding the edge of the mouth of the sea anemone usually beat from without inward thus keeping a steady stream of water flowing into the body cavity. However, if a non-nutritive substance, such as a grain of sand, is placed upon the margin of the mouth the cilia immediately reverse their motion in an effort to expell the foreign particle. Here the power of rejection is manifest.

All orifices of the body are normally self-cleansing. Their secretions are normally antiseptic and so long as their health remains unimpaired, unless overwhelmed from without, they remain clean and clear. A Diarrhea soon cleanses the digestive tract when it becomes foul.

Upon this point Dr. Oswald, said, *Natures' Household Remedies*, p. 9:

"The organism of the human body is a self-regulating apparatus. Every interruption of its normal functions excites a reaction against the disturbing cause. If a grain of caustic potash irritates the nerves of the palate, the salivary glands try to remove it by an increased secretion. The eye would wash it off by an immediate flow of tears A larger quantity of the same substance could be swallowed only under the protest of the fauces, and the digestive organs would soon find means to eject it. The bronchial tubes promptly react against the obstruction of foreign substances. The sting of an insect causes an involuntary twitching of the epidermis. If a thorn or splinter fastens itself under the skin, suppuration prepares the way for its removal. If the stomach be overloaded with food it revolts against further ingestion."

The normal undisturbed excretion of waste matter is obsolutely essential to life and health and the normal organism is capable of carrying on this process of excretion in an adequate manner so long as the normal conditions of life are present. When these conditions are only imperfectly or partially vouchsafed to the body for a length of time it gradually loses the normal energy of all its functions. The work of exretion is impeded resulting in an accumulation of toxic matter which is destructive to life and health.

Matter is constantly being formed in the body, or received into it from without, that is both useless and injurious and, if allowed to remain and clog the activities of life, would produce disease or death. If the urine is suppressed for 52 hours, death results; if the skin of a man be varnished so that elimination through it is inhibited, death comes within a few hours. The carbon dioxide exhaled in a day would kill many times over if retained. If a wound is obstructed so that drainage is stopped, septicemia and probably death soon result. There is not a moment of life, from birth to death, that the body's processes of purification are not busily engaged in eliminating all wastes and toxins from the system.

The organism, being unable to get rid of these toxins in a normal manner is forced to resort to some abnormal means to accomplish its purification. These abnormal efforts of organic house cleaning or reactions against the toxins are termed *disease.* The examples given elsewhere of the eruptive fevers should convince any reasoning mind of the truth of this assertion. The fact that inflammation is resorted to not only in healing a broken bone or flesh wound, but also in resisting and removing toxins and foreign bodies, shots, slivers, parasites, etc., together with the most obvious fact that vomiting, diarrhea, colds, all forms of catarrh, night sweats, etc., are all forms of elimination demonstrate still more convincingly, the truth that disease is a curative process. *It is the cure!*

If a poison, such as epicec, or epsom salts, be taken into the stomach it is followed immediately by vomiting, or diarrhea. These actions are, obviously intended to expell the poison. If a gnat is drawn into the nostrils sneezing immediately follows. If a piece of bread or other food is drawn into the trachea (wind pipe) coughing follows. The same is true if mucous is excreted here in quantities. Both sneezing and coughing are intended to expell the offending matter. Dr. Jennings used to say that disease is "right action," and we can all agree that sneezing or coughing or vomiting or diarrhea are all "right actions" under the conditions named. Is not inflammation "right action" in those conditions under which it develops? Are not the eruptions in scarlet fever, measles, etc., "right action" under those conditions in which they develop?

Closely wrapped up with and inseparable from this power of *rejection* is the power of the living organism to detoxify, through chemicalization, all waste and toxins that are formed in it as a result of the normal processes of life or all organic poisons that gain an entrance into it from without. This detoxifying work is accomplished largely in the liver and lymphatic glands or nodes including, also, such lymphoid structures as the tonsils, adenoids (which are also tonsils) peyres patches in the small intestines and the vermiform appendix.

In a marvelous manner these glands enlarge (hypertrophy) to enable them to meet the extra demand made upon them when the toxins in the body are in excess of their normal capacity to meet and destroy. This enlargement often takes place in a very short time and may be noted by everyone following the bite of poisonous insects or reptiles or following infection. When they enlarge this increases their capacity for work.

The liver appears to be the chief organ of the body engaged in the production of urea. Urea is manufactured out of certain compounds that result from the break down of protein substances and which are constantly present in the blood, coming either from the regular wear and tear of the body due to its activities or from the intestines.

Destructive diseases of the liver—acute yellow atrophy, suppuration, cirrhosis, etc., and acute phophorus poisoning—largely diminish the production of urea but increase the quantities of the cell wastes from which urea is produced. This work of the liver in preparing cellular waste for excretion is an exceedingly important one, as, upon the successful accomplishment of this work depends, to a great extent, the success of the kidneys in their work of excretion.

Very similar to and closely associated with *urea formation* is the conversion, by the liver, of toxic compounds, products of putrefaction of proteins, into non-toxic compounds. These substances—indol, skatol, phenol, and cresol—are absorbed from the intestine and carried to the liver through the portal vein. The cells thus depriving them of their toxicity, after which they are allowed to enter the blood from whence they are excreted by the kidneys. Other toxic substances, as, for instance, alcohol, are likewise reduced in toxicity in the liver. However, the methods by which this is accomplished vary with the varying natures of the compounds. The liver thus forms a chemical laboratory and presents a chemical defense against the entrance into the blood and general circulation, of agents that are more or less toxic.

In this connection, also, may be mentioned the power of the living body to manufacture or secrete protective substances. Pour common salt over a shell-less land-snail or gastropod (slug) and it will instantly secrete a substance that rapidly diffuses throughout the salt giving it the appearance of finely ground egg yolk that had been boiled hard previous to grinding. Poisonous and irritating substances coming in contact with the lining membranes of the hollow organs of the body or gaining access to the eye, are met with an immediate out-pouring of mucous or tears which both envelops and dilutes these, rendering them more or less inert, and then washes them away.

The whole of the modern medical practice of vaccine, serum and antitoxin therapy is based upon the supposition that the body manufactures substances called anti-toxins, anti-bodies, antigens, etc., which are capable of meeting and destroying toxins that get into the body. The idea seems to be sound, although it is possible that the work of destroying such toxins is that of detoxification carried on by the liver, lymph glands, etc. Anti-toxins, anti-bodies, antigens, etc., have never been isolated. They have only been hypothicated, while the practice based upon their assumed existence has been both a failure and a disaster. However, this may not be due to their non-existence. If they exist it is impossible to separate them from the proteins of the animal's blood and these proteins when injected directly into the blood of another animal are very poisonous. Besides this, there is no evidence that the anti-toxins of one species can be made use of by another species. Where vaccines are employed, it constitutes the introduction of the actual disease matter into the blood. That is, the supposed causitive germs or some product of the disease is introduced into the body. The consequences are often terrible. Real benefits are never observed. If the hypothesis that the body manufactures, anti-toxins anti-bodies,etc., is correct it still remains to be proven that the body ever manufactures these greatly in excess of the need for them. It cannot be shown that "FREE" anti-toxins, anti-bodies, etc., are suspended in the blood serum and can therefore be transferred to another animal in sufficient quantities to be of use to the receiving animal. In keeping with a general law of life it is very probable that the body does manufacture an excess of anti-bodies but it cannot be shown that it retains these after the need for them has ceased On the contrary, in keeping with another general law of life, it is very probable that the body begins to get rid of them the very instant the need for them ceases. If they exist they are chemical substances produced to meet an emergency and will be cast out as soon as the emergency ceases to exist.

Another feature of this power of *rejection* is the ability of the organism to envelop and deposit out of the general circulation and at the farthest remove from the more vital structures, toxins, particularly inorganic toxins, which it is unable to eliminate. Dr. Rausse advanced the theory that drug poisons such as mercury which the body eliminates with difficulty are enveloped in mucous and deposited in the tissues. That they are deposited, whether in mucous or not, and are frequently retained in the body for years is shown by various facts.

1—People who have taken considerable mercury become walking barometers. They are very sensitive to weather changes, often being able to "feel" the change a day or more ahead of normal individuals. This condition lasts for years perhaps for life.

2—People who have taken mercury years before often undergo a severe mercurial crisis when undergoing natural renovation. The old cold-water hydropaths used to have to contend with this very often in the days when mercury was dispensed so often, so freely and in such large doses. Such patients develop mercurial stomatitis (salivation), and mercurial eruptions on the skin.

31

3—Other drugs like the bromids, coal-tar products, etc., after several years have elapsed will show up in the skin where they are eliminated by means of eruptions.

This subject will be covered more fully in a later chapter.

6—THE POWER AND ABILITY OF THE LIVING ORGANISM TO SO ORDER AND ARRANGE ITS FUNCTIONS AND PROCESSES AS TO ENABLE IT TO WITHSTAND THE ACTION OF PATHOFERIC AGENTS AND INFLUENCES WITH THE LEAST AMOUNT OF WEAR AND TEAR TO ITSELF AND TO STAY ITS INEVITABLE DISSOLUTION FOR THE LONGEST POSSIBLE TIME WHERE THESE AGENTS AND INFLUENCES ARE TOO POWERFUL FOR IT TO OVERCOME. One of the most familiar examples of this power is that by which the body quickly accomodates or adapts itself to changed conditions or to various poisonous drugs. One's first chew or smoke is met by a violent systemic reaction against the poison. If such reactions were evoked by every chew or smoke they would soon exhaust and kill the organism. Adaptation follows to prolong life as much as possible in spite of the tobacco poisoning. The same is true of other drug poisons. The power of compensation also comes under this head and will be more fully covered in a special chapter.

Another familiar example is that of suspended animation. This is more often met with among the lower forms of animal life although many cases among human beigns are on record. In the latter such cases usually lead to premature burial, although some few have revived in time to save themselves. Suspended animation is simply a state into which the living orgnaism goes under those conditions that are not favorable for continued active life and is a means which enables it to resist those conditions and preserve the *status quo*. Perhaps more such occurrences would be recorded were it not for the "*sustaining*" or stimulating practices in vogue. These practices prevent the full institution of this means of defense and render recovery from it impossible. They exhaust the powers of life while the suspension of animal function is intended to conserve these. This will be more fully discussed in another chapter.

In every disease we observe the living organism altering its functions to meet existing conditions. The reactive symptoms of disease may be broadly divided into two general classes—namely, those represented by reduced or suspended function, and those represented by accelerated function. As these will be dealt with more in detail in another chapter we will no more than mention them here. Suspended or reduced function is intended to conserve power while accelerated function is intended to actively meet and overcome the foes of life. The study of these phenomena is one of the most interesting studies in the whole realm of biology, although, at present, its surface has only been scratched.

As a means of adjustment and adaptation which enables the body to prolong its life NATURE ALWAYS FAVORS THE MOST VITAL ORGANS. This is as it should be. Life would not last long under many conditions if nature treated all organs alike and caused each organ to suffer equally under those conditions. If the heart or brain for instance were not given preference over the hair or nails, if the hair and nails were treated as though they were of equal importance as the heart and lungs, man would perish in many conditions through which he now passes with a minimum amount of harm.

The more important organs are securely packed away in places of greatest safety and every possible safeguard thrown around them. The brain is carefully wrapped in two delicate membraneous covers between which is a serous fluid which serves as a shock absorber and all this is encased in a hard bony safe which protects from all ordinary influences.

The gray matter of the spinal cord after being carefully wrapped in membraneous sheaths and protected by the spinal fluid is also encased in a flexible column of bone and cartilage. Its branches, the spinal nerves, are carefully cushioned in a fine mesh-work of connective tissue, the meshes of which are filled with a semi-fluid fat. The spinal column is so constructed that it combines great strength with a maximum of flexibility and the articulations are such that no luxations or sub-luxations are possible without such violence that there is a tearing of ligaments and cartilage and a breaking of the articulating processes of the vertebrae. No vertebrae can touch the spinal nerves. Our admiration for the wisdom of the Great Designer is greatly enhanced by our contemplation of the marvelous construction of the spinal column. To serve as a further shock absorber, preventing jarring of the brain from running or walking, the spinal column is normally curved in three places so that it acts much as the springs on a automobile.

The heart and lungs are carefully protected by being enclosed in a bony cage made up of the ribs, spinal column and sternum. Nature fortifies and places all the vital organs in the least exposed and most inaccessable parts of the body.

When short of nutritive material nature nourishes the most vital organs first. In fasting, or in starvation the fat is consumed first and then the other tissues in the inverse order of their usefulness and importance. In death from starvation the loss to the nervous system is almost immeasurally small. Given rest and sleep and the nerves seem able to maintain their substance without injury through the most prolonged fast.

During a fast the diseased tissues are broken down and absorbed. Deposits, exudates, effusions, infiltrations and even growths are absorbed and either used as food or excreted. We have seen numerous small tumors entirely absorbed during a fast and many large ones markedly reduced.

In fevers, when nutrition is at a low ebb, the hair often falls out and the nails lose much of their substance. The nutrition that normally goes to these is being utilized by the other organs.

During pregnancy, if the diet is deficient, nature first sacrifices the most dispensible portions of the mother's body—the teeth, hair, nails etc.,—to supply nutritive material to the developing embryo. The more vital organs do not suffer until the less vital have first been sacrificed. Sylvester Graham admirably expressed these facts in the following words:—

"It is a general law of the vital economy, that when by any means the general function of decomposition exceeds that of composition or nutrition, the decomposing absorbents always first lay hold of and remove those substances which are of least use to the economy; and hence all morbid accumulations, such as wens, tumors, abscesses, etc., are rapidly diminished and sometimes wholly removed under severe and protracted abstinence and fasting. When by an excess of the general function of composition more nutrition is received into the vital domain than the wants of the vital economy demand, and more than its powers can regularly dispose of, and this excess has been deposited in the cellular tissue and it cannot be eliminated from the vital domain as fast as it is received. In this exigency it must be disposed of in the safest manner possible, as a temporary resource. The cellular tissue, we have seen, is the lowest order of animal structure; the lowest in vital endowment and functional character; and of all the forms of this general structure, that in which the adipose matter is deposited, is the lowest species. In the cells of this loose tissue, which is simply employed as a kind of web to connect other and more important tissues and parts, the vital economy, therefore, may, with greatest safety, in its particular emergencies, deposit for a time whatever substance it is obliged to dispose of in the most expeditious and convenient manner, and which it is not able to eliminate from the vital domain; for in these cells, such substances are deposited in this tissue; and some of these substances which are deposited here, and in some cases retained for years, are of the most deleterious character***** temporarily deposited in the cellular tissue as a necessary expedient of the vital economy in its emergency."—*Science of Human Life*, p. 194.

"Therefore, if active exercise be considerably increased, or the quantity of food be considerably diminished, the decomposing and eliminating organs of the system by all that their functions are relatively increased upon that of nutrition, will be employed in first removing the adipose matter, in order to restore the system to the most perfectly healthy condition."—*Science of Human Life*, p. 195.

It will be noticed in all the examples given of the power of self-repair that no special condition or treatment is required—just the normal or ordinary conditions of plant and animal life. Take the case of the begonia leaf; all that is required for the development of a plant from the fragment of a leaf are those same conditions required for the daily growth and sustenance of the plant, or for its development from the seed—suitable soil, water, air, warmth and sunlight. In a word, *hygienic* conditions, not *therapeutics,* are all that are required and development, regeneration, repair and cure follow spontaneously and *independently of art.* It is worthy of special notice, as well, that these follow even under unfavorable conditions and often in spite of actual hindrances. This will be made more clear in another chapter.

Cure or healing is the restoration to normal function and the repair of damaged structure. These are accomplished by the same powers, processes and agents that maintain health. The same power that determines the development of the embryo from the germ or ovum, is identical with that which is the source of the constant preservation, and renovation, purification and reparation, development and growth of the organism after birth. The generation of new structures to supplant the dead and dying ones, is due to cell multiplication, and involves the same creative forces that operate in the body of the growing, developing, unborn babe. By these processes normal health is maintained and if health is impaired, restored. As Dr. Walter was so fond of saying, the power of cure is the power of repair and the power of repair is the power of reproduction.

When the cells of the lungs are injured or sick they repair and cure themselves. Sick and damaged kidney cells cure and repair themselves. Sick and damaged stomach cells or brain cells or liver cells or muscles cells cure and repair themselves. All of this is accomplished, not with drugs and treatments, but by virtue of the cell's own inherent powers of self-cure and self-repair and is accomplished by the use of the same light and air and water and food—cell substances— that are used in building new cells. As Dr. Moras so well said (Autology) :—

"But, as air is air, and as such is not a cure; and as water is water, and as such is not a cure; and as food is food, and as such is not a cure, therefore, 'cure' is not a thing that exists outside of, or distinct from the particular tissue-cells in whose 'bosom' it (the cure) originally was (preformed and pre-ordained by nature) and is again re-formed with the elements derived from air, water, light and foods."

Cure begins and ends in the cells, organs, tissues and fluids of the body and is accomplished by the self-same functions and processes and by the use of the self-same materials, agents and forces with which nature builds and maintains the body in health. In other words, cure is simply healthy function working under a handicap.

"And that cure," says Dr. Moras (Autology), "is Nature-made and Nature-pre-ordained, and resides in the cell-matter unknown as life, but recognized as function, in the heart-granules of the tissue-cells.

"It is that thing which we call 'function or nutrition,' which enables a kidney-cell to manufacture kidney-tissue and urine with the same air and water and food stuffs with which brain cells manufacture brain-tissue and thoughts," or, with which liver-cells manufacture liver-tissue and bile, and gonads manufacture gonad-tissue and spermatazoa and ova.

These are the fundamental processes of life. Their constant and successful performance depends upon the ordinary conditions and requirements of life, and not upon some therapeutic measure.

IS DISEASE FRIEND OR FOE

Chapter IV

HOWEVER much physicians of all schools and all ages may have differed about the cause of disease, there is one thing upon which they have all been agreed; namely, that disease, is itself an unmitigated evil, every symptom of which is destructive in its tendency and puropse and must be suppressed or "cured," else life will be destroyed. With this view in mind, the practices of the various schools of medicine have been nothing more than a grotesque symptom hunt. They have been and are possessed of a real symptophobia (fear of symptoms), and their chief function is and has been that of going after each symptom as it appears with hammer and tongs. For, those who have not regarded disease as the work of some malicious entity, have looked upon the sick body as a kind of ill-mannered child that has broken away from all parental authority and restaint and must be coerced back into the path of physiological rectitude.

Innumerable have been and are the incongruous and fantastic methods and systems that have been and are being used by the different schools of medicine to force the sick body to behave in the manner the physician thinks it should act. If there has been any conception of law and order in the vital realm, when disease is present, this conception has been rather hazy and ill-defined. Disease has simply been a destructive and anarchistic manifestation which must be combatted and subdued before it kills the patient.

That this conception of disease is wholly at variance with all the facts of the case is easily shown and I shall present enough evidence in this chapter to convince the thinking reader of the truth of this statement.

If disease is an antagonistic element of any nature, and has succeeded in making a successful "attack" upon the body and obtained so firm a hold that the powers of life are unable to throw it off; if, from this time onward, from day to day, it should contiue to grow stronger, and extend its dominion deeper and wider, while the powers of life are, to the same extent, overpowered and driven before it, until there is the merest breath of life left, and in some cases hardly that, what possible chance would there be for the little remnant of life that remains to rally and regain its so thoroughly devastated dominion? Obviously there would not be the slightest chance for recovery in the absence of saving treatment, and yet, if such cases ever recover, it is after hope is abandoned and treatment forsaken.

Nearly eighty years since, Dr. Hawthorn, a standard medical author of that day, in a treatise on Epidemic Cholera, after recommending much and varied heroic treatment for the prevention of collapse, admitted that patients did occasionally revive and return to health after this stage has been reached, but added: "Almost all the recoveries from collapse I have ever witnessed, were of persons who refused to take any medicine whatever, and who recovered through the *Vis Medicatrix Naturae—healing power of nature.*"

If there was a "tendency to death" in those cases, if cholera is a real antagonistic principle, which carries on a relentless warfare against the powers of life, why did it yield the conflict and permit its victims to escape, when they were so completely in its power? How, if disease is antagonistic to life, did patients who were already in a state of collapse, rally the forces of life and, unaided by treatment of any kind, throw off their foes and return to health? If the current theories of disease are correct, it should be obvious to the least discerning that such recoveries would be impossible.

A few concrete examples will aid the reader in grasping the full significance of the stupendous truth the above facts demonstrate. In giving these, I shall begin with cases that shared in the work of launching the Nature Cure or Orthopathic movement.

The first cases I shall present were under Dr. Jennings' care, in Oberlin, Ohio, and caused him to abandon the drugs he had employed for twenty years and launch out into a new and hitherto untried field. Dr. Jennings shall tell his case in his own words, as follow:—

"Mr. Isaac Treat, some thirty-five years of age, previously of good constitution, by occupation a farmer, sickened with typhus fever. From the alarming aspect of the case, at its commencement, my highly esteemed friend Dr. Dowe, of New Haven, was in daily consultation with me during much of the progress of the disease to its crisis. Among the most urgent symptoms for a number of days, were great prostration of strength, general uneasiness, pain and soreness in the chest, and short difficult breathing; and in our prescriptions we had particular reference to these, but with very partial success. Under these circumstances, Mr. Treat inquired of us whether it would do for him to take brandy, expressing a belief that it would help him. We objected at first, from a conviction, that alcohol in any form, was contra-indicated by a quick pulse, great continued heat, dryness of the skin, and tightness or stricture and soreness of the chest.

"However, after some further fruitless efforts to relieve him by diffusible stimulants in a variety of forms, we yielded to his importunity. The first drink of brandy told upon the poor sufferer. In the language of our patient, 'It was just the thing, it went right to the spot.' To our surprise it acted like a charm in diminishing the frequency and quickness of the pulse, removing the heat and dryness of the skin, and the tenseness and soreness of the chest, relieving the difficulty of breathing, and general uneasiness, improving the secretions, opening and lighting up the countenance, imparting fresh life and animation; and in short, making him appear and feel like a new man. For eight or ten days the brandy held its sway, and all other medicines were laid aside. It was found necessary, however, to increase very considerably the quantity of brandy to obtain the same amount of relief; and in the course of three or four days, he was taking at the rate of two quarts of old and very strong brandy in twenty-four hours.

"At length this potent remedy lost its influence over the vital machinery, palled upon the nerves, its very name was loathed by the patient, and of course its use was discontinued.

"We had nothing now by which we could rally the vital forces, or make any impression upon the disease, but was obliged to stand powerlessly before it. Not an arrow in our quiver that could reach it. Our patient soon fell into a death-like coma or stupor, entirely insensible to all that was passing around him; the extremities grew cold, pulse failed at the wrist, the bowels became tympanitic or tensely bloated, the power of swallowing was suspended and hope departed.

"These symptoms, hopeless as they appeared, continued with perceptible declination, excepting occasionally very slight temporary improvements, for three days, when to the great joy of his friends, reanimation commenced that went very gradually but steadily forward to a comfortable state of health."

Let us pause a minute and look into this case. Here was a man afflicted with typhus fever, a disease that is supposed to be more deadly than war, treated by two well trained physicians of wide experience, and who had also had much experience in treating typhus. They had exhausted all the "hand grenades" and "Big Berthas" then employed by the medical profession to storm the enemies' lines, and their patient had grown steadily worse until, finally, they were at a loss as to what to do next.

Unfortunately, the patient insisted on brandy and this was given him in amount. At first it appeared that the "right remedy" had been struck upon, for the patient appeared to grow better immediately. But, as is true of all stimulants, the brandy only took away what it appeared to give, so that the patient grew steadily worse and progressively larger doses were required to secure the desired stimulation. Slowly (or, was it rapidly), but surely, the patient's vitality was being stimulated away. The organism rebelled. It refused to take more brandy. Henceforth, it would conduct its own affairs in its own inimitable way, and without the interference of the stimulant. The reader will bear in mind that alcohol only stimulates reflexly by its irritating effects upon the nerves of the stomach. It is really a depressant.

When the stimulant was withdrawn the forces of life seemed to sink. In the absence of the goad, the true condition of the patient became manifest. The patient collapsed and death seemed inevitable. Treatment had failed, the disease had apparently vanquished the powers of life; recovery without the aid of some powerful treatment would seem impossible. The extremities grew cold. The pulse was no longer perceptible at the wrist. Surely death was upon the patient. The bowels became tympanitic. Hope was abandoned and treatment as well.

But hold! The patient continues to live! He does not die! He is beginning to improve! Treatment was abandoned and the patient improved! Improved! Yea! recovered and returned to the plough! Here was another such case as Dr. Hawthorn spoke of when he said almost all cases of recovery from collapse he had ever seen had been in cases where no drugs were used. The cure was accomplished by the healing power of nature.

Gentle reader, think it over, and answer for yourself the question: If disease is antagonistic to life, and life is just about extinct, how can the healing power of nature rally and overcome the foe of life?

The second of Dr. Jennings' remarkable cases of that year, (1822), cases that blasted the old medical notions of the nature of disease out of his mind forever, was that of a Mrs. Wm. J. French who lived in an opposite part of the town some three or four miles distant from the home of Mr. Treat. This case occurred while Mr. Treat's case was in progress. Dr. Jennings recounts it as follows:—

"Within the compass of a few weeks, nine cases of Typhus Fever occurred in this family, most of them in a severe form, namely, Mr. and Mrs. French, five sons and one daughter, and a sister of Mrs. French. Mr. F. and three sons had been hard sick a number of days, when Mrs. F. failed. Worn down with labor, care and anxiety, she sunk rapidly in the first stage of the disease. The most distressing and alarming symptoms were, great prostration of strength, and extreme irritability of the stomach, with constant inclination to vomit. A great variety of means, internal and external, mild and severe, were used to allay the irritability of the stomach, but they seemed rather to aggravate than mitigate the difficulty; the symptoms on the whole becoming more distressing and alarming. Calling in one morning to see Mrs. F., about the fourth day of the disease, I was greatly pained and alarmed at her dejected and distressed appearance. I took a walk into a neighboring secluded field, that I might the better command my thoughts, and went through with a minute and thorough review of the whole case, to discover, if possible, what more could be done with promise of relief, but could think of nothing that offered sufficient inducement for trial. I returned to the house, and inquired of the nurse what, if anything Mrs. F. had taken, seemed to agree best with the stomach.

"The reply was, 'Very little difference in anything except water; when she takes that—and she wants it right from the well—it stays on the stomach, and nothing else does, no matter what it is.' My mind was soon made up on a prescription for the day. Returning to my promenade in the field, where there was a fine spring of pure soft water, I took a vial from my pocket, discharged its contents, rinsed it thoroughly, filled it with the spring water, returned to the house, and called for a clean vial, into which I turned some of the *aqua fontana pura*, and directed four drops of it to be given once in four hours in a teaspoonful of water directly from the well, and gave a strict charge that nothing but the drops should go into her mouth during the day, except water, of which she might drink to her pleasure.

"I also directed that she should be kept quiet, her room ventilated and kept clean, and all her little wants promptly attended to. I called at the house in the evening, and in answer to the inquiry, 'How is Mrs. French?' the reply was, 'Quite comfortable; you have at last hit upon the right medicine. *The drops are just the thing for her.* She has had no sickness of the stomach since she began with them, and but little distress; she has slept some, and has had a comfortable day.'

"This case gave me no farther trouble. The drops, with a little other placebo medicine, finished the cure, as far as medicine was concerned.

"In these cases, 'The impotence of our art was very manifest and considerable,' and in Mr. Treat's case especially, we were obliged to 'admit the *vis medicatrix naturae*, in practice,' and nobly did she meet and sustain the responsibility.

"For six years I had been in the habit of admitting this principle in practice, except in 'extreme cases,' and with overwhelming evidence of its superiority as a practical maxim to anything else that I had seen developed in any other mode of practice with which I had been conversant.

"Here was an 'extreme case,' the tumid state of the bowels, coldness of the extremities, pallidness of the countenance, almost total cessation of arterial action and respiration, and the cadaverous aspect and odor of the body, seemed to preclude all idea and hope of recovery; and yet the vital forces, few and feeble as they were, when left to the freedom of their own laws and modes of operating, recruit themselves, and then urge on the renovating process; they remove the superincumbent mass of effete and oppressive matter, build anew the waste places, re-endow the organism with motive power, and restore the man to himself, his family, and his friends."

The reader who is still wading around in the muddy waters of ancient superstitions about disease will be forcefully struck with the thought that if disease is essentially destructive in its nature, this case could not have recovered, after it had become so bad, unless something more powerful and effective than a few drops of water be used in treatment. Is there, then, any wonder that Dr. Jennings remarks:—

"It was under circumstances like these, that I was forced into a deep rooted and firm conviction that there was a radical defect in the general science and art of medicine; that physicians had no correct knowledge of general pathology; that they knew nothing of the true nature of disease; and that, consequently, their practice must be merely at haphazard, and exceedingly jeopardous and deplorable in its results."

Two further cases recorded by Dr. Jennings will further strengthen the case against the prevailing notion of the nature of disease. It should be borne in mind, in reading these cases that they represent extreme cases and were chosen by him for this reason. For, if one recovered from a condition which was not extreme it might be argued that the patient was not very sick anyway. If he can recover from extreme conditions without remedial aid, and these extremes are so great that life is despaired of, then it becomes increasingly evident that the prevailing view of disease is a mistaken one.

"Case VIII.—During an epidemic of scarlet fever which prevailed extensively in Derby, affecting all of the children in many families, there were five cases in the family of Mrs. Wm. Stone; three and all of her own children, and two little daughters of a Mrs. Heinaman from the South, who was spending the season with Mrs. Stone The youngest of the two children, between two and three years of age, had the disease in the most malignant form, with deep extensive ulceration of the mouth and throat. For a number of days it was tended on a pillow in the nurse's lap, emaciated, perfectly unconscious, eyes half closed and set, pale as a corpse, and with but just the breath of life in it.

"While in this state its father arrived from the South, and on learning the facts respecting the no-medicine treatment, became almost frantic with emotion, and inquired where a physician could be found that would *do something*. He was informed that there were quite a number of that character in New Haven, nine miles off, and was furnished with a list of the names of some of the most prominent medical men of that place, and an individual was sent out to dispatch a messenger to the city to bring out one of the physicians whose names were on the list. But on a little reflection Mr. Heinaman came to me and said: 'Doctor, it is impossible for this child to live by any mode of treatment with which I am acquainted, and if you think your method of management will afford a chance for its life, pursue it;' and the sending to New Haven was dispensed with.

"When the grand object for which the main body of organic forces had been drawn off behind the curtain was so far accomplished, that the attractive power in that quarter began to yield to the strong retractive claims of the visible functions, they were drawn thither again in small detachments, and their resuscitating influence was manifested by a resumption or extension of arterial action, rekindling of the eye, and general reanimation. When the child had so far recovered that it could take a little nourishment, it was the merest skeleton that ever breathed;—a frightful looking little piece of humanity. The injury done the system by the scarlet fever virus, or the subtile agency that laid the foundation for the derangement which was called scarlet fever, had been so deep and pervading, that the fabric had to be taken to pieces and thrown away, except the frame-work and covering. But in a few weeks the dilapidated parts were replaced with new, well-wrought material; and in lieu of the hideous looking skeleton, we had a plump bright black-eyed, handsome and doubly interesting little girl.

"There were a number of hard cases of scarlet fever in this epidemic, but no deaths. A young child of Mr. Abel Holbrook, on Great Hill, sunk nearly as low as the Heinaman child, and recovered, but with some defect of hearing, which is not wholly effaced in the attainment of adult age."

"Case X.—Mr. Agur Gilbert, whose case follows, was about twenty-five years of age, at the time of his sickness; of good habits and good constitution.

"The special object in noticing this case, is to call attention to one feature of the disease, to wit: the suspension of the peristaltic, or natural downward motion of the bowels, for the long period of three weeks. The disease, though of considerable length and attended with a good deal of general debility, was on the whole a mild one. There was but little pain during the progress of the disease; the general train of symptoms was regular from day to day, and pretty uniform. The stomach and bowels were quiet, the former calling for nothing but water, and the latter manifesting not the least tendency to motion for twenty days. On the twentieth day of their fasting and resting, there was clearly an incipient revival of action in most of the great functions of the body.

"On first entering the room, I perceived a little brightening of the countenance; the mouth showed a slight improvement in the secretions; the skin was a little less dry and husky; the pulse a little slower, fuller and softer; there was a little sense of motion in the bowels; and the patient began to think that ere long he might relish some kind of food. The next day the symptoms were still more improved, and there was a small evacuation of the bowels, of natural appearance;—from this time there was a steady upward and onward progress to confirmed health.

"Some of the friends of Mr. G. felt a concern for the quiet state of the bowels, and for this concern I prescribed some pills which I knew 'would do no hurt, if they did no good.' For myself, I had no fear about the bowels, and should have had none if they had been kept at rest three weeks longer, if there had been no other sign of danger. There was no necessity for action by the intestinal canal; for there was nothing to be carried off by them, and it would have been a work of supererogation in them to keep up their natural motion. A special and strong requisition had been made for organic forces in another direction; and to meet this requisition it was necessary to deprive the whole system of voluntary muscles of power to act, and to suspend the action of the nutritive system, including the vast chain of secretory and assimilatory agency. Present safety of course demanded that all parts should retain force enough to guard them against the action of inorganic affinities. It was a favorable indication, and one on which my prognosis of a happy issue of the case was mainly based, that the controlling power of the motor nerves was so generally in the ascendency, as to be able to maintain an almost universal state of rest. With this state of things, general debility, or loss of muscular tonicity—in the absence of serious organic affection—must have run very low indeed, or have been long continued, to destroy my confidence in a final recovery. I have had patients lie for days together so feeble that they could scarcely move a finger, or whisper so as to be understood, for whose safety I entertained but little doubt.

"Many practitioners deprecate protracted inaction of the bowels in adynamic diseases, because they fear that deleterious gasses or subtile vicious exhalations will be taken up and sent through the system. But these fears are groundless; for the inaction extends to the absorbents of the bowels, as well as to the bowels themselves: and besides, the contents of the bowels in such cases are kept sufficiently vitalized to prevent impure exhalations. In the case above stated there was no unusual odor attending the passage after twenty days confinement."

For another illustration of the great principle I am trying to unfold, I will come down to a little nearer our day and let Dr. Dewey tell of a case that set him upon the fasting cure and caused him to abandon drugs. He says:—

"I was called one day to one of the families of the poorest of the poor, where I found a sick case that for once in my life set me to thinking. The patient was a sallow, overgrown girl in early maturity, with a history of several months of digestive and other troubles. I found a very sick patient, so sick that for a period of three weeks not even one drink of water was retained, not one dose of medicine, and it was not until several more days that water could be borne. When finally water could be retained my patient seemed brighter in mind, the complexion was clearer, and she seemed actually stronger. As for the tongue, which at first was heavily coated, the improvement was striking: while the breath, utterly foul at first, was strikingly less offensive. In every way the patient was very much better.

"I was so surprised at this that I determined at once to let the good work go on, on Nature's own terms, and so it did until about the thirty-fifth day, when there was a call, not for the undertaker, but for food, a call that marked the close of the disease. The pulse and temperature had become normal, and there was a tongue as clean as the tongue of a nursing infant.

"Up to this time this was the most severely sick case I ever had that recovered, and yet with not apparently more wasting of the body than with other cases of as protracted sickness in which more or less food was given and retained. And all this with only water for thirst until hunger came and a *complete cure!*

"Such ignoring of medical faith and practice, of the accumulated wisdom and experience of all medical history, I had never seen before. Had the patient been able to take both food and medicine, and I had prohibited, and by chance death had occurred, I would have been guilty of actually putting the patient to death—death from starvation. Feed, feed the sick whether or not, say all the books, to support strength or to keep life in the body, and yet Nature was absurd enough to ignore all human practice evolved from experience, and in her own way to support vital power while curing the disease."

The reader may well imagine Dr. Dewey's surprise when the "most severely sick case" he "ever saw recover," recovered without drugs, food or water But when we review this case, we are again brought face to face with Dr. Jennings' old question: If disease is antagonistic to life and has secured a strangle hold upon the forces of the body and has choked it into unconsciousness and insensibility, how is that patient to recover, unless immediate and heroic remedies are used? And yet Nature refused all proffered aid! Refused drugs, water, food! She served notice that she was conducting the affairs of that organsim and knew better how to conduct them than all the doctors of all the earth in all the ages.

In his excellent little Monograph on Typhoid, Dr. John H Tilden, records a case of typhoid fever which recovered without treatment, after the physicians in charge had abandoned the case. They had let the family know that the case was hopeless and Dr. Tilden remarks that he found it in as unfavorable condition as possible. He says:—

"I arrived at the bedside of Mr. M at 2:00 P. M., July 13, 1906, and found the situation as follows: Male; age 48; height 5 feet 6 inches; weight, before he was taken sick, 215 pounds; business merchant; habits generous liver and given to periodic alcoholic indulgences, or what is called moderate drinking. He was two weeks coming down with the disease, had taken his bed one week before I saw him, and was under the care of the most reputable physicians in the state of Kansas. His symptoms were as follows: Muttering delirium; pulse, 92; temperature, 104.4 degrees; bowels greatly distended with gas—tympanitic; very restless; urine dark colored; involuntary discharge from bowels and bladder. He had a chill a few minutes after I saw him, due probably to hemorrhage as there had been several hemorrhages in the thirty-six hours preceding my arrival: the bowel discharges were very offensive and mixed with blood."

At this point Dr. Tilden reproduces the nurse's chart for the period from July 7 to July 13 which shows the temperature and pulse to go up and down as he was given stimulants and anti-pyretics He was given strychnine, alcohol rubs, colon flushings, sulphonal powder, morphine, liquid peptonoids, saline laxatives, gastric lavages, ice baths, enemas of tannic acid, quinine, and other fever medicines. After the first few doses the strychnine was given hypodermically. He was fed at regular intervals. For instance, he was fed five times on July 8th, five times on July 9th, eight times on July 10th, six times on July 11th, seven times on July 12th. The feeding was done at all hours of the day and night and in all conditions of the patient. Milk, butter milk, malted milk, and beef juice were the chief foods given. Ice to the head and abdomen, cold sponge baths, lasting often an hour and other abuses were heaped upon the man. Dr. Tilden well asks:—

"Suppose a well man should be put to bed and punished, as this man was the first seven days of his illness, what would happen? Is there any wonder that the man was sick unto death? Are there people idiotic enough to believe a sick man can stand a treatment that would kill a well man?"

All medication and feeding were stopped. A little orange juice or lemon juice in water was given every three to four hours, and all the water desired. Enemas were given. The spine was sponged.

As a natural reaction from the cessation of stimulants, the pulse rose 98, 104, and then, after a few hours, settled back into the nineties. Dr. Tilden says of this:—

"This is a positive refutation of the profession's constantly reiterated declaration that the heart must be sustained. Reader, please bear in mind that this man had been on heart tonics for one week and had been constantly fed, yet he did not collapse when deprived of them.

"I not only refuse to sustain the heart and give food for bodily nourishment in all diseases, from the start to the finish, but I unhesitatingly take any case that has been held up for a week, or any length of time, and without scruple remove the props, and if the profession's theory of a sustaining treatment were correct, such cases ought to go down and out; but on the contrary my experience is, and has been, exactly the reverse of this time honored teaching."

This case recovered and as Dr. Tilden says: "Taking into consideration the desperate condition in which I found him he made a very rapid recovery."

Further commenting upon this case and the regular treatment of fevers, Dr. Tilden says:—

"This was a case in which *scientific medicine* declared strychnine necessary to keep up heart action, and *scientific medicine* had been giving it for a week.

"If the theory advanced by the profession regarding the sustaining of the heart in fevers were correct, what would have happened to this man when I took him off of his heart tonics? He ought to have had heart failure; and his heart collapse should have taken place more surely—in fact without delay—because he had been taking the heart tonic for one week, and, if there were anything in the theory, the need was increased. Bear in mind, readers, here was a man whom the profession declared in need of a heart tonic one week before I was called, and the tonic had been given; the fever had also been ravaging the system, further weakening the heart, and in addition to all this he had been having bowel hemorrhages for two or three days, which, according to this same theory, added very seriously to the heart weakness; but in spite of all this evidence that the heart was overburdened and needed careful watching and all the stimulants and tonics possible to keep it from collapsing, I unhesitatingly cut off everything of a so-called sustaining nature—food, drugs, ice packs, and unnecessary nursing.

"I had proven to my complete satisfaction twenty years before that the theory of heart stimulation advocated and practiced by the leading professional men of the world was false—and I have ever since been unhesitatingly stopping the use of heart remedies in every *desperate* case to which I have been called as consultant, or to succeed other physicians, and instead of the patients *going to pieces*—instead of the heart collapsing—the heart invariably improves, and the improvement is immediate and continuous.

"If the theory, which is believed in by the whole profession, is true, why didn't this patient die?

"What kept his heart regular and strong? If quinine will break a fever, why did this man's fever grow steadily worse under its influence? If there is danger that fever patients will starve to death, why did not this patient starve to death? The fact is, the whole theory of sustaining treatment is absolutely unworthy of this age.

"I say boldly and with all due regard for truth, that this patient's disease would have been a very trivial affair if it had not been built to its desperate state by the treatment. Look at the first night's report, look at every day's and night's report!

"What does common sense say the treatment of a sick person should be? Isn't it a fact that all nature cries out in no uncertain voice, *Give the sick rest.* Rest to the body and mind; rest to the nutrition; rest to the nerves! Is constant attendance with the giving of drugs, food, stimulants, taking the temperature, counting the pulse and doing a thousand and one other little, annoying, useless and senseless things, giving a patient rest?

"Isn't it a burlesque to point to the regular practice of medicine and name it, *The Science and Practice of Medicine?*

"The treatment from beginning to end is a crazy, senseless regime, devoid of poise—hysterical.

"This man was fed from the first hour the medical man was called. Why? Because he was in danger of starving to death; *he only weighed 215 pounds!* It is to laugh!

"All such cases as this should be entirely rid of fever in from one week to ten days, followed by a quick convalescence. When they are complicated, as this case was ,they do well to recover at all and when they do recover it takes weeks to become normal. If the plan of treatment that I found the patient under had been continued, the prognosis that had been made by the physicians in attendance would surely have been fulfilled, namely: 'The patient can't live twenty-four hours.' When the neighbors heard that I was giving neither drugs nor food the shout went up: 'If Dr. Tilden isn't giving food or drugs, what is he doing?' Doing! Do something is the demand! Nature says, 'Do nothing.' My answer in such cases is: I am standing guard to keep medical vandalism from destroying the patient.

"My treatment is a 'do nothing treatment' according to the minds of those educated to the customs of this age of medical practice. The idea that drugs cure disease has taken such a hold on the minds of doctors and their patients that such a thought as, 'possibly nature can do something for herself if given a chance,' never crosses the threshold of their understanding. The fact is, nature does all the curing that is done; there is not, never was, nor ever will be a drug that will cure a disease. Drugs will kill pain, but they cannot cure it. There are thousands of medical excuses for giving drugs; the one that assumes the dignity of a plausible excuse is that pain kills unless relieved, but this can be offset by the truth that drugs do not save as many lives by relieving pain as they kill in the attempts at securing relief, and if there are lives saved by drugs, which is questionable, the drug-relieved disease is not a cured disease."

Coming still nearer to the present, about five years ago, a little boy in Waco, Texas, became sick with typhoid fever. A physician was called. He came and for several days hurled all the shot and shell of the Allopathic armamentarium into the camp of the enemy and used every means known to "science" to sustain the life of the little fellow. But there was no use. He grew steadily worse. Finally, after a consultation in which the wise men shook their empty heads and elongated their faces until they resembled a deacon at a funeral, a verdict was returned. It was that old familiar tune: "Everything known to 'science' has been done. There is no hope. The boy will die."

But the boy did not die. At least, he isn't dead yet. In fact, those who look upon him cannot tell that he was ever sick. What actually happened was this: The doctors left and a *Christian Science* practitioner was called. She poured out the drugs and that very day the boy began to improve. He improved rapidly and was soon back at play. Another recovery after treatment was abandoned; another apparently hopeless case returned to health after "science" ceased to combat the "enemy" and ceased to "sustain" the life of the patient! It does seem strange in the light of prevailing theories of the nature of disease; doesn't it? Strange as it may appear, medical history, past and present, is replete with such instances.

It should be needless for me to remind my readers that together with many others, including Dr. Tilden, who are now living, I have handled many cases of acute and chronic disease without resort to treatment and in seven years of practice, I have had but two deaths. One of the most severely sick cases of disease I have ever handled was that of acute inflammation of the brain and optic nerve in a young girl of fourteen years. Beginning with malaise, a cold, and a slight headache, this case progressed, within a few hours, to a point where the pains in the eyes and head were intense. Fever was 102 degrees Visual disturbances began with everything appearing to be upside down and progressed to complete blindness. Unconsciousness soon followed which lasted three days. During this period there was delirium. The patient screamaed with pain, tore at her face, and hair, and tore the bed clothes, with her hands, tossed to and fro on her bed and talked of people and incidents long dead and past. Her heart action was rapid and fluctuating.

I had with me on this case an experienced medical nurse who had assisted in caring for a few similar cases. She insisted that a medical man be called to administer a drug to relieve pain and declared the case would die. However, to her great surprise the case completely recovered in a few days. Convalescence was short and rapid.

Aside from three enemas and a few attempts to relieve the patient's suffering by hydropathic methods, this patient received nothing but watchful waiting. She was given no food, no drugs and no treatments. The hot baths employed at the start relieved her for a few minutes when the pain would return with renewed intensity. For this reason they were abandoned.

If the ancient and prevailing theory of the nature of disease were correct, the recovery of this case, in the absence of saving treatment, cannot be explained. This patient was prostrated, unconscious, delerious and nothing was done to sustain or support her.

Now for a case of a somewhat different character which will help us to understand these other cases. A few years ago the good Queen Victoria died. One day the bulletins announced:—

"The queen is sinking. She is unable to take nourishment. Her medical attendants declare that she can live but a few hours."

Next morning:—

"The queen has rallied and is able to take nourishment. The doctors declare that there is a chance for her recovery, barring complications."

A few hours later:—

"The queen is sinking. The rally of this morning was followed by a sinking spell, and she is again unable to take nourishment. Heart tonics given hypodermically keep what little life there is from ebbing away. Only the superhuman skill of the doctors prevents death from claiming the great woman as its bride."

"Superhuman skill of the doctors!" Did the reader, in his wildest moments, ever dream that physicians possess superhuman skill? They kept death from claiming the great woman as its bride. Such collossal conceit! A school boy can see that they killed her. They built the complications that prevented her recovery. They did it keeping her life from ebbing away by hypodermic injections of poisons.

Next morning:—

"During the night the doctors watched at the bedside of the distinguished patient, watching with bated breath the ebb and flow of the declining energies. Once or twice the family was arroused to view the grand queen and mother of the greatest empire on earth, while there was still a little life left in her body. All efforts at keeping life in the aged queen was abandoned at midnight."

After these fellows with the superhuman skill abandoned their efforts at "keeping life in the aged queen" she should have died without further ado. But she didn't. A little later the bulletins announced:—

"Most extraordinary, the unexpected happened! The queen rallied, and at this cabling is taking nourishment. The doctors, fear, however, on account of the queen's great age and the weakness of her heart, that the rally will only be temporary. Sir John Blatherskite, an eminent heart specialist, was called in consultation, and favors strychnine for the heart. This heart tonic will be given in the place of digitalis, which has served long and well."

The rally WAS only temporary. It could not have been otherwise. The scientific damphools would not permit it to be otherwise. Any schoolboy, in reading these bulletins, can see that the queen rallied every time feeding and drugging were abandoned and that she began sinking immediately upon their resumption. Medical men think that if their patient is able to take nourishment without dying outright, there is hope of recovery. If ability to take "nourishment" is absent, the patient is in great danger. No greater delusion was ever entertained unless it is the stimulant delusion. The more heart tonics were given, the weaker grew her heart. When they were discontinued the wonderful organ improved. More tonics and down it went again.

If these great specialists had not been so scientific, if they had not been possessed of "superhuman skill," perhaps they would have been able to see the grotesque folly of their efforts to "keep what little life there is from ebbing away." If they had not had all their common sense clubbed out of them by "science" they could have reasoned that the rallies always followed the cessation of their efforts to save life and the sinking always resulted from their "superhuman efforts" to *sustain* her. If the queen, who was given up as beyond recall, could rally without food and treatment and always grew worse with food and treatment, these superhuman, scientific idiots should have realized that their great skill in "keeping life in the body" was the very thing that was killing their distinguished patient. They stimulated her life away and announced that she was "sinking." They ceased their foolish efforts and she revived. Then these learned ignoramuses began all over again to "sustain" her heart and keep her life in her body by their diabolical skill in stimulating it away. Rest! rest! not stimulation, with air, warmth and occasionally a little water as instinct directed, was all she needed to recover.

If Blatherskite had been a Jennings or a Dewey; if he had had enough intelligence to cast not only digitalis, but strychnine and food as well, to the dogs; and stepped back and permitted the patient to recover; if instead of nourishment and stimulants, the queen had been allowed to rest in ease and quiet, then, the story would have been different.

But this could not be. Disease is a frightful monster that throws itself upon our defenseless bodies to devour and destroy them. It is the function of the doctor to route the enemy. So he stands, armor in hand, and beats down every symptom as it appears. This is true of the symptophobic members of all schools. Their methods may differ, but their principles and practices are ever and always the same.

Had Dr. Jennings resumed the brandy or resorted to strychnine or digitalis and feeding when Mr. Treat rallied, he too, would have gone as the good Queen went. Had the *Christian Scientist* continued poisoning the little boy in Waco instead of pouring out the drugs, the little lad would now be sleeping beneath a marble slab upon which loving hearts have engraved their last tribute to their dear departed. The kind preacher would have repeated that old hypocritical cant about the Lord's will, and the verdict of infallible "science" would have been justified.

If disease is an enemy and drugs and food are necessary to defeat it, why did the Queen not rally when these were used and sink when they were abandoned? Will some of the "scientific" please answer. If a patient is so near death that he no longer "responds" to treatment and hope is abandoned with the treatment – if such a patient rallies and progresses to recovery without treatment, is not the treatment a greater foe than the disease? Is there any wonder Dr. Hawthorn saw recoveries from collapse almost wholly in cases where drugs were abandoned? The drugs are the cause of the collapse.

Dr. Jennings relates a very similar case to that of the Queen:—

"A number of years since, I attended a young lady in Oberlin, sick with a typhoid affection, to whom I gave simple hygienic treatment while she was under my care. She ran down pretty low, with temporary suspension of the mental function; was taken from under my charge and put under the care of another physician. Active medication soon demonstrated by a general improvement of symptoms that there was still a good stock of restorative energy at, or that should have been left at the disposal of the vital economy for renovating purposes. After a few days, however, the symptoms declined, and on Saturday the case was given over as hopeless; and medicine withheld, as there seemed to be no support for treatment—no favorable response was received from medicine. Through Sunday there was but little change. On Monday there was an encouraging revival of symptoms, and medicine was resumed. On Thursday the young lady died."—*Tree of Life*, pp. 172.

If, as we claim, disease is a curative process that needs only to be permitted to consumate its work, is not treatment the thing that destroys the lives of the sick? When the doctors stand by to suppress and thwart, hinder and subvert (stimulate every reduced and inhibit every accelerated function), on the absurd theory that they are combatting the enemy, they kill more patients every year than ever die from any other cause in the same time. They drive the body with stimulants and lessen its activities with sedatives or inhibiting methods, as, in their infallible opinions, should be done Not once does it ever occur to them that they do not know how the body should conduct its affairs and that no living organism can ever act other than for its own interest. Thus they seek to "cure" disease, which means they combat and suppress the very measures that life has initiated to save itself. They attempt to club it back into its regular channels. The effort to cure disease has been, without a doubt, the greatest curse that has ever been perpetrated upon the human race. The idea that disease is something that must be cured, the idea that it is something that can be cured, must be eradicated from the human mind before we can ever hope to arrive at a rational solution of our health problems.

ORTHOPATHIC IDEAS OF THE NATURE OF DISEASE

Chapter V

"CONTRARY to the teachings of the standard medical books of allopathic, homeopathic, and eclectic schools," Trall declared, "we must ever bear in mind that disease is never a *positive entity*, but always a *negative quality*; it is the absence of health, or of the state, circumstances, and actions which constitute that balance of functional duty we call health. By referring to the misuse or abuse of some one or more of the hygienic agencies we find the *cause* or *causes* of those deviations from the *normal* state, which constitute the abnormal state, and which we call disease."—*Hydropathic Encyclopedia*, Vol. 2, p. 4.

"A disease, however much its cause may be adverse to the human body, is nothing more than an effort of Nature, who strains with might and main to restore the health of the patient by the elimination of the morbific matter." Thomas Sydenham, the English Hippocrates, in Vol. 1, p. 29, Edition of the Sydenham Society, 1848.

Sydenham was a keen observer and was possessed of an analytical mind, but, although he recognized, at least partially, the essential nature of disease, and was responsible for many almost revolutionary changes in medical practice, failed in establishing a true science of health and disease, a true science of living because he believed in cures.

Jennings went far beyond Sydenham when he declared, *Treatise on Medical Reform*, p. 310:—

"Accustom yourself in all your little pains and aches, and also in all your grave and more distressing affections, to regard the movement concerned in them in a friendly aspect—designed for and tending to the removal of a difficulty of whose existence you were before unaware, and which, if suffered to remain and accumulate, might prove the destruction of the house you live in—and that, instead of it needing to be 'cured,' it is itself a curative operation; and that what should be called *disease* lies back of the symptoms which, in fact, are made for the express purpose of removing the real disorder or difficulty."

He looked upon disease as *impaired health* and repeatedly referred to it in these words. For instance in *Philosophy of Human Life* (p. 18-19) he refers to "the phenomena of impaired healthy action," "disease, which is but partial health, feeble vitality," "the impaired, feeble and deranged action of the vital forces," while on page 36 he declares of disease that "what we had been puzzling ourselves about was a mere negation of or impaired health, feeble vitality, a crippled, disabled and tired state of the vital machinery," (p. 82) "an enervated physical system." On page 98 he declares: "The shortest definition that can be given of disease Orthopathically is, negation of or impaired health; feeble vitality," while on the following page, in discussing enervation, he says, "a low state of vitality, or extreme disease is never reached abruptly, except by a stroke of lightning" or other powerful overwhelming forces. His definition of Orthopathy given in the introduction of this book declares his view of disease fully, however, we shall permit him to explain it more in detail here. He declares:—

"It is unequivocally taken for granted that disease is a something that will certainly depredate on the body if left to itself, and should, therefore, be early 'discerned, distinguished, and prevented' from getting a foothold, if it can be; if not, it should be laid siege to and 'cured.' "—*Tree of Life*, p. 144-5. And that "they have impliedly assumed that in some mysterious manner, the current of healthy action and of healthy condition has been checked and turned backwards; that in some inexplicable way a tendency in the vital economy to death has been induced, which, if not seasonably checked by art, may prove an over match for the powers of life."—*Philosophy of Human Life*, (p. 97-8).

It has before been noted that Jennings regarded disease as *right action*, (Orthopathic) in contradistinction to the Heteropathic view that it is *wrong action*. In discussing this he says, *Philosophy of Human Life*, (p. 36-7):—

"In the improved light of human physiology, reason and experience conspired to show that the common idea of disease was a great bug-bear, an illusory figment of the darkest portion of the dark ages; and that the combined expedition of medicine of all ages, all countries, and of all descriptions, that had been, and is yet arrayed against this spectre, and in hot pursuit of it, through veritable living human flesh and blood, was the most tremendous and quixotic movement that had ever been engaged in by deluded mortals; that what we had been puzzling ourselves about was mere negation of, or impaired health, feeble vitality, a crippled, disabled and tired state of the vital machinery; that life was a unit, the organized mechanism one, the motive power by which it was worked, in its general character and tendency one, and the law which governed its every movement one and immutable;—that in virtue of the law of animal economy, the tendency of all vital action *must be* to protect, advance and perfect the vital organism; that as long as any measure of the principle of life continues, there *must be* as much life and health maintained as possible under the circumstances: that human skill and means can neither give nor increase the *direct* ability of, or tendency to right or healthy action; that these were made and adapted to the end for which they were designed by infinite wisdom and benevolence, and cannot be improved by art; that the latter may often, and when it can, always should remove obstacles out of the way of feeble vitality, and make the circumstances under which it is laboring, more favorable for the prolongation of life and the promotion of health, but it can never increase the vital power or disposition to do either; and that, therefore, as a general proposition, there can be no such thing as wrong action any more than there can be such a thing as water running up hill self-moved, or from its own inherent propensity or tendency."

The oneness and sameness of healthy action and "morbid" action, that disease-action is but impaired healthy action serving the same physiological or biological purposes, and cannot be added to nor directed by art or therapeutics is forcefully stated in the above quotation by Jennings. Dr. Page agreed in general with this principle, saying, *The Natural Cure*, (p. 112-13) :—

"What are commonly called diseases are in reality cures; and the common practice, with drug doctors, of 'controlling the symptoms,' is like answering the cries and gesticulations of a drowning man with a knock on the head."

Florence Nightingale, who frequently found herself opposed to medical opinions, begins her *Notes on Nursing*, (1860), in these words:—

"Shall we begin by taking it as a general principle—that all disease, at some period or other of its course, is more or less a reparative process, not necessarily accompanied with suffering: an effort of nature to remedy a process of poisoning or of decay, which has taken place weeks, months, sometimes years, beforehand, unnoticed, the termination of the disease being then, while the antecedent process was going on, determined.**** In watching diseases, both in private houses and in public hospitals, the thing which strikes the experienced observer most forcibly is this, that the symptoms of the sufferings generally considered to be inevitable and incident to the disease are very often not symptoms of the disease at all, but of something quite different—of the want of fresh air, or of light, or of warmth, or of quiet, or of cleanliness, or of punctuality and care in the administration of diet, of each or all of these.**** The reparative process which nature has instituted and which we call disease, has been hindered by some want of knowledge or attention, in one or all of these things, and pain, suffering, or interruption of the whole process sets in."

In what follows from Sylvester Graham's *Science of Human Life*, he explains both the essential nature of acute disease and that chronic disease is the same thing plus, in chronic disease toleration in a weaker organism:

"While the system is in a pure state, and the organs are undepraved, the alimentary canal will always promptly detect the presence of any morbific or disturbing cause, and with perfect integrity exhibit the most distinct and unequivocal symptoms of morbid conditions and affections, or functional derangements. But when the natural sensibilities and sympathies of the system have been depraved and crippled by habitual violations of the laws of constitution and relation, the alimentary canal is robbed of its power to appreciate discriminately the character of such causes, and to awaken such sympathetic manifestations as distinctly indicate its disturbances and its diseases; and therefore, like an individual who has been deprived of his eyes or tongue, it necessarily submits to the gradual and continual encroachments of depraving and diseasing causes, without the power to perceive or tell what harms it, till the accumulation of wrongs becomes too great for vital endurance, and the general indignation of the system is aroused into an acute disease, which either throws off the oppression, or the vital powers sink under the conflict, and death ensues; or else the alimentary canal, or some other part are debilitated or morbidly predisposed, becomes the seat of slowly progressing local disease. When the lungs, liver, or any other organ whose natural sensibilities are less depraved than those of the alimentary canal, becomes the seat of local chronic disease, the symptoms of such disease are always less obscure and equivocal; but when the stomach and intestinal canal become the seat of chronic diseases, not induced by any one violent cause, but by the constant and long-continued irritations almost universal in civic life, and indeed throughout the human world, the depraved and crippled organ has no power to announce its difficulties in distinct and unequivocal symptoms.

"It is true that symptoms of disease somewhere within the vital domain might be detected by an accurate observer; but these are often so purely sympathetic, and so remote from the real seat of the disease, and so ambiguous in their character, that it is impossible to derive any correct and definite information from them. It is true also, that when long continued abuses accumulate oppression upon the system, till the diseased organ can no longer bear it quietly, morbid sympathies are aroused, and all the instinctive energies of organic life are sometimes thrown into a blind and terrible agony to remove the oppression; and in some cases, the powers of animal life are to a considerable extent, or even totally involved; so that spasms, cramps, convulsions, delirium, and even an entire suspension of animal life result. But these symptoms, though dreadfully violent, do not by any means distinctly indicate local disease, and still less do they point out the seat of such disease. Thus, by violating all the constitutional laws of relation in regard to the alimentary canal, we not only destroy its integrity in health, but also take away its power to make known its morbid conditions, and thereby the vital interests of our bodies are doubly endangered."—*Science of Human Life*, pp. 196-7.

Again:—

"****Indeed, disease itself, as a general fact, may be said to be, in its incipient state, nothing more than an excess of healthy action to resist morbific causes; and this excess being carried too far, and continued too long, the overacting parts are brought into a morbid condition, and perhaps, involve the whole system in sympathetic irritation.****

"****But the main difference between acute and chronic disease is the degree of the morbid activity of the vital powers;****"—*Science of Human Life*, pp. 425 and 441.

The following quotations from Dr. Trall clearly emphasize and partially explain the curative nature of disease and its oneness with health. If the student once gets this fact of the oneness of health and disease firmly fixed in his mind, all the practices of Orthopathy fall easily and naturally into line.

"All morbid actions are evidences of the remedial efforts of nature to overcome morbid conditions or expel morbid materials. All that any truly philosophical system of medication can do, or should attempt to do, is to place the organism under the best possible circumstances, for the favorable operation of those efforts. We may thwart, embarrass, interrupt, or suppress them, as is usually the case with allopathic practice, or we may direct, modify, intnesify, and accelerate them as is the legitimate province of hydropathic practice. But we must confess to the parodoxical proposition, that the symptoms of disease are the evidences of restorative effort; the effort, however, may be assisted by removing obstacles, diverting irritation, etc."—*Hydropathic Encyclopedia*. Vol. 2, P. 64.

Medical men speak of drugs which act on the bowels (produce diarrhea), drugs which act on the kidneys (occasion urination), etc. Reasoning, as they always do from the wrong end of the matter they attribute the powers of action and of selective action to the lifeless drug, instead of to the living body. Trall combatted this fallacy as follows, and incidentally demonstrated the essential nature of disease:—

"A knowledge of the law of vitality would teach medical men that only living structures have inherent powers to act; that all dead things, in relation to living, are entirely passive; and that the only property they possess is inertia, which is the tendency to remain quiescent until disturbed by something else—the power to do nothing.

"The living system acts on food to appropriate it to the formation and replenishment of its organs and tissues. This is digestion and assimilation—the nutritive process. And the living system acts on drugs, medicines, poisons, impurities, effete matters, miasma, contagions, infections—on everything not useful or usable in the organic domain—to resist them; to expel them; to get rid of them; purify itself of their presence through the channel or outlet best adapted to the purpose under the circumstances.

"And herein is the explanation of the classes of medicines; the rationale of the action of medicines, which has so puzzled the brains of medical philosophers in all ages.

"Emetics do not act on the stomach, but are ejected by the stomach. Purgatives do not act on the bowels, but are expelled through the bowels. Diaphoretics, instead of acting on the skin, are sent off in that direction. Diuretics do not act on the kidneys, but the poisonous drugs are got rid of through that emunctory, etc.

"And this equally mysterious disease! Is not its essential nature sufficiently apparent? The disease is the process of getting the poisons out of the system; and so this perplexing problem is also solved.

"That the explanation I have given of the nature of disease and the modus operandi of medicines is the true one, may be demonstrated in this way. We can take all the medicines of the pharmacopoeia, and produce all the diseases of the nosology. Thus certain combinations of brandy, cayenne pepper, and quinine will produce, in a healthy person, inflammatory fever; calomel, nitra, and opium, typhus or typhoid fever; gamboge, scammony and ipecac, cholera morbus; nitre, antimony and digitalis, the Asiatic or spasmodic cholera; cod-liver oil, salt and sulphur, the scurvey, etc. Castor oil, epsom salts, and a hundred other articles called cathartics, will occasion diarrhea; lobelia, Indian hemp, tobacco, and many other drugs, will induce vomiting. And what in the name of medical science and the healing art are the diarrhea and the vomiting except efforts of the living system to expel the poisons—purifying processes, diseases?

"Any person who can explain the philosophy of sneezing, has the key which may be applied to all the problems before us. Does the dust or the snuff sneeze the nose, or does the nose sneeze the dust or the snuff? Which is acted on or expelled, and what acts? Is sneezing a healthy or a morbid process? No one will pretend that it is normal or physiological. No one ever sneezes unless there is something abnormal in or about the nasal organ. Then sneezing is a remedial effort, a purifying process, a disease, as much as is a diarrhea, a cholera, or a fever."—*True Healing Art.*

"Perhaps I can give an illustration of the leading problems of my subject still more obvious and satisfactory. I read in a newspaper the other day, that a boa-contrictor, while on exhibition in one of the theatres in Paris, having been kept without food for a long time,

'Began to feel, as well he might,
the keen demands of appetite.'

and took it into his fancy to swallow a bed-blanket. The snake was two or three days in getting the blanket down; and after retaining it for some four or five weeks, the blanket, after another two or three days struggle, was found in its former position, and not much the worse for the vain attempt of the monster to digest it.

"Now the questions to be answered are: Did the blanket act on the snake, or did the snake act on the blanket? Again, to expel a bed-blanket from the stomach is not physiological. No boa-constrictor in the normal state ever did it. Then it must be pathological, and pathology is disease. The blanket was the cause of the disease—the obstructing material, and the disease itself was the process—the vomiting, which expelled it. Should this process of ejecting the blanket have been counteracted, suppressed, or subdued, or killed, or cured; or regulated and directed?

49

"All the functions of vitality may be resolved into two sets of processes: one transforms the elements of food into tissue, and throws off the waste matters; this is Health—Physiology. The other expels extraneous or foreign substances and repairs damages; this is Disease—Pathology. Is this not all plain enough?"—*True Healing Art.*

'In concluding this chapter I believe it appropriate to quote the following from the *Natural Cure of Disease.* (p. 10), by Bernarr Macfadden:

"It is disease that saves life. It is disease that actually cures the body. By means of disease poisons are eliminated, which might have caused death, had they been allowed to remain."

ACUTE DISEASE A CURATIVE PROCESS

Chapter VI

SINCE the days of I-em-Hetep the medical professions have sought to explain the essential nature of disease but were always forced to admit that they knew nothing of its nature—they never even dared suggest that it served an end or purpose. Today it is admitted that the nature of disease is unknown. For instance, Stenhouse says in his "Pathology" (Medical Epitome Series):

"To the man born blind the idea of light has no meaning; so all that is implied in the words life, disease, and death is not yet known, and they still await a satisfactory definition."

The Standard Dictionary defines disease as:

"Disturbed or abnormal physiological action in the living organism. A morbid condition resulting from such disturbance. Uneasiness; inconvenience; discomfort."

The Medical Dictionary defines disease as:

"Any departure from a state of health; an illness; more frequently the genus or kind of disturbance of health to which any particular case of sickness may be assigned."

These definitions merely say disease is disease and drop the matter. The nature of disease is not even hinted at. The medical dictionary does mention different genuses. A genus is an order or class (in zoology and botany) embracing subordinate classes or species. This idea of classing disease as orders, genera, species, etc., will be dealt with in a later chapter.

A medical writer in *American Medicine* (New York) in 1924 declares:

"Take two, simple, disturbing maladies, boils and colds. Mankind has been suffering from these so-called 'minor ailments' ever since the world began, but there seems to be little unanimity of opinion as to what a boil or cold really is, and there is no standard procedure for their treatment."

Sir Wm. Osler declared:

"Of disease we know nothing at all."

Dr. Curtis of the Physio-Medical or reformed Botanic School declared:

"We all believe that disease tends to death."

Samuel Hahnemann, founder of Homeopathy, said:

"To the physician, whose province it is to vanquish the disease that brings its victim to the very borders of corporeal dissolution."

Dr. Drake, a prominent early Homeopath, declared:

"Disease is wrong action, or it is subversive, and therefore wrong action."

Disease is simply *wrong action* and that settles the matter. Having settled this problem the various cults in medicine now devote all their attention to changing the action and "obviating the tendency to death," as Cullen decreed. On this assumption, as a foundation, the whole fabric of medicine, in all its multitudinous and diabolical forms, has ever rested. The correctness of this assumption was seldom, if ever, questioned until a little over a hundred years ago.

Disease, they think, is a positive and organized enemy—a devouring monster which attacks and destroys the body and mind—and, against which, they must put forth every effort to defeat. This idea has been handed down from ancient times when nothing was known of either physiology or pathology. The ancients conceived of disease as an entity, usually an evil spirit, which entered the body from the outside. The symptoms of disease were thought to be, necessarily, and invariably, evidences of a destructive process going on in the system, and therefore to be combatted and suppressed else life will be the forfeit.

Through all the ages that have passed, physicians, medicine men, magi, priests, alchemists, the gods and saints have all battled against this dreaded enemy of life and used every conceivable means to suppress and subdue it. From the merest infancy of therapeutics to now, whatever the form medical practice may have been, there has been a constant uniformity of views respecting the destructive nature and life destroying tendency of disease.

51

The rules of the physicians of all schools of all ages have been to "take disease by storm," or to "nip disease in the bud," or, to "take the bull by the horns." Due to this assumption and the rule that grew out of it, physicians have always wanted to "DO SOMETHING." It seems not to have mattered much what they did so long as they did SOMETHING. Even those who adopted the expectant attitude of Hippocrates held that disease is the foe of life and that something must be done if life is to be saved.

This idea is the exact opposite of the truth as will be plainly shown. Disease instead of being an entity and an enemy is a friendly process designed to save life. The fact that every cell and organ in the living body is constantly and ceaselssly striving for self-preservation and putting forth its every effort to maintain itself in as ideal a condition as possible has been previously emphasized. That they do so under all circumstances is certain. They strive always toward health because they are constituted that way—they cannot do otherwise. Disease is a consequence of the inherited and indwelling properties of the cell or of the complex organism.

The vital activities of cells are of a threefold kind. They are directed in part toward their self-preservation, in part toward propagation, and in part toward the ordering of their outward relations. To a limited extent the cell may exist unaffected by the influence of its environment by virtue of its own inherent properties, but this range of independence is very limited. If the external conditions deviate from the natural more than a certain small amount disturbances of the cell-functions at once manifest. Such disturbances may amount to the complete arrest of all signs of life, or even in the total destruction of the cell. If these influences are not powerful enough to arrest the activities of life the cell is capable of heightening its functions above the normal physiological standard or of lowering them below the standard to meet, defensively, unfavorable influences. By disease, in the cell, is meant, then, a deviation from the normal, of some of the vital activities, in order to protect itself from inimical external conditions.

What has just been said applies primarily to the unicelled organism. However, there is no reason to suppose that what is true of a single cell is not also true of the various cell-groups composing a multicelled organism. As disease of the unicellular organism is but abnormal action of a single cell, so human disease is but abnormal action of a multiplicity of cells. But it is more than mere abnormal action—*it is abnormal action with a purpose.*

Health is the normal operation of the organs and tissues of the body; disease is a departure from this normal standard. Life is a condition in which animals and plants exist with the capacity of exercising their functions. Health and disease are simply two conditions of life. The signs of health represent the conduct of the natural functions of life under normal conditions; the symptoms of disease represent the conduct of these same natural functions under handicap. The actions and functions, in either case are the actions and functions of the living organism and represent an effort, constant and ceaseless as the march of the seasons, to maintain the living state in as ideal a condition as possible. In disease, acute or chronic, life is struggling to throw off the thing that is handicapping its functions. The severity of the symptoms indicates the intensity of the struggle.

This is in perfect harmony with the laws of vital action explained in another chapter. The primary controlling law of life is self-preservation. All action occurring in living organisms as the result of extraneous influences is vital action, that is, action of and by the living thing, and is always directed to ordering the outward relations and adjusting the inward relations of the living thing for purposes of self-defense and self-preservation.

An organism is either alive or dead. If alive it is either in good health or poor health. If in good health, all its functions are being performed well; if in poor health, all its functions are being performed abnormally. All function whether healthy or unhealthy is function of the living organism and serves the same purpose. In health the function is carried on under normal conditions and is therefore easy and normal. When handicapped by abnormal conditions function becomes abnormal. The living organism seeks to perpetuate itself, to maintain its structural and functional integrity by repairing its structure and defending itself against harmful influences. Its functions, in health or in disease, are all designed and intended to maintain life and health. Disease action is defensive action—vital action under control of the law of *self-preservation*.

We presented evidence in the previous chapter that there is something wrong with the prevailing view of disease. We have shown that recovery from "disease" has often occurred after all hope of saving life has been given up and all treatment abandoned. Without going into great detail, on this point, let us point to another fact of even greater importance; namely, all down the ages, untold thousands have recovered from serious diseases who were treated by methods that were positively harmful and destructive. Many were killed by such methods, who would otherwise have recovered, but the fact still remains that a majority so treated did return to health. This is a fact that will not be disputed by any semi-honest member of any school of medicine now in existence.

If disease is an enemy and the treatment employed to combat it is a worse enemy, that is, of a more destructive nature, how does a patient ever recover? Could more eloquent testimony of the marvelous curative powers of the body be offered? If treatment that will kill a man in the possession of vigorous health and normal strength is administered to a patient who is battling against typhoid, typhus, pneumonia or the plague, and the patient recovers, can disease really be so great an enemy to life as it is popularly and "scientifically" supposed to be? These questions are at least thought provoking and should cause the reader to pause in his activities and give some consideration to the problems they present.

What is disease? Is it the friend or foe of life? Does it kill or preserve us? Must we seek to suppress and subdue it, or shall we let it alone and permit it to consumate its work?

These questions must arise in the minds of everyone who gives any consideration to the facts that have gone before. Although these facts seem to indicate that disease is not the foe but the friend of life, perhaps our questions are best answered by an appeal to a different set of facts. In this appeal, I shall confine myself to simple facts that can be understood by the average man untrained in the mysteries of physiology and pathology.

A few years ago a well known Naturopath wrote as follows:

"A baby is born into the world—and what happened?

"When it had been here a little while it developed, we'll say, an intestinal disturbance.

"Mothers—what was the diarrhea for?

"Did baby's intestines go on a rampage for pure and simple cussedness or was there a reason?

"Why did nature want to get the morbid mass from the little one?

"Can you imagine health and such material in the same body?

"That's the why.

"Baby's body was not pure, so nature tried to purify it."

Surely every one who reads these lines will agree that the foul disgusting mass of fermenting, putrefying food, that was cast out by means of the diarrhea, was not compatible with health. Well, the body had the same view of the matter and cast it out. How was it done? By increasing certain activities of the intestines and bowels. The diarrhea was not morbid action; it was simply an excess of healthy action. It was a work of elimination, of purification, of self-defense. You and the doctors call the diarrhea disease or a symptom of disease.

The same thing occurs when calomel or epsom salts or other poisonous and irritating substances find their way into the digestive tract. Large quantities of mucous are poured out to envelop them, and render them as harmless as possible, while they are hurried on through the intestines and bowels and expelled. This is called the purgative or laxative action of the drugs. It is not drug action at all. From first to last, it has been the living body and not the lifeless, inert drug that acted.

Calomel (mercury) is a powerful poison and produces many destructive effects if allowed to remain in the body. This is the reason the body expels the drug. Calomel is not a disease. It is popularly and "scientifically" considered to be a remedy for disease. It occasions an excess of healthy bowel action—a diarrhea—and the diarrhea is considered to be a perfectly normal, wholesome thing. In fact, the physician often administers this or some other drug for no other purpose than to produce a diarrhea.

If a diarrhea induced by the physician's dose is not a disease, why is the diarrhea induced by gastro-intestinal putrefaction and fermentation a disease? If the diarrhea induced by the physician is wholesome, why is not the diarrhea occasioned by the rotting food also wholesome? The one expells the poisonous drug to prevent it from injuring the body, the other expells the poisonous products of fermentation and putrefaction to prevent these from injuring the body. The action in both cases is vital or physiological action and serves the same purpose—namely, to protect the body from injury.

Emerson, after telling how foods often cause diarrhea, adds:

"In these cases the food is an irritant and causes irritation and increased peristalsis of the bowels. Then, increased peristalsis may be caused by true poisons, such as arsenic, mercury, etc. Changes in the weather will give some persons diarrhea especially if the weather changes suddenly to cold."

He then tells how some have "nervous diarrhea" and adds: "Some have one or two fluid movements after any mental excitement or emotion."

The protective character of diarrhea is here fully shown. The sudden drop in temperature causes diarrhea because it takes nervous energy away from the digestive organs to be used in resisting cold. The food is not digested and a diarrhea results.

In Asiatic cholera the fluid from the bowels comes largely from the blood and tissues. In dysentary (inflammation of the bowels) the stools are often made up almost wholly of blood, pus, and mucous. In both these diseases as well as in fevers the protective and purifying character of the diarrhea is apparent. Its true nature cannot be mistaken. Dr. Tilden has admirably expressed this fact as follows:

"Influences that might create pneumonia in the winter time will pass off as diarrhea in the summer time.

"Intestinal diseases are either acute or chronic and are usually named acute catarrh or chronic catarrh. For instance, an acute attack of gastritis is named acute cattarrh of the stomach, and the chronic form is known as chronic gastritis or chronic catarrh of the stomach. If the inflammation is in the colon it will be either acute or chronic, and will be spoken of as catarrh of the large intestines or colitis.

"Diarrhea will sometimes pass off in a few hours or a day. This is really not a disease, as it is caused by irritating foods, for instance; if one eats very freely of spinach, it may act on the bowels in two or three hours, casuing one or several liquid discharges then the effect is gone. There is no catarrh about this; it is simply a little local irritation, the same as would occur to the nose after inhaling pepper or snuff; so long as the irritation of the pepper or snuff continued there would be an extra amount of secretion thrown out. This is nature's way of protecting the mucous surfaces from irritation. If the irritation comes from decomposed food, and this decomposition is continuous day after day, at first it creates irritation of the mucous membrane, and finally it becomes a chronic inflammation or catarrh. If an irritation is very great there may be a chill caused by the blood being drawn from the surface of the body to the mucous membrane in the bowels, for it must not be forgotten that there are antibodies in the circulating medium; they are the natural defenders of the body, and when there is a threatened absorption in the intestines of a toxic material, nature in self-defense calls an extra amount of blood to the mucous membrane; this causes a pouring out of a great amount of secretion into the bowels. This secretion antidotes the poison and causes such an accumulation of fluid to take place in the bowels that it passes out as a diarrhea.

"In cholera nature's efforts are so great at flooding and washing out of the alimentary canal the poison that threatens absorption that there is copious discharge into the bowels of the serum of the blood. This serum is thrown into the intestines through the mucous membrane which is being irritated by the toxic material, and if it were not for this copious outpouring of fluid, the poison would be absorbed.

"Sometimes the effort on the part of the system to rid itself of a poison is so great that the subject will die of collapse, brought on from the tremendous loss of the fluids of the body. This is a case of an overworked conservative measure, or, in other words, nature kills herself in her efforts at saving herself. The chill that is experienced is very much on the order of the chill that is experienced when tonsilitis or diphtheria begins. The surface of the body is deprived of the circulating fluid and as a result of that there is deficient oxidation and a consequent chilling.

"As I explained in my first volume under the head of tonsilitis, the congestion of a mucous membrane or catarrh, is a conservative effort on the part of the system to prevent absorption of materials that threaten the integrity of the organism, and so long as the defense is required—so long as it is necessary for nature to keep her defenders at certain points in the alimentary canal to prevent absorption—the catarrhal state will be continued in spite of all treatment, except that of removing the necessity for this standing army of defense "

Should the diarrhea be checked; should it be subdued and suppressed? Or, should it be permitted to consumate its work? Suppose the diarrhea that is intended to expel the mercury is checked and the drug is permitted to enter the body, there to work havoc throughout the whole system. Would this not be the same as if the diarrhea which is intended to expel the rotting food is suppressed and absorption of the poisons formed by the rotting food is forced? In combating what the physician, his patient and the friends and relatives of the patient consider to be disease, or a symptom of disease, is not the whole combat waged against the body itself?

Not every drug that goes into the stomach produces a diarrhea. Often they are vomited. Calomel, epsom salts, strychnin, epicec, common table salt, and many other drugs occasion vomiting. If a dose of strychnin is swallowed and the stomach immediately casts it up, can anyone mistake this as any other than an action of self-defense? Yet, vomiting is considered to be a disease, or at least, a symptom of disease. In this case, it is obviously an act of self-preservation. It is no less so when table salt or epsom salts are vomited. Any stomach that has not built toleration for the inorganic substance called table salt will reject it immediately if the drug is swallowed.

When a drug occasions vomiting it is called an emetic. These are, or were, said to act on the stomach. The reverse is true—the action is organic. The drug is acted upon—it is the living body that acts and in self-defense. The body rejects poisons and irritants by vomiting, but, except under certain circumstances, does not reject wholesome substances in this manner The undepraved stomach rejects table salt, but not spinach or celery. It will cast up calomel or strychnin, but not bread or cabbage nor apples or oranges. Such "abnormal" actions are directed against the foes of life, not against her friends.

Emerson, in describing *acute gastritis* (Essentials of Medicine) says:

"The gastric mucous membrane of such a stomach is red and swollen, it secretes little gastric juice, and this contains very little acid but much mucous. The patient has uncomfortable feelings in his abdomen, with headache, lassitude, some nausea, often vomiting. The vomiting relieves him considerably, for it removes the irritating substance. The tongue is coated, and the flow of saliva is increased. If this decomposing, fermenting, irritating mass is not vomited, but reaches the bowel, colic and diarrhea are the result. As a rule the patient is well in about one day, although he may not have very much appetite for the next two or three days."

Here is a distinct theoretical recognition of the protective office of both vomiting and diarrhea with proof also that lack of appetite is defensive in such cases. He tells us that acute gastritis is due to abuse of the stomach through dietetic errors, alcohol and may also be the first sign of an acute fever, i. e. typhoid. Digestion is impaired. Secretion is scanty and of poor quality. The food ferments and putrefies instead of being digested. The appetite is cut off to prevent the intake of more food. Vomiting and diarrhea expel the decomposing mass of food already present. The lack of appetite for two or three days after the patient is "well" is due to the fact that it requires this length of time for the stomach and other organs involved to get back into working order. They are not prepared to take up the work of digestion as soon as the decomposing food is thrown out. The presence of this condition of the stomach in fevers should prevent physicians from feeding in such diseases.

In cases of bowel obstruction the peristaltic wave, from the point of obstruction forward to the mouth, is reversed, and the feces are vomited. This is an extraordinary and unusual effort on the part of the body to defend itself and preserve its integrity—an effort that would probably succeed more often than it does, did physicians but stop foolishly forcing more food upon such patients.

Sometimes one vomits his meal. This is a frequent occurrence when the sick are fed. A wound will often cause vomiting. I have seen vomiting result from a slight wound to the finger. Great grief may cause vomiting. Often those who do heavy manual labor in the hot summer's sun will, especially if they have taken a heavy meal, vomit their meal. Why are these things so? The reason is simple—the state of the body called disease, the wound, grief, heavy work and intense heat and other causes have suspended digestion and nature, or the body, throws out the food to prevent it from rotting and causing harm. Vomiting is a defensive action following the intake of a drug and it is the same when an undesirable meal is cast up.

In all acute diseases, appetite or hunger is lacking. In most chronic disease appetite is poor. This lack of appetite has been dignified by the euphonious title of anorexia and is considered as a disease, or rather a symptom of disease. There is no appetite following the ingestion of a meal and this absence of desire for food is considered normal. Under other conditions, absence of desire for food is considered abnormal. But is it? Desire or lack of desire for food depends upon conditions. There is naturally and normally a lack of desire for food when no food is required by the body and there is NATURALLY and NORMALLY an absence of appetite when there is lack of ability to digest the food.

If the reader will pardon a personal reference, I will draw upon my own experience to make this matter clear. On occasions I have been forced to be up all night without sleep. The next day I had little or no desire for food. Dr. Dewey used to say that sweet, restful sleep is not a hunger producer, and it is not. But neither is lack of sleep. Lack of sleep prevents recuperation and lessens digestive power. There is no appetite. Is this a symptom of disease? Should an appetite be stimulated under such conditions? Should one eat anyway?

I recall on two different occasions a few summers since, I was forced to be up with patients practically all night. Each time, for a period of about a week, I secured about one hour's sleep in each twenty-four. My desire for food gradually waned. If I ate much food it caused distress and discomfort. A half a head of lettuce or a canteloupe twice a day was about all I could eat without producing distress. I was also constipated during these periods. Were the constipation and anorexia evidences that I was in the grip of some devouring monster—some disease? Did I need tonics or bitters and purgatives and enemas? Was the lack of appetite normal or abnormal under these circumstances?

What was my trouble? Simply lack of functional power (enervation) due to a lack of recuperation—a lack of rest and sleep. My "disease" was not a positive entity but a negative quantity. I did not need treatment, but rest and sleep. I gave no attention to my bowels. I took no purgative or enemas or other goad to action. I needed no tonics nor bitters—I took none. All I needed was an opportunity for recuperation and when I received this my digestion and bowel action was soon going along as nicely and smoothly as ever. Had I taken tonics and bitters and forced myself to eat and had I resorted to goads to force my bowels to act, I would simply have brought on a more profound state of enervation and produced a condition requiring an acute disease to remedy. Rest is the great representive restorative process—stimulation is a wasteful process.

There is a lack of appetite—anorexia—in acute disease. Why? Because secretion has been suspended and digestion is not possible. The power to digest is lacking just as it was lacking in my case when I lost so much sleep, and an absence of all desire for food under such circumstances is normal and natural. It is a conservative measure. Nature resorts to this as a means of conserving the energy ordinarily expended in digestion and assimilation. Appetite is cut off if one receives a severe wound or is in deep grief or sorrow. It is a conservative measure. It is in no sense an enemy of life. It should not be combated or subdued. Appetite will return as soon as normal secretion is re-established and this will occur as soon as the work of disease has been accomplished and recuperation has taken place.

Those who are acutely ill are said to be prostrated. This is to say, they are extremely weak and unable to be up and around. Sometimes they are too weak to stand or even to sit. They move their limbs or turn over in bed with great difficulty. All muscular power is practically lost. Muscular action is suspended, just as digestive activities are suspended. Mental and sensory activities and power are also greatly reduced. But little energy is expended through any of the voluntary functions. Except that consciousness and sensibilities are not lost, the condition closely resembles that of sleep.

Who has not dozed off to sleep and been suddenly aroused, before becoming soundly asleep, and found themselves almost too weak to rise. There did not seem to be any power in the muscles. Although, a few minutes or seconds before, no feeling of weakness was felt. The usual power and vigor were present. Activity or stimulation, a cold bath perhaps, soon restored the normal feeling of strength. This apparent weakness was not due to lack of power, but to withdrawal of power from the voluntary functions. The body seems to have some way of switching its power on and off as electricity is switched on or off.

The condition of prostration in disease or following a shock is not lack of power but withdrawal of power. A man is ploughing in the field. He is feeling fine. Suddenly everything darkens. He falls (collapses) and is carried to the house. He develops typhoid or typhus or pneumonia. Was his sudden collapse due to sudden loss of power or sudden exhaustion of power, or was it due to sudden withdrawal of power? I am convinced it was withdrawal of power and that this is a wise provision designed to conserve the energy that is ordinarily and regularly expendid through the voluntary channels in order that it may be used to meet more urgent needs.

The body cannot speed up one function without slowing down another. You cannot engage in intense mental work and carry on physical work at the same time. You must give your whole attention to the mental work. Try working an intricate problem in mathematics while doing a hundred yard dash and you will get my meaning. The common expression "breathless attention" is not without foundation. Breathing is greatly lessened when one is engaged in mental effort. If a heavy meal is eaten there is a marked falling off in mental efficiency and a decided disinclination to do physical work. While engaged in the work of digestion blood and energy are required in extra quantities in the digestive organs.

An electric light burns brightly when it alone is receiving the electrical current. But if another light in another room, or if an electric iron is switched on the same current the lessening brilliancy of the light may be seen at once. If, then, the iron or second light are turned off, the first light will instantly brighten. This same thing is true of all power machines. POWER CANNOT BE EXPANDED WITH EQUAL INTENSITY IN ALL DIRECTIONS AT ONCE.

In the work of acute disease the operation of this principle is seen in all of its perfection. First nature suspends the voluntary functions in order that the power ordinarily employed by these in doing work may be utilized through other channels in the work of elimination. Nature sends us to bed to rest. We find it painful, even impossible to be up and around; much less can we work. Mental work is well nigh impossible. Even the senses rest. The physician says we are prostrated and there is a sense in which we are. BY THIS ENFORCED MENTAL AND PHYSICAL REST, NATURE IS ENABLED TO USE THE ENERGY ORDINARILY EXPENDED IN MENTAL AND PHYSICAL WORK IN HER WORK OF ELIMINATION, REPAIR AND CURE.

Nature does not stop with enforcing mental and physical rest. The work of digestion and assimilation are suspendid. Secretion is reduced to a minimum or suspended altogether in some glands. Every function that can safely be reduced is reduced. Thus by enforcing *physiological rest* much energy is saved for the work of elimination and cure. ALL THE ENERGY THAT IS SAVED FROM ONE

CLASS OF WORK MAY BE EMPLOYED IN CARRYING ON ANOTHER CLASS OF WORK. These are wise, conservative measures without which life would soon end, although, they are considered to be symptoms of disease and to be combatted.

You walk along the roadside on a beautiful spring morning enjoying the song of birds and the rich aroma of the myriads of beautiful flowers that bedeck the fields on each side of the road. You take a long, deep breath which draws a passing gnat into your nostrils where he lodges and irritates their lining membranes. You sneeze; perhaps you sneeze again. The gnat is gone, the nose is clear once more. You are eating a cake that crumbles easily and someone tells a funny story that evokes a laugh from you. A small particle of cake is drawn down into your bronchial tube. Almost instantly violent coughing ensues, which continues until the cake is expelled. You breathe easily once again.

Sneezing and coughing are very much alike, only the first is directed at obstructing and irritating particles in the upper air passages, while the latter is directed at similar things in the lower air passages. They are intended to expel these things and are usually, if not always, successful.

Burton-Opitz, in his *Elimentary Manual of Physiology*, says:

"It is also to be observed that the respiratory movements are inhibited during the act of swallowing, so that the food cannot be drawn into the larynx. When, however, the acts of swallowing and inspiration are not properly correlated, small particles of food and liquids may be diverted into the respiratory channel and give rise to an intense irritation of its lining membrane. This excitation induces the act of coughing, a reflex contraction of the expiratory muscles furnishing a powerful blast of air which is forced through the cavity of the mouth. *Its purpose is the dislodgement of the irritating particle.* The same principle is involved in the act of sneezing. In this case, however, the air is diverted through the nasal cavity." (italics mine.)

What are these two actions? They are considered to be symptoms or parts of disease. Every cold announces its presence by a few preliminary sneezes. If it is lower down in the respiratory passages there is coughing. Every acute disease usually begins with symptoms of a cold. Coughing and sneezing are considered as symptoms of disease. Are they? Actually, they are forceful or exaggerated expirations and are accomplished by the same power and mechanism that attends to what is called normal expiration. There is a more forceful and vigorous contraction of the chest walls and the diaphram than in ordinary expiration. It is not the action of some enemy of life, but is the action of the living organism itself. In the case of the inspired gnat or cake crumb, the sneezing and coughing are obviously normal and are defensive efforts. Why should they be considered as other than this when it is mucous they are directed against as in a cold, a bronchitis, or a pneumonia? They should not.

Dr. August F. Deinhold pointed out, *Omega Reprint*, that the coughing and expectoration accompanying tuberculosis of the lungs are curative or eliminating processes. He said:

"That tuberculosis is a healing process, is proved by every symptom: by the consumptive's cough, his expectoration, high temperature, lack of appetite, night sweats, diarrhea, etc. The cough proves the presence of abnormal material, which the system tries to dislodge by the expulsive efforts of the lungs to exhale. This is called a 'coughing' spell. If successful, the expectorated mass demonstrates that it obstructs free respiration. Thus 'coughing' is one of the cleansing processes, selected by Nature to purify the system."

The discharge, through coughing and expectoration, of the mucous and other abnormal substances in the lungs, clears them out of the system. Whether "morbid matter" is sent out through the lungs or by means of skin eruptions the cleansing process is salutary.

Inflammation supplies us with an ingenuous example of the defensive powers of the body. It, like coughing, sneezing, vomiting, diarrhea, etc., is confined wholly to the living realm. There is nothing even analogous to it in the dead and lifeless world. It is wholly a vital manifestation and, true to the laws of life, is a preservative and reparative function. Since a chapter is to be devoted to this subject and it will also be dealth with in the chapter dealing with the crisis, no details of inflammation will be given at this place.

Fever, which will also be dealt with in a future chapter, is nothing more nor less than an increase in the ordinary temperature of the body and serves a very definite and very necessary function—that of accelerating the activities of the cells of the body in order that they may accomplish their work more effectively. That it is a distinctly conservative reaction and not dangerous will be shown later.

Foot sweats, the profuse and toxic sweating that accompanies some stages of disease and the night sweats that accompany tuberculosis and other diseases are simply processes of elimination. They differ from ordinary sweating (they are ordinary sweating), only in that they contain more toxic matter. In acute rheumatism sweating is profuse and highly toxic.

Dr. Reinhold said of night sweats in tuberculosis, *Omega Reprint*:

"Night sweats are frequent concomitants of tuberculosis. At night the body rests better; less impressions from without are felt; vital power is saved, recuperates, and thereby sufficiently strengthened to make a new effort at elimination; thus night sweats appear."

Here is an unconscious recognition of the fact that rest and sleep are the most effective means of stimulating elimination. This fact will be made more clear in a future chapter. I need only say at this point that what is true of night sweats in tuberculosis is also true of night sweats in other wasting diseases.

Pain is a symptom of disease. What is pain? Simply sensation or feeling so intensified as to be uncomfortable. Things that give pleasure can be carried far enough so that the pleasurable sensation passes into pain. It is excess feeling and serves a very useful protective purpose. A large part of the practice of medicine, among all schools, has always been directed to suppressing pain—not by removing its cause, but by overcoming the power of the nerves to feel. It has been a killing practice. Pain is really one of man's best friends. It is the warning voice of nature telling us that something is wrong or that the thing we are doing is harmful. It is nature's "*thou shalt not*." Dr. Oswald rightly likened the suppression of pain to "muffling the alarm bells during a conflagration." But it is worse than this. Suppression of pain not only muffles the alarm bells, it cripples the firemen.

It is literally true that the capacity of an organism for enjoyment can be measured by its capacity to suffer. The more elevated is an animal in the scale of life—the more highly organized its nervous system—the greater are its capacities for pleasure and pain.

Suffering, that is the capacity to suffer, is absolutely necessary for our protection and preservation and, to this extent, in both the moral and utilitarian sense, pain is good and not evil. Enjoyment comes from obedience to the laws of being and suffering from violating these laws. Fixed laws of life are essential. They work injury only when violated, and the consequent suffering acts as a school master to compel man to behave himself.

Suffering is an incentive to man to adjust himself to the laws of life, to adapt himself to his natural environment, or to adapt his unnatural environment to his needs. Without hunger to drive an animal to eat he would starve; without thirst he would perish in the presence of water; without pain from cold he would freeze without ever knowing the cause; without suffering from heat he would be consumed by fire; without pain from pressure his body would be crushed without warning. Pain from disease and injury is an evidence of a need for rest and a change of life. The gratification of desire becomes painful when carried to excess, and pain in such cases is necessary to prevent complete exhaustion and death. If man was capable of pleasure only and not of pain he would speedily exhaust the powers of life. Pain is a very effectual check to conduct which would otherwise lead to destruction. *The office of pain is not to destroy us, but to save us.*

All of man's powers are intended for good and serve good purposes when used in harmony with their primitive constitution. Man can govern his powers and use them rightly or wrongly. If he uses them wrongly, pain and suffering call a halt.

Man's appetites and passions stand on a lower plane than his higher mental faculties. When these passions and appetites are governed by will and reason in harmony with their primitive purposes and are not permitted to become masters over the higher powers, they serve noble ends. But when they become masters and the higher powers are made slaves to them, human nature is debased. From this, it will be seen that man should control and direct his appetites and passions aright and not attempt to eradicate them as certain Eastern religions demand. Their proper exercise brings pleasure. Their wrongful exercise brings pain and the pain is commensurate with the pleasure their right exercise affords. *Pain is life's guardian angel.*

The gratification of desire becomes painful if pushed to excess. All pleasures become painful if pushed beyond the limits of safety. The intensest pleasures are the costliest and occasion the most pain if over-indulged. Pain is a very effectual check to conduct that would otherwise lead to swift destruction. This is the reason that relief of pain is an evil. It checks Natures' check. It enables us to go on heedless of the price we are paying. It is one thing to silence the outcry of nature with pain killers, but quite another to correct and remove the conditions that give rise to it.

A common cold furnishes us with another excellent example of Nature's defensive action. Mucous is a normal secretion of the mucous membrane of the nose and throat, or of all mucous membrane for that matter. When one has a "cold" there is a very profuse secretion or, more properly, excretion of mucous. This mucous is not only greater in quantity but inferior in quality. It does not serve the same purpose as normal mucous which is intended to moisten and lubricate the channels and passages lined by the mucous membrane.

Under certain conditions the eliminating organs of the body are unable to keep the blood free of waste and impurities. The body's mucous surfaces, especially those of the nose and throat, are forced to aid in purifying the blood. They are forced to compensate for the failure of the eliminating organs. We have a "cold." Perhaps we say we "caught" cold. Caught it, indeed! Instead of catching something we are getting rid of something and that something is too hot and feverish to be called cold. We may attribute the cold to a "slight exposure" or to "getting our feet wet" or some other convenient bugaboo. These things can no more cause a cold in the man who is not prepared for one than the fall of the hammer can send a bullet from an unloaded gun. Just as the fall of the hammer is only the occasion and not the cause of the bullet's flight from the loaded gun, so the slight exposure is only the occasion and not the cause of the cold. Without the slight exposure, the cold may not have come when it did, but it would have come, anyway. The cold is a process of compensatory elimination as will be shown.

As an example, let us suppose that at this point, you are exposed to the cold and skin action is temporarily suspended. The amount of poisons and impurities that were previously being thrown out through the skin are now held up in the blood. The lungs and kidneys, already having all the work they can do, are unable to excrete the additional amount of retained waste and poison. It must, therefore, be eliminated through some other channel.

The prevalent, widespread fear of colds, the opinion that if they are not "broken up" or "thrown off" they will "throw" one into pneumonia or consumption is a delusion. The tendency of a cold is to "throw" one directly the other way. If colds are let alone and not suppressed or interfered with they will be shorter in duration, more regular in their course, will leave the system in an improved condition and develop less often. Anyone may test this for himself.

Catarrh is but a chronic "cold" of the lining membrane of one or more of the organs of the body. It acts as a constant *safety valve,* by which, the body, heavily encumbered with pathoferic matter, relieves itself of that portion which the normal channels of elimination are unable to get rid of. Practically every one in civilized life is afflicted, more or less with catarrh. This attests the fact that we are all living unnaturally. For, while disease is the natural result of our present mode of life, the diseased state is not the natural state of man.

Confirmatory of the above Burton-Opitz says:—

"Cilia are found in the respiratory passage, where they beat towards the outside. Their function is to move the particles of dust into the pharnyx, whence they are flushed into the stomach by saliva. It is true, however, that a certain proportion of dust always gets beyond these ciliated regions into the finer bronchioles and alveoli of the lungs. Thus, the domestic animals and inhabitants of the cities commonly present lungs considerably stained with dust. It is true, however, that a much greater amount of this foreign material would be able to enter if these tubules were not ciliated.

"Particularly heavy depositions of dust are frequently found in the lungs of coal miners and marble cutters. *Nature eventually endeavors to dislodge them by a catarrhal inflammatory reaction which may at times assume the general character of tuberculosis*" (Italics mine.)

We might go on naming and discussing symptoms of disease but we would find nearly all of them to be efforts of the body to purify and protect itself. The few exceptions are those symptoms that are obviously the destructive work of the poisons the body is trying to eliminate and are found chiefly in chronic disease. Chronic disease is a state of weakness in which the body has learned to tolerate the toxins to a greater or less degree and in which it lacks power to rise to an acute eliminative effort. This part of our subject will be discussed elsewhere.

The facts enumerated plainly show that fever, pain, coughing, sneezing, vomiting, diarrhea, inflammation, eruptions, night sweats, etc., are vital phenomena and demonstrate conclusively that disease has no individual factor-entities other than those that sustain life in general and in particular. The symptoms of disease depend upon the same power and functions that produce the signs of health. Health and disease are the same thing—vital action intended to preserve, maintain and protect the body. If this view is correct, and who will question it, there is no more reason for treating disease than there is for treating health. The body slides easily into *disease* when conditions warrant and glides as easily back into *health* when conditions justify.

Orthopathy recognizes the essential unity of *healthy* and *morbid* phenomena and sees in each a lawful and orderly adjusting of the internal and external relations of the organism. Sir John Forbes long ago partially recognized this fact of the unity of these phenomena but he did not fully comprehend the beneficient nature of the *morbid* phenomena. The same may be said of M. Gubler, of France. These men saw that what we term diseases are not things different from or external to the living body, but rather particular conditions of the body, or modified phases of the vital manifestations. They are essentially vital or biological, are processes of the living organism. All *morbid* action is but a modification of the normal functions and processes of the body and all the physical results making up *morbid* structural alterations are simply modifications of natural or normal textures, produced from the same materials and by the same vital processes. When disease results in changes in the structures of the body, or in the functional products of the body, the constituents of these changed structures and products consist of materials identical with the normal or healthy constituents of the body and are aggregated, arranged and elaborated by the very same organic or physiological processes that operate in normal health. These are all the result of the same fundamental processes and functions of nutrition, elimination, reproduction, etc

Dr. Moras gives us an excellent example of this fact in the following quotation from his *Autology:*

"If now you will investigate the products or by-products of the organs and tissues of your body, in health and in sickness, you will readily recognize that there is no real, distinctive difference between any given 'healthy' product and its corresponding 'sickly' product, aside from the difference in the quality or (adulteration) of the two—I mean the 'healthy' and the 'sickly.' For instance, the so-called pale, watery blood of anemia is just as much blood as the red, plastic blood of plethora, except in the proportion of the white and red corpuscles and the richness of the serum. So with the saliva, gastric and intestinal juices, cerebrospinal fluids, genito-urinary secretions or excretions of these two individuals. It's only a difference in the 'grade'—not in the 'stuff' itself. The 'mucous' secretion of the mucous membranes anywhere in the bodies of these two individuals—one 'healthy' and the other 'sickly'—is exactly the same slime and lubricant; only this: that the sickly kind is more diluted or less oily, or more 'ropy' and less watery, than the healthy kind. That's all."

Again he says:

"You understand that all 'symptoms'—such as fever, pain, redness, swelling, etc.,—are phenomena manifested by each and every organ or tissue in conditions of impairment or disease; and that there is no real difference between the 'sickly' symptoms and the 'healthy' signs manifested by the organs or tissues in sickness and in health, aside from a mere difference in the degree of heat (fever), or sensation (pain), or color (redness), or size (swelling)."

Disease is no new thing superadded to the living organism but is a mere "complex" or aggregation of modifications of structures already existing and of functions and processes always going on in the living economy. The disease is always a product of the vital actions and is in no sense an entity or new and novel condition of structure and function. *Disease* is as truly natural as *health* and is constituted and maintained by the same vital powers, functions and structures as those which constitute and regulate the conditions of normal, as distinguished from impaired, health.

The *healing power of nature* is inherent in the living organism. It is not a special or unique power, nor is it a single power. It is simply the ordinary vital powers by which we live and grow. How true were Dr. Trall's remarks in his famous lecture on *The True Healing Art:*

"What is the *vis medicatrix naturoe?* It is the vital struggle in self-defense; *it is the disease itself.* So far from disease and the *vis medicatrix naturoe* being antagonistic entities or forces at war with each other, they are one and the same. And if this be the true solution of the problem, it is clear enough that the whole plan of subduing or 'curing' disease with drugs is but a process of subduing and *killing* the vitality. We see, now, the rationale of the truth of the remark of Professor Clark: 'Every dose diminishes the vitality of the patient.'

"The announcement of the doctrine that the remedial powers of Nature and the disease are the same; that the *vis medicatrix naturae* which saves and the morbid action which destroys are identical, may sound strangely at first; and so do all new truths which are in opposition to doctrines long entertained and universally believed. It seems exceedingly difficult, and in many cases utterly impossible, for medical men to get hold of this idea, so contrary is it to all their habits of thought, and all the theories of their books and schools. Their minds have been so long wedded to the dogma, that disease and the *vis medicatrix naturoe* are in some inexplicable way hostile powers, that after I have talked with them for hours on the subject, answered all their criticisms, and silenced every one of their objections, they cannot overcome their prejudices and prepossessions sufficiently to comprehend it And some of my medical students have revolved, and pondered, and criticized, and controverted this idea for months before they fully understood it. But it is true, nevertheless:"

Health is not a fixed state. It is a constantly varying condition of the organism ranging all the way from almost ideal health to the lowest depth of impaired health. But it is always health. Nor is *disease* a fixed state. It is a condition of impaired health and partakes of the same natural variations as does good health. Good health and poor health (disease) are but varying conditions of life. They are not antagonistic entities but different degrees of the same thing. The oneness and sameness of health and disease is as certain as that a bright light and a dim light are both light.

Heat and cold are relative terms. If we assume that heat is the positive condition, then cold is only a little less amount of heat. The hypothelical *absolute zero* is nothing more than a mere convenience of thought or of measurement. Wealth and poverty are relative terms. If wealth is assumed to be the positive condition, then poverty is only a little less wealth. So, health and disease are relative terms. Health is the positive condition; disease is only a little less health. There are not many kinds of health or specific forms of health; so there are not many kinds of disease or specific forms of disease. Disease is a unit just as health is a unit and health and disease are a unit. There is only one life, only one health, only one disease. But, just as there are many manifestations of life and many manifestations of health, so there are many manifestations of disease.

Health and disease shade off into each other by insensible gradations so that it is difficult to say where one begins and the other ends; just as it would be difficult to say at what point on the thermometer heat ends and cold begins. In health and disease we are not dealing with antagonistic entities but different degrees of the same thing—*Life*; just as with heat and cold we are not dealing with antagonistic entities but with different degrees of the same thing—TEMPERATURE. Health is not a fixed state. It varies with the varying conditions under which life exists. Health and disease shade so insensibly into one another that no differential criteria can be offered to distinguish the one from the other, that can be exact or invariable. It is difficult to say just when a rapid heart, for instance, is to be considered a sign of disease or a flushed skin an evidence of congestion. A rapid heart may be due to effort or excitement or stimulation and a flushed skin may be due to heat or cold or to embarrassment, as in blushing. Blanched cheeks may be due to fear.

The body is an organic whole. Its diseases are one. They are departures from "normal" conditions. We may say it is more or less "accidental," although this word does not correctly express the facts of the case, whether this that or the other organ suffers since its sufferings, are local effects of a general or systematic derangement.

Dr. Densmore rightly defined disease in these words:

"Disease always ensues upon the disturbance of the conditions of life natural to the animal, and is an unfailing and friendly expression on the part of the system of an effort to rid itself of conditions and substances inimical to health."

Disease is the process of cure—it is a means of saving life. It is not something to be cured—it is the cure. This is why my good friend, Dr. B. S. Claunch, declares that it would break a law of nature if acute disease were to kill one man or woman. It is just as reasonable for us to expect a curative process to kill as for us to expect a killing process to cure. We should know that the organs of the body can no more function in any other than the life preserving and life protecting way for which they are constituted than gravitation can send bolders upward or cohesive attraction split rocks. They cannot transgress the laws that govern them. Only in our voluntary actions are we capable of placing ourselves in opposition to the laws of being.

In considering the above proof that disease is a curative process we find two general classes of phenomena to be present in all acute disease—namely, (1) increase of function, and (2) decrease of function. There is, in other words, an elevation of some of the most important functions of life, with diminution of others. Representing the first group, we have:

1. Increase of temperature.
2. Rapid pulse and rapid heart action.
3. Pain—excess of feeling.
4. Inflammation.
5. Flushed skin.
6. Quickened respiration.
7. Coughing and sneezing.
8. Increased action of the mucous membranes.
9. Often increased action of the skin and kidneys.
10. Increased bowel action—diarrhea.
11. Vomiting.

Representing the second group are:

1. Lack of appetite.
2. Absence of secretions.
3. Dry mouth and skin.
4. Suspension of digestion.
5. Often inactive bowels.
6. General "prostration" of voluntary functions.

We have grouped these two classes as eliminative and conservative. The increase of some functions is intended to expel the poisons from the body. The diminution of other functions conserves vitality so that it may be used through other channels—that is, energy conserved by diminished action in one direction is available for expenditure in accelerated function in the work of cure.

In this work, the body acts as though guided by some unseen intelligence which knows just what to do and when to do it. Under those conditions that necessitate disease for their correction every province in the vital domain, from the least to the greatest is put under the most severe and rigid contribution to the end of saving life.

In proportion to the need to conserve energy are the various functions of the body suspended and guarded with just enough vitality to maintain their continuity and preserve them in a state of resuscitability. With the suspension of the nutritive functions and the muscles of voluntary motion at rest, there is little action in the system generally, and consequently little wear and tear, so that the cost of maintenance is almost nothing. Perfect economy is everywhere exercised in the appropriation and use of the vital energies, and the whole process is conducted under perfect law which nicely and minutely adapts the means to the end.

The following quotation from Jennings well illustrates the principle of conservation of power we are here attempting to make clear:

"In the course of my 'let alone' practice, I have many times been astonished to see to what lengths the economy of life would carry the reduction of active processes, and yet restore the machine to new and vigorous animation. Many times have I stood by my patients and seen their eyes closed apparently in death, and yet had the satisfaction of witnessing their return to life and health. To what extent it might be expedient and practicable, in some cases, under the most favorable circumstances, for the vital economy to carry this suspension of all vital action within the scope of human ken, and then have it issue in reanimation, it is of course impossible for any man, with his present limited means of knowledge on the subject, to form even a satisfactory conjecture. But I have no doubt that if the theory of unity of vital action prevails, and the practice of leaving the work of renovating the human system in the hands of nature, under such circumstances as further light and experience shall dictate, it will be found to occur occasionally that persons will lie for days and even weeks, to all human appearance within the cold domains of death, and after all be restored to their friends and society on earth. Under the present system of managing disease and interments, it is no unheard of thing for persons to be apparently dead for some length of time, and resuscitate. The following scrap, cut recently from a weekly periodical, is calculated to excite interest and awaken inquiry on this momentous subject.

"'BURIED ALIVE.—We have often thought that some provision should be made by the government against the possibility of living interments. Death and the funeral follow each other so closely that we have no doubt many persons are buried alive. An exchange paper states that since 1833, accidental circumstances have prevented ninety-four persons from being buried alive. Of these, thirty-five have recovered spontaneously from their lethargy, at the moment when the funeral ceremonies were about taking place; thirteen were aroused by the stimulus of busy love and grief above them; nine by the pricking of the flesh in sewing the shroud; five by the sense of suffocation in their coffins; nineteen by accidental delays which occurred in their interments; and six by voluntary delays suggested by doubts as to their deaths.'"— *Medical Reform*, pp. 294-5.

It is quite evident that delay, whether accidental or voluntary, is not a cause of recovery. The twenty-five recoveries attributed to this were spontaneous recoveries. And if these, why not also those due to "busy love and grief above them"? Indeed, are not all of them spontaneous recoveries? What is there in the falling of a coffin, the prick of a needle or a sense of suffocation to restore a man to health?

The body that is struggling against powerful toxins and attempting to repair great and vital damages must of necessity save, if possible, the more vital organs first. This repair and cure can only be done by the vital processes, and in carrying forward these processes, it is necessary for nature to make certain developments, that is, produce what are commonly called signs and symptoms of disease. There is no other way by which she can accomplish her object.

The body is a very complex organism, composed of many organs, all of them dependent upon a common source of power. When danger threatens the body, although it is already greatly enervated and its functions all more or less impaired, there will be increased action in some parts and decreased action in others. Organs with dual functions may have one function increased and the other decreased. Jointly considered, the power of the body is insufficient for the purpose of maintaining healthy action in all the organs. When there is a departure from the highest standard of healthy action or condition in the individual, the parts concerned fail in their functions and in maintaining their healthful conditions, not from any want of disposition or tendency to do right, but for want of sufficient power to do what they would do if they could. They do the best they can with the power at their disposal.

If there is not power enough in reserve to carry on the restorative operations and, at the same time, continue all the functions of life in their full vigor, the *Law of Limitation* enforces such curtailments as the exigencies of the case calls for, and the power witheld from one organ is supplied to another to accomplish a more urgent and more necessary work. Power is witheld from the digestive organs, the appetite for food is cut off, and the power thus saved is used by the organs that are doing the work of elimination or that are repairing their injuries. The voluntary muscles are deprived of power, the sick man is thrown upon his back (prostrated) in bed, and is unable to help himself. What power the body possesses is used, under the direction of eternal and immutable law, to the best possible advantage, just where it is needed and the curtailment of function is carried just as far as, but no further than, the emergency demands.

When we once grasp the significance of the universal and unfailing upward tendency of vital action, the now universally prevalent delusion, that any "unnatural" or unusual action or lack of action of the human oragnism is an unfriendly one, hostile to the best interests of the body, will be relegated to a belated oblivion.

Nature never wantonly turns aside from her habitual course of action to throw her complex machinery into disorder and give it suicidal motion and tendency There is always an imperative necessity for her actions and her operation. The work of preserving life devolves upon the vital economy and this economy does not require to be reminded of its duties. Nature does not withdraw power from an organ to *destroy* life, but to *save* it. She gives us the strongest possible guarantee that all available power will be put in requisition, and expended most economically in her work of cure and reparation. Her action can never be wrong.

The tendency of all the movements of life, in *disease*, is to save life as far as that may be in danger and especially to avert threatened injury to any particular organ. The first object nature aims at in her work is to shut down all unnecessary waste-gates for the needless expenditure of power in order that those organs that must accomplish the greater part of the work of cure may have power with which to do their work. There is no man living who is wise enough to determine just which functions should be diminished and which accelerated. The organism is itself the best judge in the matter. In other words, just as the organism alone can safely manage its functions in *health*, so it alone can safely manage is affairs in *disease*.

Dr. Jennings well says:

"There is no danger in the symptoms, singly or collectively. The danger lies back of the symptoms; it existed in all its extent before the process which is now going on in the system commenced. This is a recuperative or restorative operation. It was called for by the state of the system. It is, therefore, a gross libel upon the economy of life to call it a wrong condition—or wrong action!" *Medical Reform*, p. 145.

In truth alone is unity and agreement. But present day so-called science robed in learned subtilty has so automationized the people that they readily believe the puppet in the professional chair in the face of the most obvious errors and disagreement. It has, therefore, been almost impossible to convince the mass of mankind that disease —that thing they have always been taught to consider their worst foe—is in its very nature their best friend under certain circumstances; that it is, in reality, not more nor less than the inevitable reaction of their own organism against the foes of life.

Perhaps this latter statement should be qualified a bit. Symptoms of disease are of two classes—namely, those that are the result of the organic struggle against the toxins that are endangering life, and those that are the result of the destructive effects of the toxins, upon the body. The first of these were classified by Rausse as "*symptoms of reaction*" the second he called "*symptoms of destruction*." He also pointed out that the "symptoms of reaction" in their perfection, totality and greatest strength are only to be found in acute, or as he called them, the "*primary or healing diseases*," but that they exist although in lessened strength and perfection in the chronic or "*destroying diseases*."

When a poison, mercury for instance, is taken into the system two sets of effects are observable—first, the reaction of the system against the drug, and second, the destructive effect of the drug upon the tissues fluids and organs of the body. If the drug is taken in by way of the mouth vomiting or diarrhea follows. These are organic reactions against the drug—*efforts at elimination.* When the drug gets into the blood it begins a work of destruction that may end only in the death of the victim. Just to mention one of its destructive effects, it destroys the tissues and cells of the kidneys, where it is taken for elimination, and produces "Bright's Disease." The part it plays in destroying the functioning cells of other organs of the body and thus producing other degenerative diseases—diabetes, diseases of the heart and arteries for instance—will be discussed later. That it does destroy bone and nerve substances, gland substance and the structures of the hollow organs of the body as well as the skin and mucous membrane is well known. Insanity, paresis, paralysis, locomotor ataxia and other forms of nervous disease as well as gumma of bones and arteries are also well known effects of this deadly mineral.

What is true of mercury is more or less true of every other poison whether taken into the body from without or formed within the body itself. Cirrhosis of the liver, for instance, is due in almost every instance to alcohol. Alcohol formed by carbohydrate fermentation in the digestive tract is equally as destructive as an equal amount taken from a bottle. Not understanding the nature and purpose of disease, and either not knowing the body's powers of self-cure or being content to ignore these, the many healing cults that have arisen and flourished since the dawn of history have sought to suppress the symptoms of reaction by almost every conceivable means, often by means of powerful poisons that, themselves, are chiefly responsible for the destroying symptoms the chronic sufferer carries around with him.

Observe that Rausse's symptoms of reaction include both the conserving reduction and suspension of functions and the actively resisting acceleration of functions. In other words the symptoms of reaction may be subdivided into these two classes.

Diseases with all their many labels, are simply complexes or aggregates of the symptoms we have been discussing and a few more like them. Each symptom complex is given a different name, as though it were something distinct from other symptom complexes. Glance briefly at so-called measles: It begins with catarrhal disturbances (cold) accompanied with fever, chilliness, sneezing, coughing and headache followed by skin eruption. There is lack of appetite, malaise and even prostration, often diarrhea and usually unusual kidney action. Every symptom present belongs under the classification of *symptoms of reaction.* The disease is a process of cure every symptom of which is beneficial under the circumstances.

There is no danger in the symptoms, singly or combined, of so-called disease. The danger lies back of the symptoms. It existed in it's greatest extent before the process which we call disease began. It grows less and less as this process continues and grows less in proportion to the severity of the symptoms—this is to ay, THE MORE ACUTE THE DISEASE THE MORE RAPID WILL RECOVERY BE.

The recuperative or renovating work never begins but once—with the beginning of life—and it never ends until life ends. There is but one difference between this work in disease and in health. In health there are sufficient vital energies to sustain all the organs and functions of the body while in disease, there is not sufficient energies to sustain all these functions adequately to meet the ordinary demands of life. And this lack of power, or disproportion between work to be done and ability to work is the fundamental reason for disease.

The laws or principles on which disease action is conducted are precisely the same as those upon which healthy action depends—namely, to use what power the system possesses, be it much or little, in the highest interest of the organism. This principle will not permit a single function, however small or relatively unimportant, to be unnecessarily reduced or disturbed in its conduct. So long as it can repair damages and waste without depriving the cardinal organs of sufficient force to conduct their work, it will do so. But should it become necessary to enforce the *Law of Limitation* in respect to these organs and diminish their power so that their action is enfeebled, in order that the power may be used elsewhere, the change will be cautiously made and conducted with the greatest regularity if not interfered with. The "old order" will be restored in the same lawful and orderly manner, as soon as the end for which the change was made has been attained.

When an extremity necessitates bold and decisive movements, these will be made in any and every direction and to the extent demanded by the exigencies of the case, without regard to the temporary suffering and impairment that may result in other parts of the body.

It makes no difference whether the end for which these changes are made is attainable or not. If the heart, for instance, is injured beyond the possibility of recovery, unless the injury proves immediately fatal, so as to preclude all attempts at repair, a reparative process will be immediately begun and prosecuted in the same manner and with the same vigor as if the case were a curable one.

Suppose a man is wounded in some vital spot, is pierced by a bayonet or gun shot, or is poisoned by arsenic or other deadly agent, not immediately fatal, but of such a nature and extent that recovery is not possible. In spite of this nature will put forth every possible effort to repair the damage and restore soundness to the injured organ or organs. And she will pursue precisely the same course in such a case as she would have pursued had the injury done been reparable and recoverable from.

The sick body musters all its forces and expends them with a most rigid economy in an effort to repair damages and perpetuate its existence, and even when the saving work is beyond their power of achievement, or the interference interposed by treatment renders it impossible for them to accomplish their work, and they must fall, they continue, to the last to attempt to repair damages and eke out their existence.

In conclusion, every part of man's body, is designed for a particular function, and is controlled by laws that are as immutable as the law of gravitation. These laws are designed to govern the body's actions and preserve its integrity.

Every involuntary power exhibited in man's body constantly and ceaselessly obeys these laws. In the very nature of things it could not be otherwise. The organs must perform the functions for which they are designed. They must obey the laws of their constitution. They can no more do otherwise than the earth can reverse its motion, or stones cast themselves upward. When cohesive attraction splits rocks and magnetism arranges needles parallel to the equator, then may we expect to see organs of man's body disobey the laws of their constitution and perform functions for which they are not designed.

So long as our organs act, they must act lawfully. The action must be upward and right. Their action can never be downward and wrong. In disease, as in health, all the actions of the body are according to immutable law. Every organ and function performs the work for which it is designed. Every action is correct, upward, and designed to save, improve, and perpetuate life.

There are no amendments to the constitution of Nature. None of her laws have been repealed. They cannot be broken, but men may break themselves in the attempt to break them. The damage is to the man, and not the law. And it is only in our voluntary actions that we are capable of setting ourselves in opposition to the laws of our being. Every time that we do this, the laws inflict a certain penalty. There is no escape from the penalty.

This is a Universe of law and order. Every law is the expression of a Force behind it. Every force must act lawfully, being unable to act in any other way. The laws and forces controlling the body are the same in disease as in health, and their action is always for the same purpose—harmony, betterment, improvement.

Disease action, no less than health action is right action; yet it occasions suffering because of adverse conditions that have been imposed upon the body. So, by the term ORTHOPATHY we mean RIGHT SUFFERING. The individual suffers, not because the action of the body is wrong, but because the body under control of law, is struggling in the only way it can struggle, to free itself from impending dangers resulting from bad habits—misuse and abuse.

Let no man deceive you; let no man lead you astray. The actions of the body are always right, and in disease are as true to the pole-star of health as the needle is to the magnetic pole. The so-called symptoms of disease, which puzzle physicians, are not destructive processes; they are not evils to be resisted, combatted, suppressed, subdued, or subverted. They are merely external evidences of a body's striving under control of law to preserve its integrity and existence; and the physician who regards them as anything else, reveals his abject ignorance of the most fundamental facts of life.

SELF-LIMITED DISEASES

Chapter VII

MEDICAL men say that most if not all acute diseases are self-limited. They explain this term to mean that the disease persists until the body cures itself by forming a sufficiency of immune substances. Man gets well when his body has manufactured enough antitoxin to counteract the bacterial toxins that are held to be responsible for the disease. It is generally admitted by medical men that they have no treatment that will cure pneumonia or which will shorten its course by one day. But they say it is self-limited. Typhoid fever is said to be a self-limited disease but "there is scarcely an acute disease in which relapses are so common," (Emerson). Four or five relapses may occur and prolong the disease for six months. Diphtheria is a self-limited disease. The person sick with this disease is said to get well as soon as "enough antitoxin has been manufactured."

If this theory is a correct one, the question remains to be answered: Why do relapses occur? If enough "immune substances" have been produced to *cure* the disease, and the patient is convalescing, how does he relapse? Does he suddenly lose his "immune substances?" Is he suddenly invaded by an army of germ recruits that call for more antitoxin than he possesses? If either of these latter are correct answers how may man be assured immunity to disease by manufacturing antitoxins or by being inoculated with animal "antitoxins"—serum and pus? If the man who has had a disease is unable to manufacture or retain enough "immune substances" to protect him, how is the well man to be protected?

But it is only in a few diseases that these "immune substances" are held to establish immunity. Even in these, two or more "attacks" are more frequent than is commonly supposed. Cases of men having had smallpox five different times are on record. One may have typhoid more than once. Pneumonia may be had many times. Colds are frequent. Tonsilitis is equally so. Influenza may also be had many times. So with acute rheumatism and this may even become chronic. This list might easily be greatly enlarged and extended to include all acute "diseases."

Colds and tonsilitis, both of them self-limited, may follow one "attack" after another for a whole year or more. Then, should they cease, from whatever cause, it is assumed that immunity has been established.

This theory, it is not proven and is, therefore, only a theory, does not satisfy a reasoning mind. We are willing to recognize the so-called self-limiting nature of acute disease, but must reject the medical explanation. So far as I am aware, none of the drugless schools attempt to explain the fact.

This theory assumes at the outset that acute disease is caused by germs. It assumes that it is not caused by anything else. It ignores the detoxifying work of the liver, lymph glands, tonsils, etc., and the eliminating work of the kidneys, skin, bowels, lungs, etc., and assumes that cure can only result through the process of antitoxin manufacture. It is unable to build immunity upon a basis of health but must secure it at the cost of disease. In this it reverses the whole order of nature and secures health and immunity to disease by employing the causes of disease.

One other objection, and a powerful one, may yet be offered to this theory, it assumes that an acute disease, say typhoid, runs a more or less definite length of time and that recovery is not possible before this time has expired. It attempts to "support" the body with stimulants, suppress the symptoms in various ways, and increase the body's "resistance" by heavy feeding. Now, as a matter of fact, no disease ever lasts nearly so long as it is supposed to, when cared for orthopathically. Measles lasts four to five days, scarlet fever three to four days, typhoid fever seven to eight, rarely fifteen days. Pneumonia quickly ends—often as early as the fifth day. And all this on a diametrically opposite plan of care.

No food is given to "increase resistance." No stimulants are administered to "sustain" the patient or to "sustain" the heart. No efforts are made to suppress or combat the symptoms. Under such a plan recoveries are more frequent, more rapid and uniform and more complete. Relapses are exceedingly rare, complications and sequelea seldom met with and the patient is better after than before he had the disease.

In what respect does disease differ from health? There is no sudden cessation of the "healthy action" and immediately subsequent establishment of "diseased action," or of an action the tendency of which is adverse to health. There is no reversal of the laws of life, no confusion of the vital forces, no assumption by the organs of the body, of functions or actions for which they were not designed and constituted. The organs of the body, have not (and cannot) taken on wrong action. They must obey the laws of their constitution, and so long as they have power to act at all, act correctly. The action of any part of the body in disease, is the same as its action in health. Its action may be impaired, but it is not changed.

Whether we have rapid breathing or slow breathing, it is still breathing. Whether heart action is slow or rapid, it is still heart action. Breathing and heart action are slow when we are lying down; they are rapid when we run. But neither of these represent wrong action. On the contrary we all recognize these as right actions. Why not in disease, also. Healthy action and sickly action are all vital action—ALL ONE. Health and disease are the same thing differing only in degree. We have previously learned how natural a thing *disease* is—how natural a thing is recovery.

The very same phenomena, the same actions, and the same powers as are natural to the body, and which when manifesting easily and smoothly constitute the state of *Health*, are the same powers and phenomena, these latter slightly modified, that are observed in *disease*. The state of disease implies no new or additional powers, no action or phenomena other than those that belong to the organism in *health*.

Health and *disease* are *relative states* of the living body. They are both, in the truest meaning of the term *natural* conditions of the living organism. Not being different *things*, but only variations and natural variations of one and the same thing, no successfull effort to set a precise boundry between health and disease is possible. The *normal* passes so gradually into the *abnormal* and the *abnormal* repasses so gradually back into the *normal* that is not possible to say where one begins and the other ends.

Disease is so like health that the powers concerned in it are themselves adequate to the cure of it. The living organism is a *unity*; and its vital powers are the same in *Health* and in *Disease*,—the same also in *Recovery*, which is *Health* regained by the operation of these powers.

The habitual tendency of all the vital operations is ever and always in the direction of the highest degree of health. This is the inherent *bent* or *propension* of all the vital powers and processes of the living organism. All the energies of the body are always directed toward health. This is equally as true of their actions in *disease* as in *health*. Disease action is not a mere haphazzard process, but serves a distinct and a useful purpose or end—the removal of offenses.

Acute disease is a temporary, an evanescent, state. It arises under those conditions, as before explained, when unusual defensive action is required if life is to be preserved. The occasion or cause of disease removed or corrected, so that it is no longer operative, the organism quickly subsides into its usual tranquil state. This is to say, as soon as the body, by means of the disease, has succeeded in freeing itself of danger, it returns to its normal state of ease and equilibrium.

In certain "diseases" there occur changes which, if permitted to remain, would endanger life. The organism possesses power to effect the removal and correction of these, and bring about a more or less completely natural condition in the parts. As an example notice the retrograde changes which occur in the absorption of the exuded serum in the lungs in pneumonia, and the restoration of normal circulation through the lungs. The limit of this condition is determined by the power of the body to remove it. The exudate is not self-limited.

If there is no necessity for a protracted disease—a prolonged renovating process—the vital forces can be driven into one only by care and treatment that produce such a necessity. If a cold is all that is required to cleanse the organism, a pneumonia, pleurisy, smallpox or measles, etc., will not be developed. Only such disease manifestations are developed as are needed. What is more, once these operations have thoroughly completed their work, the body cannot be driven again through the same train of symptoms until the foundation is again laid for them. Relapses can come only where there has been suppression.

In discussing the absurd notions entertained by Dr. Jacob Bigelow, of Boston, and others regarding what they termed self-limited disease, Trall declared, *The Hygienic System*:—

"The theory of disease which I advocate, and which, so far as I know, I was the first to entertain and advocate, disposes of self-limited diseases, and a hundred other vexed questions relating to the nature, forms, phenomena, and tendencies, of particular diseases, in few words. Disease being itself remedial effort, all diseases are limited, in degree or severity, to the ability of the living system to make the remedial effort more or less vigorously; and in duration, to the time required, under the circumstances, for the system to rid itself of the impurities (the *causes* of disease), and to repair, as well as may be, the damages which have been occasioned by the presence of the impurities and the vital struggle to expel them."

A disease is "self-limited," said Jennings, "not by anything peculiar to the morbid condition of the part or parts affected, but by the extent of the lesion in the injured parts, and the amount of recuperative energy that can be controlled by the parts for their recovery; just as the jobs of the mechanics are 'self-limited' by the quantity of work that is to be done in each job and the amount of force that can be appropriated for its accomplishment."—*Tree of Life*, p. 184.

Dr. Tilden declares: "That diseases are self-limited—that every definite or specific cause must have a definite or specific effect—there can be no question, and that there must be a limit to an effect is another fact. It is self-evident that every cause and every effect must be self-limited; it is really a platitude to make such a statement about anything pertaining to disease. If there is ever an excuse for a doubt to arise regarding the eternal fixity of this law of limitation, it must be in those diseases where there is a multiplicity of causes and some or all of them obscure, for it must not be forgotten that there is no such thing as a mono—or unitary—cause to be found in the whole field of medical nomenclature or nosology."—*Criticisms of the Practice of Medicine*, Vol. 2, p. 243.

These three quotations all agree in one thing—namely, that diseases are limited because their causes are limited. There are no limitless causes—there can be no limitless effects.

Jennings and Trall both agree that another factor enters to determine the limits of a disease—namely, that of the power of the body to throw off the cause and repair damages. Not only are the causes of disease limited but the powers of the body are also limited. The more power there is in reserve the more intense or vigorous will be the *symptoms of reaction* and the sooner will the curative work be accomplished.

The temporary duration of all acute disease actions may be said to be a rule of pathology. Coexisting with this is the fact that the intensity and degree of this action is, while it lasts, always within the limits of *safety* or, within the body's powers of endurance—for the reason that *the power of the disease is also the power of life.*

Where the powers of life are inadequate to the work of cure, or where the body's curative efforts are suppressed by treatment, death or chronic disease result. The acute process cannot be continued indefinitely. Accomodation and a subdued struggle against cause must occur, if death does not result before this can take place. Chronic disease is continuous because its cause is continuous—it is a protest against chronic provocation.

THE RATIONALE OF INFLAMMATION

Chapter VIII

IN a previous chapter we presented evidence that it is a definite property of all living things that repair takes place following injury and that the process of repair is accomplished almost wholly by an accentuation of the ordinary processes of life—nutrition, drainage, growth and maintenance. A very remarkable example of this fact is presented to us by the phenomenon of inflammation. We shall here glance briefly at this manifestation of life and note its protective purpose.

Until about thirty years ago the medical profession regarded inflammation as an evil and spent much time endeavoring to determine whether it was due to excess action or deficient action in the inflamed parts. Regardless of which theory they held, they all agreed that it should be suppressed and employed the same means with which to suppress it. In 1897 Prof. G. Bier presented his paper on inflammation as a constructive process after which the fact began slowly to be accepted theoretically, although it continues to be dismissed and ignored in practice, and every effort is still made to suppress it. But the beneficent office of inflammation has been proclaimed outside the field of medicine for over a hundred years.

Samuel Thompson, founder of the Physio-Medical School, who lived in the closing years of the Eighteenth Centry, apparently taught this fact. Certain it is that his followers of seventy-five years ago proclaimed it. Prof. Curtis, for instance, in his Medical Criticisms, (p. 176) says:—

"Before the present centry (the 19th), Samuel Thompson, of Alsted, New Hampshire, discovered *that law, the primitive fact,* and expressed it in the language that 'fever is a friend to the System and not an enemy; and should be aided, not opposed,' in its effort to remove disease or its causes. Such is his doctrine, also, of *irritation and inflammation.* But learned men do not love to look in the lower walks of society (Thompson was an uneducated farmer) for men who will unfold to them the Mysteries of Nature."

Curtis, (Medical Criticisms, p. 24), also quotes a Prof. Watson, of this same school, as saying:—

"It is by inflammation that wounds are closed, and broken bones repaired, and that foreign and hurtful bodies are carried out of the body safely. A cut finger, a deep saber wound, alike require inflammation to reunite the divided parts."

J. S. Thomas, M.D., in his work: "Physio-Medicalism," (1870), says:—

"No laceration of the flesh can be healed without the aid of that physiological operation termed inflammation, which together with fever they (the Allopaths) treat as 'disease.'" p. 162.

In his "Philosophy of Human Life," (1852), Dr. Jennings records a case of *"Inflammation of the eyes, with general inflammatory affection,"* in which his partner in practice became alarmed and insisted that medicines be used, saying: "You will lose your patient if you do not do something to purpose soon; the eyes are already gone past redemption." Dr. Jennings replied:—

"This is not a freak of nature**** There was an imperative necessity for just the series of developments in this case that have been and yet are to be made."

He explained also that "Inflammatory heat never rises high enough to do positive harm," and used to refer to a man who was laid up with any disease but particularly with an inflammatory disease as having been "Suddenly laid aside for repairing purposes." He regarded inflammation in any part of the body as a process of repair and strengthening. It was particularly, he thought, a means by which the body strengthened weakened parts and fortified all parts against irritation.

In explaining the *"Rational of inflammation,"* Dr. Trall said, *Hydropathic Encyclopedia,* 1851, Vol. 2, p. 108:—

"Inflammation, as well as fever, is the effort of the vital powers to protect the organism from injurious mechanical, chemical, or vital irritants, or to expel morbific materials. This is proved by the phenomena of a multitude of morbid conditions. When a part of the body becomes grangrenous or dead, the living parts, provided there is sufficient vitality remaining in them, immediately form a line of demarcation, and the dead portion is soon separated from the living; this process is called *sloughing*. When a chemical or mechanical body is imbedded in the flesh too firmly to be removed by absorption, as a bullett or a splinter, purulent matter is formed around it, and its further action, on the parts is partially or wholly prevented by inclosing it in an abscess. When a grain of calomel gets into the lacteal vessels, the mesentric glands, which may be regarded as organic inspection officers, receive an increased determination of blood, swell up, or inflame, and thus retard the contraband article, until it can be more or less modified or destroyed by the vital powers. When a structure is divided, as by an incised wound, coagulable lymph is poured into the wound, forming, as it were, a bed for the newly formed vessels to reunite the part—a process called *adhesive inflammation*. And when a portion of flesh is torn away by violence, or decomposed by corrosives, or burned out with fire, a covering of purulent matter is thrown over the exposed surface, beneath which granulations—a new growth of substances—gradually fills up the cavity."

Emmett Densmore in "*How Nature Cures*," (1892), p. 5, after describing the processes of healing a cut, a broken bone and of expelling a sliver that has become imbedded in the flesh, says:—

"These everyday occurrences are as familiar to the layman as to the physician; but the strange part of it is the fact that almost no one—layman or physicians—seems to understand *that these and like processes of nature are all the healing force there is*."

Again, (Page 7):—

"The feat of engineering performed by the ruling force of the organism in building a bone ring support around adjacent ends of a broken bone may very properly be defined as a *curative action* on the part of this ruling force. The inflammation and pain consequent upon the presence of a sliver or any foreign body in the flesh, the formation of pus, and the subsequent expulsion from the body of both the pus and the foreign body which caused it, are further expressions of curative action. It is one of the objects of this publication to adduce conclusive proofs that disease and all manifestations of disease are friendly efforts and curative actions made by the organism in its efforts to restore the condtions of health."

In his "*Vital Science*," (1899), pp. 280-281, Dr. Robert Walter says:—

"The living organism is hourly in process of repair and waste. Waste and repair are facts of Life which are always being carried forward in the animal economy, at least. And this is a fact of physiology,—a process of health. But extraordinary processes of repair may also be necessary at times, and these are often painful, laborious, and exhaustive. They cannot be called healthful. They are pathological processes, and, therefore, diseases. They are abnormal in answer to abnormal conditions, but they are curative all the same. In the emergencies of life, if a wound is suffered, Nature at once begins a process of repair. At first it is naturally a process of resistance to further injury. It is called irritation, and soon becomes inflammation, which is the immediate process of healing. Then follows, in many cases, a process of purification. The parts are liquified in order to expulsion; and this is called suppuration. By and by granulation appears; and this is the ultimate process of healing. The process is a disease process, every step in it having an object in view. The symptoms are the symptoms of disease. The heat is increased because of increased activity in the nutritive processes. There is abnormal redness for the same reason that there is increase of heat. And there is swelling, due to the increase of nutritive material in the parts. Pain also is usually present because of pressure on sensitive nerves or from excessive labor. But the process is a process of healing, which is properly called inflammation, a real disease.

"****Suppuration, we have said, is a cleansing process. It seldom occurs except where contact with the external world has introduced foul matters which must be eliminated. A broken bone, for instance, if there is no external wound, seldom suppurates. Never does so unless the blood is very foul and itself introduces impurities into the wound. Nor does fever, any more than inflammation, ever proceed to destructive processes except because of exceeding foulness within."

I have, in the above quotations, only touched the high spots of the past. I need hardly add that all nature cure or hygienic or orthopathic as well as all hydropathic and physio-medical practitioners have regarded inflammation as a curative process and many of them have acted upon this. In short, holding that disease and every manifestation of disease is a beneficient effort to restore health, they have from the start regarded inflammation in the same light. As before stated, this fact has now found its way into medical theory, although it is ignored in medical practice. For instance, Lipshutz, a standard medical author, says:—

"Inflammation is a manifestation of the effort made by a given organism to rid itself of, or render inert, certain obnoxious irritants arising from within or introduced from without."

This definition does not differ from that given by Dr. Trall seventy-five years ago at which time the medical profession scoffed at the idea and called all who then believed such "nonsense" quacks, charlatans, and other such pleasing terms. Calling one's unnecessary opponents ugly names is not a monopoly of street urchins and theologians. Scientists and pretended scientists also indulge quite freely in this unproductive folly.

Before inflammation can arise there must be a cause or necessity for it, in the form of some agent or influence inimical to health and life, either of the whole body or of some part of it. Such causes may be chemical (poisons), thermic (burns and freezing), mechanical, (cuts, buises, particles of iron, wood, bone, etc.), electrical, or vital (parasites, etc.) and mental (as in hypnosis). The process of inflammation will differ in degree and character depending on the nature of the injurious agent, the intensity of its action, the character of the tissue affected, and the condition of the individual affected. Examples of the different reactions of different tissues to the same causes are common. A blow which would not effect the general surface of the body may easily produce serious results if it strikes the eye. Many substances that produce no perceptible irritation when applied to the skin produce intense irritation if dropped into the eye or taken into the mouth. Traumatic injuries produce less serious results, in healthy, robust individuals than in the weak and ailing. A cut that at one time heals rapidly without suppuration, may under different conditions of the system, heal slowly and form pus. Cuts and bruises heal more readily in the young than in the aged.

Dr. Jennings observed:—

"It is common for physicians to estimate the danger in inflammatory affections, by the degree of violence or force of inflammatory action, and hence they are solicitous to keep down the action to obviate the danger. Now admitting, for arguments sake, that the danger in these affections lies somewhere in the *symptoms*, it is still far from being true that the danger is to be measured by the degree of violence or strength of inflammatory action; for it is not uncommon to see pure inflammation of any and every part of the system, susceptible of such action, run very high, and yet terminate kindly by what physicians term resolution; while other cases, with little pure inflammatory action, often end in effusion of water, producing dropsies; in exudation of lymph, causing adhesions of contiguous surfaces; thickening of the lens, or other opacity of the eye, occasioning partial or complete blindness; in schirus, or induration, of gland; or in mortification. From these facts it is obvious that if deranged action in general produces the evils that follow such action, the evils that follow inflammatory action are not attributable to that action according to the amount of pure inflammation, or excessive action, but considerably, if not principally, to some other circumstances connected with it.

"These remarks are made in reference to spontaneous inflammations, or such as arise from remote causes, where an interval of time has intervened, sufficient to allow the animal economy an opportunity to accomodate parts that have been injured, to the unavoidable changes through which they must pass immediately by surgical operations, blows, and other injuries."—*Philosophy of Human Life*, p. 72.

Evils that follow inflammation are not to be attributed to the inflammation, but to the thing that occasioned the inflammation. The impairment in a lung that has been wounded is not to be attributed to the inflammation that healed it but to the thing that caused the wound. The evils that follow vaccination are not to be attributed to the inflammatory process by which the body resists and casts off the septic matter but to the pus that the physician infects the victim with.

The violence of the inflammation depends on the extent and nature of the injury or poison, the purity or foulness of the blood and lymph and the reactive powers of the individual. It is well known that wounds heal more quickly and with less inflammation in those of pure blood than in those of foul blood. There is also far less likelihood of suppuration in the individual of pure blood. Healing, ultimately, is more perfect and satisfactory. Broken bones, too heal more quickly in those of pure blood. It has long been known to surgeons that vegetarians recover from wounds and operations much more quickly and satisfactorily than meat eaters. Indians, living outdoors, their nude bodies exposed to the direct rays of the sun, recover from wounds with remarkable rapidity.

Many of the changes that occur in a tissue after injury may be watched under the microscope. If the thin membrane between the toes of a living frog be placed under the microscope and then injured by pricking it, or by putting some irritating substance upon it, changes begin, quickly, to occur in the circulation.

The arteries and veins dilate and the circulation is quickened. After a brief time the rate of circulation in the dilated vessels slows down until it is slower than normal. The web becomes swollen from the increased amount of fluid and blood corpuscles that are forced out of the blood vessels into the tissues in and around the injured section. The injured point becomes very sensitive, even painful and hot. This gives us the four cardinal symptoms of inflammation—redness, heat, pain and swelling—to which a fifth has been added—more or less complete loss of function. All of these symptoms are due to the unusual amount of blood and blood plasma in the tissues. The increased temperature is due to the increased amount of blood in the parts, the redness is due to the same cause, as is the swelling and pain—the pain being due chiefly to the increased pressure upon the sensory nerves.

The increased blood sent to the injured part serves as food to be used in repairing damages and serves also protective purposes in meeting and decomposing drugs or infectious matters.

The life of cells in a complex body depends upon the circulation of its blood and lymph. There exists a definite relationship between the blood supply of a part and the activity of its cells. The action of muscles calls for a greater supply of blood to these. The digestion of a meal calls for an increased amount of blood to the organs of digestion. Thinking demands more blood to the brain. The ripening of an ovum demands that more blood be sent to the ovaries. The repair of an injury calls for extra blood at the point of injury. Microscopic examination of an inflammed section shows all the cells in that area, even those forming the walls of the blood vessels, to be swollen, while their nuclei contain chromatin. There are changes in the nuclei which indicate that the cells are multiplying. There is every indication of a more active life within the section.

So greatly does the increased cellular activity necessary for repair depend upon an increased blood supply that new blood vessels frequently develop. In this way the capacity for nutrition is greatly increased. An excellent example of this is seen in the eye. The cornea of the eye contains no blood vessels. Its cells are nourished from the lymph which comes to it from the tissues at its outside. If the center of the cornea is injured, the cells of the blood vessels surrounding the cornea multiply and form new vessels. These appear as a pink fringe around the corneal periphery. When the process of repair is completed the new blood vessels disappear.

Under abnormal conditions, the usual activities of the injured cells are not sufficient to restore the integrity of the injured tissue. It is essential that the processes of cell-formation and repair be accelerated and all injurious substances removed, or else such changes must take place in the cells as will adapt it to new conditions of life. The blood vessels dilate and new vessels are formed thus carrying more nutritive material to the part. This excess nutritive material exudes into the tissues surrounding the point of injury as well as into the injured section. This serves several purposes.

It dilutes any injurious substance that may have found its way into the tissue. Drop a crystal of salt into your eye. It is highly irritating. Dilute such a crystal in a small amount of water and the solution produces little or no irritation. Drugs, bacterial exccretions, etc., are diluted and carried away from the point of injury. Or, the character of such poisons may be so changed as to render them less harmful or not harmful at all.

Not only is the nutritive material sent to the part in greater abundance than under normal conditions, but its character differs somewhat. Ordinarily, those substances upon which coagulation of the blood depends pass out through the walls of the blood vessels to a very slight extent. But in cases of injury the coagulable substance may be present in such amounts that the exudate easily clots. Calcification, granulation, fibrin formation, etc., result. These arc all defense measures.

The white blood corpuscles arc seen in the exudate in greater abundance than under normal circumstances. These cells are credited with wonderful powers of destroying germs, particles of dead matter, etc. Some of these are credited with great germ killing powers and have been named phagocytes. Others that are said to have but little phagocytic powers, and called by Metschnikoff, macrophages, are said to be chiefly responsible for the removal of non-bacterial substances. They are said to often contain dead cells, fragments of cells. Granules of pigment which get into the tissues when a hemorrhage into the tissues occurs, are said to be removed by this class of cells. They are described as often joining together, thus forming connected masses around a hair, or around a thread placed in a wound by a surgeon, in their efforts to remove these. They are also credited with power to destroy living cells when these arc too great in number in some part, and thus they tend to restore cell equilibrium.

This view of the nature and function of the white blood corpuscles is rejected by many. The late Dr. Thomas Powell contended that these are not true cells but that they represent decaying particles of protein matter. He claimed that their increase was the cause of disease and not a means of overcoming disease. He gave them the name pathogen—disease producer.

This view was accepted by the late Dr. Henry Lindlahr and many others. The future will have to decide which view is correct. The view that their increase is the cause of disease is not illogical. The view that their increase is a means of defense is not out of harmony with what we know of the body. It is a definite property of all living organisms that repair occurs following injury and most of the changes that take place in the work of repair are merely modifications and accentuations of the ordinary processes of normal life.

We have our point of injury now to a point of almost feverish activity. There is an excess of fluid pouring into it. The cells are dilated and multiplying. Blood vessels are also dilated and, perhaps, multiplied. The cells in the injured area are actively engaged in repairing damages. This feverish activity continues until the injury is repaired, or so long as the cause producing the injury operates, after which it gradually returns to normal. Then a reverse process begins.

The excess of fluid is removed by increasing the outflow until this exceeds the inflow. The excess of cells are removed. Part of them are removed with the fluid. Others undergo solution while others are claimed to be devoured by the other cells, particularly, by the white corpuscles. The blood vessels return to their normal size, the newly formed vessels atrophy and disappear in the same manner as the excess cells. The exudate is absorbed, the swelling goes down, pain ceases, the color becomes normal and function returns to its normal standard.

When the changes which an injured part undergoes are closely analyzed they are seen to be purposeful. They all serve definite ends and these ends are all beneficient. They are each and every one, without exception, designed to restore the integrity of the living organism and protect it from further injury. What has happened?

A broken bone has been repaired; or a cut has been healed; or a foreign body has been removed from the flesh; or toxins have been diluted, altered and cast out; the threatened danger to the life of the organism or its part has been overcome. This is the work of inflammation. Truly, as Jennings said, there is "order in disorder" in the workings of nature even in the most violent stages of disease. As Jennings remarked of a case of inflammation:—

"This is not a freak of nature. She does not wantonly turn aside from the natural and habitual course of action, and throw her complex machinery into disorder, and give it suicidal motion and tendency. There was an imperative necessity for just the series of developments in this case that have been and are yet to be made."—*Philosophy of Human Life*, pp. 162-163.

He also remarked:—

"Inflammatory heat never rises high enough to do positive harm. (He is here combatting the suggestion that cold water be applied to the inflammed area.—author). It is not the *cause* of the distress or any other accompanying symptom, but a concomitant effect (and an actual necessity to the rapid work of repair that is going on.—author.) with them of a common occasion, which will remove when the occasion removes."—*Philosophy of Human Life*, p. 167.

A mere brief notice of a few examples of the work accomplished by inflammation must suffice at this place as other chapters of this work are replete with such examples. A sliver becomes imbedded in the flesh and is not removed. Inflammation sets up at this point. The tissues around it are liquified and formed into pus. The fester thus formed bursts and the pus runs out carrying the sliver along with it. The place is then healed and forgotten. By inflammation a bruise, as from a blow, a cut, a burn, etc., is repaired and healed. Any irritating substance, as mustard, Spanish fly (Cantharis), and other drugs, when applied to the surface of the body, or when taken internally are met and overcome by inflammation. And bites, bee stings, the bite of insects, snakes, and other poisonous animals, and the poisons of plants are all met and overcome by inflammation.

Cyanide of potassium, an excellent Allopathic *remedy*, if applied "*locally causes* inflammation of the skin with an exzematous eruption, and if applied in quantity to an abraded surface will produce fatal effects." The inflammation and eruption, which is also a form of inflammation, are simply means of expelling the poison.

Inflammation follows the forcible infection of a person by what is called vaccine. Vaccine is pus and is septic. Syphilitic infection takes place in the same manner. Septic matter comes in contact with an abraded surface and infection follows. In both cases, inflammation with ulceration follow, as a means of preventing the entrance of the septic matter into the general circulation and as a means of expelling it from the system. In inflammation, there is a large increase of blood to the affected part. This overcomes osmosis and prevents absorption.

Similar to the exzematous eruption produced by cyanide are the secondary eruptions—vaccina and secondary syphilis—often following vaccination and so-called syphilitic infection. These eruptions serve the same eliminative and protective purposes.

The primary stage of syphilis, like that of vaccination, consists of an initial ulcer which forms at the point of infection. The ulcer is usually single, as in vaccination, and is hard at its base. It is accompanied by enlargement and enduration (hardening) of the near-by lymph glands. It is simply an enduration following local irritation and infection. The irritation produces inflammation which is the same as any other inflammation and is of a defensive character. It means that more material is carried to the point of inflammation than can be used or carried away by the veins. This prevents absorption and dilutes the infection. The thickening and hardening overcome *osmosis*. Just as in a pus sac, or abscess, the wall of which is thick and endurated, the escape of pus into the surrounding tissue is prevented, so, in the so-called syphilitic ulcer, or chancre, the hardening at its base prevents absorption of the septic matter into the system. Upon this point Dr. Tilden has the following to say:—

"Nature is always busy fortifying against invasion, and when a mucous surface cannot be healed it is utilized as an *exit for waste products*. In thus utilizing a broken surface two important objects are attained: First, it should be understood that a broken surface is a menace to life so long as the parts are raw, for absorption takes place very readily in a fresh wound; hence, to obviate this danger and furnish healing material, there is set up at once a rushing to the wound of a lot of plastic material, which soon covers and protects the surface. Through this provision of nature's a raw surface is soon fortified against the possibility of a foreign substance coming immediately in contact with it; this coating also protects from the air, and prevents absorption, even if the wound does not heal. The rushing forward of the plastic material for primary protection will end in developing a secondary protection if the parts refuse to heal, which is the second object referred to above. It consists of a gradual thickening and hardening of the tissues, because more material is being taken into the tissues of the injured parts than is utilized, and it is not carried back by the return circulation, which means that there is a greater quantity of material taken to such a surface than can be used in healing, and it is either thrown out—exuded—excreted—or retained in the tissues; this causes accumulation—a thickening and hardening of the edges of the wound—the material that is taken there primarily for healing is used secondarily for fortifying and preventing the entrance of unfriendly and detrimental material. Please understand that nature, in this operation, is *destroying the possibility of molecular attraction—overcoming the law of osmosis.*

"Nature is never engaged in a senseless and purposeless work of any kind. I do not infer that there is a ratiocinative guidance; simply the adjusting of needs to ends, the laws for which are resident and imminent in the needs. This no one should know or recognize sooner than the physician; hence, he whose business it is to watch nature in her operations should know that the thickening and hardening at any point of inflammation is for a purpose, and that purpose is to overcome the carrying out of the laws of osmosis and molecular attraction, which, under normal conditions is necessary for the ready exchange of fluids in the body. When a raw surface is made to come in contact with environments containing materials that will be injurious to the body if they gain entrance, nature begins at once to destroy the possibility of exchange, and her plan is to build an indurated wall about the wound. And what does induration mean? It means that more material is taken in than is taken out; it means that the pressure from within is greater than from without; and such a thing as germ absorption can not take place in a fortified surface, the profession's opinion to the contrary notwithstanding. It should not be forgotten that nature is constantly fortifying against invasion. Sometimes she outreaches herself, and fortifies so extensively that her fortifications degenerate, because the induration becomes so solid that the capillary arteries fail to carry enough oxygen to the interior of her breastworks to keep them alive; hence degeneration takes place, and unless drainage is established septic infection will quickly end the life of the victim.

"I have gone into this explanation rather extensively to show that it is contrary to all the laws governing bodily development for germs to enter our bodies when and where they please. If the profession's belief regarding germs and their absorption were true the world would be depopulated.

"Think for a moment of a pus sac. The walls are thick and indurated. Blood and building material are taken to, in and through this fortification, but nothing is allowed to cross the dead line from the pus sac to the tissues outside or in the body. The only way the pus can get into the body is for the sac to be broken.

"I want to go on record as declaring that germs can not cross any of nature's fortifications unless the hand of man has broken her safeguards. I want to say that it is absurd, unscientific, and positively in opposition to biological as well as pathological science, to say that the 'tonsils and lymphatic tissues act as portals of entry for micro-organisms.'"

The enlargement of the lymph glands in all infections—syphilitic, vaccinal, or from a corpse or beef,—and from insect bites, and in colds, etc., is a means of arresting and destroying toxins of an organic nature that find their way into the lymph. It is a defensive measure.

In an abscess, in appendicitis and similar internal conditions, inflammation serves the same defensive and reparative purposes as when it is developed in the superficial structures of the body. It is never anything to combat. IT IS THE COMBAT.

Nature always localizes inflammation wherever possible and this is usually possible. If resistance is low, if the blood is foul, or if meddlesome methods of treatment are resorted to, the inflammation may spread. It is seldom that the primary cause of inflammation is sufficient to cause more than a local inflammation. Even in so-called syphilitic infection, the primary ulcer is usually the end of the trouble.

Inflammation is roughly divided into acute and chronic. If the changes take place rapidly the inflammation is said to be acute. Its intensity will depend on the amount and character of the injury or the concentration and virulence of the irritant or poison, the length of time through which it acts and the condition or susceptibility of the individual. The stronger the irritant and the greater the reactive powers of the individual the more apparent will be the reaction. The healthier the individual, however, the less will be the time required to overcome the irritation or repair the injury.

Chronic inflammation is met with more often in old age rather than in the young; and is seen more often in the weak than in the strong. It is more complex than acute inflammation and presents more variations in single conditions. Its chronicity may be due to a number of conditions, such as the persistence of cause, (chronic disease is due to chronic provocation), imperfect healing, due to a depraved condition of the system, etc.

An example given by Dr. Tilden makes clear the relation of the systemic condition to healing:—

"Mothers of such children (sickly children) have no resistance, or very little, and their systems are kept at the saturation point—full of by-products seeking every opportunity for *vicarious excretion*. The following facts are worthy of the reader's most careful attention: If these mothers suffer laceration at childbirth, an accident they can't well avoid, because the children are overweight, and their systemic perversion renders their tissues unyielding, the tear will not heal. Instead of closing up or healing over, the raw surface drops down into a low grade granular inflammation, which is called catarrh, or catarrhal inflammation.

"When a physician examines a case of this kind a few months after childbirth he will find a tear, not necesarily large; the edges will be thick and granular, and for some distance back, in what was once normal tissue, there is infiltration, causing thickening and induration; the parts are several times larger than normal, and the catarrhal inflammation extends through the neck into the womb. This desease is what is called endocervicitis and metritis (inflammation of the lining membrane of the neck and body of the womb). Why did the tear in the neck and the bruise in the uterus not heal? This is exactly what should and would have taken place if the woman had been normal, but she was not normal; her body was charged with waste products, so that the plastic material thrown out for healing these wounds was of such a low grade, and the tissues were so devitalized, that healing could not take place. When such a state of the fluids and solids as this obtains healing is very slow, if it takes place at all, and when it does not all such raw, denuded surfaces are utilized as *portals of exit*, rather than portals of entry. This is contrary to current and general professional opinion."

A chronic inflammation may be nothing more than an almost continuous series of acute inflammations. Repair, in such cases, is continuously less perfect.

Where the irritant is mild, or if it is powerful but introduced in minute quantities over a long period of time, much connective tissue is formed at the site of irritation. This is seen in cirrhosis of the liver, harnening (sclerois) of the arteries and in the so-called "replacement" fibrosis of nerve degeneration. In such cases, it appears that the poison is incompatible with the life of the higher cells so that these are destroyed and their places filled by tissue of lower grade but more resistant qualities.

Different types of inflammation are described by their most prominent features, as follows:—

CATARRHAL or MUCOUS INLAMMATION or catarrh occurs on mucous surfaces in all parts of the body that are lined with this membrane, as in bronchitis, coryza, diarrhea, gastritis, etc. Accompanying inflammation of this type there is increased secretion of mucous of an altered character.

FIBRINOUS (Croupous) INFLAMMATION develops particularly on the serous surfaces of the body. It is seen in peritonitis and sometimes in the substance of tissues. In the corium (of the skin) for instance, in severe erysipelas. It sometimes occurs in the larnyx and bronchi and in such acute diseases as smallpox, typhoid, pyemia and in the lung in pneumonia. This form is characterized by a thick deposit of fibrin on the inflammed part.

DIPHTHERIC INFLAMMATION is a more severe form of the preceding variety. In addition to the fibrinous deposit there is necrosis (death) of the mucous membrane. This is seen in diphtheria and in typhoid.

SEROUS INFLAMMATION is inflammation of the serous membranes of the body and is marked by an effusion of serous fluid into the tissues and cavities, as in inflammation of the joints, or of the pleura or peritoneum.

PURULENT INFLAMMATION is inflammation accompanied with the formation of pus. It is seen in septic infections, as in vaccination; while, in foul conditions of the system, simple inflammations anywhere may become purulent.

The above forms of inflammation may be combined as *seropurulent, mucopurulent, serofibrinous* inflammations, etc.

PARCENCHYMATOUS INFLAMMATION is the term applied to inflammation of the functioning cells of an organ as in *parenchymatous nephritis*. This is accompanied with more or less destruction of the active cells of the organ.

INTERSTITIAL INFLAMMATION is the term employed to designate inflammation of the supporting framework of the inflammed organ, as in interstitial nephritis. Repeated "attacks" of this kind result in an overgrowth of connective tissue in an organ resulting in *cirrhosis, fibrosis,* or *induration*.

It is well to note that the cardinal symptoms of inflammation and the essential changes and activites which occur in the blood vessels and tissues involved are the same in all these varieties of inflammation. The process and purpose of inflammation is the same in each variety. The essential nature of inflammation remains unchanged. The distinguishing characteristics of the different varieties are largely those of degree and of the structures involved. Thus, *mucous inflammation* is inflammation in a mucous membrane while *serous inflammation* is inflammation of a serous membrane. The structure involved determines the type of exudate. Likewise the degree of the inflammation and the condition of the system determine the differences in the exudate. *Diphtheric inflammation* is simply a greater degree of *fibrious inflammation*. The necrosis is also due to the severity of the condition. The character and extent of the cause also aids in determining the type. *Purulent inflammation* is a breaking down of tissue for the removal of infectious matter or foreign bodies. INFLAMMATION IN WHATEVER PART OF THE BODY IT IS LOCATED AND WHATEVER ITS CAUSE, IS ESSENTIALLY A UNIT.

In simple cases of inflammation where there is no breaking down of tissue, the exudate is absorbed and the tissue is left apparently as it was with, perhaps, a deposit of pigment or a slight growth of new connective tissue or a thickening of the skin. Where there has been tissue destruction and its removal, as in an abscess, the gap is filled with granulation tissue. The surplus exudate in such cases is discharged as pus. A little more detail about suppurative and septic inflammatory processes is desirable.

Dr. Walter brought to our attention, in a former quotation, that inflammation does not proceed to a destructive stage unless foul matter has obtained entrance into the inflammed section either from without or from the blood. Dr. Tilden explained that in cases of foulness of the system nature utilizes the wound or suppurating process as a "portal of exit" or, to use the words of Dr. Lindlahr, "discharges and ulcers act as fontanels to the system." That this is so is unintentionally corroborated by orthodox testimony. (See chapter on "Crisis.")

The repair of injury requires extra nutrition. Nature sends great quantites of this to the injured section. In a wound, the exposed surface is sealed up by the coagulation of the exudate and healing proceeds. But where the waste is retained, that is where drainage is not perfect, microbic fermentaiton, as distinguished from enzymic fermentation, occurs. This changes the chemistry of the exudate and decomposition or pus formation supplants healing.

Germs must be pent up in the wound or abscess before they can set up a morbid process. Nature is not afraid of dust or germs or air. Dr. Tilden rightly says:—

"The whole question of wound infection hinges on drainage. Any wound that drains well may be smeared with the most virulent septic poison without infection. The infecting agent must be rubbed into the wound so that it will be pushed into, or below, the granular surface. The infecting material must find a lodgment so secure that the flushing—enzymic—serums cannot dissolve and wash away.

"Injuries in canals, tubes, ducts and air-passages will heal normally if drainage is not obstructed; but when obstructed, the usual conservative measures of nature may further obstruct, and death may result from a rational therapeutic measure mechanically obstructed in its execution."

Again:—

"The cell-building elements cover the cut or mutilated surface, and crowd the border so much that there is a heavy discharge through the drain, if the wound has been properly dressed or has been left open. Where drainage is unobstructed, the healing behind the barrage of nutritive material thrown out moves along without a halt. The proportion of enzymes and nutritive material furnished by a healthy, not overfed, wounded individual insures rapid renewal of tissue. If obstruction takes place, microbic fermentation is set up in the pent-up surplus. This is a conservative process; for it thins the discharge, irritates the wound, and causes an extra amount of serum to be exuded. The purpose is to melt down any incrustations and new-made tissue that is obstructing drainage."

Serious trouble may occur if this fails. Microbic fermentation gains the mastery over enzymic fermentation, sepsis is evolved and, unless walled off, may cause death.

If inflammation is due to a virulent irritant which is incompatible with the life and integrity of the tissues, these undergo retrograde charges, cloudy swelling, fatty degeneration, and complete necrosis, finally forming, in union with the decomposed serum, blood cells, etc., pus which breaks through on a nearby surface and runs out, or is walled off as in an abscess.

The irritation of an open wound caused by the air acts to accelerate the flow of nutritive material to the wound. The air dries up and coagulates the discharge of serum and thus it is sealed up so that healing can go on behind the protection. The dry covering "acts as a stay or fixation expediency, to secure the necessary quiet for healing." If the wound is too closely sealed in and danger of infection threatens, itching sets in causing rubbing and scratching thus breaking enough of the covering to permit the washing out or escape of the pent-up pus and waste matter.

A wound that is not thoroughly cleaned and that is bandaged up so that drainage is imperfect, suppurates. Decomposition and infection end repair and cause sloughing. Sloughing re-establishes drainage and the work of healing is resumed. If sloughing does not occur so that drainage is not established and the normal reciprocal balance between the organized ferments (germs) and unorganized ferments (enzymes) is not established, sepsis is generated and this may end in death. One of the greatest surgeons of all time, Sir Wm. Arbuthnot Lane, of London, declared, that where drainage is perfect there is no death. As Dr. Tilden remarks:—

"Every conservative provision of nature can be, and sometimes is, overcome; but this does not alter the fact that nature places a special guard over each one of the body's vital functions, the normal action of each being necessary to total health of the body, and that each gaurd must be vanquished before the function over which it presides can be deranged or checked."

If the surfaces of a wound are brought together and held there healing must be completed sooner than if nature must build up a bridge of tissue to span the gap. But bringing these edges together interferes more or less with drainage and if means for drainage is not supplied may result seriously. Again, healing is interfered with by the causes that lead to the inflammation. Inflammation is slight when the wound is in a state of health. Dr. Tilden says of the exudate in inflammation:—

"There can be no rest or standing still; the exudates must be execreted, thrown out, or re-absorbed. To fit these exudates for absorption, they must be treated with enzymes, in order to fit them to re-enter the circulation. If there is enervation and lack of enzymes, then it will be 'up to' bacterial fermentation to prepare the exudate for expulsion from the body. If there is no break in continuity—if there is no open wound—then the bacterially treated exudate must be absorbed into the general circulation, causing infection; or the infection will be corralled by walling in the devitalized territory and lining the inclosure with an impervious pyrogenic membrane.

The pus that forms is retained—not allowed to escape into the general circulation; for, if it should, it would cause pyemia. If the body's natural resistance is too low to fortify it in this way—if it cannot localize and immunize the infecting material—then general infection takes place and the victim dies of septicemia."

It is not correct to limit the disposal of pus in a closed inflammation to absorption or abscess formation. The process of inflammation and suppuration more often extends, along lines of least resistance, through neighboring healthy tissue, until the abscess points at some surface. The pointing thins and liquifies the overlying tissues which finally ruptures allowing a spontaneous evacuation of the abscess to occur. Every one has seen this in boils or furuncules. However, in these liquification is only partial. The dead tissue sloughs *en masse*, as the "core" of the boil. Of internal exudates Dr. Tilden explains:—

"If the point of irritation is the pleura, the exudate may accumulate, and, from lack of bacterial influence, the fluid is neither digested and absorbed, nor decomposed and converted into an abscess of the pleura, nor absorbed, creating septic fever and death; but remains a bland, innoxious fluid in the pleura."

Tissues which have been killed by injury or by inflammatory processes and inflammatory exudations are no longer parts of the body. They are foreign substances and act as such. They act like foreign bodies thrust into the tissues from without. They cause inflammation in their neighborhood. The fact that they once belonged to the body makes no difference to the tissues they affect. In such cases there is in addition to the ordinary phenomena of a simple inflammation, processes the object of which is the removal of the foreign substance.

If a foreign substance is soluble or destructible these are attacked and dissolved and carried out of the system. If the substance is not soluble as, for instance, necrosed bone, compact hemorrhagic patches, infarcts, coagulated or condensed exudations, necrotic cheesy masses, leaden bullets, ivory pegs, ligatures, drainage tubes, etc., the process is a bit different. Inflammation and infiltration are followed by the formation of granulation tissue and later fibrous tissue around the foreign body. If it cannot be absorbed or sent out by suppuration it becomes encapsulated.

Pieces of dead flesh and bone are sure, sooner or later, to be dissolved and carried away. In every case the process of absorption and encapsulation is carried out with the purpose of either ridding the body of a substance that is foreign and useless to it and, perhaps, also harmful; or of encasing it and rendering it harmless. Every movement of the body in the highest stages of health and in the lowest depths of disease is intended to preserve the vital integrity.

Inflammation is said to end in (1) regeneration or resolution; (2) due to destruction and infection (a) repair or scar tissue, (b) suppuration, (c) ulceration, (d) abscess, (e) extentive necrosis or gangrene.

RESOLUTION:—Pneumonia and pleurisy and arthritis each offer excellent examples of this. In each of these there are exudation products to be removed and disposed of. In the former the exudate is in the lungs and pleural cavity. In the latter, in the joint cavity. The exudate or serum is rapidly absorbed and removed. In the so-called second or *hepatization* stage of pneumonia, the exudate in the lungs becomes more or less solidified, forming a liver-like consistency. In the so-called third stage, or that of *Resolution*, the exuadte normally undergoes liquification and absorption. This is the return to health. If the body is unable, due to weakness or suppression, to liquify and absorb the exudate this undergoes destructive changes, producing chronic pneumonia, gangrene, abscess, or death.

REPAIR BY SCAR TISSUE is healing by *second intention or union by granulation* and occurs when there is an abscess or wound the edges of which are far apart and there is a large amount of exudate present.

SUPPURATION occurs when there are poisons as in vaccination, or an inert body as a sliver, to be removed, or when drainage is blocked so that the exudate becomes foul, or, when the blood is foul as when gastro-intestinal putrefaction and fermentation fill the blood with putrescence. Ulceration is simply a suppurating process upon a free surface.

AN ABSCESS occurs when the inflammatory area is walled off. It is a circumscribed cavity containing pus. Suppuration begins at the center of irritant action and extends to the surrounding uninvolved tissues. The extension follows the line of least resistance, until the abscess *points* ("comes to a head") at some surface. The overlying tissue is thinned and liquified and spontaneous evacuation of the abscess occurs. The fibroblastic layer forming its walls are now supplied with blood vessels, the walls are converted into granulation tissue, and, beginning at the bottom, this granulation tissue fills up the cavity. This is healing.

GANGRENE is the death of a tissue followed by its putrefaction while it is yet in the body. NECROSIS is the same process confined to the bones.

The condition is considered to be due to (1) such great devitalization of the cells that they are unable to assimilate nutriment; and (2) circulatory impairment or blockage so that the tissues do not receive sufficient nutriment. One or both of these conditions may result in *gangrene or necrosis.* Various kinds of gangrene are named, depending on the conditions causing it. These distinctions are unimportant. *Dry gangrene* occurs where the arteries become blocked but the veins remain open so that the tissues are drained. *Moist gangrene* occurs where both arteries and veins are blocked. In the first the tissues become dry, hard and shriveled. Sepsis is absent. A line of demarcation or ulceration forms at the expense of the dead tissue. It does not spread. In the second the parts are purple, or greenish and become covered with blisters. The adjacent tissues undergo an inflammatory reaction. Symptoms of toxemia with fever are present. A line of demarcation or ulceration forms at the expense of the living tissue.

We get sick and we either live or die. The doctors of all schools can help us die. But the doctors of no school can help us live. The sick man, woman or child fights a lone battle in disease and succeeds or fails without aid, but usually with much interference.

The most trying ordeal through which the author ever passed was that of standing by the bedside of a dying baby while listening to the distracted mother implore him to save her child. No doctor can save a patient. The patient is able to save himself or he is not. If he is not he dies. Only in rare cases where surgery may remove a deadly secondary cause, is outside effort of aid. There may even be doubts about this kind of aid.

Every disease is a curative process, but not all diseases are devoid of danger. One of the things inflammation does is to cripple or suspend the function of the inflammed parts. The process is protective, curative, first, last and all the time, but its location is often an element of grave danger. Inflammation of the brain or spinal cord may involve certain vital centers to such an extent that some vital function is suspended. The respiratory center may be involved and respiration supended. Death follows. The cardiac center may be involved and heart action suspended. Death results. A bee sting on the eye lid closes the eye but is of no serious consequence. In a day or two the inflammation is gone and the eye open. A bee sting on the glottis would quickly close the air passage, with no more inflammation than that which the sting causes on the eye lid, and the victim would die of suffocation. Not the nature and extent of the inflammation, but its location is the measure of its gravity. Bees do not sting the glottis but worse things than a bee sting may happen to it.

Inflammation of the heart may become so great that heart action ceases. Inflammation of the lungs may become so great that respiraiton ceases, or, the lungs may fill up with exudate. In diphtheria or membraneous croup, the false membrane may extend down into the bronchial tube and cut off breathing. Inflammation of the kidneys may become so great as to suspend the function of these and death from uremic poisoning result. In all this the inflammation is a curative process but accidentally located in a place that makes it a potential danger to life.

Inflammation must develop where it is needed—whether in the hand or eyes, the lungs or brain, the heart or kidneys. It must become as great as the necessities of the case demand. Nature always tries to localize inflammation. She usually succeeds. Failure is due to feeding and drugging usually. All feeding should be stopped at the outset of any trouble. A few days of feeding when the trouble is only mild may be enough to cause death. Life is too precious to throw away for a few unwanted, unneeded and unenjoyed meals.

There is always danger in inflammation of the lungs of aged persons whose lungs are perhaps greatly weakened, or are very faulty in spots. This is the reason absolute rest and quiet are so essential in pneumonia. Getting out of bed too soon may result in death. There is also danger in these people when inflammation develops in any of the vital organs that may be structurally unsound. Even in young people there may be unsound organs that may break under the strain.

THE RATIONALE OF FEVER

Chapter IX

IN his now famous lecture on "The True Healing Art," delivered in the Smithsonian Institute in Feb. 1862, Dr. Trall declared:—

"Fever has no seat; fever is an action. Do not forget the primary question, what is disease? Fever is one form of disease; and as disease is a process of purification, fever must be one of the methods in which the system relieves itself of morbid matter.

"How much longer will medical men expend brain and labor, and waste pen, ink, and paper, in looking for a *thing which is no thing* at all, and in trying to find a seat for a disease which has no localized existence."

The idea here expressed, that fever is but a part of the general process of purification and reconstruction that is disease, and that fever is salubrious or beneficial, has been held by Orthopaths, Hydropaths and Naturopaths as well as by the Physio-medicalists from their origin. The idea was ridiculed by the "regular" profession, but, as will be shown later, they are now begining to accept this view. Hippocrates, indeed, is declared to have said: "give me fever and I can cure any disease," but Hippocrates cannot be classed as a regular. He was a cross between a modern hydropath, and a physio-medicalist.

The physio-medicalists' idea of fever may be seen from the following quotation from J. S. Thomas, M.D. (Physio-medicalism, p. 145):—

"We contend now from what we have said that *disease is a condition that diminishes the energy of that power which sustains and preserves* life, and that *irritation, inflammation, and fever* are simply manifestations of the vital power to restore lost action."

Again:—

"These vital actions (the actions of disease) are all friends to the patient, and should be aided, not subdued. *The lost function of the surface before an ague* (chill) cannot be *restored without fever*, and no laceration of the flesh can be healed without the aid of that physiological operation termed inflammation, which together with fever, they (the Allopaths and Homeopaths) treat as 'disease.'"

Dr. Joel Shew in *The Hydropathic Family Physician*, (1854) declares: (pp. 45-46):—

"Whatever may be true in regard to the nature and general tendency of fever, it is to be remarked that patients, when properly treated, and not injured by harsh and injudicious measures, are often found better after an attack. This happens even after certain fevers which have had their origin in malaria, or some other poisons."

It has been said that "Inflammation is a local fever and fever is a general inflammation." If by this is meant, that they are both parts of the same healing process we do not object. But a general inflammation could not exist because of lack of sufficient blood in the body to produce it. Fever is rather a general systemic reaction where irritation and inflammation are great and affect the internal organs to some extent.

It is the rule that fevers are preceded by a chill. The chill is due to the withdrawal of the blood from the surface of the body and the chill causes a suspension of skin radiation, and fever follows due to the suspension of skin radiation. Fever not only enables the cells on the interior of the body to accelerate their activities but also assures the warmth of the surface of the body which would otherwise remain cold.

The cells in all the tissues and fluids affected in fevers and inflammation are enlarged. There is always an increased exudation of fluid from the blood in the affected parts resulting in increased nutrition and more rapid growth. This elevation in body heat in inflammations and fevers is constant and it is impossible for these to occur without a temporary increase in the amount of living matter in the affected areas. The cells always experience increased nutrition.

Perhaps we can best get a picture of the rationale of fever by observing the movements of an amoeba under varying conditions of temperature. Autonomous as this single celled creature may seem, it is unable, without outside influence, to raise its functions above the physiological standard, or, on the other hand, to check or suppress them. If the temperature, in which it exists is raised a few degrees its movements, previously perhaps slow and languid, immediately become more lively—the vital activity of the cell is increased. *An increase in temperature is necessary to an increase of vital activity.*

A decrease in temperature has the opposite effect. If the liquid in which the amoeba exists, is gradually cooled the cell gradually ceases its movements and activities and becomes, finally, a mere inert globule which is capable of resuming its former activities only after its temperature is raised. *Reduction of temperature reduces cellular activity.*

If the temperature is raised too high the movements of the cell gradually cease. At a certain degree of warmth the cell becomes still and stiff and can resume its actions only after its temperature has been allowed to fall. *Excess warmth stops cell activity.*

We can raise the temperature of the amoeba as high as we like for we supply the heat from the outside. It is not a product of the cells own activity. In the body, in fever, this is not so. The heat is the result of the body's own activity and if it goes beyond a certain point cell activity is automatically lowered and heat production lessened. *There is then, an automatic check to the height fever may rise.*

One of the chief functions of the skin is to regulate body temperature. Heat is radiated through the skin, chiefly through sweating. The body is cooled by evaporation of perspiration. Any fluid, in evaporating, takes up heat. The sweat, in evaporating extracts heat from the body.

By regulating the amount of blood that reaches the skin the escape of heat from the body is controlled. The more blood there is in the skin the more heat there is radiated from the body. If the body is chilled the blood vessels in the skin contract. This forces the blood away from the surface into the interior of the body and conserves its heat. When the body is hot, its surface vessels dilate. This allows larger quantities of blood to reach the skin and dissipates more of its heat.

Two sets of nerves are concerned in the regulation of heat conservation and heat radiation. The vasomotor which control the size of the blood vessels and thus control the blood supply, and the secretor which stimulate the activities of the gland cells. Generally an increased blood flow and accelerated glandular action exist together. It sometimes happens in cases of shock or in nervous individuals that a profuse clammy perspiration occurs with a decrease in the blood supply. The excretion of sweat is regulated by the nervous system. The sweat centers, located in the medulla and spinal cord are aroused into action by exercise, changes in external temperature, mental emotions, many drugs and often by an increase in the temperature of the blood circulating in the medulla and cord.

The body not only regulates the radiation of heat but also regulates the production and distribution of heat. It often happens in people of low vitality, or in shock that the body's ability to produce or conserve its heat is reduced so that its temperature is below normal. In most stages of acute disease the temperature is above normal and the patient is said to have fever. *Fever is simply a few degrees more of the ordinary temperature of the body.*

In fever there is usually a greater production of heat than under the usual conditions of life, but heat production is not nearly so great as in violent exercise. The reason for fever is not so much an increased production of heat, but a lessened radiation of heat. Skin radiation is suspended. Fever is not always accompanied with increased heat production.

Fever often synchronizes with impaired respiratory functions, as in pneumonia, and the introduction into the blood of far less oxygen than when normal and the subsequent formation and removal of less than the normal proportion of carbonic acid. Inflammation and fever do not necessarily depend on increased oxidation. Fever is not a process of "burning." It neither burns up the body nor the causes of disease. It is an essential part of an acute disease, however.

Slight fevers and inflammations do not necessarily result in permanent tissue changes. Many leave no traces behind them. There may be no degeneration of any tissue in the body, no structural change, no evidence left of the struggle. After a fever or inflammation the organism may be left precisely as it was before the struggle occurred; or, as is the case where suppression is not resorted to, the organism is renovated, cleansed and renewed.

Where damage to the body or parts of it follow fever it is the cause of, or, more properly, the occasion for, the fever or the suppressive measures employed, and not the fever itself, which works harm to the body, so that no good whatsoever is accomplished by suppressing the fever, as is the usual practice among all schools of "healing." The fever itself is an essential part of the acute process, is salutary and constructive in its office, and itself is never fatal or injurious. The presence of fever is both a sign of returning health and an evidence that the body still possesses sufficient vital vigor to put up a stiff fight against the foes of life.

The *crisis* or turn of a *fever* is usually characterized by a resumption of sweating, which had previously been suspended, and a consequent reduction of the temperature of the body. In fevers the skin is usually dry.

When there is infection in the intestine, for instance, as in typhoid fever, requiring that large quantities of blood be sent to the intestine, the blood is drawn away from the surface of the body, resulting in a chill. The "onset" of fevers is preceded by a chill. The chill serves the definite end of suspending surface radiation. During the chill, although the surface temperature of the body may be normal, the temperature of the interior of the body is above normal.

The withdrawal of blood from the surface of the body and its concentration in the interior unbalances the circulation and disutrbs blood pressure. Automatically, this increases the rapidity of the heart's action and this in turn increases respiration. Thus, as will be seen later, two other essentials of the work of cure are automatically cared for.

The height of the fever will be determined by:—1. The reactive power of the sick man or woman, and 2. The virulence and amount of the toxin against which the forces of life are pitted. Of these two factors, the reactive power of the sick person is the greater factor in raising the temperature. Young and vigorous individuals easily develop a high fever in response to minor causes, whereas, the old or feeble are often unable to develop fever in defense against the most virulent toxins. The fact that fever serves a definitely beneficial end has begun to percolate through the craniums of the Heteropathic professions. Even staid old Allopathy, or the "regular" or "scientific" school is beginning to recognize this fact.

Before giving any medical testimony on this point I desire to quote Dr. Shew, *Hydropathic Family Physician,* p. 51:—

"The danger in fevers is not in proportion to the heat and excitement present, as many suppose, but to the debility. The evidences of debility, are great rapidity and weakness of the pulse, as well as weakness of the body generally. If the pulse remains long as frequent as 140 or 150, there cannot be much ground for recovery. Recovery has been known to take place when the pulse has been as high as 160, although it must be admitted that such occurrences with adults are rare. Dr. Heberden knew a case of recovery from fever even after the pulse had been at 180. Facts of this kind should be known both for the encouragement of the patient and the physician."

Coming now to medical testimony, an European authority, F. A. Rizquez, declares (General Pathology):—

"Fever is a reaction of organic defense, and as such, it should be protected, rather than opposed. Generalized febrile infections are more dangerous when they develop themselves apyretically (without fever), as, for instance, pneumonia in old people, cholera, diphtheria, etc."

Schiller declared "a fever which does not kill, invigorates."

The Literary Digest, June 14, 1924, quotes Dr. Oliver Heath as saying in the *Lancet,* a leading British medical journal:—

"For many years a heightened temperature was regarded as evil in itself— very much as a heightened blood pressure quite usually is now—and in the treatment of febrile conditions the main line of attack was directed toward its reduction.

"Experience of anti-pyretic drugs led to some doubts as to the actual benefit to be expected from a mere lowering of temperature, and experimental work showed that in infectious conditions some degree was certainly beneficial; animals kept at fever heat were able to withstand infections fatal to normal control."

The absurdities of the "quacks" and "fanatics" have again triumphed. Fever that every "scientific" physician knew to be an evil that must be suppressed turned out, after all was said and done, to be the benefit the "lunatic fringe" declared it to be, and its suppression proved to be a veritable slaughter, as we have declared for over a hundred years. Orthopathy will yet find its way into the very citadel of Heteropathy and wreck its elaborate structures and prove its bombast and pretended science to be east wind. Human progress has never come from entrenched institutions nor from the forces of exploitation. The "lunatic fringe" is the source of progress— always.

Emerson, who considers fever to be a protective measure, declares:—

"It may be said, in general, that the height of temperature is really no index to the severity of the case. The highest temperatures occur in the least serious fevers, such as relapsing fever and malaria, while in the severest fevers, the rapidly fatal infections, there may be no rise of temperature at all. In the latter case it seems as if the body were unable to make a febrile defense against the infection."

From our viewpoint the height of the temperature is an index to the reactive powers of the body. It is an index of his fighting powers. "Rapidly fatal infections" are such because there is no fighting power and this is also the reason the powers of life are so depressed by the infection that little or no fever develops.

Summing up what has just been said: FEVER IS A NECESSARY INCREASE IN BODY TEMPERATURE DESIGNED TO ENABLE THE BODY OR SOME PART OR PARTS OF IT TO EFFECTIVELY MEET AND DESTROY SOME FOE OF LIFE THAT IS THREATENING THE BODY AND TO REPAIR DAMAGES.

It is absolutely essential to the acute process and does not rise beyond the point of safety. In order to have fever two things are essential:

1. Suspension of heat radiation through the skin, and:—
2. Increased production of heat in the body.

Increased heat production demands increased oxidation. This calls for more oxygen and a more rapid circulation. In order to meet these two demands there is increased respiration and increased heart action in acute disease. Thus it will readily be seen that these two "symptoms of disease,"—rapid heart action and accelerated breathing—each serve definitely beneficial ends.

Heat production is not as great during fever as while running or during other vigorous physical activities; but heat radiation is suspended so that the heat is retained in the body. Breathing and heart action are not as rapid during fevers as when running. When engaged in vigorous effort sweating carries away heat from the body and thus prevents the temperature from running up. Suspension of skin radiation is, therefore, the most essential thing in the production of fever.

At the expense of repitition I take the liberty to quote the following from the pen of Dr. Wm. F. Havard, one of the world's leading naturopaths:—

"There are three cardinal features or symptoms in all acute diseases—increased temperature, increased heart rate or pulse beat, and increased respiration. The increased activity of the cells indicates that there is a demand for an increased amount of oxygen. This is supplied through a more rapid circulation of blood and a more rapid action on the part of the lungs. There is a lower degree of skin activity during the earlier stages of an acute reaction because of the necessity for circulatory compensation. The excessive dilation of the internal arteries necessitates the constriction of the blood vesels of the skin. This reduces heat radiation, which coupled with the increased heat production in the body, produces fever.

"Fever plays an important role in the maintenance of the acute reaction. All matter manifests more molecular activity as its temperature is increased. Protoplasm, the living substance of which cells are composed, is no exception to this. It is normal in activity, in the human body, when maintained at a temperature of about 99 degrees Fahrenheit. Its activity decreases proportionately as the temperature is lowered below this point. If its temperature is brought too far below the normal, its life processes cease and death ensues. The molecular activity of protoplasm increases proportionately with a rise in its temperature until a point of maximum activity is reached. If carried beyond this point, the activity decreases because of too rapid disintegration of the protoplasm. In fevers, where the increased temperature is due to greater combustion taking place in the cells, it is impossible for the temperature to be carried to a point where it would cripple the cells. When the maximum activity is reached, any tendency to push it beyond this point results in decreased activity of the cells, consequently decreasing combustion and lowering temperature immediately. The action is automatic and needs no regulation from outside influences.

"No one ever died of fever. Some observers record temperatures in acute diseases of well over 108 degrees Fahrenheit, with complete recovery of the patients. The greater the reactive power of the body, the higher the temperature is likely to rise during a crisis of this nature. Children, in whom the natural vitality has not been worn down by abuse, are prone to manifest a higher temperature in reactions than adults. This would tend to prove that the fever is an index to the reactive power of the body. It is almost impossible for a person of very low vitality to have an acute disease. (This agrees with the statement made by one of the earlier Orthopaths, Felix Oswald, M.D., in his Physical Education; to wit: "A man may be too tired to sleep and too weak to be sick. Bleeding, for the time being, may 'break up' an inflammatory disease, the system must regain some little strength before it can resume the work of reconstruction." Author.)

* * *

"The temperature of the body is maintained normally at about 99 degrees. Heat is generated as a result of combustion—burning up of carbonaceous matter (sugar and fats)—which takes place in the cells. Heat is distributed by the blood and is radiated from the surface of the body and from the lungs. The degree of heat radiation depends on the quantity produced, but must always be sufficient to keep the temperature from rising above 99 degree F. The temperature of the external atmosphere has considerable bearing on heat dissipation. If the external atmosphere rises, either heat production within the body must decrease or heat radiation must increase. Heat production cannot always be reduced immediately, but heat radiation can be readily increased by a dilation of the blood vessels of the skin. The blood vessels of the skin, when dilated, will hold at least one-third, possibly one-half, of all the blood in the body. The greater the amount of blood flowing through these vessels, the greater will be the heat radiation. Persons with inactive skins secure the increased degree of heat radiation through the dilation of the blood vesesls of the membranes of the respiratory tract. This causes overheating of these membranes, and is responsible for much catarrhal trouble. Nasal and bronchial catarrh are always associated with dry, inactive skins.

"The balance between heat production and heat radiation is maintained through the activity of a very delicate nervous mechanism, which is influenced by the thermosensory nerves of the skin and the temperature of the blood which comes in contact with it. This heat center, or heat regulating mechanism, is located in the medulla, and communicates directly with the mechanism controlling the circulation and distribution of the blood, namely the vaso-motor mechanism. A chilling of the surface of the body thus produces a constriction of its vessels, the internal blood vessels are compelled to dilate. This increases heat production. If the surface of the body is heated, the reverse takes place.

"If combustion in the cells is excessive, due to irritation or a preponderance of sugar, fats, or proteins in the blood, the temperature of the body tends to rise, and would rise were it not for the fact that the heat center in the brain senses the condition and, by reflecting its findings to the vaso-motor mechanism, brings about a dilation of the skin vessels. If the body or blood temperature has a tendency to fall due to low heat production the skin vessels are immediately constricted to conserve the heat. Heat production should be greater in winter and lesser in summer. From these facts it is seen that heat regulations are automatic within a normal range and are successful in maintaining an even temperature.

"In acute diseases heat production is, and of necessity must be, excessive in order to keep up the greater activity in the cells. Heat dissipation is therefore reduced sufficiently to maintain the higher temperature. Fever is natural in acute disease. In fact, there would (could) be no acute disease without it.

"If we regard the body as an automatic, compensating machine, with all parts and functions bearing a true relationship to each other, we will immediately see that increased cellular activity (molecular activity of the protoplasm) calls for an increased quantity of blood, demanding many alterations in functional activity. Oxygen is demanded in greater quantities to support the combustion occurring in the cells, which can only be supplied by bringing extra blood to the cells. This can be partly accomplished through the dilation of the blood vessels, but inasmuch as this very action reduces the blood pressure (the constriction of the skin vessels affording insufficient compensation), and would cause the blood to flow at a slower rate, the heart is compelled to beat with greater rapidity. The blood flows through the pulmonary vessels at the same rate that it goes through the systemic vessels, consequently the respiratory movement must increase in proportion to the heart beat, in order to insure sufficient oxygen to the blood. Thus we find that the cells' demand for more oxygen causes a dilation of the internal blood vessels, an increased heart rate, and a more rapid respiratory movement. In acute diseases the temperature, pulse, and respiration are all increased proportionately, the degree of increase depending on the activity of the cells and the extent of compensation.

"Inflammation is a state or condition produced by increased circulation and oxidation. It has five cardinal features—(1) heat, (2) redness, (3) swelling, (4) pain, and (5) alteration of function. This is the marvelous manner in which Nature proceeds to remedy injuries and to correct abnormal conditions, and that is why inflammation is present in all acute diseases, being greater in the part or parts of the body where the irritants causing the disorder are concentrated, or from which they are distributed.

"Orthopathy and Allopathy take two different and very opposing views of the subject. Admitting that an individual may be poisoned and a reaction produced by infection, Orthopathy regards this reaction (acute disease) as a process of Nature by which poisons, already accumulated in the system, are driven to a focus for the sole purpose of being destroyed and eliminated.

"Orthopathy, therefore, makes a distinction between acute disease, in which the whole body is reacting to accumulated poisons, and local inflammation the causes of which are essentially traumatic.

"A cinder in the eye will cause a local inflammation of that organ. Remove the cinder and the inflammation gradually disappears. Red pepper or any other irritant taken into the stomach with food, will produce local inflammation which will subside and disappear when the irritant is removed or disposed of. Gases breathed into the lungs, will cause irritation and even inflammation of the respiratory membranes. In fact, any irritant, whether mechanical, thermal, chemical, or electrical, will cause inflammation of the part of the body to which it is applied.

"Inflammation is a constructive and protective process. The blood contains all the healing and repairing elements, and wherever tissues are irritated or damaged, the vital fluid is rushed there in abnormal quantities to carry off the debris and repair the damaged part. This causes (1) abnormal heat (fever), (2) redness, (3) swelling, (4) pain, and (5) alteration of function, all of which subside and disappear when the work has been done—when the dangerous irritant has been removed and the injury repaired. This is accomplished quickly by a pure blood-stream, but if the river of life is loaded with foul waste matter, you can readily see that is very poor repair material, and it often happens that a local injury produces a focus very similar to that of an acute disease, because of the excess of impurities concentrated by the inflammation at the point of injury."

LIFE'S ENGINEERING

Chapter X

THE greatest engineering feat of which we know anything is the building of a complex animal organism from a microscopic ovum. Think, for instance, of the marvels of the human body with its pulleys and levers to perform mechanical work, its channels for distribution of food and drainage of sewage, its means of regulating its temperature and adapting its actions and functions to its varied environments and needs. Its nervous system and the eyes, ears, etc., are constant sources of wonder. We regard the radio as a wonderful invention, as indeed it is, but we are all equipped with more wonderful "sending" and "receiving" sets than any radio manufacturer will ever produce. All human inventions have their prototypes in the animal body.

In studying the wonders of the human body, its structures, functions, development, growth, and its varied powers and capacities, it is well to keep in mind that the building and preservation of all these things is from within. The power, force or intelligence that evolves the adult body from the fertilized ovum is in the body, is part of it and is in constant and unceasing control of all its activities. Whether it is an intelligent power or a blind energy, it works determinately toward the latest results in complexity of structure and function. In development and maintenance; health and disease, the movements of life appear to be guided by intelligence greater often than the conscious intelligence of man. Indeed, unless we grant that something can come out of nothing, that intelligence can come out of that which has no intelligence, we must believe that the conscious intelligence of man is a subordinate part of that broader intelligence that evolves his body and which inheres in it.

If we view a few of the engineering feats performed by the body in cases of injury and disease we are forcibly struck with the truth of Graham's remark: "*In all these operations the organic instincts act determinately, and, as it were, rationally, with reference to a final cause of good, viz., the removal of the offending cause.*" Some of these wonderful feats have been presented to you in previous chapters. We will here present a few of a different class.

To begin with let us consider the natural healing of a wound, scratch or broken skin. We have become so accustomed to this familiar phenomenon that we have come to regard it as an almost mechanical process. But a close examination of the process shows us the presence of that same marvelous intelligence that builded the body from a tiny microscopic speck of protoplasm to its present state.

Whenever the skin, and maybe the deeper tissue, is broken or cut, there is an exudation of blood which coagulates and forms an air-tight scab. This scab serves as a protection to the wound, and remains for a shorter or longer time as is needed.

Underneath this scab a wonderful thing occurs. Blood is rushed to the injured part in large quantities. The tissues, nerve and muscle cells, etc., on each side of the wound start multiplying rapidly, and build a "cell-bridge" across the gap until the severed edges of the wound are reunited. But this is no mere haphazard process. Everywhere is apparent the presence of directing law and order. The newly formed cells of the blood vessels unite with their brothers on the other side so that in an orderly and evenly manner the channels of circulation are re-established. In this same lawful and orderly manner the connective tissues reunite. Skillfully, and just as a lineman repairs a telegraph system, do the nerve cells repair their broken line. Muscles and other tissues are repaired in a similar manner. And what is a wonderfully, marvelous fact to observe, no mistakes are made in this connecting process—muscles do not connect with nerve or blood vessels, or with connective tissue, but each tissue connects with its kind.

After the wound is healed, when a new skin has been formed, so that there is no longer any need for the protecting scab, nature proceeds to undermine and get rid of it. As long as the scab was useful it was firmly attached to the skin so that it was not easy to pull it off, but when there was no longer need for it, it was undermined so that it fell off of its own weight.

What more evidence than this does one require to know that the same intelligent power that built our bodies is also the power that heals it? What better evidence do we want that the healing process is accomplished in the same orderly manner and by means of the same functions with which the body is built and maintained, modified, of course, to meet the present needs.

We get, if possible, a still more wonderful view of how nature performs her work, if we observe the healing of a fractured or broken bone. If an arm or leg be broken, this same marvelous intelligence that has brought us from ovum to adulthood, immediately sets about to repair the damage done. A liquid substance is secreted and deposited over the entire surface of the bone in each direction from the point of fracture. This secretion quickly hardens into a bone-like substance and is firmly attached to the two sections of the bone. Until nature can repair the damage this "bone ring" forms the chief support whereby the limb can be used. By the same process of cell multiplication which we saw in the healing of the wound, the ends of the bone are reunited. The circulatory channels are re-established through the part. It is then that the "bone ring" support is softened and absorbed, except about an eight to a quarter of an inch about the point of fracture.

You strike your finger with a hammer. A very painful bruise is the result. There is an effusion of blood under the surface, with inflammation and discoloration. The tissues are mangled, the cells are broken, and many of them are killed. But does the thumb always remain so? No. As time passes, new tissues are formed to replace the dead ones, the dead cells and the dark, wasted blood, is absorbed and carried away. The inflammation subsides, the pain ceases, the bruise is cured, and soon forgotten. Thus again is manifested the marvelous intelligence of the power that superintends the workshop, which we call our body. Once, again, we watch his work and see his marvelous efficiency as a workman.

A similar manifestation of the body's self-healing, self-adjusting, self-repairing powers is seen in the common accident whereby a sliver becomes embedded in the flesh. If it is not removed immediately, nature, or vital force, does a skillful little piece of engineering and removes it for us. Pain and inflammation are soon followed by the formation of pus, which breaks down the tissues towards the surface of the body. Gradually increasing in amount, the pus finally breaks through the overlying skin and runs out, carrying the sliver along as a souvenir.

A remarkable engineering feat is presented to us in abscess formations. Ordinarily the abscess is limited by a thick protective wall of granulation tissue, which prevents the abscess from spreading and prevents rapid escape of the puss into the circulation.

In appendicitis the loops of the bowels around the appendix form friendly adhesions. They adhere together and form a strong wall against further spread of the trouble. Within this enclosure the abscesses form. The line of least resistance normally is into the bowels so that practically every case, if not interfered with by meddlesome doctors, will rupture into the bowels and the pus will pass out with the stools.

Where the ice bag is employed for one or two days prior to the usual operations in these cases there is a noticable lack of effort on the part of nature to wall off the appendix from the rest of the abdominal cavity whereas, where the ice bag has not been employed a distinct walling off of the acutely inflamed and gangrenous appendix from the general peritoneal cavity is found. So greatly does the ice-bag interfere with the curative and protective operations of Nature that one of the leading abdominal surgeons of this country declares: "I have entirely discarded the use of the ice bag, and in cases brought to me in which it has been used I always announce beforehand that I expect to find a gangrenous appendix, and am seldom disappointed. *Clearly the ice bag should never be used in cases of actual or suspected appendicitis.*" Nature can do her own work in her own way and all our so-called aiding nature amounts to nothing more than meddlesome and pernicious interference.

Acute inflammation of the liver usually terminates in resolution, but sometimes in suppuration with abscess formation. This is more apt to be the case in hot climates. The amount of matter discharged from an abscess of the liver is sometimes enormous and it is wonderful to see in what ways nature operates in getting rid of it.

There are several channels through which the pus may be sent out of the system. The inflammation may extend upward until an adhesion to the diaphram is accomplished. A dense wall of scar tissue is first formed around the abscess. The abscess then extends through the diaphram to the lungs which become adherent to the diaphram. Liver, diaphram and lungs form one solid piece. A tight union of these organs prevents the pus from pouring into the peritoneal or pleural cavaties. A hole is eaten through the lung, the pus is poured into a bronchial tube, is coughed up emptying the abscess and leaving a clean hole. The wall of scar tissue thrown up around the path of the abscess grows stronger and contracts until, finally, only the scar remains, it having closed the hole, and the patient is well.

The abscess may be directed downward or to the side of the liver. In such a case the process is the same, except the liver becomes united by adhesions produced by inflammation, to the stomach or intestines or to the wall of the abdomen. If it adheres to the stomach or intestine the abscess will perforate into these and the pus pass out in the stools. If it becomes abherent to the wall of the abdomen the abscess will "come to a head" under the skin and the pus will be discharged on the surface of the body. In either case cicatrization follows and the patient is well. In some cases the abscess discharges into the gall-bladder and passes from here into the intestine. It has also been known to "point" on the back.

It sometimes happens in weak individuals that nature is not able to make proper connections along the line of march and the pus finds its way into the pleural cavity causing empyema; or into the abdominal cavity where it results in peritonitis and, usually, death.

Another daring engineering feat is often accomplished by nature in the case of gall stones that are too large to pass through the bile duct directly into the small intestine. She frequently causes the gall bladder to adhere, by means of inflammation, to the wall of the intestine. An ulcer forms making a hole through both the wall of the gall bladder and the wall of the intestine. The stone slips through into the intestine and passes out with the stools. The hole heals up and all is well again. In other cases the stone may be sent out through the abdominal wall and skin, on the outside of the body.

An unusual piece of engineering which shows, in a remarkable manner, the ingenuity of nature in her efforts at prolonging life in spite of every obstacle, is recorded by J. F. Baldwin, A.M., M.D., F.A.C.S., in a surgical paper dealing with blood transfusions. He performed an operation on a middle aged woman who had been having frequent hemorrhages from her bowels for several years. He says:

"At the operation I removed a snarl of small bowel, making the usual anastamosis. Examination of this snarl showed that there had been an intestinal obstruction, but Nature had overcome it by ulceration between adherent loops of the bowel above and below the obstruction. The ulcer persisted, however, and it was its persistent bleeding that caused her anemia. She made an excellent recovery and got fat and hearty."

It looks like a real intelligence at work when nature causes two folds of the bowels to adhere together and then ulcerates through them in order to make a passage around an obstruction. There can not be the slightest doubt that the ulcer would have healed, leaving a passage, and the bleeding stopped, had the opportunity been afforded it. Nature probably cried out day after day in unmistakable language for the cessation of feeding long enough for her to complete her engineering feat. But this was never given her. The ulcerated surface was kept constantly irritated with food, and drugs as well.

Abscesses everywhere in the body are limited and walled off by the formation of a thick wall of granulation tissue. Gangrene is also walled off in the same manner The necrosed portion then sloughs off, nature grows new tissue to take the place of the destroyed tissue and the place is healed.

Encapulation is the process of surrounding a body or substance with a capsule. A cyst or capsule consists of a cavity lined according to its origin by endothelium (in preexisting cavities of connective tissue—exudation cysts) or epithelium (in pre-existing epithelial cavities—retention cysts) with a fluid or semi-fluid content.

Those of chief interest to us here are known as DISTENSION CYSTS and are divided into:

(a) RETENTION CYSTS; which are due to the obstruction of the excretory ducts of glands. The cavity becomes filled with the secretion of the gland which later becomes altered and circumscribed by a fibrous wall. These may develop in any glandular structure, as pancreas, kidneys, salivary glands, mammary glands, sebaceous glands (wens).

(b) EXUDATION CYSTS; which arise in cavities having no excretory duct. These occur in bursae, tendon sheath, thyroid, ovary, tunica vaginalis (hycdocele), canal of neck, certain ganglia, hygroma and the central canal of the spinal cord.

The effusion in pleurisy sometimes becomes circumscribed by adhesions, or it may be encapsulated to the diaphram.

(c) EXTRAVASION CYSTS; which result from a collection of blood in a pre-existing cavity, e. g., tunica vaginalis, pelvis, arachnoid cyst.

Cysts also form around foreign bodies and around parasites. The most common parasitic cysts are hydated cysts due to the small tape worm, *Tearia echinococcus*. These get into the body in food and drink and their larva find lodgement in the tissues. A wall of fibro-cicatricial tissue is formed around them. Such a cyst may become inflammed, suppurate or rupture. If the parasite dies the cyst may became thickened by absorption.

CYSTS OF DISINTEGRATION form around disintegrating tissues as in the brain, in tumors, etc.

Around a foreign body such as a bullet such a capsule forms. There is first inflammation and perhaps suppuration. But if this fails to remove the bullet a capsule of tissue in which is also fluid, is formed and the bullet rendered innoctious. A similar thing frequently happens in the lungs in the case of germs. Rausse thought this fluid was a variety of mucous and thought that chemical or drug poisons were enveloped in this same "mucous" to render them harmless, and that they were then deposited in the tissues. He says with regard to the fact that this theory cannot at present be demonstrated:

"This theory is founded upon the incontrovertable principle of nature in the elimentary and organic world, that nature operates similarly under similar circumstances. Hence, the theory here offered loses none of its certainty, because we are unable to recognize with the unaided eye, on account of their minuteness, the inimical atoms and the minute net-work around them, and to exhibit them by section."—*Water Cure Manual*, p. 92, 1845.

The encapsulation of exudates, excretions, extravasions, disintegrating tissues, germs, parasites, bullets and other foreign bodies renders them harmless. The process and structures it evolves are plainly defensive measures. They once more remind us of the many and varied emergency measures the body has at its command.

The formation of gall stones, and other stones, is, in itself, an engineering feat that serves a useful purpose, and, perhaps, saves life. In the lungs, for instance, in those who have tuberculosis, the affected spots are often the seat of the formation of stones. When this takes place, the disease, in that part, ends. Medical authorities consider that nature employs this means to wall up the tubercle bacilli.

The formation of stones in the gall-bladder and kidneys, just as in the lungs is the end-result of inflammation and undoubtedly serves a definite and useful purpose. Sometimes, it is true, they are made so large that they are the source of much trouble, but it is safe to assume that they are never made larger than the gravity of the situation demands. Most gall stones are small enough that they pass out without causing pain and the individual is never aware that he or she has had them. A large number of people examined at autopsies are found to have gall stones in the gall bladder and were never aware that they had them. They never cause trouble until they go to pass out and, only then, if they are small enough to get into the gall duct but too large to make the entire passage. A stone that may easily travel through the common duct may be forced, with extreme difficulty, through the small opening of the duct into the intestine. This causes severe pain. As soon as the stone is forced through the pain ceases. The sufferer is then sure that it was the last treatment he employed that relieved the pain and cured his troubles.

A *thrombus* is a small blood-clot formed inside of a blood vessel. The condition is called *thrombosis* and the vessel is said to be *thrombosed*. They are the result of injury and inflammation and may completely plug the vessel.

In the intestines are many small glands composed of lymphoid structure just as are the tonsils of the throat, and known as Pyer's patches. In typhoid fever these patches are swollen or enlarged (hypertrophied) and frequently they suppurate. They may slough off. This peeling off may result in a hemorrhage or it may not depending on whether or not all the vessels in that locality are tightly *thrombosed*. If they are all tightly *thrombosed* no hemorrhage occurs. If the work of sealing the vessel is not complete or perfect then a hemorrhage occurs with more or less loss of blood before it finally ceases. This is but another evidence of nature's engineering work. These *thrombi* may later be swept into the general circulation and carried to some vital spot where they are too large to pass through the artery and may there cut off the blood to parts of the organ causing it to die of starvation. Starvation would only occur in cases of stopping of an "end-artery." "Anastamosing" arteries would soon establish sufficient collateral or compensatory criculation to supply the part with blood.

If heat or friction is applied to the skin of sufficient intensity and duration a blister forms. That is, a watery exudate or serum is poured out of the surrounding tissues and circulation into the "space" between the dermis and epidermis and detaches the dermis from this raising it up and thus protecting the tissues beneath. The accumulated fluid holds back the heat or, in the case of sun burn, the actinic rays, and protects from the friction. This little piece of engineering work is quite obviously a defensive work. In both burns and sun-burn inflammation and healing follow the blister and, in the case of sun-burn, pigmentation to protect from future sun-burn.

Of a similarly defensive nature are corns and callouses that form on the feet and hands or any other surface of the body that is subjected to constant friction. The young clerk who deserts the store for manual labor finds his hands are tender and blister easily when he handles tools. However, before many days have passed the skin on his hands has become thickened and hardened, ultimately becoming almost horn like. When this occurs he finds that no reasonable amount of hard work blisters his hands.

Tumors likely begin in this same manner. They probably begin as hardening and thickening of the tissues at a point of irritation as a means of defense.

Hardening and thickening of the tissues occurs in any and all parts of the body to resist constant irritation. This can be seen in the mouth and throat of those who employ tobacco in any form. It is seen in the mouth, stomach and intestines of those who employ salt and condiments. It is seen in the constant use of drugs. Silver nitrate, for instance, if repeatedly employed converts the mucous surface upon which it is used into a kind of half-living leather. Other organs harden and thicken as a result of toxic irritation. Toxemia with or without the aid of external irritation often necessitates, at certain points of the body, the erection of greater than ordinary barriers against it. When the normal cells of a local spot become so impaired that they no longer successfully resist the encroachment of toxins, not only are the usual defense processes brought into activity, but also, since a more than usual condition is to be met, nature calls into play her heavier battalions. She begins by erecting a barrier of connective tissue cells. Then, with a slowly yielding fight against the toxins, she continues to erect her barriers. This may continue until the tumor becomes so large as to constitute a source of danger itself. Were it not for the erection of this barrier, the causes against which it is erected would destroy life long before they ultimately do. The tumor actually prolongs life.

A process similar to this is seen in plants that have been invaded by parasites. The large, rough excrescenses seen on oak trees form about the larva of a certain fly. This fly lays its eggs beneath the bark of the tree. The larva which develop from the eggs secret a substance that results in the formation of the huge tumorous mass. Large tumor-like masses form on the roots and stalks of cabbages as a result of parasitic invasion. The olive tree also develops tumors from a similar cause; while, cedar trees present peculiar growths, called "witches' brooms," as a result of a fungus growing on them. There are many other examples and they are all quite obviously protective measures. Tumor formation is undoubtedly due to a variation in the complex relations determining normal growth and is of a distinctively protective nature. A tumor is not a source of danger until it beigns to break down.

In inflammation of the kidneys, due to the impairment of kidney function the normal constituents of the urine are decreased. They remain in the blood instead of being eliminated. Due to the necessity of removing from the circulation, the salts, etc., that are normally eliminated through the kidneys, and to the necessity, also, of keeping these in dilute solution so long as they remain in the body, and to the equal necessity of removing them from the circulation, dropsy develops in various portions of the body, but particularly in the tissues immediately under the skin. It may also collect in the cavities of the body. When kidney function is restored the dropsical fluid is gradually absorbed into the circulation and eliminated.

An *aneurism* is an inflated portion of an artery. If the walls of an artery become weak at a given place, they either burst, or some of its coats are strengthened, or else it becomes bulged out due to the pressure of the blood from within. The body at once sets about to protect itself by forming a wall of new tissue around the *aneurism*. Should it rupture so that the blood finds its way along between other organs, a wall of scar tissue is thrown up around the *aneurism* to limit the escape of blood. This is called a *dissecting aneurism*.

Thus we might continue giving example after example of the wonderful engineering feats of the body and show with what marvelous powers and works it meets emergencies and protects its own vital interests. When we consider the wonderful mechanism of the human body, the certainty with which all organs perform their allotted work, the marvelous ingenuity with which the body meets emergencies, its almost limitless powers of repair and recuperation, we develop a large respect and admiration for the curative power of the body and learn to view, with contempt and disgust the means that man employs in his unintelligent efforts to cure.

Well did Jennings affirm:

"But at every step of her (nature's) downward progress (in the face of pathoferic causes she cannot overcome), her tendency and effort have been to ascend and remount the pinnacle of her greatness; and even now, in the depth of her degradation, the tendency of all that remains of her, of principle or law, power and action, is still upwards."

PHYSIOLOGICAL COMPENSATION

Chapter XI

WE should not think of the body as a mere assemblage of organs and parts like a machine. Its organs are not independent entities without vital connection. Rather, the body is a unit. It is an organism all parts of which are so firmly bound together both in structure and function that no part suffers without involving the whole in the consequences. It is a closely grouped community of inter-related organs and parts, every one of which serves a definite and useful function.

There exists a great amount of reciprocity among the various tissues and organs of the body. In the case of loss or impairment of organs, the loss or impairment of one can be made good by increased size and activity of the remaining ones. Certain of the tissues of the body are so nearly alike in function that the loss of one is compensated for by the increase or modification of function of a closely related organ or part. Instances of such compensation are numerous.

The destruction of single cells in the Kidneys is quickly made good by the formation of new ones, but the loss of an area of tissue cannot be restored. This loss involves an increase in the amount of work the remaining cells must accomplish. They promptly increase their activities and perhaps enlarge in order to meet the extra demands made upon them. If one Kidney is removed, as in a surgical operation, the remaining Kidney greatly enlarges (hypertrophies) to do the work formerly accomplished by the excised kidney.

In chronic inflammation of the Kidneys there is a gradual degeneration and destruction of the functioning tissues of the Kidneys. Their places are taken by connective tissue, which is not a functioning tissue, but is capable of living on much less food and under conditions in which the functioning tissues cannot continue to exist. It serves merely to fill up the breach or patch up the hole. As the death of the Kidney cells continues and the growth of scar tissue procedes, the actual functioning tissue of the Kidneys grows progressively less and less, until there is but little left. The Kidneys may be reduced to about one-fifth their normal size. The cortex shrinks to from one-third to one-sixth its normal thickness, or even disappears entirely in places. Many of the glomeruli and convoluted tubules are destroyed. That so small an amount of Kidney tissue as remains can come so near to protecting the body proves conclusively that the normal Kidneys are capable of doing many times the amount of work that a normal life demands of them. Great and long continued abuse of the body is required before the normal Kidney is broken down.

Patients in advanced stages of this disease may go for extended periods without any symptoms at all, thus showing that even the small amount of functioning tissue that remains would be capable of maintaining a fair degree of health if the patient learned to live properly. A similar fact is seen in cirrhosis of the liver, where large areas of the hepatic cells are destroyed and their places filled by fibrous tissue. A considerable portion of the liver may thus be destroyed, and yet the remaining portions be able to do the normal work of the organism so long as nerve force is adequate.

Reciprocity exists between the Kidneys and the skin. For instance, when through exposure to cold, or due to shock, skin elimination is suspended, the kidneys increase their activities and eliminate the water and waste ordinarily eliminated through the skin. In cases of suppressed urine, that is, when Kidney action is impaired, the skin eliminates large quantities of matter that should have passed out through the Kidneys. In Bright's disease the skin may get rid of some of the nitrogenous waste. Near death in this disease urea sometimes crystalized out on the skin as "urea-frost," as nature makes one last desperate effort to save life These urea crystals form little solid masses about the size of a pinhead, thickly clustered over the skin of the face.

Both the skin and Kidneys do extra duty in individuals suffering from constipation. The foul odor eminating from the bodies of constipated individuals is due to the "feces" eliminated through the skin. The intestine is also an excreting surface, and in Bright's disease is able to aid the Kidneys.

A very remarkable reciprocity of function exists between the skin and the mucous membranes of the body. Indeed, the skin and mucous membranes are continuous structures. The mucous membrane lines all hollow organs and ducts that communicate either directly or indirectly with the outside world and may be rightly termed the *internal skin*. The frequency with which "colds" follow temporary suspension of elimination through the skin will serve to show the close reciprocity of these two surfaces. A "cold" in any part of the mucous surfaces is a process of compensatory elimination and is made necessary by the inadequacy of the normal channels of elimination in keeping the systemic toxemia at or below the toleration point. Catarrh, wherever its location, is also a process of compensatory elimination. The skin converts the body waste into sweat, the Kidneys convert them into urine, the mucous membranes convert them into mucous. Each tissue turns out its own products and by-products from the same material.

Sylvester Graham wrote upon this point:

"The depurating organs, as I have stated, reciprocate with each other in function to a considerable extent, even in the healthy state of the body, and in a diseased condition vicarious function is often attempted. Copious perspiration diminishes the secretion of the Kidneys, and on the other hand, a suppression of the cutaneous function generally increases that of the Kidneys. The skin and lungs reciprocate in the same manner. Excessive exhalations and excretions of the alimentary canal also frequently result from the suppression of the function of the skin and, by watever cause induced, they are always attended with cutaneous depression. *But the welfare of the particular parts, as well as of the whole system, requires that each organ should uniformly and vigorously perform the full measure of its own duty, because frequent excesses arising from undue determination of fluids to any one part, lead to debility of the part, and often result in impaired function, imperfect assimilation, local diseases, and general injury and death.* In this manner, sudden suppressions of the functions of the skin often lead to diabetes and pulmonary consumption, by causing undue determination to the kidneys, (In Graham's day diabetes was thought to be a disease of the kidneys.— Author), and lungs, and inducing inflammation and permanent disease in these organs. The liver also suffers from all want of integrity in the other depurating organs, and its derangements compel the skin, and indeed the whole system, to make an effort to throw off the matter which it should have eliminated. Still more excessively morbid and extravagant attempts at vicarious function take place when the mammary glands and other organs endeavor to perform the duties of the kidneys. But cases of this kind are very rare; frequent enough, however, to show the wonderful resources of the vital economy in extreme emergencies, and also to demonstrate the great importance of health and integrity in each and every organ." (Italics mine) *Science of Human Life,* pp. 197-198.

The symptoms associated with atrophic cirrhosis of the liver, a condition in which the functioning liver cells have been destroyed by alcohol and other toxins and have been replaced by scar tissue, do not result from the diminished amount of liver cells, but from obstruction of the portal circulation caused by shrinkage of the scar tissue. But a small amount of the liver is sufficient to perform the sugar and urea functions under all ordinary circumstances. In the normal liver is a great reserve of functioning power, more than enough to meet the emergencies of a normal life.

The entire destruction of the pancreas by disease or its removal by surgery destroys the body's ability to oxidize sugar. It has been found, however, that if but a little piece of that organ is successfully grafted in any part of the body, under the skin of an animal from which the pancreas has been removed, the work of this small piece of transplanted organ will be enough to save the animal from diabetes. It is evident from this that in the normal pancreas also there is a great reserve of power, more than enough to meet any emergency of life. It is equally evident from this that diabetes in those who still have a functioning pancreas would be cured if the enervating mode of living was corrected.

Cases of compensation that are commonly known are the increased acuteness of one ear accompanying deafness in the other, or, the increased sight in one eye following destruction of the other. A few blind individuals have learned to distinguish colors by means of the sense of touch. Armless individuals are often able to do with their feet and legs what their arms should have done. The increase of the size of the lobes of the lungs following destruction of one or more lobes is also a compensatory measure.

The destruction or removal of one testicle in man or of one ovary in woman is followed by an increase in the size of the remaining testicle or ovary. In certain toxic states of the body the thyroid gland enlarges producing hyperthyroidism or goitre. Removal of part of the gland is followed by enlargement of the remaining portion. Situated by and closely associated with the thyroid gland are a number of little structures known as the para-thyroids. Removal of part of these is followed by an increase in size of the remaining ones.

Enlargement of an organ is of two kinds. First there is an increase in the size of its cells. This is called *hypertrophy*. If this is not sufficient to accomplish the extra work, there follows an increase in the number of its cells. This is called *hyperplasia*. Both of these (*hypertrophy* and *hyperplasia*) are means of increasing the capacity and efficiency of the organ in order that it may meet the added demands that are being made upon it. I may here remark that these two processes are added evidence of the correctness of our claim that disease is a curative process.

A common example of hypertrophy is seen in the enlargement of the lymph glands in various regions of the body following infections. An excellent example of this is seen in the enlargement of the glands of the arm pit, chest and neck following vaccination. Vaccine is septic matter and when forcibly introduced into the body results in a whole series of pathological manifestations included under the term *vaccina*, and frequently in many evils not included under this term. The vaccine finds its way into the lymph and is conveyed along the lymph channels to the lymph nodes or glands where the work of destroying it begins. These glands are forced to enlarge to meet the demands placed upon them by this extra poison. If they are still unable to accomplish this work general septicemia and death may follow.

Professor W. T. Councilman, A.M., M.D., LL.D., of Harvard University, relates a story of two people, a physician and a nurse, becoming infected from handling parts of the body of a dead man. Both the physician and the nurse had skin abrasions on their fingers. In the course of a few hours the wound on the fingers of each of them became inflamed and very painful with red lines extending up their arms along the course of the lymphatic vessels. There was high fever and great prostration. The lymph glands in the arm pit of the physician became greatly enlarged and even suppurated. However he recovered. In the case of the nurse, all the lymph nodes in her armpit and near by had previously been removed by operation so that the infection was not held up at the armpits. General infection took place followed by death in a few days.

In what is wrongly called syphilitic infection there is a similar enlargement of the lymph glands in the groins. In a cold the glands in the neck enlarge. Enlargement of the tonsils and adenoids is the same phenomena and is intended to serve the same purpose.

Serious injury or destruction of the brain or spinal cord is never regenerated. However, adjustment to the condition is often effected by reciprocity of function. Other cells of the brain or cord take up the functions of those that are destroyed.

It not infrequently happens in cases of wounds and destruction of tissues that new blood vessels are formed to assist in carrying the extra nutriment to the injured part. After the part is repaired and there is no longer any need for the extra supply of nutrient material the newly formed vessels disappear.

A remarkable example of compensation is often seen in cases of cirrhosis of the liver. Practically all of the blood from the digestive organs is collected by the portal vein and conveyed to the liver. In cirrhosis the normal channels of circulation are more or less obstructed so that the blood is dammed back into the digestive organs interfering with their functions and causing various troubles in these organs. Now, at certain points in the abdomen the portal circulation anastomoses with the general circulation so that some of the portal flow can reach the heart without passing through the liver. The anastamosis of veins throughout the body is to enable the blood to choose between two channels should one channel become obstructed. There are more veins in the body than are really required to carry the blood under ordinary conditions. There is here, also, a sufficient reserve for all ordinary emergencies. There are several channels through which a compensatory circulation may be established in cases of cirrhosis of the liver. If the cirrhosis is not great compensation will take care of it. Otherwise ascites and death follow.

A similar example is seen in cases where an artery is obstructed by a blood clot. Arteries are divided into two classes—*end arteries* and *anastamosing arteries.* *Anastamosing arteries* are two small arteries which are connected with each other by small communicating branches. An *end artery* is a small artery that possesses no communicating branches. These are few in number.

When an end artery becomes obstructed by a blood clot (Thrombus) the tissues fed by this artery must die. The dead area is known as an *infarct.* But, if the clogged artery is not an *end artery* the communicating artery will send enough blood through its communicating branches to maintain the circulation and thus feed the tissues of that area. They do not die. The small communicating or *anastamosing* arteries become larger and larger until a sufficient collateral circulation is developed to carry the blood necessary.

What is called vicarious menstruation, or xenomenia, is probably not properly so classed at all. A little explanation should make this clear. In order to ripen the ovum and cause the ova sac to rupture and discharge the ovum an added supply of blood must be sent to the ovaries. In order to bring this about, there normally occurs at regular intervals an increased tension in the blood vessels through the body, except in the pelvis. This forces the blood into the pelvic organs producing *pelvic hyperemia.* There is commonly, though not always, a discharge of blood from the uterus at this time producing what is called menstruation. The blood is forced through the walls of the blood vessels and leaks out of the body. If the walls of these vessels are strong and elastic there is no necessary flow.

It often happens in such cases, however, that the blood vessels in some other part of the body are weakened and the increased tension put upon them causes bleeding at that point. Thus, what is called vicarious menstruation has been known to occur in the stomach, lungs, breasts, nose, in the armpits and elsewhere. It should be regarded as an evidence of weakness of the blood vessels in these parts rather than as a vicarious menstruation. This is so because: (1) menstruation is not necessary to ovulation and is probably not normal: (2) the so-called vicarious menstruation does not accompany more than a fraction of "suppressed" menses; and (3) it may occur from any cause that increases blood pressure, even in males.

What is called "*supplementary menstruation*" is probably also nothing more than a sign of weakness. It is a hemorrhage from any part of the mucous membrane of the body coincident with the usual discharge of blood from the sex organs. I regard it as evidence of weakness of the walls of the blood vessels in that area which permits them to rupture with the increased blood-pressure during the period of ovalation. I do not think that loss of blood is really an essential of ovulation.

However, what may truly be regarded as a compensatory measure—a conservative measure of great importance—is the absence of menstruation and even ovulation (this latter resulting in sterilty) for longer or shorter periods of time in cases of extreme weakness, and in wasting diseases. Strange reasoning in the past has often considered the absence of menstruation to be the cause of the wasting disease.

The stomach provides secretions to meet the usual demands of digestion. However, it is normally able to take care of an unusual amount of food. The skin is able to greatly increase its output of sweat when the external temperature or one's muscular exertion increases the need for surface radiation.

The power of the heart in meeting the many and various conditions it is called upon to meet is marvelous. Under conditions that would be ruinous to a machine it continues to throw three and one-half ounces of blood seventy to eighty times per minute against nine feet of water pressure. Its size is influenced by the size and occupation of its owner. It is larger in large individuals than in small, and is larger in the active and vigorous than in the inactive.

In some diseased conditions of the heart the orifice of the heart into the aorta becomes narrowed. Under such conditions the heart can send into the aorta a given amount of blood in a given time only by contracting with greater force and thus giving a greater rapidity to the stream passing through the orifice. In other disease conditions the valve becomes incapable of fully closing so that some of the blood, after being forced out of the heart regurgitates back into it. The orifice in such conditions may also be narrowed. The heart must then, in order to keep up the necessary pressure in the aorta and give to the blood-stream the needed rapidity of flow and compensate for the blood that flows back into the heart through the but partially closed valve, contract with greater force upon a greater volume of blood. The heart cavity becomes larger in order to receive the greater quantity of blood.

In women the additional burden which pregnancy places upon the heart may be sufficient to overcome a crippled heart, or if the heart is not too bady damaged it may be just enough to cause the heart to be greatly strengthened and improved.

The work of the heart may be doubled by severe muscular exertion as in running or lifting. It meets this extra demand by an increased force and rapidity of contraction. If the exertion is repeated habitually the heart becomes larger and stronger just as the muscles of the arm or leg are made larger and stronger by exercise.

All this is made possible, because the heart, like all other organs of the body, possesses a large reserve force which enables it, even suddenly, to meet demands that are double or more than double the usual demands made upon it. Under the usual conditions of life the body always possesses a store of reserve force. No tissue of the body is worked to its fullest capacity.

If circulation is to be carried on without embarrassing the heart there must be just enough blood to completely fill the circulatory system. If there is vaso-dilation (dilation of the blood vessels), in one part of the body there must be a compensatory vaso-constriction in another part of the body—or if a hyperemia exists in one part of the body a compensatory anemia must exist elsewhere and vice versa—if blood pressure is to be maintained. For instance, in digestion there is hyperemia of the stomach with anemia of the brain. We thus find thinking difficult after a full meal. If the skeletal muscles are active, as in work, play or exercise, there is vaso-constriction in the viscera and vaso-dilation in the muscles—thus digestion proceeds less rapidly during work or exercise. During menstruation there is congestion of the pelvic organs because of vaso-dilation in these with vaso-constriction in the rest of the body. During sleep there is an anemia of the brain, skin and skeletal muscles with hyperemia of the viscera. Digestion is better. This precise adjustment of the blood flow to the changing needs and conditions of the body and its parts is controlled by the autonomic nervous system. Two sets of nervous fibers (vaso-motor nerves) known as the vaso-dilators and vaso-constrictors so balance each other, normally, that this compensation takes place so smoothly and easily that the individual is never aware of it.

If you buy an automobile you get a high powered car—say sixty horse power. You may not need more than thirty horse, but you like to feel that the extra power is there in reserve to be used in emergency or in climbing a steep hill. The added power is there to meet unusual demands. The same is true with regard to the body. Nature has prepared us to meet unusual demands. Unlike the engine, the increased demand for activity of the heart, for example, causes it to become larger and stronger, the reserve force rising with the load to be carried. However, the ratio of reserve force is diminished.

Loss brought about by injuries, destruction of tissues as in disease or by surgical mutilations, etc., can be compensated for, even where healing is imperfect, by increased function in similar tissues of the body.

There is, however, a limit to the body's compensating powers and when this limit is reached any added burden must produce serious damage. With every increased demand for work there is a gradual diminution of the body's reserve force so that as time passes the ability to compensate for the added work gradually diminishes.

Compensation may be gained in other ways. The demand made upon the heart, for instance, may be reduced by changing the mode of life—by reducing the amount of physical activity, by avoiding stimulants, by correcting gluttenous habits, by avoiding excitement and other conditions that put extra work upon the heart.

It is the power of compensation or the reserve force back of it that enables the young man to live a life of reckless dissipation for a considerable time without apparent harm. It is compensation that enables a man or woman to go on living, for years, perhaps, after the surgeon has left him or her a mere hull of his or her former self. It is compensation that enables the diabetic patient or the sufferer from Bright's disease to go on living in spite of the destruction of the tissues of the pancreas or the Kidneys. It is this same compensation that will enable these same patients to live many years if they will only learn how to live in order not to overburden the compensation. In modern life compensation keeps most of us alive many years longer than we would live were we devoid of such a power. Modern living places a tremendous constant tax upon the whole organism of man. Were it not for their marvelous reserve powers few men and women in modern life would ever reach maturity.

In all these and similar cases of compensation there exists an imperious necessity for vicarious action, and those organs and parts which engage in it do so on the principle of self-preservation, and manifest thereby a previous adaptation to the work. Compensatory or vicarious action can in no sense be considered *fortuitous* or *wrong* action, but becomes, under the circumstances, the appropriate duty of the organ which performs it, and is the only course of action that would or could be *right*. Such actions show unmistakably the *unity of action* of the organs of the human body in a common cause and for a common end. They illustrate the remarkable supervision which the vital forces and vital laws exercise over the functions of the body and should lead us to exercise the greatest caution in our attempts to repair an organism which so nicely and minutely adapts means to ends, lest in our efforts to counteract what we conceive to be *wrong action* we make war upon the forces of life and injure rather than help the body.

LIFE'S STRATEGIC RETREAT

Chapter XII

ORDINARILY we say that living organisms are distinguishable from dead organisms by certain criteria. But we must not forget that such criteria are not infallible. There are stages in the life of the living organism when all the life processes seem not to exist; life remains *dormant* from lack of appropriate stimuli, or condition, or from some unexplained pecularity. Broadly speaking, we may say that we know two kinds of life, that is:

1. Passive or quiscient life, and
2. Active life.

Passive life is common to plants and animals, alike, and is considered as a state in which the living organism becomes capable of withstanding conditions unfavorable to activity. The organism is maintained in *status quo*. Seeds for instance may lie dormant for years. Eggs of some insects lie dormant through a long winter and withstand the cold. Some animals have been observed to lie in this dormant condition for periods up to fourteen years.

During this dormant stage there is nothing that will distinguish the living organism from a dead one. The processes and functions of life, are, so far as is discernable, wholly inactive. However, when such organisms are introduced into conditions favorable to active life, they become active Dormant seeds or eggs begin to germinate and grow. Dormant plants put forth leaves and grow. Animals in a state of suspended animation revive and become active. Active life is dependent upon certain factors, chief among which are warmth, air, water, food and light. Factors that tend to induce the passive state are cold, dryness, darkness, quiet, lack of food, etc.

Force preserves as well as produces. It must exist before it can become active and before it becomes active it is passive. All forces are both *passive* and *active*. They are active to do work and passive to preserve. When vital action ceases, it is commonly thought that life has ceased, but this is not essentially so. We are too prone to regard life as activity, because it is so connected with action and unobservable except when in action. Still, there are inumerable facts to show that this is a delusion of the senses—a delusion to those who live in the appearance of things and who never dream of their realities. We must learn that all vital inaction does not constitute death—it may equally constitute preservation.

Jordon and Kellogg say, in *Animal Life:*—

"Of death we know the essential meaning. Life ceases and can never be renewed in the body of the dead animal. It is important that we include the words 'can never be renewed,' for to say simply that 'life ceases,' that is, that the performance of the life processes or functions ceases, is not really death. It is easy to distinguish in most cases between life and death, between a live animal and a dead one, yet there are cases of apparent death or a semblance of death which are very puzzling. The test of life is usually taken to be the performance of life functions, the assimilation of food and excretion of waste, the breathing in of oxygen, and breathing out of carbonic-acid gas, movement, feeling, etc. But some animals can actually suspend all of these functions, or at least reduce them to such a minimum that they can not be perceived by the strictest examination, and yet not be dead. That is, they can renew again the performance of the life processes. Bears and some other animals, among them many insects, spend the winter in a state of death-like sleep. Perhaps it is but sleep; and yet hibernating insects can be frozen solid and remain frozen for weeks and months, and still retain the power of actively living again in the following spring. Even more remarkable is the case of certain minute animals called *Rotatoria* and of others called *Tardigrada*, or bear-animalcules. These bear-animalcules live in water. If the water dries up, the animalcules dry up too: they shrivel up into formelss little masses and become desicated. They are thus simply dried-up bits of organic matter; they are organic dust. Now, if after a long time—years even—one of these organic dust particles, one of these dried-up bear-animalcules is put into water, a strange thing happens. The body swells and stretches out, the skin becomes smooth instead of all wrinkled and folded, and the legs appear in normal shape. The body is again as it was years before, and after a quarter of an hour to several hours (depending on the length of time the animal has lain dormant and dried) slow movements of the body parts begin, and soon the animal-cule crawls about, begins again its life where it had been interrupted. Various other small animals, such as vinegar eels and certain Protozoa, show similar powers. Certainly here is an interesting problem in life and death."

Rotatoria have been dried and resuscitated many time in succession. In the dried state life is passive to preserve the *status quo*. Many forms of bacteria in addition to the usual mode of multiplication form what are known as spores, (these being what Beauchamp called microzima) which are analagous to the seeds of plants, only they are much more resistant than such seeds. They endure boiling or even higher degrees of dry heat for some time before they are destroyed. When placed in conditions favor-able for bacterial life, they form bacteria which grow and develop in the usual manner.

They are produced when conditions are unfavorable to bacterial life. In this changed form and under natural conditions the germs are almost indestructable and await better conditions when they again blossom forth into active bacterial life.

Drysdale and Dallinger showed that the germs of Infusoria cannot be destroyed by the heat of boiling water, but live when the thermometer shows a temperature of 300 degrees F. These germs, dried and floating in the air, will revive on the accession of water.

Many cold-blooded animals may be frozen and retained in a dormant state through-out the whole of Winter and, upon being thawed out, resume their activities where they left off at the time of being frozen. Freezing does not destroy germ life but merely suspends it until the germ is thawed out. Pieces of human tissues have been preserved in cold storage for some time and then grfated on a living man or woman where they readily grew.

Usually, it is not difficult to recognize a dead body. However, in many instances, the heart's action is so feeble that the pulse cannot be felt nor its action detected by means of the stethescope. Respiration is so feeble that the current of expired air is not sufficient to disturbe a feather held to the nostrils, or cloud the surface of a mirror by the precipitation of moisture upon it. The patient is unconscious, the temperature of the body is below normal, the muscles seem paralyzed. This condition closely simulates death and has often been mistaken for death. There are numerous reports of people being pronounced dead by the physician and all preparation for the funeral being made only to have the supposed dead person revive. There is ample evidence to prove that many have been buried in this condition and have revived after "death." One instance will show what I mean. A man "died" of penumonia. He was buried. A short time later the grave was opened to move him. He was found turned over in his coffin, much of his hair torn out and much hair grasped in each hand. The grave and coffin had not been disturbed.

Examples of trances or apparent death which have lasted considerable time are numerous. The Fakirs of India have voluntarily induced such a state and have per-mitted themselves to be buried for long periods of time and have, upon being taken out, returned to active life, apparently none the worse for their experience. It is as-sumed that in such cases all the activities of the body are reduced to the utmost and that an imperceptible respiration and circulation are sufficient to keep the cells living. Rescusitation from drowning after all demonstratable vital activity has ceased is quite common.

These facts, to which more will be added later, prove that suspended animation is possible for man. This, I believe, will not be denied. What may be questioned is the interpretation I shall place upon this phenomenon. I told you before that biologists looked upon this state in animals, plants, bacteria and seed as a state in which the living organism becomes capable of maintaining the *status quo* in the face of condi-tions unfavorable to active life. I shall maintain that this is exactly what it is in man also when it occurs in disease. In other words, I shall maintain that it is a means of pas-sive defense. This is in perfect harmony with the facts about disease which we learned in Chapter 6. We learned that:

1. In disease, every function that can be temporaily dispensed with is either greatly reduced or suspended altogether.

2. The various functions and activities of the body are reduced or are suspended in proportion to the need to conserve energy.

3. The less action there is in the body, the less is the wear and tear and therefore the less is the cost of maintenance.

4. Perfect economy is everywhere exercised in the appropriation and use of the vital energies.

5. Nature never wantonly turns aside from her habitual course of action to throw her complex machinery into disorder and give it suicidal motion and tendency. There is always an imperative necessity for her actions and operations. The work of preserving life devolves upon the vital economy and this economy does not require to be reminded of its duties. Nature does not withdraw power from an organ to *destroy* life, but to *save* it. She gives us the best possible assurance that all available power will be put in requisition, and expended most economically in her work of cure and reparation.

The state of coma produced by anesthetics is a near approach to suspended animation. Indeed, there is often an actual state of suspended animation produced, with subsequent recovery even without efforts to save life. At first the body violently resists the anesthetic, but, being overpowered gradually sinks to stupor then coma. But in this state it successfuly resists and throws off the anesthetic and revives. It actually accomplishes in this passive state what it failed to accomplish by its first violent resistance. The success of its work is *inversely as to the degree of activity.*

Coma produced by asphyxiation and drowning are speedily overcome if their causes are removed before actual death is produced.

Closely analagous to suspended animation is sleep. During sleep all the voluntary functions are suspended. The mind and special senses are dormant. The voluntary muscles are inactive. The grand purpose served by sleep and repose is reparation, restoration, recuperation. It is a significant fact that the *deeper* or more *sound* is sleep, the more refreshing and invigorating it is. Disturbed and *shallow* sleep leaves one more or less tired and depressed. In disease, the more sleep one secures the more rapidly does he recover. In infancy the child that sleeps most grows fastest.

Activity expends energy, consumes substance and produces exhaustion. Rest and sleep enable the body to recuperate its energies and repair its substances. A wound or broken bone requires rest to heal. The acutely sick require rest if they are to recover. In chronic disease, the "rest cure" accomplishes more than any other measure. People often make wonderful improvement while undergoing a "rest cure" in spite of bad food, bad environment, tobacco and drugs.

All such facts tend to establish that part of Dr. Robert Walter's "Law of Life" which he expressed in these words:

"The success of whose (the vital force) work is directly proportioned to the amount of the force, and inversely to the degree of its activity."

"Certainly," he declares, "inversely as the degree of activity is frought with immense consequences to human health and life. It makes all the difference whether we are *increasing* or *reducing* vital power by increasing vitay activity**** Vital activity expends power or increases it; if the latter, rest and sleep are waste of time and opportunity (and should shorten life. Author); if the former, the medical practice of our day is engaged in exhausting vital power."—*Life's Great Law.*

If the success of the work of an organism in repairing and restoring itself is inversely to the degree of its activities, as we have shown, why then should it seem strange that suspended animation is a saving measure? To the writer, the saving office of this state is self-evident.

Dr. Joel Shew stated:

"There is an old saying, 'that while there is life there is hope'; and every physician who has had some experience, can readily call to mind cases in which he thought it was not possible for the patient to survive, and in which he did finally recover. And more, he may, in some cases, have supposed a patient actually dead—the vital principle wholly extinct—and the patient did yet recover, spontaneously, in spite of doctors and drugs.' Such cases certainly have occurred. I have myself seen at least two within the past six years: one, of a gentleman who had been for a long time delirious in fever, and before I had seen him; the other, a child that had cholera, and appeared to be dead, but which lived. The older a physician becomes, the less willing will he be to prognosticate *positively* in any given case."—*Hydropathic Family Physician*, p. 40, 1854.

At this point it may be well to introduce a few cases by way of illustration. To Jennings, again, shall we give the honor of supplying the first cases.

"Case 111.—Mr. Birmingham, gardener, complained a few days of slight turns of dizziness of the head, and on going out to work one morning, staggered and fell, a compainion by his side breaking the fall. He was conducted back to his lodgings, and by lying still on his back, with his head and shoulders a little dependent, he recovered and retained his consciousness, and suffered but little pain. He remained in this condition for a week, with no appetite for food, and took none. The whole alimentary canal was inactive, and there was but little power of voluntary motion, with a constant tendency to faintness or giddiness on raising the head. At the expiration of a week he began gradually to recover, and in due process of time re-enjoyed his usual good health."

"Case IV.—A RELAPSE AND PECULIARLY ALARMING CASE OF AGUE AND FEVER. In the summer and autumn of 1844, Mr. William Hosford, of Michigan, had a long and severe turn of the ague and fever, but enjoyed a tolerable respite from it during the ensuing winter and spring.

"In the succeeding summer he visited Oberlin, Ohio, partly on account of his health, as it was still rather feeble, and soon suffered a relapse in his complaint. After running down pretty rapidly for two or three weeks with regular every other-day paroxysms, he sunk into a profound lethargic state, and remained senseless and motionless for nearly three days; after which he rose, slowly at first, and returned home, had no more of the ague and fever, and has since enjoyed uninterrupted good health.

"At Michigan, during the first season of the Ague and fever, Mr. Hosford had the advantage of thorough medication under Allopathic supervision. At Oberlin, in pursuance of his own free and deliberate choice, while reason was on the throne, nature was permitted to manage her own concerns in her own way, with Orthopathy for her handmaid, or general supervisor of her affairs."

"Case IX.—Subject, Capt. C. Elliott of Huntington, opposite Derby Narrows, my then place of residence. In consequence of a rapid rise in the Housatonic river which flowed between us, I did not see this patient till the latter part of the night, when the case had been a number of hours in hasty progress, and seemed drawing fast to a fatal close. The extremities were cold, pulse gone at the wrist, strength prostrate and tendency to faint. As I entered the room, I was told that immediate and active means must be used, or the Captain would die. To quiet mental disturbance and apprehension, pills, powders and drops were administered; while the real physical disturbance was left entirely to the freedom of natural law. The extreme point of the recuperative work was reached about the time that I began to dispense the representatives of medicine, and in a short time there was an evident abatement of the disorder, and of course the little pills, powders and drops took the credit of the cure. A few hours after I made the Captain a second visit and found him sitting up, quite comfortable and in fine spirits. 'Well, now, Doctor,' said the Captain, 'you see that medicine is sometimes necessary in "extreme cases," I could not have lived without it.'

"At Westfield, Chautauqua Co., a young lady was supposed to have died of dysentery, on Saturday afternoon, and on Sunday, after having been prepared for burial, she came to life, spoke, and is likely to recover. So says an exchange!

"If there was a 'tendency to death' in these cases, a real antagonistic principle, distinct from the pestilential causes, and superinduced by them, which was warring against the vital economy, in what did it consist, and why did it yield the conflict and suffer its victims to escape, when they were so completely in its power? There *had* been an enemy in the field, a potent one, and it had done its dreadful work, struck its almost fatal blow in an unguarded moment, and in that act had spent itself, and was no longer an object of terror or regard. Not so its effects; those remained and were to be recovered from, or all was lost; and there was but one way in which this end could be secured, and that was by withholding the remnant of vital forces from all the coarser or visible parts of the system, and concentrating them upon the more attenuated or finer portions that lay beyond the ken of man, leaving only a sufficient number of sentinels in the open field to prevent the intrusion of inorganic or disorganizing forces. And the fact that precaution was taken to guard every tissue of the body with vital force sufficient to keep them in a salvable state for so long a time, under an extremity that required the suspension of every visible function to meet the exigencies of these remarkable cases, leaving nothing to human view but the cold semblance of death, is a strong argument in favor of Orthopathic theory. For in any case if a single essential organ had been left *entirely* destitute of the vital principle but for a short time, through lack either of forecast, or ability to supply it, the inorganic affinities would have at once seized upon that organ, and spoiled it for further organic use, and the whole organism of which it was a member, would have fallen an easy prey to the principle or law of decomposition. Will Heteropathy—any branch of it—be kind and candid enough to tell us how an accurrence of this kind is explicable on its principles? The pulse ceases to beat, the lungs to heave, and every fibre within the purview of human cognition is gelid, apparently, in death; and yet without any medicinal or artificial interposition, life is restored. Now the question is, if there was no real necessity for this retrogression of life, under the circumstances; if no good purpose could be answered thereby, but on the contrary, the retrogressive powers were acting a suicidal part, subverting their own habitation and themselves, how when the work of destruction was apparently complete, was reanimation effected? There was no wrong or subversive action, or wrong tendency in these cases. The movements were wisely devised, arranged and executed. There was a deep necessity for holding back the organic forces until life seemed extinct in order to save it. Neither in these or other cases is life suffered to wane further than its safety or greatest good demands, within the scope and ability of the life-sustaining principle. When this principle, let it consist in what it may, is generated, elaborated, evolved or any how furnished, and becomes free to move and act, it is constrained by inexorable law to take its position and expend itself when and where it can accomplish the most for the safety and highest well being of the whole system. And this constraining influence is enhanced in direct proportion to the general destitution of sustaining energy; that is, every part of the system has its wants, and has a way of expressing them; and in proportion as its necessities rise above its supply, in just that proportion does it call with increased importunity for help."

"The fact that extremely low diseased states of the system have been recovered from by the unaided operations of nature, not only militates against the Heteropathic doctrines, of disease, but actually demolishes it. . . . And yet the instances have been very numerous, in which spontaneous recoveries have taken place from under circumstances apparently the most forlorn and unpromising.

"When Mr. Wm. Hosford, whose case is mentioned in part third of this work, was lying in the deep collapse of a typhoid intermittent, his son, the Rev. Oromel Hosford, who had the care of his father, and was carrying out his wishes, which were made known while the father's rational voluntary powers were in active exercise, was beset with much ardor by a number of prominent citizens to have speedy and thorough medication employed for the relief of his honored patient, and was told that he was assuming a fearful responsibility in the course which he was pursuing. 'Why,' said they, 'how is it *possible* that your father can live, borne down as he is, to the very border of the grave, without the use of the proper remedial means?' Sure enough, what possible chance was there for the man's life under the let-alone treatment, if the nature of disease is what Heteropathy has taken it to be? And the recovery of Mr. Hosford ought to have led those men to reverse their opinion of disease, and taught them its true Orthopathic character as clearly as a mirror would have shown them that they had noses on their faces. Many cases of resuscitation from *apparent death*, with cholera and other diseases, have been reported in different parts of the world, and in some instances a number of hours elapsed between expiration and resuscitation.

"Some cases of this kind occurred in this country during the late prevalence of the cholera One of these took place in Cincinnati. The body of a man, a number of

107

hours after the apparent extinction of life, was put into a coffin and laid in a vault for the purpose of being conveyed home on the arrival of his friends, who lived at some distance. On opening the coffin, it was found that the man had come to, turned partly over, gnawed some of the flesh off his fingers, and exhibited a ghastly appearance."

"In the fall of 1822, Miss Ann Hurd, with genuine typhus fever, that continued for a number of weeks, became exceedingly debilitated, and for a week was scarcely able to move a limb, and twice in twenty-four hours would seem just on the point of entering the dark valley.

"The most alarming of these sinking turns occurred about midnight; and in one of these, to all human appearance, she passed away from earth, I closed her eyes, the family turned away weeping, and Mrs. Pool, her nurse, said, 'I am glad to see her die so gently.' In a few moments I perceived a light heaving of the breast. Breathing returned, and from that time, gradually for awhile, she rose to her former good health."

With these cases we leave Dr. Jennings to let Dr. J. H. Tilden present one case. He says:

"This patient, a boy about thirteen years old; quiet, frail looking; nervous-mental temperament; had been in the mountains on a vacation trip, camping out, fishing and hunting He had not been in camp more than two weeks when he began to feel ill. He was too tired and weak to do much fishing; every day he thought he would be better, but every day found him weaker and feeling a little more uncomfortable until at the end of a week of ill-feeling his friends decided to break camp and bring him home.

"I was called to see him in the evening of the day he returned home. I found him a little feverish, temperature 101.5° F., pulse 110, tongue slightly coated, rather long, edges and tip somewhat red; headache, bad taste in mouth and no appetite. He had been eating with more or less relish until this date.

"My diagnosis was typhoid fever and my prescription was: Be quiet, eat no food, drink all the water desired and wash bowels with enema night and morning; bind wet towel on bowels, towel to be wet in cold water night and morning.

"Before 9:00 A. M. the next morning, when I was to call, I was sent for in great haste; the messenger informed me that the patient was in a very desperate state from hemorrhage of the bowels. I had but a block and a half to go, hence I was at the boy's bedside very soon after the hemorrhage, and I took in the situation at a glance. I do not think I have ever seen a more profound collapse than that boy was in. His pulse was not countable on account of its weakness and frequency. As near as I could make out the rate was near 180, temperature below normal.

"I took the pillow from under his head, elevated the foot of the bed six inches and ordered absolute quiet. No one was to go into his room except the nurse, and I forbade her speaking to him. She was instructed to keep his feet warm and take water to him occasionally, but never speak nor ask him a question. She was to put the spoon with water to his mouth and repeat as often as he would swallow it.

"Here was a typical case for hypodermics of heart tonics, general stimulation, nutritive enemas, scientific madcap endeavors at restoration and all sort of subdued whisperings and crazy attempts at revival, but nothing was done except what I have related above. The parents wanted to know how soon I thought he should take nourishment. This was after I had explained to them that I did not intend to use stimulants, heart tonics nor food in any shape, or form, and that if they thought I was not doing enough, they were welcome to send for someone who would; that I did not intend to give drugs at any time and as for food, I should wait for full reaction, which I did and it came the eleventh day. The pulse was not countable for several days, but it did grow stronger and more regular, and finally it came down to 110, after which I prescribed a very light food and increased it daily as the pulse grew stronger.

"Here was a case of almost fatal hemorrhage; the exhaustion was so great that the boy could not lift his head, hand or foot, and this frightful weakness continued with but very slight improvement for four or five days. The improvement was not enough to justify feeding before the eleventh day.

"This case refutes the professional idea of the necessity of heart tonics, food, etc. I insist that this boy would have died if he had been interfered with in any way."

In comparison with the amount of work to be done, the vital energies are few and feeble, and all that can be accomplished, even under the most favorable conditions, is to save enough of the old fabric to build upon anew. To this end a great economy is exercised. There is a general concentration of the forces of life upon its most essential organs with only enough left in the other organs to maintain them in a salvable condition. This work is accomplished, where it is not opposed and counteracted by treatment with the greatest regularity, and with as little haste as is compatible with final safety. In this retrocession of power from the organs of the body, the voluntary motions are usually the first to lose functional power. The digestive apparatus is the next to follow. Then the mind is put at rest. In some cases the need for conservation is so great that the heart is slowed down till it shows but the feeblest signs of life, respiration becomes almost imperceptible, temperature falls below normal and death seems imminent. But nature has succeeded in her main object. She has brought the expenditure of power within the limits of the available supply, after having appropriated sufficient to the organs essential to life to maintain them in a restorable condition ready for replenishment and use as the replenishment of power warrants. Although death seems imminent, there is hope in such cases.

Space does not permit giving more such cases. Let us come now to the practical conclusions the facts presented justify.

First, they demonstrate that the sick require rest in order that they may recover. They show beyond the shadow of a doubt that the sicker an organism is, the greater is the need for rest. The weaker is the patient, the greater is the need for *doing nothing*. These conclusions are opposed to the prevailing practice of stimulation. The weaker a patient grows under the prevailing practices the more he is stimulated and the more he is stimulated the weaker he grows.

Dr. Walter well observed:—

"As therefore activity expends and exhausts, while passivity recuperates and preserves, and the power of life being the all important consideration, it follows that the recovery of health, preservation of life, and the cure of disease, take place and must be calculated *directly as the amount of the power and inversely as the degree of its activity*. The inactivity of sleep, not the strength of stimulation, is the great representative process of recuperation and health, and all treatments that should be successful with the enfeebled and chronically ailing, no less than with the acutely sick, must operate as sleep does. It must reduce activity and increase power, instead of increasing activity and reducing power, as is the plan everywhere in vogue."

Any mode of living that is not based upon the conservation of the body's powers, rather than their dissipation, must sooner or later lead to weakness, disease and premature death. It matters not whether your energies are wasted by thrills and excitement, or by drugs and mechanical stimulants, sexual excesses, worry, anger, tenseness, loss of sleep, and dissipations and excesses of various kinds, the ultimate results are all the same.

Any method of caring for the sick that does not aim at conserving the patient's powers must result in much needless suffering and many premature deaths. Work exhausts, whether it is work of one organ or of the whole body,—rest is the condition of recuperation. Rest for each organ is as important as rest for the whole organism. Whether it be calomel for the liver, salts for the bowels, digitalis for the heart, or whiskey or hot and cold baths and tonics for the general system, whatever arouses or increases vital activity, and particularly vital resistance, exhausts the patient's powers and hinders or prevents recovery. Promoting increased action in the present necessitates reduced action in the future. The future reduction must necessarily be commensurate with the present increase—"*action and reaction are equal but opposite*."

We are influenced too much by appearances. We must learn to distinguish between processes of expenditure and processes of recuperation. Prevailing modes of medical practice produce the diseases they seek to cure and exhaust the powers they seek to sustain because men are content to be guided by appearances. A more enlightened age will look back upon the practices of the present schools of healing (killing) with greater horror than that with which we now look back upon the practices of a thousand or two thousand years ago.

109

THE RATIONALE OF CRISES

Chapter XIII

REMEDIAL efforts are always going on in the organism when it is in any way morbidly affected. This is true even in those cases where the morbid influence is unknown to the individual and its effects are so slight as to be unrecognized by him. When these morbid influences are greater than the organism can overcome their effects accumulate until a formidable pathological condition develops. When this stage is reached some unusual effort is required to preserve vital integrity. It is then that the efforts of the vital organism are disproportionately manifest in one or more parts of the body or at one or more of the eliminating organs, and we call this *disease*.

That the living organism, by virtue of its own inherent powers, does purge itself of impurities and repair its damages is no longer a matter of doubt. That its curative efforts are sometimes disproportionately directed to one or more organs of the body and is accompanied with more or less systemic commotion is equally certain. In the preceding chapters we have presented ample proof that disease is a curative process. In this chapter we propose to develop this fact a bit further, and incidentally, supply more proof of this principle.

In doing this we cannot do better than discuss a few acute diseases and show from ascertained and admitted facts that acute diseases, at least, do accomplish a curative work. We might begin, innocently, with typhoid. Dr. Richard C. Cabot, one of the highest authorities in medicine, says:—

"One of the curious things about typhoid is that people are sometimes healthier after an attack than before, people who are thin are especially apt to be stouter, not merely for the first few weeks but for life."

Emerson says (Essentials of Medicine), of typhoid fever:—

"After the fever has gone, convalescence begins. The patient is at first thin and weak, but he slowly returns to good health or to even better health than he formerly had."

If *disease* is really *something* that "attacks" the body, if it were of a destructive nature, improved health could not be one of the results of its devastating ravages. The improved health can only be explained on the ground that the pain, fever, prostration, lack of desire for food and lack of digestive power, profuse sweating, diarrhea, vomiting, unusual kidney action, skin eruption, etc., accomplish a curative work. To medical authorities, this improved health may be a "curious thing;" to us, it is fraught with much meaning.

In describing the symptoms of gout, Dayton's "Practice of Medicine" remarks: "*After the attack the general health may be improved.*"

An improvement in the health of the sufferer, following an "attack" of gout, proves beyond a doubt that the pain, fever, inflammation, profuse acid sweating, elimination of large quantities of highly acid urine, the lessened or suspended food intake, enforced rest, etc., have accomplished a cleanisng, purifying work.

Cyanide of potassium, an excellent allopathic "remedy," if "applied locally causes inflammation of the skin with an eczematous eruption, and if applied in quantity to an abraded surface will produce fatal effects." The inflammation and eruption, which is also a form of inflammation, are means of expelling the poison. The true character of inflammation has already been shown. Similar to these eruptions are those that follow the swallowing, inhalation, absorption or injection of various drugs, such, for instance, as bromide, mercury, etc., and serums. They are means by which these poisonous substances are thrown off.

Of a similar nature to the eruptions produced by cyanide of potassium and other drugs and serums are the secondary eruptions which often follow vaccination and so-called syphilitic infection—generalized vaccina and secondary syphilis. These eruptions serve the same eliminative and protective purposes. An excellent example of this same phenomenon is furnished us by the exanthematous or eruptive diseases.

Gould and Pyle say, *Cyclopedia of Medicine and Surgery*, second edition:—

"The pre-eruptive stage of an exanthematous disease, especially scarlet fever, is sometimes ushered in by one or two convulsions followed by coma. The temperature is high, the pulse is rapid, and the respirations are frequent. *The coma disappears with the appearance of the eruption.*" (Italics mine.)

These same authorities say of smallpox:—

"The fever rises rapidly from 103° to 104° F., within 48 hours, where it remains until the third or fourth day, or until papular eruption appears, when it falls several degrees"

The lesson of these two cases is obvious. The eruption rids the system of the poisons that are endangering life. The high temperature, convulsions and coma in the first case and the high fever in the second are preliminary preparations for the eruptions. The eruptions serve the same purpose of *elimination*, they do in generalized vaccina and secondary syphilis. That this is so is evidenced by the ending of the coma and the decline of the temperature immediately upon the appearance of the eruption. Thus is manifest the truth of the oft repeated assertions of Louis Kuhne, when dealing with smallpox, measles, scarlet-fever, and other eruptive diseases that "the more profuse the eruption the less is the child's life endangered. The less abundant and slighter the eruption, on the other hand, the greater is the danger." "The smaller that portion of the skin which co-operates in expelling the morbid matter, by admitting and eruption to break out, the greater the danger." "As soon as the rash is fully developed, vital danger is over in *most cases*." This may be questioned by some because confluent smallpox is more severe than the discrete form. But this is only an apparent contradiction. Such cases represent, it is true, more severe forms of the disease but the greater severity is not due to more rash but to more cause for the rash. The fact still stands, I believe, that the greater the area co-operating in the work of elimination (eruptions) in these cases, the less is the danger to life in the individual case.

A young boy was all his life, up to six and one-half years, in poor health. He was underweight, suffered with frequent nose bleeds, with the beginning of each spring had bronchitis, and had gone the usual round of treatment and operations. Tonsils and adenoids had been removed. He had been carried from one hospital to another and had had his lungs X-Rayed a number of times in search of evidence of tuberculosis.

At six and one-half years of age he developed a very severe case of scarlet fever. His life was dispaired of. The eruption was great and scaling afterwards was as great. But after this the whole condition of the boy changed. His weight became normal, his nose bleeds ceased, he had no more bronchitis, and, upon being examined at school, was given a health percentage of perfect.

If this were an isolated case, it might be regarded as proving nothing. But it is not an isolated case. This improved health follows all eruptive diseases if they are not suppressed by the treatment. A few years ago a brilliant young English Nature Cure physician showed from the official statistics of that country that wherever an epidemic of smallpox had existed it was always followed, in that locality, by a falling off in the cancer rate. The rate of falling off in cancer was far in excess of the number of deaths that occurred during the smallpox. Previous to this, however, a Dr. Wallace in a work entitled "Cholera," and in another entitled "Necessity for Smallpox," had shown that acute diseases have saved many lives. An acquaintance of the present author was always in very poor health until he had a case of smallpox. For many years thereafter he enjoyed excellent health. Is there any wonder Dr. Claunch declares smallpox to be almost a cure-all. There is no means of estimating how many people are saved from tumors and cancers and other degenerative diseases by the cleansing and reconstructive work accomplished by acute disease. Were it not for acute disease, man's present mode of living would produce far more physical degeneracy than exists at present, and would produce it much earlier in life.

In speaking of smallpox, medical men frequently say: "The chief difficulty in diagnosis lies in those cases where the disease is so virulent that the patient dies before the eruption develops." This statement confirms Kuhne's statements in that it reveals that death is not due to smallpox, but to the failure of smallpox—that is, the body was unable to develop the disease, particularly the eruption, and was forced to succumb to the poisons it sought to eliminate. The patient was not killed by disease but by the poisons. He died because the disease failed. A successful acute *disease* would have *preserved life.*

In this connection a description of hermorrhagic smallpox by Chas. P. Emerson, M.D. ("*Essentials of Medicine*"), is of interest. He says:—

"The 'hemorrhagic' smallpox is a very virulent type. In some cases there are only little hemorrhages into the vesicles, but the true hemmorrhagic form, 'black small-pox,' is from the first exceedingly severe. On the second or third day appears an extensive rash of hemorrhages under the skin and even into the eyes. The patient bleeds from the mouth, nose, lungs, rectum, kidneys, etc. He is a frightful object, with skin of a deep purple color, the eyes bloody, the face swollen, etc. *These cases die early, even on the third day, before any papules have appeared.*" (Italics mine.)

Chicken-pox or "varicella" is a similar disease to discrete smallpox but not so severe. In this disease the rash appears in the first twenty-four hours of the fever. It is our belief that this is the chief difference between chicken-pox and smallpox—the fact that the body gets the rash out early. We are convinced that the earlier in the disease the rash develops the less severe the disease will be. Even under medical mis-management chicken-pox seldom proves fatal.

Emerson says of measles (Essentials of Medicine) :—

"In very severe cases, usually fatal, the rash consists not of little red papules which disappear on pressure, but of minute hemorrhages under the skin (black measles). The patients thus affected may bleed from the mouth also, the bowels, etc."

Consider the above facts in the light of all that has gone before and they take on a significance that the medical world (I include all schools and cults) has never dared to face. Emerson does indeed recognize this principle in relation to fever. He says: (*Essentials of Medicine*) :—

"While these toxins of germs may be called the "cause' of the elevation of temperature, yet the word 'reason' (we would say *occasion*) is better. Fever seems to be one of the protective measures of the body, a means to an end, and that end is a fight against the *germ*. The body seems to fight the germ better at a higher than at a normal temperature, and so the fever is really rather a part of the defense than a direct result of the toxin in the sense in which the headache is such a result. We emphasize this point because so many persons think the fever an evil and try to lower it by drugs. They can do this easily, but with no benefit—perhaps always with injury—to the patient."

Perhaps more direct proof of the curative nature of acute disease is contained in the well known fact that chronic disease is often cured by an acute disease. Within the last few years we have heard much of the malaria "cure" for paresis and syphilis. This "cure" constists in producing an acute disease in a man or woman suffering from one or the other of these maladies. The supposed causitive agents of malaria are introduced into the victim's body. A temperature of 105° F. is often maintained for from five to seven hours and in some cases for seventeen to eighteen hours.

Professor Wagner von Jauregg, of Vienna, who is responsible for this method of "cure" observed that victims of paralysis showed improvement after fever diseases— not just one fever disease, but *after several of the fever diseases.*

In an article in the *Medical Journal and Record*, April 1, 1925, Herman Goodman, M.D., (New York City), says:—

"It has been known for a long time that remissions of chronic disease may occur after an acute specific fever, or a long continued suppurative process."

Again:—

"As early as 1816 it was noted that cases of general paralysis frequently showed remissions of symptoms, and that often apparent cures were established following febrile diseases."

The "Practical Medine Series, 1924," says:—

"Viacuska reports two cases, one occuring in his own practice, in which patients suffering from syphilis developed typhus fever. In both cases a positive Wassermann remained after vigorous therapy (which means, from their point of view that "vigorous therapy" failed to cure the patient. Author), but after typhus fever the blood showed a negative Wassermann reaction, and to all appearances there was a cure of the syphilis "

The cure of chronic disease by various fevers (acute disease) confirms in a very positive manner our contention for over a hundred years that the fevers are curative processes. The cure of chronic disease by a "long continued suppurative process" confirms in an equally positive manner our equally old claim that the body often establishes a fontanel or makes use of a wound as such, for the purpose of pouring out of the system toxins and accumulations that are interfering with the life processes and impairing health. Every acute disease from a cold to typhus fever or bubonic plague is a curative process. So is chronic disease a curative process, although, not so efficient as acute disease. It is not so efficient due to vital exhaustion—indeed, if the reactive power was present it would be an acute and not a chronic disease. Chronic disease also represents a contending against chronic provocation to which accomodation or toleration has been established.

These facts bring up the questions: What is disease? If acute disease cures a chronic disease, is acute disease the friend or foe of life? Upon the correct answer to these questions the future will build an enduring and dependable system of caring for the sick.

In strictest accuracy, disease is neither the friend nor the foe of life. It is the action of life in defending itself against its foes. The organs of the body are constituted for health. They are governed, in their actions, by laws as fixed and eternal as the law of gravitation and can no more disobey these laws than stones can fly upward or than a man can lift himself by pulling at his boot straps. Their action is always healthward, and, in the very nature of things, can never be in any other direction. Whether in the most violent stages of acute disease or in the lowest and most feeble stages of chronic disease, every action of every organ of the body is designed to restore and maintain health.

The human body which evolves itself from the ovum to the highest point of completion and maintains itself in health under many handicaps and adverse influences, resorts with unerring certainty to the best means for the restoration of its health when this has been impaired from whatever cause. Not only does the body choose, of its own accord, the best means for a hasty restoration of health, but it possesses as well, the capacity to order its functions and processes so as to delay, as long as possible, its ultimate destruction by inimical forces and influences which it is unable to overcome or destroy. The symptoms of disease are, therefore, either for the elimination of the immediate causes that endanger life and the repair of structural damages, or for the longest possible protraction of life in the face of the organic destruction that is gradually creeping upon the body due to pathoferic causes it is unable to destroy or overcome.

From all this it logically follows that no indication of disease, no symptom, should be removed through forcible means, but should be permitted to continue unabated until it has accomplished its work. We live in a more learned than thinking age and I can hardly expect the great majority of readers to see, in the facts above presented, confirmation of Orthopathy—that is, that disease is "right action" or a curative process.

For doctors of all schools to admit this principle is to admit that most cases of chronic disease are due to suppression of acute disease by treatment—and they are. If they admit these things it would be tantamount to the admission that the curing professions are the greatest enemies of the human race that ever existed—which they truly are. To admit that disease is a curative process (and it is) is to admit that all their combat with disease is an onslaught against the patient's life— which it is. It would be to admit that complications, sequelea and deaths are the direct results of their meddlesome intreference with the natural processes of disease—and they are. For physicians of all schools to admit these things would be to condemn themselvse and openly admit that they have no reason for existence—that both the well and the sick would be far better off without them.

Even in chronic disease crisis will often occur. Dr. Joel Shew, in his *Water Cure Manual*, published in 1847, says:—

"A crisis may be said to be a visible effort on the part of nature or the natural power of the system, to rid it of some morbid matters in it, or expelling them at some of the natural outlets of the system, as the skin, bowels and kidneys."

Dr. E. Johnson wrote:—

"That the system, by virtue of its own inherent energies sometimes purges itself of morbid matters by a crisis, that is, by establishing some temporary outlet through which such matters may and do escape, is perfeclty certain. The Aleppo boil, small-pox, measles, and many other well-known diseases, prove this to demonstration, and beyond the possibility of question."

These crises take various forms and are named by medical men according to the form as different diseases. Crises may come on without any accidental or unusual exposure or gross dietetic error, etc., or they may be incited by such external factors. If the former, the living power or nature, as we often call it, arouses itself against the disease influence for the same reason and in the same way that it arouses itself following the exposure to external factors. In the latter case the external factors are to be regarded as the straw that breaks the camel's back and forces a reaction against the disease influence, while the crisis of "disease" which occurs without the influence of the final straw has been made necessary by conditions in the organism that have reached the breaking point.

An acute reaction against a morbid influence, a crisis or acute disease, is then some unusual vital action in self defense. If, however, due to the reasons already enumerated, the body is not able to overcome or destroy the unatural or morbid conditions which have been imposed upon it then the body is forced, in self-defense, to accomodate or adapt itself to the condition as far as possible.

The body accomodates itself to the habitual use of tobacco, alcohol, opium, etc., to the extent of its ability to do so, but this does not prevent these substances from slowly and gradually undermining the constitution and finally resulting in disease and death.

Likewise, the unnatural and morbid conditions which have been imposed upon the system, which it has not been able to overcome but has been compelled to accommodate itself to, also, gradually and insidously undermine the system, resulting in disease. If the body is able by means of a crisis to overcome the disease influence then health is the result of disease. But if it is unable to overcome such influences and is not destroyed by them, it is forced to settle back into its accustomed quiet and make the condition as bearable as possible. This gives us chronic disease.

Even in chronic disease the periodic return of crises is very common. These may take the form of boils, eruptions, diarrhea, sweatings, mucous and bloody discharges, discharge of highly colored urine, feverishness etc. Under natural living conditions, where enervating influences are removed and the organism is gradually strengthened the body, not infrequently, arouses itself to acute eliminating efforts or crises. These, too, occur, apparently, in accord with the law of periodicity and are similar to all other crises. Crises usually last until the disease producing factors have been reduced to the toleration point. This point varies with the individual and with the varying conditions of the individual. Thus the greater the amount of vitality one possesses, the less morbid matter will his system tolerate, and as the vitality of one with chronic disease is gradually raised, his toleration point also rises so that crises occur.

There is much difference of opinion about the necessity of crises in the recovery from chronic disease. Some authorities maintain that complete recovery from chronic conditions can be accomplished only through crises. Dr. Trall wrote in his *Hydropathic Encyclopedia*, Vol. 2, p. 62:—

"It is perfectly certain that many bad cases of chronic disease are cured without any appearance of crises whatever; it is equally certain, in my judgment, that some few cases are utterly incurable without the production of a decided crisis—and I am fully convinced that in many cases crises are rendered unnecessarily and even dangerously severe by excessive or injudicious treatment."

Dr. Tilden says that while crises are very common during the process of recovery from chronic conditions, these are not absolutely essential to recovery in every case. Even Dr. Lindlahr finally admitted that many do recover without marked crises.

It is the authors opinion that crises are often forced by harsh treatment. In those institutions where the idea seems to prevail that the more the body is tortured the quicker will be the recovery, it is no uncommon thing for a patient of low resistance to be kept in a cold bath for long periods, or to be given such baths too frequently. Or, patients are forced to stay in the scorching sun until their bodies are burned and blistered from head to foot. Such treatments may easily force a reaction or crisis. Again, I am convinced that in many cases a prolonged fast can be made to accomplish the work of crises, although I am aware that crises often develop during a fast.

Crises develop in keeping with the diathetic tendencies of the individual. This is the explanation for the fact that "healing crises," as they have been called, often come in the same form and at the same location as that of some previous acute "disease." There is no difference in the essential nature of the "healing" crisis, and the "disease" crisis. This classification is wholly arbitrary. A "healing" crisis is one in which the vital powers are strong and voluntarily start a house cleaning when there may be no immediate danger to life. In this case the organism is on the aggressive. "Disease" crises develop under conditions in which the disease influence is great enough to be an immediate danger to life. The organism is forced to undertake the house cleaning; it is on the defensive. The tendency of both is towards recovery. They are essentially one and the same process.

Dr. Jennings used to refer to those with acute disease as having been "*suddenly laid aside for repairing purposes*" and connected with this both in acute and chronic disease what he called a "*rotary renovating operation*," and which he declared is "constantly going forward among the numerous organs of the body while in an imperfect state " The idea back of this was that in an enervated body all parts could not be maintained in perfect repair at all times so nature repaired the organs one or two at a time, always concentrating her energies upon those organs that were most in need of repairs He said:—

"The rotary tendency or alternating law of the animal economy, for the government of pathological movements, under a complication of ills, may readily be observed and learned by anyone who is subject to a variety of complaints of any kind. At one time he may have a headache, toothache, or nose bleed; at another, 'crick of the back,' or lameness of a shoulder, hip or some other joint or joints, or in some muscle or muscles; or a cold, asthma, eruption or some pathological embarrassment to which he is liable and which will be passed through a cancelling process in regular order, if not injudiciously interferred with. Heavy general fits of sickness are sometimes immediately preceeded or ushered in by other affections; and sometimes, too, closed by them. Physicians speak of diseases coming in under the mask of other diseases. The Orthopathic philosophy of this is easy. In some cases where the system is laboring under a serious complication of injuries, before an essential tissue or group of organs that have been badly damaged, can be safely and conveniently put under a renovating operation, some other part must be improved in its condition. Smallpox and other heavy exanthematous diseases, are sometimes apt to be preceded by fits, particularly in children. Physicians also speak of critical termination of disease, and some practitioners try to bring on the condition that they have known or heard of being the closing part of a disease, as if this would be a cure for the whole malady. The affections that mark the winding up of general curative efforts are numerous, such as eruptions, diarrhea, small spontaneous bleedings, as a few drops of blood from the nose, sweating, gaping etc. Yawning, or gaping, is a common token of amendment. No one that is hard sick ever gapes until there is a change for the better in the specific disease through which he is then passing."—*Philosophy of Human Life*, pp. 147-8.

He records a case of pneumonia that at the end of two weeks appeared nearing recovery when a diarrhea developed. This was followed by more improvement when night-sweats developed. To the father's anxious inquiry about what he was going to do with the night sweats, he replied: "I am going to let them sweat it out." This he did and the patient went steadily forward to health.

Dr. Jennings wisely asks: "What human intellect could have foreseen the need for these renovating efforts, or having foreseen them, what earthly power or skill could have superceded the necessity of such work?" I would also ask: What earthly power or skill could have hastened or aided such work?

The doctrine of crisis is as old as Hippocrates. Crises frequently occur in acute disease and are still recognized as such, even by so artificial a system as the allopathic school. It may be well at this point, however ,to say that under orthopathic care acute diseases are generally relieved by mild, yet effectual functional efforts of all the excretory organs, unattended by any great commotion in the organism, or strong determination to anyone emunctory. There is seldom, or never, a sinking of the vital powers which can in any sense be called critical.

With chronic disease the case is often different. These, when left to nature, are frequently resolved by some external abscess or internal abscess. Many cases do recover without any disturbance which can be properly called a crisis, while, others recover only after repeated disturbances which are more or less severe and which are properly called crises.

In dealing with the forms of crises I cannot do better than to quote what Dr. Trall said of them :—

"The most common forms in which crises, or critical efforts, present themselves are diarrhea, boils, and general feverishness. Boils present all manner of appearances from the hard diffuse, inflammatory swelling, with scarcely any supporting point, to the deep, fully-matured, sub-cutaneous abscess; there may be one or several at the same time, or they may succeed each other for weeks or months, and be very painful, or scarcely troublesome. Those of full habit, saguine temperament, and active external circulation, are most subject to boils and eruptions."

"Diarrheas, when critical, come on without any accidental or unusual exposure or dietetic error, and continue with greater or less severity from three days to two weeks. There is not usually much pain, gripping, or distress of any kind in the bowels, but the evacuations are thin, watery, and frequent; generally there are from three to six or eight motions in twenty-four hours. In persons who have been most subject to piles the motions will be most frequent, and attended with considerable bearing down or dragging sensation about the lower bowel, and the discharge will exhibit a great amount of mucous or slimy matter, often intermixed with blood. A critical looseness of the bowels is not attended with debility like ordinary diarrhea; if long continued, there is, of course, some degree of languor. Those who have long labored under derange-ments of the digestive organs, and particularly those with torpid livers and constipated bowels more especially, if these conditions are complicated with pale, yellow, bloodless skin, and shrivelled, superficial, capillary vessels, are most liable to critical evacuations by the bowels; and, as far as my observation extends, they are invariably beneficial, always being succeeded by a decided sense of improvement in the patient's entire physiological condition.

"The term 'feverishness', does not very well express the other common form of critical action, but I know of no better one to employ. It is characterized by more or less of the symptoms which attend an attack of simple fever, but they appear in a more disguised and irregular form. There is chilliness and heat, languor, depression, backache, headache, general restlessness, great sensitiveness to cold, etc. etc., but, unlike the same symptoms in a paroxysm of simple fever, they do not follow each other in the order of the cold, hot and sweating stages. This febrile disturbance continues from one day to a week, when, unless aggravated by improper treatment, the body recovers its balance of action and feeling, and the patient feels himself advanced at least one step on the road to health. Other manifestations of critical disturbances, as eruptions, rashes, free evacuation of bile, etc., stiffness of the muscles, joints, fetid perspirations, do occur, but require no special management."

Boils and skin eruptions are especailly likely to occur in those who change from the conventional death dealing diet to a sensible mode of eating. Boils often come out in crops and may last for weeks. However, their appearance is always beneficial to the health of the individual. The case of a former patient of the author's will serve to illustrate this nicely. Mrs. H. of New York City was paralized from her waist to her knees. There was no power of motion in any part of the paralized regions. Medical physicians had told her that she would always be paralized. In addition to the paralysis there were severe pains in the back.

Abandoning medical treatment after her physicians had pronounced her case hopeless she resorted to natural methods: Her condition forced her to rest. A change of diet was all that was done. After a few weeks a large boil developed on her back. This was followed by others until there were thirteen in all, one appearing as the other was cured. With the appearance of each boil there was an immediate and marked improvement in her condition. With the appearance of the first boil she became able to move her thighs. Three boils enabled her to walk. By the time the thirteenth appeared she was walking as well as ever and has not had a return of her trouble. At this writing she has been well for nearly two years.

In this connection a statement made by Dr. Trall is of interest. He said:—

"Critical efforts attempt to perform a threefold duty: Eliminate morbid matters, balance the circulation of the blood, and equalize the distribution of nervous energy. This latter duty is too generally overlooked. Some authors write as though all the good effected by a crisis, a boil, for example, was the riddance of a specific quantity of morbid material; but this is a very narrow view of the subject: that is indeed one, but the least of the remedial effects accomplished. The amount of morbid matter deterged from an extraordinary boil in a week would not equal the ordinary daily elimination of morbid matter from the skin and kidneys. The greatest effect, therefore, is the restoration of some efficient vital action, the better radiation of vital power from the presiding center of organic life."

There may be truth in this theory of Dr. Trall's. However, it should not be lost sight of that the toxins eliminated through boils are in addition to those that go out through the regular channels. We should keep in mind also that the amount of toxins necessary to cause trouble is not great. Only a drop of some toxins is enough to kill. The amount of opium, for example, that is daily eliminated by the habitual user is enough, if taken by the non-user, to kill him quickly. There is, however, an improved circulation and freer distribution of nervous energy following a crisis, and this may not be wholly due to the elimination of toxins. Indeed, some crises are attended with nervous symptoms that would indicate changes going on in the nerves.

Of boils in acute diseases, Dr. Shew said, *Hydropathic Family Physicians*, p. 49:—

"A *crop of boils* is not unfrequently one of the consequences of fever**** These are, doubtless, beneficial in their effects, although they have been looked upon in a different light. Patients generally who get boils in abundance do well in the end."

Again, on pages 50 and 51 he says:—

"We sometimes see fever end in what is called a critical way. The ancients were much in the habit of looking for critical symptoms, as they were called. Such do certainly take place in some cases. There may be a discharge of blood either from the nostrils or the bowels; or there may be purging or sweating just as the disease is about to break up and leave the system. Dr. Gregory knew a case of fever to terminate by a great discharge of healthy urine. Andral knew a fever to end in a profuse expectoration, and another case with an alternation of sweating and expectoration. The formation of boils has in some cases appeared to be connected with a favorable issue of the disease."

A patient of the author's, a woman aged 56, had a place at the base of her spine about the size of a man's hand in which there was no sensation (anesthesia). She described it as being "dead." Pins could be stuck into it or it could be cut or bruised, but there was no pain or feeling. This condition had persisted for ten years. After two weeks under my directions she called me on the phone and excitedly explained that she was suffering with pains in the "dead spot." I said "good." "Doctor," she replied, "I am serious, I am not joking." "Neither am I joking," I replied. "I, too, am serious. When the pain ceases, sensation will again be normal in that area." She desired to know what she could do to relieve the pain. I instructed her not to relieve it but to let it alone. Two days later when she called at my office she joyfully described how the pain did not last long and that the "dead spot" was now normal again. Sensation was normal. Here was evidently a change in the nerves and in nervous distribution

An aged woman suffered with high blood pressure. Under excitement and when suffering with gas the pressure would rise still higher, resulting in severe headache and blood-shot eyes. Then the nose would bleed and relieve her. A boy of mine had the same trouble following the wrecking of his body by vaccination. His physician seared the lining of his nose and prevented it from bleeding. One eye then began to act as a safety valve. It would bleed and relieve the pressure. But this destroyed the sight of that eye.

A young woman, apparently as strong and healthy as any woman, with no aches and pains elsewhere, had a cancer of the womb in an advanced stage. She bled continuously from the womb. By means of an ice pack her physician stopped the flow of blood. I predicted that this would kill her. In three hours she was in a septic coma from which she never recovered. She died a few hours later due to the closing of Nature's safety valve.

In his *Notes on Tumors*, a work for students of pathology, Francis Carter Wood says:—

"In a very small proportion of human malignant tumors spontaneous disappearance for longer or shorter periods has been noted. The greatest number of such disappearances has followed incomplete surgical removal of the tumor; they have occurred next in order of frequency *during some acute febrile process*, and least frequently in connection with some profound alteration of the metabolic processes of the organism, such as extreme cachexia, artificial menopause, or the puerperium."

Spontaneous disappearance of tumors in mice and rats is frequent, but in man Bashford, an authority on the subject, estimates that spontaneous recession occurs in approximately one case in one hundred thousand. Wood states, however, that only three hunderd well verified instances of recession can be found in the literature on the subject. These three hundred instances must be but a very small fraction of the number of cases that have occurred. We are not interested here in the claim, obviously false, that the greatest number of such cases follow incomplete surgical removal of the tumor. We are here interested only in the admission or recorded observation that an acute disease and other profound changes in the system frequently result in the disappearance of the malignant tumor. Wood also says that there has long been current an idea that the body may develop an immunity to tumors similar to the immunity medical men regard as existing in the so-called infectious diseases, and says that the basis for this theory is the "occasional occurrence of spontaneous disappearance of neoplasms (new growths or tumors), either following infection**** or subsequent to slight operative proceedures, or even without any outside interference at all." `

It may be stated as a general law of life that precisely in proportion as we become accustomed to the use of any substance or to any indulgence which exerts a depraving influence on the body is the power of the body to recognize and react against the substance or indulgence impaired. In other words the more tobacco you can consume without being made sick, or the more alcohol you can imbibe without being made drunk, the greater is your physiological depravity—the more depraved are your organic instincts and the farther away from the ideal are the cells of your body. I cannot too strongly impress upon your mind the fact that EVERY ADAPTATION TO ANY INIMICAL SUBSTANCE OR INFLUENCE IS ACCOMPLISHED BY CHANGES IN THE CELLS AND TISSUES WHICH ARE AWAY FROM THE IDEAL. *They represent a form of degeneration and always necessarily cripple the efficiency of those cells and tissues which have been forced to undergo the adaptative changes.* All such changes, while they are defensive in character and are necessary to protect the body against the inimical influence, ultimately shorten life. However, they prevent the inimical influence from killing you much sooner.

The power of regeneration is much stronger than the power of degeneration and more or less regeneration will take place, commencing immediately, if the inimical influence is withdrawn. If the depravity is not great, complete recovery may be expected. At any rate if you do not correct the inimical influence you will shorten your life. Often, when a bad habit, like the tobacco habit or alcohol habit, is given up the individual will lose weight and undergo crises and this will convince him that the abandonment of the bad habit was injurious. What was really happening was the tearing down and casting out of the system of the depraved tissues and substances and this is then followed by a renewal and regeneration of the body. The crises and loss of weight are beneficial measures and should be welcomed, not feared.

The headaches suffered by the coffee user when deprived of coffee, the pains suffered by the drug addict when deprived of his drug; the unsteadiness of his nerves suffered by the tobacco user when deprived of his tobacco; the depression suffered by the stimulant user when deprived of his stimulant—these are not evidences of the beneficial influences of these substances but are evidences of their deleterious character. Outraged nerves and other tissues are simply coming out from under their influence and making their true condition known. Let the habitual rum-drinker abandon his rum, and the parts of his body that have suffered most by the long continued excitement begin to cry out and make known their actual state. Greater or less suffering and discomfort which are regarded by superficial and ignorant observers as indications of an adverse change, immediately result, but the sequel is a happy issue.

The proffered opportunity to repair the injured and damaged parts is immediately siezed upon and the work of restoration begins at once. But due to the very general *apparent* detriment experienced in the initial stages of the restorative process, consequent upon the sudden cessation of the habitual excitement, this all important and beneficial process is commonly thought of as a "pulling down," or destructive, rather than a building up, or constructive, operation. People are warned not to break off their bad habits suddenly, but to "taper off" gradually. This latter plan both prolongs and increases the actual suffering that one must go through in the renovating work. One does not gain, but loses by the "tapering off" process, for the bad habit is continually interfering with the work of repair that may be begun when the amount of habitual injury is decreased. What is more, the "tapering off process seldom enables one to succeed in breaking off from a bad habit for each repetition tends to keep the habit alive.

In discussing the evidence the Orthopath offers against the medical theories of the causes and nature of disease, Dr. Wm. F. Havard says:—

"In the first place, the Orthopath can offer as evidence, the fact that patients who are given the proper care, do not die while undergoing an acute reaction to pathoferic influences. In the second place, he can conduct their convalescence in a manner to build them up into a better state of health than they enjoyed before their acute *illness,* showing that the body was improved by being purged of an accumulation of impurities. In the third place, he can prove by his experience, if it has been extensive enough, that where a patient develops an acute reaction (disease) during the course of treatment for some chronic ailment, the progress of the chronic condition is checked and a positive repair process begins. Let me cite one case as an example of this. A man of fifty-eight years, suffering from chronic articular rheumatism, presented himself for our care. He was almost a cripple and had been the despair of numerous doctors and sanitariums for fifteen years. According to his history the trouble had started shortly after a seige of malaria. The latter was *suppressed* with copious doses of quinine. After six months of Orthopathic care, with little noticeable improvement, this patient developed a typical case of malaria, which lasted six weeks. Now for the miracle! On moving about, he found that the pain had disappeared from his joints and the motion in them had increased a hundred per cent. His improvement continued, and in a short time he was actively engaged in engineering work."

Some have attempted to prove that crises develop according to what they are pleased to term the law of sevens—a subsidiary law to the law of periodicity or the rythmical ebb and flow of the forces of life. Under this so-called law, crises occur according to Dr. Henry Lindlahr, as follows:—

"When a chronic patient, whose chances of cure are good, is placed under proper (natural) conditions of living and of treatment he will, as a rule, experience five weeks of marked improvement.

"The sixth week, if conditions are favorable, usually marks the beginning of acute reactions or healing crises."

The seventh period is then a period of adjustment, reconstruction, recuperation and rest, and the beginnning of a new cycle of sevens. This is a highly fanciful theory with much plausibility but is not borne out in my experience.

There is a rythmic ebb and flow of the forces of life. This can be seen in the acutely ill, the chronically sick and in the conventionally healthy. But we cannot prove that this ebb and flow follows any septeminal law, or law of sevens.

Medical men have objected that by the use of drugs they produce crises—such, for instance, as vomiting, diarrhea, etc. They ask then, why we do not accept the drug induced crises. There are several good reasons why we do not accept such crises. The critical action, in such cases, is directed against the drug, not against the cause of the disease. The critical action represents only the primary and not the secondary effect of the drug. The secondary and lasting effect of the drug is worse disease. Lastly, the drug induced action does not secure the desired elimination of toxins. Dr. Lindlahr has well expressed this fact as follows:—

"Such enforced artificial purging may flush the drains and sewers but does not cleanse the inner chambers of the house. The cells in the interior tissues remain encumbered with morbid matter. A genuine and truly effective house-cleaning must start in the cells and must be brought about through the initiative of the vital energies in the organism, through healing crises and not through stimulation by poisonous irritants.

"When, under a natural regimen of living and of treatment, the system has been sufficiently purified, adjusted and vivified the cells themselves begin the work of elimination."

What Dr. Lindlahr and most so-called natural therapists or naturopaths do not understand is that crises forced by hot and cold baths, packs, water drinking, enemas, manipulations, electricity, and other methods and modalities of mis-called natural treatment are no more desirable or beneficial than drug induced ones. There are no natural therapeutics in the sense in which these men employ the term, while drugs, vaccines and serums are as natural as electricity, heat and cold, etc.

ACUTE DISEASE NOT A RADICAL CURE

Chapter XIV

THE fact that acute disease is a curative process is so revolutionary in its nature that its acceptance by the various schools of Heteropathic medicine would mean the complete destruction of all their laboriously constructed therapeutic systems. For this reason there has been much theoretical acceptance and practical dismissal of this great truth, such as has been accorded many other mighty principles that have been discovered to the world after much suffering and cost by a few earnest workers.

But, great as is this truth, and revolutionary as is its nature, it is not the whole truth. When the whole truth is accepted, it will work an even greater revolution in practice than any save the purest hygienists have ever visualized. Probably Dr. Jennings himself had the clearest vision of what this revolution would mean in practice.

The whole truth is that, while acute disease is a curative process, it is not a radical or complete cure. It does not apply the axe to the root of the trouble and stops far short of complete elimination of the immediate cause of disease. This is easily stated but will require considerable explanation before the reader will be able to fully understand it. The remainder of this chapter will be devoted to making the matter clear.

It is first necessary to understand why these acute reactions, which we call disease, arise and against what they are directed. Briefly, waste matter is constantly forming in the body and we are in the habit of regularly taking into the body, from without, poisons and impurities which are inimical to life and health. Normally these wastes and impurities are eliminated, but men and women so live that they weaken the functional powers of their depurating organs and this causes a retention and gradual accumulation, within the body, of these wastes and poisons. The body reacts against these poisons to expel them, and these reactions we call acute disease. The form the reaction takes depends on a number of factors which cannot be discussed here. The important fact, for the present, is that acute disease is a reaction of the organism against accumulated poisons, and in the words of Sylvester Graham: *"In all these operations the organic instincts act determinately, and, as it were, rationally, with reference to a final cause of good, viz., the removal of the offending cause."*

The whole process of acute and chronic disease is not unlike the results of the use of tobacco, and I may appropriately introduce this matter at this point. Tobacco is one of the most powerful and loathsome poisons in the whole vegetable kingdom. Therefore, when taken into the undepraved organism, its presence is met with vital resistance for the purpose of expelling it. There follows, in rapid succession, a distressing dizziness, muscular relaxation, tremor, weakness, perhaps fever, nausea, vomiting, diarrhea and convulsions. The whole system seems to be thrown into disorder, yet, through it all, law and order reign supreme, while every evidence of apparent disorder and chaos serves a definite and purposive end.

This aggregate of symptoms constitutes an acute disease and is intended to free the body of the tobacco poison. Such a reaction always follows the introduction of tobacco into the undepraved organism; and the more vigorous and undepraved the organism is, the more prompt and powerful will this reaction be. But, by commencing a career of depravity, with cautiously measured steps, we may easily break down the body's resistance to the poison and ultimately bring about a condition in which the body actually calls for and embraces, as a friend, its arch foe. The body may become so accustomed to the deadliest poisons that these may be habitually taken, in considerable quantities, and only bring about an immediate feeling of apparent well being. We have an excellent example of this in the method by which a young man *"becomes a man."* In his ignorance and inexperience he persists in his efforts to conquer Nature's stubborn resistance to the employment of the poisonous weed. Nature is then forced to swing her power of accomodation, adjustment or adaptation into operation for the purpose of conserving vital energy and maintaining existence. Once accomodation has taken place the body ceases to react so vigorously against the poison.

Upon this point Graham wrote, *Science of Human Life*, pp. 613-15 :—

"But the narcotic substances which are almost universally employed by mankind purely for stimulating and intoxicating purposes, are far more deleterious in their nature, and when used with equal freedom are much more pernicious in their effects on the human system, than salt, spices and other pungent substances ordinarily used as seasonings and condiments with food. The narcotic or intoxicating substances which have been used as means of stimulation by different portions of the human family, are somewhat numerous; but the most common in the civilized world, and especially in our country, are tea, coffee, tobacco, opium and alcohol. Alcohol, though not commonly considered a narcotic, is nevertheless properly classed with those substances, for its effects on the living body are essentially the same. It is produced, as we have seen, not by any formative process of nature, but by a process of decay, or the decomposition of the saccharine matter of organized bodies. The grand characteristic of all narcotic substances is their anti-vital or life-destroying property. When they are not so highly concentrated or energetic as to destroy life instantly, they produce the most powerful and often the most violent and distressing vital reaction, which causes a correspondent degree of exhaustion, depression, and prostration; and they often destroy life, purely by vital exhaustion in this violent and continued reaction. But when the discriminating sensibilities of the system have been depraved by the habitual use of these substances, and its powers of giving a sympathetic alarm greatly impaired, these same substances, even the most deadly in nature, if the quantity be only commensurate with the degree of physiological depravity, may be habitually introduced into the stomach, and even received into the general circulation, and diffused over the whole system, and slowly but surely destroy the constitution, and always greatly increase the liability to disease, and almost certainly create it, and invariably aggravate it, without any of those symptoms which are ordinarily considered as the evidence of the action of a poison on the living body; but, on the contrary, their simulation is attended with that pleasurable feeling and agreeable mental consciousness which lead the mind to the strongest confidence in their salutary nature and effect. Hence, there is not a poison in the vegetable or mineral kingdom which the human body, cannot by careful training, become so accustomed to, that it will receive into the stomach, at a single dose, without any immediate evidence of its deleterious effects, a quantity sufficient to kill, in a very few minutes six men who have never used it. Arsenic may be taken with food as a seasoning, as freely as table salt, with as little immediate evidence of its poisonous character; and even prussic acid, which kills instantly like lightening, where the body is wholly unaccustomed to its action, may with proper care be gradually brought to act upon the human system, till it can be used with considerable freedom as a means of exhiliration and intoxication.

"This wonderful capability of the living body to adapt itself by physiological depravity to the action of poisons of every kind, has not only led the infatuated human race to the excessive use of such substances as means of intoxication, but, almost as a necessary consequence, has also led them to the full belief that those substances are innoxious and salutary. Accordingly we find in every period in human history, in every portion of the world, that not only the ignorant multitude, but also the more intelligent, and to a great extent even the members of the medical profession itself, have stoutly denied the poisonous character of those deleterious substances which they employed as means of habitual stimulation and intoxication, on the ground that they could be habitually and freely used without producing immediate death, or any of the distressing symptoms which indicate the action of a poison; but, on the contrary, so far as the feelings can appreciate their effects; they act on the system as grateful cordials. From an experience of this kind, the poisonous character of tea, coffee, tobacco, opium, alcohol, and all other narcotic substances, has been boldly, boisteriously, and vehemently denied, by those who habitually use them as means of stimulation and intoxication. Even in our own land of boasted intelligence, in the middle of the nineteenth century of the Christian era, and in our very colleges of learning, the idea that alcohol is a poison has been treated with ridicule and contempt, as too absurd for any but a visonary fanatic to believe; and yet there is no truth in science more perfectly demonstrable than that alcohol is one of the most energetic and fatal poisons known to man; and with equal ecrtainty can it be proved that tea, coffee, tobacco, and opium, are powerful poisons to the human body.

"But this point is not in any measure to be determined by what is called experience, or the fact that these substances can be habitually used as a means of agreable stimulation without producing the immediate symptoms of the action of deadly poisons; for, as we have seen, if this be our criterion, we are forced to the fallacious conclusion that there is no such thing as a poison in nature. We have seen that the solids of the human body consist of three general tissues or forms of organic structure; that each of these tissues is endowed with peculiar vital properties, together with the vital affinities, which are under the control of the nervous power, constitute the vital forces of the organic economy, and the functional powers of the organs. Now then, whatever substance, by the action of its own intrinsic qualities, is immediately destructive to the vital properties and vital constitution of these tissues, is as certainly a poison as that two and two make four. If a real poison, in a very small quantity or a very diluted form, be brought to act on a living organ composed of these several tissues—as the stomach, for instance—the organ may, by its own peculiar economy of vital reaction, and by the cooperation of the associated organs in the general vital economy, so far protect itself and the system from the pernicious properties of the poison, as only to suffer considerable exhaustion of its vital powers and depravity of its organic sensibilities. From this state the organ may be recovered by the renovating economy of the system. But if the poison be at first received in a highly concentrated form of large quantity, it will either arrest the functions of life at once, by paralyzing the nervous power, or it will produce violent reaction, and in the terrible conflict utterly exhaust the vital properties and destroy the vital constitution of the tissues, and death will be the result! That is, therefore, the only true mode of ascertaining the properties of substances in relation to the physiological powers of the human body; and it is a matter which has been repeatedly and fully demonstrated, that all the substances which I have named contain a strong anti-vital quality,— or in other words, their effect on the living body is to destroy the vital properties and vital constitution of the tissues which compose the organs."

There is not a poison in the animal, vegetable or mineral kingdom which the human body cannot, by carefully guarded steps, be accustomed to, so that, it no longer offers any vigorous resistance to it. Arsenic may be taken as freely as table salt, with food, with no immediate evidence of its poisonous character. Prussic acid, "which kills instantly, like lightening," if introduced into the body unaccustomed to its use, may be used with considerable freedom as a means of exhiliration and intoxication, after one has carefully accustomed his body to it. The opium addict often takes enough of his favorite drug to kill several non-users outright.

This process of adaptation is a depraving process. The greater the physiological depravity, the more of the poison will be demanded, and the more that can be used. In other words, in precisely the proportion to which one becomes accustomed to the use of any deleterious substance is his system depraved and his defensive powers reduced. The small boy thinks that when he has acquired the tobacco habit, and can smoke several cigars a day, he will be a man. The fact is the reverse. The ability to consume large quantities of tobacco is an evidence of weakness and physiological depravity, not of strength and physiological fitness. Instead of being a man, he becomes a slave and Homer truly had Ulysesses to say: "Surely a man loses half the virtue of a man when he becomes a slave."

After toleration for any deleterious substance has been established, those acute reactions that followed its initial employment, arise only when one takes an unaccustomed amount of his accustomed poison. I will give a few examples from life to illustrate what I mean by this.

A young man of twenty-five years, having both smoked and chewed tobacco from childhood, made a bet that he could consume, without harm, an amount of tobacco considerably in excess of the amount he had been accustomed to taking. He consumed the tobacco, all right, but suffered all the acute symptoms of tobacco poisoning as a result. An elderly man who had smoked for a life-time attended a stockholders meeting where he smoked an unusual amount and breathed tobacco fumes through the whole of the afternoon. He suffered all the symptoms of acute nicotine poisoning as a result.

An old man who had been in the habit for years of taking strychnine as an aphrodisiac, until he was able to take rather large doses, took, by accident, a larger dose than he was accustomed to using. He suffered all the symptoms of acute strychnine poisoning in consequence. For several days it was not known whether he would live or die, and his young wife was placed in jail charged with poisoning him When, finally, he became conscious, he told the true story, and the young lady, who faced a possible hangman's noose, was freed.

A man who suffers from constipation, resorts to epsom salts to force his bowels to move. They work like a charm. He continues to use them until toleration is established and, then, finds that in order to secure the desired movement, he must increase the size of the dose. By using more salts than the body has learned to tolerate he secures bowel action. Similarly, physicians, in giving stimulants to their patients, find that they must continually increase the size of the dose, or, resort to another and unaccustomed poison, to secure the desired stimulation. The body is forced to accommodate itself to such substances, so that it no longer reacts violently against them, or else it will exhaust itself in the frequent reactions.

Common table salt will occasion vomiting, diarrhea, and increased heart action in those unaccustomed to its use. But by gradually accustoming the body to this powerful irritant, one may learn to consume considerable quantities of the mineral, after which, the above symptoms are produced only by taking an unusual or unaccustomed amount. Table salt is frequently employed as an emetic and will serve this purpose in even the most inveterate users of salt if given in sufficiently large doses.

With these facts in mind, we may proceed with our explanation of the fact that acute disease is not a radical or complete cure. Just as the body learns to tolerate tobacco, alcohol, opium, arsenic, tea, coffee, etc., so, it builds toleration for the toxins that form in the body or in the digestive tract. At first the young man's body will not tolerate more than two or three cigarettes a day, but, in the course of a few years, he is smoking two or more packages of these daily. So, in infancy and childhood, the body will not tolerate much of the toxins of disease, but develops frequent crises and throws them off. As time passes, however, more toleration is built, and crises become less frequent and less vigorous. Just as the body that is accustomed to the use of tobacco develops acute reactions against it only when it is consumed in unaccustomed amounts, so, acute reactions against the toxins of disease occur only when these toxins are raised above the toleration point. Similarly, just as the reaction against the tobacco ceases as soon as the poison is reduced to the toleration point; so, the reaction against the toxins of disease subsides when they have been reduced to the point of toleration.

I speak of the toxins of disease and tobacco poisoning separately merely for convenience in making comparison. Tobacco poisoning produces disease as truly as any other poison and is often one of the toxins that helps to produce the various diseases from which men suffer.

The tobacco, opium or arsenic user is in a state of chronic tobacco, opium or arsenical poisoning. Every one in the ordinary walks of life is in a state of chronic auto-toxemia, which has been brought on by a mode of living that has reduced the functions of the body and which impairs digestion, secretion, excretion and elimination. A toleration for these toxins is established and no acute eliminative efforts to throw them off arise, unless they accumulate above this point. The acute reaction subsides when the toxemia is reduced to the point of toleration, or slightly below, and thus, the sufferer "recovers" from the "attack" in a state of chronic toxic poisoning. He returns to his former state of health, which is a very low one, when contrasted with what man's health standard can and should be. Dr. Jennings rightly called the health standard of the average man a state of "impaired health." Indeed, he was equally correct when he repeatedly declared that what we call disease is simply a state of impaired health.

Now there is evidence that in some instances these healing crises do reduce the toxins much below the point of toleration, before they subside, but they never last

124

until the system is wholly free of its accumulated toxins. Often one's health is better following an "attack" of gout, or typhoid fever, or following a cold, than it was before these curative efforts were initiated. A similar improvement in health often follows smallpox, boils, and other forms of skin eruptions. Still, however, the body is left in a state of chronic poisoning.

The average man or woman, in the ordinary walks of life, hovers constantly near the border line of acute disease. All that is required to bring on a toxemic crisis (acute disease) in the average individual is some unusual influence or unusual amount of an accustomed influence to cause the amount of toxins in the system to rise above the point of toleration. There are many influences that may occasion such an accumulation. Any influence that calls for an unusual or added expenditure of nervous energy and thus puts an added check upon elimination, will cause a sudden rise in the amount of toxins in the body. Extremes of heat and cold, cold feet, wet feet, getting wet, fatigue, an unusual day's work, an unusual meal, loss of sleep, an unaccustomed stimulant, a little more dissipation and excitement, shock, fear, worry, sorrow, anger, and other such emotions, and many other influences lessen the powers of life and impair physiological efficiency. These are then spoken of as the causes of the trouble. They form one of the causes. They are the "last straw that breaks the camel's back." Disease is due to a multiplicity of causes. It is the final culmination, or summing up, of a long series of causes that have been operating over a longer or shorter period of time. Disease does not develop suddenly. However sudden may be the apparent "onset" of the crisis, back of this "onset" are weeks, months and even years of what Jennings called "*arrears of expurgation.*" Exposure of the body to cold temporarily suspends elimination through the skin, and if the lungs and kidneys are unable to compensate for this, causes a sudden increase in the toxins in the body. A "cold," an "influenza," or a "pneumonia" may be the result. The body that is not already saturated to the bursting point will not be harmed to any appreciable extent by such influences. These healing crises represent a culmination or summing up of a long series of bodily abuses, and no more develop suddenly than the infant reaches maturity suddenly. Many drugless physicians employ harsh treatments, such as cold baths, etc., and these force an increase in the toxemia. A crisis results and they regard it as evidence of the value of their methods. It is evidence of their harmfulness.

As before stated, toxemic crises last until the systemic toxemia is reduced to the point of toleration, or slightly below, after which they subside. This is called cure. It is really only the beginning of cure. The sick man considers himself well as soon as the acute symptoms subside. He is still chronically toxemic. He is still hovering near the borderline of acute disease. He is still greatly enervated. Most important of all, he is still living his old disease producing mode of life.

Toxemic crises come and go. They do not last. They are said to be self-limited. They are self-limited because their cause is limited. *They are processes of cure.* They last, if not suppressed by treatment, until the toxemia is reduced to the toleration point, or slightly below, after which they subside as naturally as they arose. Whatever treatment is employed coincidentally with the subsidence of the crisis receives credit for the "cure." Whatever form of treatment is employed to *suppress* a crisis is called a "cure." For these reasons almost anything appears to cure disease. DISEASE IS THE PROCESS OF CURE. The "curing" systems ride to glory on the work done by this process.

The years pass. Toxemic crises ebb and flow. More and more toleration for toxemia is built. Chronic toxemia, like chronic alcoholism, chronic nicotinism, chronic morphinism, slowly undermines the system and chronic disease develops. The essential differences between acute and chronic disease are those of time and severity of symptoms. They are essentially one and the same process, caused immediately by the same ENERVATION and TOXEMIA and remotely by the same HABITS THAT KILL.

The evil effects of a poison do not cease merely because the body has learned to tolerate it. The habitual use of a thing which is injurious in itself, does not alter its nature and render its use salutary. The habitual use of tobacco, alcohol, opium or other poisons, impairs the health, destroys the tissues of the body, creates disease, slowly and insiduously undermines the constitution and produces premature death. My good friend, Dr. Claunch, declares that toleration is the only cause for death not due to violence. By this, he means that tolerated toxins are the cause of death. I agree with him fully.

The body learns to tolerate tobacco, but its use results in nervousness, weakness, tobacco heart and a train of other affections. The body quickly learns to tolerate alcohol, but its use, even in what is called moderation, destroys more or less of the functioning tissues of all the organs of the body, producing sclerosis (hardening) of the liver, arteries, spinal cord, etc., a permanent impairment of the stomach and kidneys, delerium tremens and other nervous and mental affections. Hardening of the tissues due to such irritation interferes with cell renewal and elimination and thus results in gradual cellular death from starvation and poisoning.

In the same way, the toxins of disease, although the body learns to tolerate them, slowly but surely destroy the organs and tissues of the body and impair their functions. The powerful acids produced by fermentation and putrefaction in the digestive tract, destroy the tissues of the liver, pancreas, kidneys, lungs, etc., producing diabetes, Bright's disease, tuberculosis, and other diseases. As this destruction of cells and tissues of the body continues the body develops all those symptoms and "diseases" that are associated with "old age" and later death.

If it were not that the body learns to tolerate these toxins, if it always vigorously resisted and threw them off, then no chronic toxemia would or could ever develop. The body would either exhaust itself in its struggles against the toxins or we would be forced to reform our modes of living and conform to the laws of being. It is the power of toleration that deceives us and enables us to embrance and cherish our deadliest foes. It is the power of toleration that enables the young man to confidently assert that tobacco does not harm him. Toleration is the siren voice that leads us on to death.

A true cure is possible only after all enervating habits and influences are corrected and an opportunity for vital recuperation is afforded. This necessitates a complete revolution in our present mode of life and, in most cases, a prolonged period of mental, physical and physiological rest. Life must be ordered in conformity with physiological law and the body must be permitted to recuperate its dissipated energies. All efforts to eradicate disease, and bring about a restoration to the primitive health standard, which does not recognize the enervating factors of our present mode of life as the remote and producing causes of *impaired health*, and seek, first of all, to correct these, are doomed to failure and disappointment. At its best, such a mode of treatment is but a system of palliation, at its worst, a mode of destructive suppression, like so-called *Modern Medical Science*.

The practice here indicated is not the usual or popular one. Little or no effort is made to correct the patient's mode of life by the physicians of all schools save the ORTHOPATHIC, while the organs of the body are usually goaded on in their work, by irritants and stimulants, instead of being permitted to rest. The physician usually prescribes "plenty of good nourishing food," meaning by this, the conventional diet of meat, eggs, white bread, coffee, etc.

THE UNITY OF DISEASES AND SYMPTOMS

Chapter XV

IN *The Water-Cure Journal*, for August, 1853, (pages 28 to 32), is an article by Dr. N. Bedortha, entitled *Medical Reform*. Incidentally, this is also the title of Dr. Jennings' first book. In this article Bedortha says:—

"Thompson's theory of disease was simple, and his pratcice in harmony with that theory. He discarded the endless nosologies of medical books, and advocated the unity of disease. Under whatever form the disease might appear, his mode of practice was simple and uniform."

Again he says, in briefly recounting the development of Orthopathy:

"Disease in his, (Jennings) theory is a unit, and the manifestations of disease in the form of fever, coughs, colds, etc., are kindly efforts of nature entirely true to the laws of life and health, which cannot be aided by any system of drug medication whatever, relying solely upon the *Vis Med. Naturae*, placing the patient in what he supposes is the best possible condition by rest, pure air, and proper diet."

The Unity of Disease means simply that all "diseases" by whatever name they are called are one and the same thing. Instead of there being hundreds of diseases there are simply many variations in form and manifestation of the disease process—*the curing process*. This is a most revolutionary principle and when finally understood and acted upon will simplify medicine and result in the passing away of nearly all of what now passes for science in the realm of medicine. It is possible to see all symptoms and all symptom complexes in terms of their essential unity. We can go still farther and show that the phenomena of health and the phenomena of disease are essentially one. Instead of health and disease creating, for us, the puzzles of nosologists and epistemologists, they are but two phases of the same thing—life or living.

Jennings says: "Philosophy of Human Life," p. 18:

"The external appearances, or tokens of distress, which the vital economy is compeled to develop under the pressure of overpowering causes, and which are called diseases, are as evanescent in their general character as the morning cloud, and the early dew; and as changeable as the 'shifting figures of the magic lantern' and a numerous and multiform, as endless variety of causes and influences acting upon millions of parts, each impressible with varied action, in kind and degree, can produce. And these phenomena will vary in different countries or communities according to the nature and degree of violence done to the vital machinery, by different modes of life. Where departure from correct living is the widest and longest persevered in, the phenomena of impaired healthy action will be the most numerous, complicated and severe or aggravated; and where the laws of life are best observed, and for the longest period, these phenomena will be the fewest, least complicated and mildest."

Over against the heteropathic doctrine of disease which runs throughout the theories and practices of all schools today, Jennings placed the great fundamental fact of Orthopathy, from which the system derives its name, and which he states thus in the introduction to his "Philosophy of Human Life" (preface):

"It will be the subject of the following pages . . . to show the *unity of human physical life*; that its tendency is always upward towards the highest point of health; in the lowest as well as the highest state of the vital funds; and that what is called disease is nothing more nor less than impaired health, feeble vitality; that recovery from this state is effected, when effected at all, by a restorative principle, identical with life itself, susceptible of aid only from proper attention to air, diet, motion and rest, affections of the mind, regulation of the temperature, etc., with occasional aid from what may be justly denominated surgical operations and appliances."

Thus, at the very outset, orthopathy differs from all heteropathic systems past or present in that it regards disease as a state of health, a low state of health, in which the efforts of the body are all directed toward the normal health standard. Every action of the body is "RIGHT ACTION" instead of "WRONG ACTION" as is held by all other schools.

Casting the confusing nosologies and classifications of the schools to the wind and building upon the sure foundation of the *unity of disease* Jennings wrote, *Philosophy of Human Life:*

"Most systems of medicine, in their nosological character, are but *attempts* to classify the *phenomena* and *symptoms* of disease; and from the very nature of the subject, can be but *fruitless attempts.*"

Jennings wrote, in discussing what Heteropathy calls *Predisposition* to disease:

"Orthopathy makes this predisposition of Heteropathy, the first stage of disease, and makes no difference in any of its stages; it is all of a piece from first to last. There are different stages and degrees, and different forms, but the nature and tendency is one throughout.—*Philosophy of Human Life,* p. 111.

This "first stage of disease" he regarded as the "first grade of degeneracy, verging toward the second grade, constantly liable, from a low state of vital powers, to be hurried into it," and said of the second stage:

"In this second stage or grade of degeneracy, we have what is called functional disease—a change from the natural (normal) condition of the functions of the body or parts of it. It may be in the form of what would be called a pleurisy, fever, or other form of derangement to which the body is liable—some external or sensible manifestation of internal difficulty."—*Tree of Life,* pp. 117-118.

In discussing *idopathic* and *symptomatic* "diseases" he declared:

"There is however about as much propriety and utility in these attempts to discriminate between idiopathic and symptomatic diseases, as there would be in making a distinction between old debts and new ones. And when the vital economy is allowed the opportunity and can command the necessary means for liquidating her embarrassments, she will make about as much difference between idiopathic and symptomatic diseases, as an honest man would in the settlement of just claims against him, as he acquired the ability to do so, between old and new debts. When an individual gets largely in debt, whether from improvident husbandry, or the force of circumstances beyond his control, the extension of his indebtedness is natural and easy, if not unavoidable; and so when man's vital energies are broken down or very much impaired, it is not only natural and easy for one part after another to yield to the influence of disturbing causes, but absolutely impossible for them to do otherwise; not from sympathy, but because the overflowing scourge has at length reached them in its disolating effect, as it reached their neighbors before them; and their diseased condition is as truly idiopathic as that of the others."—*Philosophy of Human Life,* p. 134.

Discussing *General* and *Local* "diseases" he wrote:

"It has long been a mooted question with Heteropathy, whether disease could be *general* in its commencement—pervade all parts of the system at once in its onset. If the Heteropathic view of disease were true, it certainly would be difficult to conceive how it could *attack,* or *fasten upon* and develop itself in every part of the system simultaneously.

"But Orthopathy avoids all difficulty in this particular; for as it makes all disease consist in a partial exhaustion of the life and health-sustaining principle, this negative condition may be produced at the same time throughout an entire tissue or set of organs, or in some particular part of it, according as the causes operate generally or locally."—*Philosophy of Human Life,* pp. 134-5.

A brief reference to the doctrines of the *Unity of Disease* as held by Thomson and his followers is in order.

Samuel Thomson was born in New Hampshire in 1769. He early became an herb doctor and in 1822 published his "New Guide to Health" which passed through many editions and ultimately became "Thomson's Materia Medica or Botanic Family Physician." As has already been pointed out he promulgated the principle of the *unity of disease* and for many years all members of the Thomsonian and Physio-Medical school based their practice largely upon this principle. When Thomsonism became incorporated with the *eclectic system* this principle was lost. Thomson died in 1843. Prof. Curtis, in his *Theory and Practice,* declared:—

"Disease is *one,* . . . The *symptoms* are *one,* . . . and the treatment *must* be one. . . ."

128

Curtis was the leader of the Physio-Medicalists in the middle of the last century. In his *Criticisms* he declared:

"... we define the word *disease* widely different from any other 'sect'; or, in other words, we boldly pronounce 'it a *unit*.' This is remarkable, and worthy of special attention and remembrance; for industrious nosologists (or classifiers of disease) have summed up more than two thousand *different* diseases; while we say there is but one! 'All are but parts of one stupendous whole.' At least we say this: That 'disease is the inability of an organ to perform its proper functions,' and in this sense is a unit! Disease of the eye, stomach, heart, lungs and bowels are not *different* diseases, but disease in different places. This startles and confounds the learned. Meningitis (inflammation of the brain), cystitis (inflammation of the bladder), metritis (inflammation of the womb), or the inflammation of any part, as in erysipelas, small-pox, scarlet fever, and cancer, are the same, all proceeding from the action of the vital force; but the specific, exciting causes are different, each 'superadding' its own peculiarity or specific action, which gives all the different characters of the specific forms of disease."

It is evident that Prof. Curtis mixed his terms even if he was not, himself, more or less mixed on the subject. Obviously, if all diseases are part of a whole, if disease is a *unit*, there are no *specific* diseases. He again declared:

"By its forms (the forms of fever) are meant the different appearances given to it by different obstructing agents, as bilious fever, spotted fever; or the locality of the excitement, as pleuritis, the suffix, 'itis', denotes, inflammation of an organ or locality, as phrenitis, of the brain, iritis, the eye, etc. When the fever is confined to a small portion of the body it is called inflammation."

In 1835 there was published in London a little treatise under the title, *Fallacy of the Art of Physic as Taught in the Schools*. This little book, by Dr. Samuel Henry Dickson, a native of Edinburgh, a graduate of the University of Glasgow, and for several years a medical officer in India, but then residing in Cheltenham, where he was engaged in active practice, was a severe arraignment of blood-letting and heroic drugging.

"The phenomena of perfect health," he said, "consist in the regular repitition of *alternate* motions or events; ... *Disease*, under all its manifestations, is, in the first place, a simple exaggeration or diminution of the amount of the same motion or events...."

He further declared:

"It was my fate—I can scarcely call it my fortune—to make two most important discoveries in medicine, namely: The *periodicity of movement* of every organ and atom of all living tissues, and the *intermittency and unity* of all diseases, however named and however produced. To these I added a third: the *Unity of Action of Cause and Cure*; both of which involve change of temperature. Such is the groundwork of the *Chrono-Thermal System*."

In 1838 Dr. Dickson published a treatise on *The Unity of Disease*. Throughout his subsequent works among which were *Elements of Medicine* and *Fallacies of the Faculty* (1861), he defended the principle of the unity of disease. These books have long been out of print. In his *Physio-Medicalism* (1870) J. S. Thomas, M.D., gives the following brief quotation from his *Elements of Medicine:* "I regard these (the different kinds of scarlatina then recognized) as mere differences in degree of violence and intensity." In his *"Fallacies of the Faculty,"* he declared: "Properly speaking there never was a purely local disease."

In a previous chapter attention was called to the medical dictionary's definition of disease as a "genus or kind of disturbance of health." It was there noted that a genus is an order or class (in zoology and botany) embracing subordinate classes or species. Upon this point Dr. J. H. Rausse declared:—*The Water Cure*, 1845, p. 18:

"Before I attempt to define the terms health and disease, I must point out that there are in reality no species and varieties differently marked off from one another; that the individuals of every species and variety have dissimilarities among themselves; that the transitions from one species to the other are so imperceptible, that with certain individuals and concrete cases it cannot be determined with certainty to which species they belong. This is particularly the case with the different diseases, and even the line of demarcation between health and disease is in cases of reality very wavering, in a word, the denominations of species, etc., are not borrowed from reality, and from here delivered over to human ingenuity, but vice versa, have originated in the human mind, and from there have been transferred to reality, because the former cannot operate without them."

Thus, instead of there being many diseases of different orders, classes, species and genera, Rausse declared all these things to be merely conveniences of thought. The human mind must separate, classify and arrange in order that it may think. But it too easily falls into the habit of regarding its subjective taxonomic orders as objective realities of nature. Thus it regards inflammation in one part of the body as a separate disease from inflammation in another part of the body. This easily leads to confusion and ruinous practices. Witness the insurmountable confusion in theory and practice and the deadly destructiveness of the practice of what is absurdly called *Modern Medical Science*.

Florence Nightingale, who taught the English physicians and surgeons the value of cleanliness, declares in her *Notes on Nursing* (1860), pp. 32-3:

"Is it not living in a continual mistake to look upon disease, as we do now, as separate entities, which *must* exist, like cats and dogs? Instead of looking upon them as conditions, like a dirty and a clean condition, and just as much, under our own control; or rather as the reactions of kindly nature, against the conditions in which we have placed ourselves.

"I was brought up, both by scientific men and ignorant women, distinctly to believe that small-pox, for instance, was a thing of which there was once a first specimen in the world, which went on propogating itself, in a perpetual chain of descent, just as much as that there was a first dog, (or a first pair of dogs) and that small-pox would not begin itself any more than a new dog would begin without there having been a parent dog.

"Since then I have seen with my eyes and smelt with my nose small-pox growing up in first specimens, either in close rooms, or in overcrowded wards, where it could not by any possibility have been 'caught' but must have begun. (originated, Author.)

"Nay, more, I have seen diseases begin, grow up and pass into one another. Now, dogs do not pass into cats.

"I have seen, for instance, with a little overcrowding, continued fever grow up; and with a little more, typhoid fever; and with a little more, typhus, and all in the same ward or hut.

"Would it not be far better, truer, and more practical, if we looked upon disease in this light?

"For diseases, as all experience shows, are adjectives, not noun substantives."

Miss Nightingale distinctly recognized the unity of "Morbid" phenomena and saw that the names of the nosology are merely terms descriptive of varying conditions and not names for entities or *things*. She saw as well that this wealth of terms only confuses and misleads both the laity and the professions.

About 1889 or 1890 THE NEW SCIENCE OF HEALING, *or the Doctrine of the* UNITY OF DISEASE *Forming the Basis of a Uniform Mode of Cure, without Medicines and Without Operations,* by Louis Kuhne, of Germany, was first published. This book had a remarkable sale, ran through many editions, was translated into about twenty-five languages, and is still published and widely sold. So great has been and yet is the influence of this book in Europe and the two Americas that hundreds of thousands of people think that Kuhne discovered the principle of the *Unity of Disease* and that to him we owe practically all we know about this important matter. It is probable that Kuhne did arrive at his conclusions independently of those who preceded him, for, although he was acquainted with the works of Rausse, the latter had never emphasized nor developed his ideas on the unity of "morbid" phenomena and it is both possible and probable that the works of Dickson, Jennings and of the Thomsonians did not reach Germany. It is also a fact that Kuhne arrived at his conclusions by an entirely different process of reasoning.

Kuhne's theory is that disease is caused by the accumulation and deposition, in the body, of *foreign matter*. "The presence of such foreign matter in the system," he says, "is disease. This matter consists of substances of which the body has no need. . . ." "We can best designate the forms of disease resulting from such accumulation, as painless and hidden; they are essentially the same as those generally called chronic or lingering."

After developing his theory of disease as briefly skeletonized above he declares:
"From the foregoing exposition we must now draw the momentous conclusion: THERE IS ONLY ONE CAUSE OF DISEASE AND THERE IS ALSO ONLY ONE DISEASE, WHICH SHOWS ITSELF UNDER DIFFERENT FORMS. We, therefore, ought not, strictly speaking, to distinguish betkeen different diseases, but only between different forms of disease. It may be remarked in passing, that direct injuries, which are not really disease in the above sense, are not here included; I shall speak of them in detail further on when, dealing with the Treatment of Wounds."

There is an obvious difference between the unity of disease as seen by these people. Kuhne places injuries, poisoning, etc., outside the pale of *unity*, whereas Jennings included these. The reason for this difference is apparent. Jennings regarded disease (the aggregate of symptoms—pain, fever, inflammation, etc.) as a curative process and as curative regardless of the inducing causes; whereas, Kuhne defines disease as the "morbid encumberance" or "foreign matter" and not as a process at all. Kuhne really confounded the inducing causes of disease with the disease process itself.

The Physio-Medicalists, on the other hand, regarded all disease as the inability of an organ to function properly and, in this sense, all disease is a unit. They laid very little stress upon the unity of the process we call disease although they partially recognized this at times.

Jennings' conception is more in harmony with our present knowledge than that of Kuhne or the Physio-medicalists. Dickson, Rausse and Miss Nightingale may also be said to agree more closely with our present conceptions. It is the process and not the inducing cause that is the essential *unit*, as will be made clear a little later.

Dr. Benjamin Rush, who signed the Declaration of Independence, and who also insisted, when the Constitution was being framed, that provisions for medical liberty equal to that of religious and political liberty be made, also accepted the idea of the unity of disease. Dr. Rush was one of the greatest minds of the Revolutionary period, a scientist and painstaking investigator. It cannot be said whether he arrived at his convictions independently or received them from Thomson with whom he was very friendly and whose views he endorsed to a great extent. He declared:

"Much mischief has been done by the nosological arrangement of diseases. . . . Disease is as much a unit as fever. . . . Its different seats and degrees should no more be multiplied into different diseases than the numerous and different effects of heat and light upon our globe should be multiplied into a plurality of suns.

"The whole materia medica is infected with the baneful consequences of the nomenclature of disease; for every article in it is pointed only against their names. . . . By the rejection of the artificial arrangement of diseases, a revolution must follow in medicine. . . . The road to knowledge in medicine by this means will likewise be shortened; so that a young man will be able to qualify himself to practice physic at a much less expense of time and labor than formerly, as a child would learn to read and write by the help of the Roman alphabet, instead of Chinese characters.

"Science has much to deplore from the multiplication of disease. It is as repugnant to truth in medicine as polytheism is to truth in religion. The physician who considers every different affection of the different parts of the same system as distinct diseases, when they arise from one cause, resembles the Indian or African savage who considers water, dew, ice, frost, and snow as distinct essences; while the physician who considers the morbid affections of every part of the body, however diversified they may be in their form or degree, as derived from one cause, resembles the philosopher who considers dew, ice, frost, and snow as different modifications of water, and as derived simply from the absence of heat."

We agree perfectly with Dr. Rush in placing those who see in every "abnormal" manifestation of life a different and specific disease on the intellectual level of savages and those who view these different manifestations as varying expressions of one thing on the intellectual plane of the philosopher. H_2O (water) is solid (ice), liquid (water), or vapor (steam) depending on the conditions of temperature and pressure under which it exists, but it is always H_2O and one form may always be transformed into the other. So, with disease. So with the varying forms of disease.

After describing the internal condition of the sick man—with reference both to general and local enervation and to general and local toxemia—Dr. Trall says, *Hydropathic Encyclopedia*, p. 66:—

". . . it may well be supposed that the *vis medicatrix naturae* would present many phases of irregular and disorderly action; sometimes concentrating the whole remedial effort in one direction or to one outlet; sometimes making it, with more or less force, successively in various directions."

This well describes the fact of the unity of the disease process. It is the same whether "located" in one organ or part or in another organ or part.

The terms measles, typhoid fever, pneumonia, etc., only indicate a more or less distinctive group of symptoms. But these "diseases" are not as *distinctive* as we may on first thought believe. No two cases of any "disease" are exactly alike. *There are no typical cases.* Text-books of medicine describe typical cases of this or that disease but no case the practitioner ever meets ever follows these descriptions. This will largely account for the frequent mistakes in diagnosis.

A few symptoms are grouped together and called a disease. They are endowed with individuality and are given a specific name and henceforth are regarded as though they represent specific entities. But the symptoms of all "diseases" are the same. Fever is the same thing whether it is in "measles," "scarlet fever," "typhoid," "pneumonia" or "other" disease. So is pain. So is acceleration of heart action or of respiration. So is decreased function. Destruction of tissue in one organ is the same as destruction of tissue in another organ. No "disease" possesses its own symptoms. All "diseases" are merely varying groups of the same symptoms. Each "disease" is a group of symptoms that varies greatly with different patients and under different modes of treatment, or at different periods of life. The unity of phenomena is a fact even in Pathology. The nomenclature of the schools should be abolished, since it tends to confuse and mislead.

The essential unity of phenomena is a corner stone of modern science. Biological phenomena is no less a unit. The many uniform needs of the body constitute a unity of function in organs of the widest dissimilarity of form, so that that however different these may be in shape, structure or position they all serve the ends of the animal economy, and enable the body to adjust itself to the varying conditions of its environment. The forces and processes of the body are all surbordinate to a system of adaptation and adjustment.

In contemplating the vast system of adjustment that we call the Universe, we are impressed with a sense of its unity. In contemplating the almost equally intricate system of adjustment in the living organism we cannot fail to be impressed with this same sense of its unity. It is difficult to understand why the various sects of Heteropathy have not long ago sensed the essential unity of *healthy* and *morbid* phenomena and seen in each of these the orderly operations of the living system of adjustment and adaptation.

To quote Arthur Vos, M.D., B.A., a reformed medical man, *The Unity of Diseases:*

"It is indeed a strange and inexplicable fact that the regular medical profession, of all the various professions in the world today, should be the last one in point of time to recognize a unity in the phenomena of those things in which it claims to have what would almost amount to a monopoly of knowledge. . . . the regular medical profession is alone groping along in its usual experimental and haphazard way of declaring that the thousand and one diseases described in its text books are so many independent entities, having no connection either in cause or in manifestation. That a neuritis of the shoulder, for instance, has been traced to a pyorrhoea alveolaris, to a diseased condition of the tonsil, to a sinus inflammation and even to a diseased ovary and tube is an occurrence frequent enough; but that pyorrhoea, tonsilitis, sinusitis and salpingoovaritis are conditions that may have a common, unifying causative element, even though

132

such disease conditions appear remote in place and time has rarely been suspected. It seems rather contradictory and peculiar that the medical mind recognized the possibility of one disease condition arising either simultaneously with or subsequently to some other disease, commonly called complication, and yet be unable to comprehend that all such disease conditions must have a universal substratum, aside from the human body itself, to support them. It is indeed unfortunate that such a view is not generally held by the medical profession for it would add both confidence and certainty and would contribute very largely to the greater success of medical practice; . . .

"From the very time that I was taught to think in medical terms, in fact from the very day that I entered upon my duties in the Cincinnati General Hospital, the usual nosology and classification of diseases presented to my understanding a rather insuperable difficulty. I could not comprehend why such recurring ailments as sick headaches and many forms of neuralgia were not considered by the profession as standing in some causative relationship with such subsequent conditions as Bright's Disease, diabetes or cancer, which invariably terminated the lives of individuals in whom simple ailments so frequently recurred. Presented with a problem of this kind, I could not but conclude that the patient who had been afflicted with recurring colds in the head from time to time and who came to me later with hay fever and subsequently developed bronchial asthma and still later rheumatic arthritis, must have been suffering with a single constitutional condition, the various so-called simple diseases and ailments being merely so many manifestations of one fundamental and constitutional origin. However, having neither time nor inclination for formulating a philosophy on these, my observations, and being considerably disturbed because of a lack of clarity in my own ideas and understanding on the subject, I turned to the regular medical literature of the day in the hope of finding some definite and satisfactory answer to my problems. But here I was doomed to disappointment, and, not finding a satisfactory explanation of such disease phenomena that appeared to me to have some common element as their cause, I then turned to the literature of the so-called irregulars, where, much to my delight and benefit I found a theory of the unity of disease that satisfied my inquiries and gave me a safe and useful working hypothesis in the practice of my profession. The effect of this new theory of the unity of disease was revolutionary for, henceforth, all doubt as to the best method of procedure disappeared and I could ever afterwards approach the sick bed with a confidence and certainty that dispelled every misgiving as to the ultimate recovery of my patient. The singular advantage as I saw it then of a theory of the unity of disease consisted chiefly in the fact that active and successful treatment of disease could be begun in the first visit to my patient, even in those cases and under those circumstances where the diagnosis may, for a time, have been uncertain or in doubt."—*Philosophy of Health, June, 1926.*

But if disease is a unit and the disease process is the same wherever located and however far advanced, how are the apparent different diseases accounted for. This question may, at first, seem difficult to answer. However, the difficulties are more apparent than real. The so-called different diseases are disease in different organs or in different structures. The apparent differences are given to them by the differences in the affected organs and the degree of affection.

The brain can't vomit and the stomach can't become insane. The liver can't urinate and the kidneys can't produce bile. The bowels can't cough and the lungs can't give rise to a diarrhea. The heart can't sweat and the skin can't miss pulsations. Each tissue has its own work to perform and when affected or deranged gives rise to its own peculiar symptoms—that is each deranged organ speaks its own language or dialect.

The symptoms of any disease are characteristic of the part affected. The distinguishing symptoms of the "different" so-called diseases are due to the differences in the organs affected. Thus, if the meninges of the brain and cord are affected, stupor and delirium will be present; if the lungs are affected, respiratory difficulties are present; if the stomach, intestine or bowels are affected, the symptoms will be characteristic of these organs. It is the tissue that is affected and the degree of the affection that lends individuality to disease. All the specific characters of disease are derived from the tissue or organ affected and not from some specific character of the "disease" itself. Disease is not an entity.

133

The reason for calling one form of disease catarrh, another diarrhea, or appendicitis or phrenitis, or tonsilitis, or metritis, or nephritis, or asthma or headache, etc., is not because of any real essential difference in the "disease," nor even in the cause of the "disease," but rather because of the difference in location. Each organ has its own way of acting and feeling and this gives rise to "different" symptoms. The real difference in one disease and "another" disease is in the structure and function of the organ affected. All disease is essentially one, every form having essentially the same general characteristics and, at basis, due to the same causes.

In the chapter in *Inflammation* it was learned that inflammation is a unit. Names and forms relate, not to the process we call inflammation, but to the organ affected or to the stage of the process. Inflammation of the tonsils is not one disease and inflammation of the ovaries another disease. It is the same thing in different locations. Ovarities and tonsilitis are merely names denoting locations. Inflammation is the same in whatever location it is found—whether in the brain or appendix or lungs or legs. The various names given to the "inflammations" are derived from the organs or tissues inflamed.

Dr. Moras, in *Autology*, divided diseases into two general classes: Muco-purulent and Sero-purulent—depending on whether they had their local seat in a mucous membrane or in a serous membrane.

". . . These two membranes assort and refine the material offered them by the organ-cells proper, and then turn out the various grades of their respective by-products through their meshes and walls and reject the unusuable, which they must accumulate in the tissues to be burned up in 'fevers' or disposed of as 'discharges' or 'effusions,' or 'exudates' or 'dropsy' or 'catarrh,' etc."

Carrying this thought a bit further, he said:

"As the lining sac of joints is 'serous' instead of 'mucous,' it is natural that the inflammatory or excessive exudate which leaks into the joints, instead of into the bronchial tubes or throat or uterine cavity, should be 'serous' instead of 'mucous' or slimy."

If then there is inflammation in the knee joint the exudate will be serous fluid, but if the inflammation is in the bronchial tube the discharge will be mucous or catarrhal. *Serous inflammation* is inflammation in a serous membrane and it's underlying structures while *catarrhal inflammation* is inflammation in a mucous membrane and its underlying structures. The inflammation is the same in both cases. The cause may be the same in both cases. The differences in the "two diseases" are in the structures involved. Either of these "forms" of inflammation may become purulent—that is there may result a breaking down of tissue. These differently located inflammations differ only in location and exciting causes.

Catarrhal inflammation may exist in any mucous surface in the body and may be either acute or chronic. Or inflammation may begin in one mucous surface and, as time passes, extend to other mucous surfaces. Thus a woman who has catarrh of the nose and throat may develop metritis and the woman who has asthma or hay fever almost always has leucorrhea and metritis. The same constitutional derangement is at the bottom of each of these "diseases." Hay fever is but an aggravated case of catarrh. Bronchial asthma is a bronchial catarrh. The symptoms in these "diseases" are fundamentally the same. The distinguishing symptoms are those of location or structure. Asthma is a special disease only because it is located in the bronchial tubes and not in the nasal passage or colon. Dr. Tilden sagely observes that if the structural changes occurring in the nasal mucosa during an attack of hay fever or in the bronchial mucosa during an attack of asthma were also to occur in the neck of the womb their presence there would afford a complete and adequate explanation of the phenomena of dysmenorrhea or painful menstruation. "This simile," he adds: "can be carried to every passage and cavity of the human body that is lined with mucous membrane. The fact is, there is no difference between a catarrhal state of one part of the body and that of some other part."

The same blood and flesh condition that causes asthma can and does cause uterine and ovarine diseases to develop and exist at the same time the asthma exists. The asthma is not the cause of the uterine troubles nor *vice versa*. They both stem from the same fundamental cause. Osler ascribed uterine and ovarine troubles as rare causes of an attack of asthma. Dr. Tilden rightly replied that this statement "is equivalent to saying that the hair on the dog's tail causes hair to grow on his ears."

Catarrhal inflammation of the bile ducts receives one name, while catarrhal inflammation of the gall bladder receives another. These "two diseases" are obviously only one condition in two locations. Regarding them as different diseases is like regarding dirt on the parlor floor as a different disease to dirt on the bedroom floor. Catarrh of the gall bladder or bile-ducts always follows catarrh of the stomach and intestine and is an extension of this. It is but a part of gastro-intestinal catarrh, and results from the same causes. The catarrhs are not different diseases but the same condition manifested in different locations. When this fact is once fully realized the problems of disease are greatly simplified.

Thus, we might go on with "disease" after "disease" and show that disease in one organ of the body is the same as disease in another organ. Inflammation in the kidneys gives rise to different symptoms to those produced by inflammation of the liver, not because the inflammation is different, but because the liver and the kidneys differ. The cardinal symptoms of inflammation—pain, redness, swelling, heat and impaired function—remain the same in either case. A tumor or cancer in the kidneys is the same as a tumor or cancer in the liver or womb. Atrophy and degeneration of the kidneys is the same as atrophy and degeneration of the liver or heart or brain, and is due to the same causes. An abscess in one organ is the same as an abscess in another organ. Diseases are all of a piece.

The symptoms of catarrhal inflammation differ somewhat with different locations. If it is located in a narrow passage as in the bile duct, Eustachian tubes, urethra, neck of the womb or bronchial tubes, obstruction will occur and the "symptoms of obstruction will be urgent and in keeping with the importance of the passage. Inasmuch as the bronchial tubes are necessary for the admission of air into the body, anything that interferes with their lumen causes breathing to become urgent."

Tilden declares, *Criticisms of the Practice of Medicine*, Vol. 2, p. 206:—

"It is true that an inflammatory process presents symptoms a little different with each different anatomical location. Inflammation of the stomach causes vomiting of mucous, and the symptoms are nausea, pain and vomiting. In duodenitis there is usully jaundice, and not always diarrhea; this inflammation frequently follows burns to the surface of the body, and may be expected in catarrh of the gall bladder and with gall stones.

"When the inflammation is of the small intestine there will be colicy pains about the naval region and large liquid discharges, with mucous well mixed with the movement. In inflammation of the large intestine—colitis—there is much colic and the pain is lower than the naval, and if the inflammation is great there will be long, ropy discharges. Sometimes the mucous has the appearance of sloughed mucous membrane. In acute colitis and sigmoditis there are large watery discharges at times; then, again, small discharges, mixed with blood, after the disease has lasted from three to seven days. This disease is especially marked by backache and distress in the legs reaching down to the feet. A severe attack is exceedingly distressing."

Is there need to further multiply facts to show that catarrhal inflammation in one organ is the same as that in another and that the differences in symptoms are only those of degree and those supplied by the different structures involved? The inflammatory process is the same, the exudate is the same, the cause is the same.

What then of diseases of serous cavities? Are they not the same whether located in the pleura of the lungs or in the synovial membranes of the knees? The serous effusion that oozes from the pleural cavity, the ovaries and testes, or in the brain and spinal cord or in the joints or in the scrotum or in dropsy or in edema anywhere in the body is physically and chemically the same and all originates from the same blood and lymph. The same blood and flesh condition that gives rise in inflammation with effusion in one serous-lined or serous-covered organ can and does give rise to inflammation with effusion in another such organ. "Sero-purulent" diseases are a unit differing only in location and extent or degree.

The oneness and sameness of catarrhal conditions and the oneness and sameness of dropsical or edematous or serous conditions are facts which should be patent to all with intelligence enough to read English. But we go a step further. There are no differences in "muco-purulent" and "sero-purulent" diseases. The differences are in the organ or organs affected. Inflammation in the pleura does not differ from inflammation in the bronchial tube. In the one we have a serous-exudate or effusion; in the other a mucous discharge. The pleura is a serous structure and cannot secrete mucous. The lining of the bronchial tubes is a mucous structure and cannot secrete serous fluid. Each tissue turns out its own product from the same blood and lymph.

Whether catarrhal "disease" and edematous "diseases" are called acute or chronic, contagious or infectious makes no difference. They are all one and the same thing and all come from the same source and in the same way.

There is no essential difference between pneumonia and typhoid, encaphelitis or appendicitis, tonsilitis or nephritis. Whether we have one or the other depends not upon any predeliction of the toxins for the sick organ, but upon the weakness of the organ. The weaker organ is the most vulnerable. It offers least resistance to the toxins. This organic weakness that renders one organ more vulnerable to poisons is usually, if not always, a structural or anatomical weakness. Such weakness may be inherited, congenital or the result of abuse. Chronic disease is a contending against chronic provocation.

A patient once handed the writer a long report issued to her by the Life Extension Institute, after she had been examined by their physicians. A detailed report was made out for the patient and another was made out for her to give to her physician. On this latter report were listed twenty-three physical defects in various locations in her body ranging from diseased tonsils and a few bad teeth to worse conditions. The report then said to the physician:

"Minor physical impairments are listed on the detailed report but are not considered to be at present affecting the general health."

The implications of this language clearly express the up-side-down view of disease that prevails in medical circles. The twenty-three defects that were considered worthy of notice by the physician and the minor ones that were unworthy his notice are regarded as independent affections and not as depending on the same primary or basic cause, not as merely local manifestations of a general condition. On the contrary the language implies that the local trouble affects the general health; that is, the local trouble is the primary trouble, while the impairment of the general health results from this. The language also implies that the local impairment is the thing that should receive attention and that those that "are not considered to be at present affecting the general health," should be ignored until they have developed to sufficient magnitude that they do affect the general health. All of this confusion and uncertainty arises out of a view of life that regards the organs of the body as independent isonomies and its affections as independent entities. When the unity of the body and the unity of its affections are understood and accepted this uncertainty will pass away.

The difference in "Bright's disease" and "diabetes" is not a difference in the tissue destruction that has occurred, but is a difference in the tissue that is destroyed. If the same destruction occurs in the brain insanity or paralysis or both may result; if in the cord, paralysis. If the causes of disease are not corrected, if they are permitted to continue until organic change takes place, until tissue destruction occurs, the "disease" that results will depend on the organ or organs that are the subjects of greatest change. Functional disturbances can result in organic disease only if the cause is great enough or of sufficient duration. Atrophy of an organ or parts of an organ is brought about by the same causes and is part of the same process.

It will, of course, be objected that so-called veneral diseases are exceptions; that they fall outside the pale of the general unity of disease. This is not so, however. Veneral diseases do not differ from other diseases. Why is pain, inflammation, suppuration, discharges, etc., different in the sex organs? They are not. They are the same processes and serve the same purposes as when they occur in the tonsils or stomach. The sex organs cannot be separated from the rest of the body as independent isonomies. They are not governed by laws different from the laws governing the liver or lungs. They are integral parts of that structural and functional unit we call the body and are subject to the same governing principles as every other part of the body. The body is not a mere machine without vital connection between all its parts. Rather, it is an organic whole every part of which is dependent upon the whole and the whole upon every part.

It should be observed that the principle of the essential *unity of disease* does not involve the unity of cause of disease, although there is a broad general sense in which this latter unity is real. It matters not whether inflammation is directed to the repair of a wound, the destruction and removal of infection, as after vaccination, the removal of a sliver or gun shot from the flesh or a parasite from the skin or liver, it is essentially the same process and serves ultimately the same end and object. Whether it is a bee sting on the eye lid, a burn on the leg or a caustic substance in the throat that occasions the inflammation, the process is identical differing only in degree and receiving its specific character from the tissues affected and from the degree of inflammation essential to success of the work in hand.

The rule of practice that must grow out of the recognition of the unity of disease, is all "diseases" by whatever names they are called and wherever they are located are to be regarded and treated alike.

There is not one treatment for inflammation of the knee and another for inflammation of the chest or lungs. There is not one treatment for diabetes and another for Bright's disease; nor one treatment for tuberculosis and another for cancer.

To quote Moras:—

"I cannot too strongly impress on your mind this one foundation principle of Autology and Autopathy; namely, that the essential cause or blood-and-flesh condition which sickens one organ or tissue, in one person, is exactly the same as that which sickens another organ or tissue in another person. The actual or real difference is not in the ailments or sickness, but it is in the difference of the organs or tissues involved or affected and in the environments in which you live and toil and play and think.

"When once you get this 'truth and sense' fixed in your brain, you will quit trying to treat your head or nose or stomach or bowel or liver or kidneys or fevers or colds, etc., etc., but you will begin to treat the 'sound' or healthy tissues of your body in order to enable your system to throw off the 'objectionables' and to repair the 'damages'; thus re-establishing equilibrium."

Again:

"You own some prejudices about yourself and your ailments. They are a menace or a hindrance to your health. Let us get rid of them. All your prejudices amount to one. They arise from the mistaken idea that your ailment calls for a different remedy, or treatment, or diet, than somebody else's ailment calls for; or from the equally mistaken idea that you need a different remedy, or treatment, or diet, for your liver than you do for your kidneys, or for 'catarrh' than you do for 'rheumatism' or for 'constipation' than you do for 'diarrhea?' But you don't.

"Or, that any 'sick' organ or function anywhere is man's or woman's body should be treated differently than any other 'sick' organ or function anywhere else in man's or woman's body. But it shouldn't.

"At first it may seem somewhat difficult to see through this foundation-truth of Autology and Autopathy. Yet—think it over a minute. You—that's every bit of your blood and organs and tissues—were created with, and you subsist on, the same elements of light, air, water and foods that enter into the creation and composition of other people's blood and flesh. And when you were well, nature kept you 'well' with the same blood-and-flesh remedies that she keeps other people well with. So, likewise, when nature makes or keeps you sick, she does it with the same blood-and-flesh things that she makes or keeps other people sick with."

The unity of disease and the unity of cause leads inevitably to the unity of cure. This is to say, the cure of one disease is the cure of all disease. I do not, here, employ the word cure in the sense of a something that is given or done to the patient that imparts health to him or her, but rather as the natural processes and conditions that result in the spontaneous restoration of normal health.

If disease is a unit, as we have shown, and if it is, in general, the resultant of a common basic cause, as we have said and shall prove in another chapter, what

137

bearing do these facts have on specialism in medicine? Suppose, for instance, that a woman suffers with tonsilitis and metritis or ovaritis, does she need two "specialists," one a "specialist in diseases of the throat" and the other a "specialist in diseases of the genito-urinary organs?" And if she also suffers with intestinal catarrh must she call in a "specialist in intestinal diseases" to care for the third condition? Or will the "cure" of *one* disease "cure" the *other*? It should be obvious that if we do not have two diseases or three diseases, but merely the same condition in two locations or in three locations, neither of them causing the other, but all of them caused by the same primary factors, all "three" diseases would be cured by correcting or removing the primary factors. A specialist would merely treat the diseased organ that is the object of his specialty and ignore the basic cause of the trouble. In its very nature specialism in medicine is a system of tinkering and patchwork. It is a failure where it is not a disaster.

It is a commonplace fact that the specialist can find the disease that is the object of his specialism in almost every patient that comes to him. It is no uncommon thing for a patient to visit a dozen or more specialists and return with a dozen or more "diseases" and a dozen or more prescriptions. And all these specialists may be right in their diagnosis inasfar as they name the symptoms or pathology they find. They are all wrong, however, insofar as they consider each "disease" to be a separate entity, each independent of the other and insofar as they fail to recognize that these dozen or more "diseases" are merely so many local manifestations of a general or systemic derangement.

Because of it lacks unity and coherence, what is called medical science presents a pitiful spectacle of confusion, frenzy and impotency. Dr. Tilden well describes it as follows:—

"The mind without a fundamental philosophy looks about it and sees nothing but diversity; the philosophical mind sees order and unity in diversity. The doctor without philosophy sees in man a heterogeneous junk-pile of different kinds of organs, requiring a specialist for each organ; the philosophical physician sees in a deranged organ a local expression, of a constitutional perversion, and, instead of 'plucking the eye out because it offends,' the cause is removed and the eye stops offending

"Unfortunately, the professional mind runs routine on custom—professional precedent—which, with no fundamental philosophy, causes it to see in every symptom-complex an individual disease—not a clean cut individuality with a symptomatology so stable that he who runs may read. On the contrary, there is a borderland to every so-called disease, causing it to blend with other complexes or diseases, requiring the intensive farming peculiar to, and belonging to, specialism to designate—diagnose. Hence the field of symptom-complexes—diseases—has been divided into four hundred individual diseases, requiring four-hundred specialists, who in turn require clinicians to survey the field and designate what particular specialist or specialists are required. Often a patient is so honey-combed with diseases that he requires several specialists. To meet this requirement of *modern medical science*, groups of scientific experts form collation for the purpose of special examinations and final group consultations; after which even God Almighty stands abashed at the display of erudition, not even dreamed of in His philosophy"—*Philosophy of Health.*

THE CAUSES OF DISEASE

Chapter XVI

A CERTAIN fact of common observation which has been denominated *The Law of the Cell*, has been formulated in these words: "*Every cell in the body will continue to perform the functions for which it was designed throughout its entire life cycle provided its environment remains congenial to it.*"

Many experiments have shown that the cells of the animal body require, if they are to continue to live, grow and reproduce, proper nutrition, adequate drainage, a suitable temperature and protection from violence. Cells forming the bodies of the higher animals are not capable of independent existence under ordinary circumstances because of their specialized character. Once the germ cells of the developing embryo become differentiated they are incapable of returning to their former undifferentiated or germ-cell state. This is to say, muscle cells, when once they have become such, can never be anything other than muscle cells. To borrow from Delafield and Prudden "when differentiation has advanced so that such distinct types of tissue have been formed as connective tissue, epithelium, muscle, nerve, these do not again merge through metaplasia. There is no evidence that mesoblastic tissues can be converted into those of epiblastic or hypoblastic type, or vice versa." Once cells have been differentiated and dedicated to a particular function, they can never become another and distinct type of cell with other and different functions. Therefore their dependence upon the body and their helplessness when separated from it.

In experimenting, in the laboratory, with pieces of tissues from animals it has been found that if these are washed clean each day and supplied with a fresh nutrient media, they are able to live indefinitely. They grow and reproduce, old cells even regenerating and becoming young again. They do not seem to grow old in the sense that their vitality becomes diminished. Their life and health depend upon the medium in which they live and upon its being continually renewed.

The organs composing the animal body make the medium in which its cells live. The body is also capable within reasonable limits of regulating and maintaining its temperature at the desired point. Such bodies are equipped with organs whose duty it is to take crude food substances from the surrounding environment and prepare it for use by the cells. Other organs carry it to and from the cells. Other groups of organs eliminate from the body or from this medium which bathes its cells in a continuously flowing stream, all the waste and poisons that have been formed by the activities and breaking down of the cells, or which have gained an entrance into the body from without.

Under ordinary circumstances the Amoeba is supposed not to die. Barring death by violence, poisoning or starvation it is supposed to go on dividing and rediving forever. Conditionally it is supposed to be possessed of everlasting life. What are the conditions upon which life depends? So far as these are discoverable they are: Appropriate food, water and oxygen, proper temperature and freedom from poisoning and violence. We might say its life depends upon a favorable or congenial environment, and that so long as its environment remains congenial it continues to function and reproduce.

The larger plants and animals are made up of cells assembled in vast numbers. When cells are thus massed as in the body of a worm, the situation of the cell differs much from that of the cell leading an independent existence. Its environment is made up largely of other associated cells. Comparatively few are in direct contact with the outside world; the greater portion being submerged among their brothers. They are shut in from food supplies, from the oxygen of the air and from water. A cell so situated would soon perish, were no special provisions made for its needs.

The cells composing an animal body are similar to, though more complex than, the amoeba. All cells composing the body of any animal are of common descent, but they have taken on widely different characters and functions, this being made necessary by the conditions under which they are to exist. The amoeba, leading an independent existence, must perform all the activities essential to its existence—preparation of crude food, locomotion etc. In the multi-cellular animal this is changed.

139

The specialization which groups the cells of such an animal into a number of classes, each with definite work to perform, also, entails the dependence of each class upon the other. While the amoeba is self-sufficient those of the animal cannot continue to live under ordinary circumstances if separated from the body.

The association of cells into an organism necessitates the formation of special structures to perform special work and this in turn necessitates the assumption of special functions by the cells making up the various structures. Special function, as distinguished from the common or fundamental functions of cells, is the power to perform a special work in the body. Special functions are those which are not common to all cells and are not essential to the life of the cell *per se*, but are essential to the life of the organism. Special function varies greatly for the different cells, some as the bone cells serving as supports for other structures; others like the skin cells as protectors; some, like the kidney cells excrete waste matter, some of the liver cells secrete bile, others store up glycogen, etc. Fundamental functions are those that are common to all cells alike and are essential to the life of the cell *per se*.

The living thing grows, reproduces and multiplies its parts and extends itself by this repitition. To affect this it selects from matter in contact such elements as it has the capacity to arrange as parts of its own structure, and as promptly rejects and refuses all others; *a necessary condition to the maintenance of its vital integrity.* In the plant or animal, or wherever vitality reigns, assimilation and growth and refusal and rejection are its constant actions, and *the energy of these acts must bear a constant relation to each other; for the vital endowment equally seeks its own welfare in either act.* This process of self-formation from dissimilar materials which is wholly peculiar to living things, and, without which, none exist is by appropriation and transformation. Collectively this is called nutrition.

Nutrition is the sum of the processes concerned in maintaining the normal condition of the cell and includes growth and repair. So long as this is adequately accomplished, the cells and the tissues which they form are able to perform their functions and to exhibit their own characteristic activities, to develop and maintain themselves. Development is the process by which each organ of a living body is first formed; or by which one which is already incompletely formed, is so changed in form and structure as to be fitted for the functions for which it is designed. Growth, which concurs with development and continues after it, is properly, the normal increase in the size of a part by the insertion or super-addition of materials similar to those of which it already consists. In growth proper, no change of form structure or function occurs. Parts only increase in weight and size, and if they acquire more power, it is power of the same kind as before exercised. Maintenance is the process of repair and reconstruction by which the worn out or injured parts of a tissue or organ are replaced. Development, growth and maintenance are all accomplished by cell proliferation and, in the case of development, differentiation. What produces the differentiation is not known, probably never will be known, but it is known that the power that determines the development of the embryo from the germ or ovum to the nine months infant is identical with that which is the source of the constant preservation and renovation and of the development and growth of the individual after birth.

The processes of cell life are carried on ideally only in a nutritive medium which is in a state of solution, life being possible to cells only when their nourishment is in liquid form so they can assimilate it. The amoeba, as was previously stated, lives in water or substances containing liquid. The cells composing both plant and animal bodies likewise require a liquid medium in which to live.

In all the larger forms there is a moving liquid medium which flows incessantly. In animals this medium is known as the blood and lymph, in plants as sap. This medium bathes all the living cells in the body and acts as a common carrier, supplying them with food and oxygen and removing their wastes. In the higher animals the lymph only comes in direct contact with the majority of the cells. From this they draw their needful supplies of food and oxygen and into it they discharge ttheir waste. The resources of the lymph at any point is very limited and is replenished constantly from the blood stream which passes close by in rapid movement in vessels whose thin delicate walls permit the passage of material both ways. The blood exchanges its fresh oxygen which it has just brought from the lungs for the carbon dioxide from the lymph. It then carries the carbon dioxide to the lungs and exchanges this for more oxygen. At the same time it exchanges fresh food for the waste of the cells and carries these wastes to the organs of elimination for excretion.

Just as the amoeba appropriates food and oxygen from the water or slime in which it lives and moves and has its being and excretes its waste into this same water or slime, so the cells composing the organs of the animal body appropriate food from the lymph in which they live and "move" and have their being, and excrete into this same lymph their waste.

If the nerve supply to an organ or part is destroyed it loses sensation and motion and perhaps it atrophies but it does not necessarily die. From this it becomes apparent that organic function is not possible in the absence of the nerve supply. If nutrition and drainage are cut off from an organ or part its death is only a matter of minutes. This may serve to show the relative importance of nutrition and drainage as compared to innervation, but it must not be lost sight of that nutrition and drainage in the higher animals is wholly a matter of organic function and that under all ordinary circumstances normal organic function is capable of maintaining nutrition and drainage up to the standard demanded by healthy life. The preparation of food the intake of air and water and their distribution to the cells and the removal of cellular waste and toxins are all accomplished by organs, the food, air and water being passive substances under the control of these organs.

Just as life, growth and reproduction, in the tissues used in the experiments, referred to in a previous paragraph is a master drama of nutrition, drainage, and warmth under the control of the scientists in the laboratory, so, life, growth, and reproduction, to the tissues in the body, is a master drama of nutrition, drainage and warmth under the control of the nervous system and the organs by means of which it accomplishes its work. If innervation is entirely suspended it results in a train of pathological phenomena included under term death. Respiration and circulation, and through the latter, nutrition and drainage, are suspended suddenly, if the cause is applied with sufficient force. If the cause is applied more gradually so that innervation is gradually suspended, in a few days, it may be , or in a few years it may give rise to any one or a number of the many pathological phenomena that have been classified as disease and given separate names.

The tremendous importance of the nervous system and the vital organs through which it carries on the functions of animal life is thus made manifest. For it must be borne in mind that such is the interdependence of the various parts of the body upon each other that serious injury to one speedily effects the others. Nutrition and drainage are as essential to the nervous structures as to the muscular or glandular, etc. Oxygen is required by the nerves as well as the muscles. If from any cause the lungs are damaged and oxygenation of the blood impaired the whole system suffers. If breathing is stopped entirely for a few minutes death of the whole body is the result. Damage to the heart suspending the circulation results in somatic death. Yet the sole work of the heart, and its accessory organs, the vascular system, is to distribute to the various parts of the body the nutritive material. Death comes because nutrition and drainage have ceased. Destruction or serious impairment of the kidneys, for instance, soon results in death from poisoning as these fail to relieve the blood of its load of toxins before its return to the tissues. The toxins soon accumulate in such quantities as to overwhelm the cells and stop all function.

The human body is adequately equipped with special organs the functions of which it is to keep the cells supplied at all times with food, water, oxygen, warmth and to carry away from the cells and cast out of the body all waste and poisons that form therein or that gain admittance from without. That the normal organism is fully capable of supplying its cells with these conditions of continued active life requires no proof. *There is no sound reason for believing that the cells of the body could not live as long and as well in the body as in the test-tube of the scientist if the functions of life are not impaired.*

Every organ in the human body, if not impaired or defective from birth, or from causes operating after birth, is capable of performing much more work than is necessary for the life of the organism. The heart and lungs, for instance, are capable of greatly increasing their work if one is called upon to do a hundred yard dash or even a ten mile marathon with a trolley car or a bear. The kidneys are capable of increasing their activities and taking up part of the skin's work if, for any reason, the skin fails in its duties. The skin, when one is subjected to great heat or to vigorous muscular effort, is capable of increasing its activities many times. The stomach, liver, intestines, bowels, etc., are all capable of doing much more work than the actual needs of life require. The organs of a normal body are capable of carrying on the functions of life under all ordinary circumstances without strain, so long as they are not impaired by some cause or causes.

If cells that are kept clean and properly nourished never grow old in the sense that they lose their vitality, and in the human body there are organs and functions that, when normal, completely rid the body of waste and toxins; and another process that, when normal, keeps the cells supplied with a fresh supply of nutrient material, what impairs these organs and functions so that the cells do grow old, do lose their vitality and die. It is assumed by some biologists, that this impairment is a necessary result of the community action of the cells of the body.

Cells in the laboratory are killed by starvation and by poisoning. Why assume that their death in the body is due to other causes? The uneliminated products of metabolism, plus the breaking down of cells in disease, plus toxins absorbed from without, are as capable of destroying cells in the body as in the scientist's test tube. Drugs, serums, vaccines, anti-toxins, etc., that are taken into the body, in any manner, for any purpose, kill cells and cripple organs. Starvation of the cells resulting from eating denatured food or from impaired digestion and assimiltaion is capable of killing cells in the body.

In considering the causation of disease it is important that we keep in mind that the antecedents of every so-called disease are many and not just one. As an instance, it is asserted that irritation is the cause of tumors, but irritation alone will not produce a tumor while the number of sites or localities of man's or woman's bodies that are subject to constant irritation which do not develop tumors are as infinity to one, when compared with the seats of irritation which do become tumors. Irritation is *a cause* and not *the cause*. It contributes to the production of a tumor. It is but one of a number of correlated factors which collectively constitute cause. It is an erroneous practice which men indulge in when they single out one of these correlates and say that it is the cause of cancer.

Headache is a symptom that may be produced by many different causes. A cold may be due to a simple indigestion, or to exposure, or to overwork, or to loss of sleep. But a simple indigestion is alone insufficient to produce a cold. Exposure, overwork, loss of sleep; neither of these alone can produce a cold. A cold is an evolution out of a number of correlated *causes*.

It is said that a certain germ causes a certain disease. This theory will be discussed later. At this point I only desire to call your attention to the fact that if germs are *a cause* of disease, they do not constitute *the cause* of disease. There are a number of antecedent causes and their effects which must be present before the germs can enter into *the cause*. At most they are but secondary and never primary causes. If we grant them a place in the causation of disease we must recognize that they are but one of a number of correlated causes which collectively constitute *the cause*. It is a mistake to single out one particular correlate and hold it responsible for the disease.

Disease is not a simple, but a complex effect, not of one antecedent but of many It is, as Dr. Tilden declares, "the sum of a multitude of elements." Individuals differ, the combination of causes differ in each individual case of disease, and hence, each supposed specific disease differs—no two cases are alike.

Two men are out hunting and are caught in a cold rain-storm. They are drenched and are exposed to the rain and cold for hours. The following day one has pneumonia, the other arthritis. A mother dies. Her children grieve deeply and long for their mother. One of them suffers a "nervous collapse;" the other develops Bright's disease. A group of people have a feast. They eat and drink. One develops a diarrhea, one develops typhoid, another has pleurisy, still another has rheumatism and another is apparently unharmed. One man indulges his sex appetite excessively and becomes extremely nervous. Another man worries over his business and becomes equally nervous. Consider these facts and hundreds more like them and you see that different causes acting on the body may produce the same result while the same causes acting on different bodies, or on the same body at different times may produce different results. Yet these things are true only because the correlates are different. If the correlated causes were identical in a thousand cases, then a heavy meal would, in conjunction with these correlates, cause the same difficulty in each of the thousand cases. These elemental factors in the causation of disease are legion. The idea that there are specific causes for specific diseases is purely fallacious. Every so-called disease is a river the waters of which are derived from many tributaries.

This being true what is to be thought of a mode of treatment which attempts to dry up the river ("cure" the disease) by destroying one of its tributaries (causal elements)? What are we to think of the effort to find a "unitary entity" which will immunize one against a multiplicity of causes? Is it not true, as Dr. Tilden says, that "a multiple causation must be met by an opposing treatment co-equal in elemental constituents?"

With these few preliminary remarks we will address ourselves to a brief consideration of the causes of disease, making no apologies for the order in which they are treated.

ENERVATION.

Vigorous health and a sound constitution is the natural and normal condition of man. Anything below this represents a stage of degeneracy or impaired health. From the topmost peak of bodily soundness to the lowest depths of physical depravity is a long and progressive decline brought about by adequate degenerating causes. The lowest depths of physical rottenness are not reached quickly or suddenly. Over the whole decline there are a number of successive stages that have to be passed through in their natural order.

The impairment of health is due to violation of the laws of life in our voluntary habits. To make this statement clear, let me first explain that the functions of the human organism are operated by and under control of a force which we call nerve force, because it resides in and is distributed by the nervous system. Without this force, organic function is impossible. When nerve force is abundant, bodily functions are vigorous; and when it is low they are impaired.

We might compare the body to an automobile and the nervous system to its storage battery. If the storage battery is well charged and the wiring is in good order, the car has plenty of spark, bright lights and an efficient starter. But, if the battery is low and the spark is poor, the lights are dim and the starter weak. Indeed, the starter may not be able to turn the engine over, and the battery may be so low that the car cannot be run and the lights burned at the same time.

The human body is not capable of generating an unlimited supply of nervous energy. Often in modern life we consume our energies faster than we recuperate them, so that our vital or nervous batteries run low. Then, just as a low battery means poor spark, dim lights and a useless starter on our cars, so lack of nervous energies in the human body lower the functional efficiency of all its organs. Digestion is impaired, secretion and excretion are checked, elimination lags. This condition we call Enervation. produced by severe injuries, surgical operations or by strong emotions. It consists in "a relaxation or abolition of the sustaining and controlling influence that the nervous system exercises over the vital organic functions of the body." There are all degrees of shock ranging in effect from slight disturbances of function to their total or almost total abolition. Rest, quiet and warmth are the essentials of recuperation and recovery Enervation always impairs organic function An excellent example of the manner in which enervation impairs organic function is supplied us by shock. This may be from this state: Jennings declared:—

"It is true ****that life in the human body is sustained by the presence and action of a real potential principle, which has its chief seat in the brain, and is drawn forth through the medium of the nerves, to the several parts of the body by a vital affinity or in virtue of a relation which the parts and powers sustain to each other; that this principle or power becomes exhausted or used up by action, and therefore needs a constant replenishment; and that, in consequence, it is liable to rise and fall in quantity and vigor, provided the expenditure exceeds the income; that the source and income of this power is beyond the ken and control of man; while both its economical and extravagant expenditure are within his discretion, and at his pleasure; that this principle of life can never be in excess, for if it were to abound in sufficient quantity to furnish a full supply to every moving fibre, and charge the whole of the solids and fluids to their fullest capacity, it could not exceed their necessity and demand, and would only serve to secure the most perfect health and highest degree of physical well being; that, other things being equal the health and strength of the system is in proportion to its vitality."—*Philosophy of Human Life*, pp. 89.

Enervation and feeble function are not disease. The functions of an organ may be feeble from a number of circumstances. Power may be withdrawn from one organ to support another as when the voluntary muscles "collapse" in typhoid fever. But this state of "collapse" does not indicate that the muscles are damaged.

Changes of conditions, climate, work, etc., may require more power to maintain the ordinary operations of life at their previous common standard. If the power is on hand, the body will easily and quickly meet the emergency, but if power is lacking function will falter. Local abuses of the body may result in such an excessive expenditure of power in one direction that functions elsewhere in the body falter. An enforcement of the *Law of Limitation*, or shutting down of expenditures generally, for repairing and replenishing purposes, causes functions to lag.

A mere temporary or partial exhaustion of power from too long continued or excessive action is quickly recuperated from if sufficient rest and sleep are secured. If stimulants are substituted for rest and sleep, recuperation lags and finally, function falters.

Many people in modern life so prodigally waste their powers that there is just enough for the steady maintainence of the structures and functions of the body at their common standard without leaving a balance as an accumulating fund for emergencies so that under ordinary circumstances the current expenditure of power by many people, while not enough to produce noticeable impairment of the body, leaves them with but a "pinching scantiness of motive power," so that, when unusual conditions or emergencies arise, there is not the power in reserve to meet the extra demands made upon the organism. A period of life is finally reached in which there is an accumulation of "pathological embarrassments" and those "organs standing foremost on the table of insolvency" are the first to falter and complain.

If there is a leak in a dam and it is not repaired it continues to grow larger until the existence of the dam is threatened. If there is a leak in the powers of the body and this is not corrected, its powers grow less and less each day until the stability and integrity of the body are threatened. If a man's life-blood is running away he makes an effort to stop the leak. If his nerve force is being leaked away day by day he should also make an effort to stop this leak.

In many ways men and women waste the forces of their bodies and deplete their vital reservoirs. Day by day their precious reserve funds are being eaten away and sooner or later a time is reached when the overdraft on the vital funds threatens the very foundations of their existence. Functional collapse forces a halt. Anorexia, nausea, vomiting, prostration, etc., put them in bed for repairs.

Under a full tide of the vital energies, with all the organs sound, function is perfect and a high standard of health is maintained. But with power low, functional efficiency is impaired.

Occasional causes of impaired function may or may not be connected with any structural defect or even with a low state of the vital funds. These may only cause a temporary expenditure of power beyond the immediately available supply and may occur in those of sound constitution, although this may more easily occur in impaired organisms. Such a tired, weary, faltering condition of the body is soon overcome by a night of sleep.

The difference between enervation and such a condition is one of degree and duration and not of kind. All impaired functions whether local or general, little or much, is due primarily to a tired state of the body or of the organs—to lessened power. The causes that use up power have operated so long and to such a degree, and recuperation has not kept pace with expenditure, that the enervation is constant.

When enervation has already been brought on it requires but a little more of debilitating agency or influence to place one on the sick list. The foundation for every disease is an exhausted state of the sub-treasury of life. If the funds on hand are low an unusual draught will necessitate a retrenchment of the vital forces for purposes of recuperation. Functions falter and discomforts develop. Dr. Oswald gives us an excellent example of this in dealing with asthma. He says:—

"Any waste of vital power may bring on a fit of spasmodic asthma, and the aggravating effect of *incontinence* is so prompt and so unmistakable that experience generally suffices to correct a *penchant* to errors in that respect. Like gout, asthma is a moral censor, but its reproofs do not so often come too late."

Any influence that places a little more tax upon the powers of the body may be enough to bring on a crisis in the feeble organism. By checking elimination and increasing the amount of systemic toxemia a crisis becomes necessary.

It should be known and borne in mind that the occasion for a crisis is entirely distinct from its *cause*, or rather its *causes*. The causes, by a little by little process, cripple and impair the organs of the body and thus lay the foundation on which the aggregate of symptoms, by whatever name they are called, rest.

The state of the body, therefore, more than anything else, determines the severity and duration of a disease. The common cold may be used as an admirable illustration of this.

Not infrequently a person will feel, in the evening, like he is developing a severe cold, and on awakening in the morning, find every vestige of it gone. Colds may last from a few minutes to a few weeks. Every one has his remedy for colds, and as these complaints usually get well of themselves in a very short time, whatever the "remedy" employed, these "remedies" are given full credit for recovery. It is thus that there is such a great variety of cold cures, all of which are of good reputation. Occasionally, however, a severe cold holds on for weeks or months and all the "cold cures" fail.

What causes enervation? Briefly, any act, habit, agent, influence, or indulgence that uses up nerve force in excess, or that prevents thorough recuperation from the daily activites. Let us glance briefly as some of these.

MENTAL CAUSES.

The destructive effects upon the body of certain states of mind are as interesting as they are evident. The effect is often like an electric shock altering the feelings, deranging the body's functions and affecting the individual's sanity as certainly as alcohol or opium.

Many people, particularly women, have a very bad habit of allowing their emotions to run away with them. Indeed, they seem to derive a kind of false pleasure out of the sham emotions which they purposely work up. A sham emotion is an impulse or sensation which is cultivated for its own sake. It is not intended to be translated into actions. Emotionalism is, indeed, a variety of intoxication, or, perhaps it is more correctly described as hysteria. Emotions or sensations should normally be translated into action. If they are cultivated for their own sake, with no purpose beyond this, they weaken and destroy both the mind and body. Intense emotions and sentimentalism work in much the same way as liquor and have very much the same evil results.

Religious emotions, often used as a source of pleasureable thrills, are very destructive to the nervous system. They have resulted in insanity in many instances. Any religion which leads to emotionalism, hysteria, trance, catelepsy, etc., is not religion, but mania. St. Paul admonished all Christians to exercise the "spirit of a sound mind."

Self-control is the great law of mental hygiene and he who has not learned to control his emotions is permitting these to cut short his life. Bear in mind that sham emotions, whether of art, music, love, or of some other nature are as weakening as religious emotions.

Fear is the most destructive of all emotions. It benumbs and paralizes the body and wastes nerve energy as few other things do It has often been the cause of sudden death in weak individuals. There is a striking similarity between great fear and freezing. In both cases the face is blanched, the teeth chatter, the body trembles (shivers), becomes cramped and bent, the chest is contracted, breathing is slow and comes in short gasps.

Fear greatly affects the heart. In one case of death of an animal, through fear, witnessed by me, the heart was ruptured.

The stomach ceases to function under fear. Dr. Cannon, noted investigator of the physiology and pathology of digestion, was once watching the movements of the intestines of a cat by means of the X-ray. One day during the course of his observations a dog barked near the laboratory, frightening the cat. The cat's intestines immediately became rigid and immobile, forcing him to discontinue his experiment for several hours. Fear had caused the rhythmic muscular motions of the cat's intestines to cease altogether. Many experiments have shown that these same influences interfere with and impair the functions of the glands that secrete the digestive juices. Note the dryness of the mouth, because of suspended salivary secretion, in fear.

Not only are the muscles and glands involved in digestion impaired by fear, but the muscles and glands of the whole body are impaired. Human beings, due to their more highly organized nervous systems, are more quickly and more profoundly affected by emotions than are cats or other animals and the results are more far reaching.

As another example of the effects of fear upon the secretion, there is the well known graying of the hair in those who have been profoundly shocked through fear, or by some great horror. Men sentenced to death often become gray haired in a few days. I saw young men go to France with hair as black as graphite and return a few months later as gray haired as aged men. This loss of color by the hair is due to the suspension of the secretion of minute glands at the roots of the hair. Fear caused the suspension. Fear often results in a sudden and involuntary discharge of the contents of the bowels and bladder. Apprehension causes frequent urination and often produces a diarrhea.

Worry is a baby fear. It impairs secretion and excretion and depresses all the functions of the body. The secretions are altered and nutrition is impaired. Poisons accumulate in the body. The victim gradually wastes away. None of the functions of the body are carried on properly under such a state of mind. The appetite is impaired and digestion is weakened. Every time there is a panic in the stock market the stock brokers rush to their physicians to be cured of constipation or of a functional glycosuria (sugar in the urine).

Jealousy is a curious combination of fear, anger and the desire to have and to hold. There is no doubt that it is a strictly natural, normal manifestation and it is met with among the lower animals. It is truly, as Mr. Macfadden has termed it: "the green-eyed guardian of the family honor." It is this so long as it does not dethrone reason and intelligence. If it dethrones these it is a devastating pestilence.

Some one has called self-pity, mental consumption. It is the dry-rot of the soul. We frequently meet whining, complaining individuals who feel that life has not given them a square deal. Instead of buckling down to hard work and earning the rewards of life, they sit around and feel sorry for themselves. Every such person feels that his lot in life is the worst that anyone ever had. I say "feel" advisedly for this class of people seldom think.

The mental state of such "lone, lorn creatures" is difficult to describe, but its effects on the body are readily apparent. They do not regain their health until they are educated out of their self-pity. They do not enjoy life. They do not relish their foods. Everything they eat disagrees with them. Their bowels never function properly. They never sleep well. They are victims of constant introspection. They are continually discovering new symptoms, new pains, new worries. They lead a miserable life, indeed. And their misery is all due to the fact that they feel sorry for themselves and desire that others also feel sorry for them.

Grief is among the mental states that exert the most profound, far-reaching and powerful effects upon the body. It takes away the appetite instantly. Intense grief often kills outright. As in fear, in grief also, the hair has been changed from black to grey in a few days. The secretion of the mother's milk is checked and altered as surely and quickly by grief as by lack of or by a change of food. Indeed, one of the immediate effects of grief is to reduce and impair secretion and function. Sorrow, as in disappointed love, often produces a wasted, weakened state of the body resembling consumption. Blighted love constitutes one of the most fruitful sources of indisposition.

Secretion and excretion are impaired, elimination is checked, digestion is deranged, nutrition is perverted, profound enervation is produced and toxemia grows daily. Weight is lost. Appetite is lacking. Disease and death may easily result.

Lying, stealing, cheating, gambling and all forms of dishonesty, produce enervation and hardening of the arteries. In all of these there is the fear of being found out. In gambling there is the tension and fear of losing. Before conscience becomes hardened there is the stinging lash of remorse and loss of self-respect.

Violent fits of passion will often arrest, alter or derange the functions of the body as quickly as an electric shock. Digestion may be wholly suspended by a profound state of fear, worry, anxiety or suspense. Fright, anxiety or even sudden joy are often immediately followed by diarrhea. Many students who have been exceedingly anxious about their examinations have experienced a diarrhea as a result. These same mental influences have all been observed to cause the appearance of sugar in the urine.

Mental shocks, anger, melancholy and all disagreeable or abnormal mental conditions render the secretions of the body more or less morbid. Anger quickly modifies the bile; grief arrests the secretion of the gastric juices; violent rage makes the saliva poisonous. Fear relaxes the bowels. It is claimed that many mothers have injured, and even killed, their nursing infants by furious emotions, which alter their milk. It is known that such emotions as fear, worry, jealousy, anger, anxiety, etc., will reduce the secretion of milk and impair its food value to such an extent that the infant does not thrive on it.

These things should serve to emphasize for us the fact that the functions of the body are all under nervous control and make us see that any influence that impairs the nervous system or wastes nerve force will bring on disease and death.

Such mental habits and mental states may be appropriately termed HABITS that KILL, for they do shorten life and often kill quickly. Learn, then to control your emotions. Self-control is the great law of mental hygiene. Cultivate poise, cheer and contentment. Be of good courage. Cast fear and worry aside. Learn to love your fellow men. Be not quick to anger. Dismiss your troubles and think upon the better things of life. By so doing your health will be improved and your life prolonged.

POISON HABITS.

All normal individuals are possessed of a natural repugnance to poisonous and injurious substances. The instinctive aversion to any kind of poison may be perverted into an unnatural craving after that poison. Instinct is plastic. If the warnings of the organic instincts are unheeded, and the offending substance is again and again forced upon the body, nature, true to the law of self-preservation, seeks to prolong life by adapting the body to poison.

All poison habits are progressive. The slave of a poison is conscious of a peculiar craving which is entirely distinct from a healthy appetite; an uncompromising craving for a once repulsive substance, each gratification of which renders it more irresistible. Only natural appetites have natural limitations. An appetite for peaches may be satisfied with strawberries, but an appetite for tobacco can be satisfied only with tobacco.

The seductiveness of every poison habit acquires strength with each indulgence, and that power is proportioned to the original repulsiveness of the poison. The opium habit holds its victims in a stronger grip than the coffee habit. Hashheesh is a more powerful master than tobacco. Tobacco is a more imperious master than tea.

But all these are progressive. The longer they are used the more is required to satisfy. Each indulgence is followed by a depressing reaction. The feeling of exhaustion is also steadily progressive and causes a correspondingly increased craving for a repitition of the stimulating dose, which forces the user either to increase the quantity of the poison used or else resort to a stronger poison. This is why abstinence is easier than "moderation." This is the reason one poison habit often leads to others. This is the reason, too, that one poison habit cannot be broken by substituting another and weaker poison for the one used, and supplies the reason why "tapering off" on a poison habit is a failure.

Tobacco produces enervation by overstimulation—poisoning. The use of tobacco will cut down one's vitality twenty-five to fifty per cent. In any of its forms, the tobacco habit is a foe to the user. It is a virulent posion—nicotine ranking next to prussic acid in its deadliness—and kills those not accustomed to its use when given in small doses. Its habitual use plays havoc with the nerves, unsteadying the hand and eye, impairing hearing and reducing efficiency. It stunts growth in the young, impairs digestion and produces "tobacco heart" in adults, and reduces strength and endurance in all. Due to this latter fact, athletes abstain from its use during periods of training for a contest. Repeated tests have shown that the use of tobacco lowers mental efficiency.

The lining membranes of the mouth, throat and lungs become hardened, thickened and reddened from the use of tobacco. This hardening, toughening and thickening is the means resorted to to protect against poisons and irritations. It is part of the process of adaptation and really cripples the efficiency of the organs thus hardened. ADAPTATION TO ANY HARMFUL INFLUENCE IS ALWAYS AC-COMPLISHED BY BODY CHANGES THAT ARE AWAY FROM THE IDEAL.

Many have the vulgar habit of smoking in the house. The walls, curtains, rugs, carpets, bedding, closets, etc., become saturated with tobacco poisoning and those who live in the house, the wife or mother, the children, are forced to breathe day and night, air laden with tobacco. Their health suffers as a result.

Alcohol is a strong poison and its use in any form is inimical to the human body as, indeed, it is to every organized thing in existence. It is a product of the decay of organic matter occasioned by bacterial action. Only a small percentage of it is required to arrest the action of the bacteria themselves. It is for this reason that it is employed as a preservative.

Whether ardent spirits, malt liquors, wines, cider or other alcoholic drinks are used, the alcohol they contain is poisonous. In small doses it acts as a stimulant, in larger doses its effects are those of a depressant. It is highly irritating to every organ and tissue of the body and there is not one of them that is immune to its destructive influence. It coagulates the protoplasm of the cells of the body, just as it coagulates, or cooks, the white of an egg. This coagulation impairs and destroys the cells.

The normal cells are then replaced by a substitute of connective tissue cells forming what is called "scar-tissue." This may occur in the brain and spinal cord resulting in paresis, paralysis, insanity and other nervous disease; in the liver producing sclerosis and ascites; in the heart and arteries producing hardening and other troubles in these; or it may occur in the lungs, kidneys, muscles or any other organ of the body. The functioning powers of these organs are gradually destroyed and the individual's resistance to other disease influences is lowered. The death rate and case rate in pneumonia is much higher in alcohol addicts than among abstainers.

"Moderate" drinkers are not immune to these effects. They receive their full share of them. In fact, the habitual "moderate" drinker receives more injury from alcohol than the occasional drinker who gets drunk when he does drink. It is used as a stimulant to digestion, but finally wrecks digestion.

Tea, coffee, cocoa and chocolate shall all be considered together because they all contain very much the same active principles and have very much the same effects. Neither of them have the slightest excuse for existences as beverages. Tea and coffee contain no food value, while the unaltered flavors of all of them are obnoxious to every unperverted taste. Cocoa-cola which contains caffine might also be included in this list.

They act primarily as stimulants and secondarily as depressants, or sedatives. Like tobacco, opium, and alcohol they are habit forming, and they are habit forming to exactly the degree in which they are stimulating. And they are stimulating in the degree to which they are poisonous and unfitted for the real needs of the body. The bitter, nauseous tastes of all these substances require the addition of sugar or other substances before they can be used by the undepraved taste.

It is the curse of all stimulants that they enable one to work beyond his normal strength. That is, they enable him to keep on working long after nature has called for rest. They do this, not by adding to the powers of the body, but by calling out the powers held in reserve. They act in the same way a spur does on a tired horse. Slowly, but surely, the reserve powers of the body are consumed under the influence of stimulants and physical bankrupcy follows. Coffee, tea, coca-cola, cocoa and chocolate, because of their almost universal use, are great offenders in this respect. They produce ENERVATION and sleeplessness in proportion to their use. Those who use them become coffee and tea or cocoa inebriates. They are addicts as truly as the opium user. The habitual user of tea or coffee is tired, listless, irritable and suffers with headache and other discomforts when deprived of his habitual cup. Nervous diseases result from the employment of such nervines.

Give a stimulant to a man of full-resistance and he reacts to it with increased activity and an increased feeling of well-being. When the period of increased activity ends there sets in, due to the excessive expenditure of energy and substance, a period of depression. Rest soon restores full health. All stimulation is followed by a period of depression equal in duration and intensity to the period of stimulation. Keep up this stimulation by habitual repetition and renewal of nerve energy fags. A permanent depression—a profound enervation—which forms the foundation for the development of any disease of the nosology, follows. There is a slowing down of the functions of the body. The processes of nutrition and elimination fail to meet physiological needs.

Stimulants stand at the head of the many causes of excessive expenditure of nervous energy. The increased feeling of strength which follows their use is due to the expenditure of power which they occasion and not to any power which they add. We are conscious of power only in its expenditure. A pure or uncompensated stimulant is any agent or influence that occasions or induces an increase in the activities of the body or any of its organs without supplying any real need of the body. All such stimulants should be avoided.

There are many very popular drug habits. Thousands daily take a purgative or a laxative to induce bowel action. Many thousands more employ drugs to aid digestion, or to brace up their nerves, or to tone up their system, or purify their blood. Many use patent medicines, others use proprietary remedies or their physicians' prescriptions. The patent medicines are almost, if not quite, as bad as those prescribed by the physician and should be avoided along with the rest.

There never was a drug or drug remedy that had any business in the human body. Speaking generally, drugs either destroy more or less of the tissues of the body or they occasion a needless and wasteful expenditure of its vital energies. Most of them do both these things. Their effects upon the system are not altered, because they are prescribed by a physician. It makes no difference once the drug is in the system who prescribed it; the effects are the same.

I shall pass over the opium, morphine, heroin and such debasing drug habits— not because they are unimportant, but because no one doubts their destructive offices —and shall pass to more common drug habits that are supposed by many to be beneficial. Among these is the use of headache remedies.

The habit of taking headache "remedies" is becoming a national pastime. The average person, apparently, suffers from frequent headaches, and, judging by the readiness with which they resort to the "remedies" they fear a few minutes of slight pain more than the deadly drugs they introduce into their system.

They do not realize what a terrible price they pay for this short respite from pain and for the restless stupor, miscalled sleep, which they secure through hypnotic or narcotic drugs. Deadening sensation does not cure disease; pain is never cured by deadening the nerves. Cause is never corrected in such manner. The reader should know that there is no cure outside of correction of cause.

Every dose of such drugs lessens nerve force and thereby impairs the various functions of the body. When nerve force is lessened there is always necessarily a checking of elimination resulting in a retention within the body of part of its waste products. And these produce disease and death. Every headache "remedy" interferes with elimination, and thus perpetuates the condition for which it is given. They are also habit forming, and many of them have a very deleterious influence upon the heart and other organs.

Anything that "relieves" pain without correcting its cause does so by diminishing the power of the nerves to feel. It is the part of wisdom to find out what is causing the trouble and correct this.

EXCESSES.

Man is adapted to his natural environment. He possesses a great power of resistance. He weakens his resistance by certain habits that have a debilitating effect upon him. Those who possess strong resistance may so weaken it that they fall easy prey to any unfavorable influence in their environment. Weather changes that have no appreciable effect upon the robust and strong occasion all manners of disagreeable symptoms and increase the severity of already existing ones in the sick and those of low resistance. The normal body, if not abused, is capable of adjusting itself to all ordinary conditions of nature. The author of nature did not intend that man, any more than the lower animals, should be the helpless victim of his natural environment. That delicacy which like the house plant, is injured by every breath of air, and that rottenness of constitution which is the effect of indolence, intemperance and debauchery was never intended by the Author of Nature, and lays the foundation for numerous diseases and premature death.

All excess is harmful. Exess means over-indulgence in the normal or wholesome things of life. The word excess is not correctly applied when used in reference to tobacco, opium, alcohol, etc., for this would imply that the use of these up to a certain point is normal and wholesome. Excess is more than the needs of the mind and body. It cannot be said that anything over the normal needs of the mind and body for tobacco, alcohol, etc., is excess for the mind and body have no normal needs for these things. Their use in any quantity is simply an unmitigated evil.

The human body is very largely a self-regulating organism. It is so constructed and arranged that if excessive demands are made upon it during youth and middle age, provisions for supplying these demands are made, so that there seems to be no injury done to the body. No generally recognized sign is given that the demands upon the body's forces are in excess and that its reserve fund is being slowly consumed. The greater the demands made upon the forces of life, apparently the greater the supply. However, no truth is more certain than that expressed by Sylvester Graham when he declared that: "An *intensive* life is not compatible with an *extensive* life."

What is called overwork is excess. We work or play until we grow tired. If we do not stop and rest we soon become so tired we cannot continue. Nature has wisely arranged that under ordinary circumstances we cannot use up all the energy we possess. She holds back a reserve fund for emergencies. If we always rest when tired, there will always be a surplus of reserve energy to be used under stress or to maintain good health.

When nature demands rest it is the custom to give her a stimulant. Overwork is really overstimulation. Fatigue is a demand for rest just as thirst is a call for water and hunger is a demand for food. Stimulants of all kinds overwork the organs of the body, prevent sleep and enable us to go on with our work long after nature has hung out her fatigue sign.

Those who disregard nature's call for rest, and go on in spite of it, are overworked. Ambition, the desire for fame, place, power and pelf, drives many to overstep the limits of fatigue and wreck their health in the pursuit of these baubles. The pursuit of happiness, or as it is practiced, the pursuit of thrills and excitement, overworks many more. Economic necessity goads many others onward into overwork. In any case, overwork is the result of forcing oneself to work when nature calls for rest, or, to put it differently, it is failure to secure sufficient rest and sleep to completely recuperate from one's daily activities.

Another form of overwork is that of keeping the body or parts of it tense at all times. To be constantly tensed in body, and perhaps in mind as well, constitutes a ceaseless drain upon your nervous energies, and is often largely responsible for the troubles for which people run to doctors. Many people are so tense and nervous that they do not fully relax when they go to sleep. This prevents them from falling asleep quickly and prevents sound restful sleep when they do fall asleep. As a consequence they do not awake refreshed in the morning. The tensed person is always tired and exhausted.

America is a busy world. We are always rushing, hustling, trying to get somewhere before we get started. This constant state of tension constitutes a terrible drain upon our nervous energies. Conservation is the secret of power. Relaxation is the means of conservation. Tension is a waste of power. Your reserve gone, you collapse just when it is most important that you hold up. Learn to relax—LET GO.

Another favorite form of excess is that of overeating. This is an almost universal practice It usually begins in infancy when children, due to the ignorance of doctors, nurses and mothers, are fed too much and too often. As the child grows older the almost continuous eating is kept up. An imperious appetite is thus built up out of the early perversion of normal hunger and only rarely does anyone ever escape from its grip.

Eating beyond physiological requirements is a most prolific source of weakness disease and premature death. Those who preach and practice the belly's doctrine of three squares plus and go by your appetite are always ailing.

Overeating is a form of overwork. It overworks the entire digestive system in the effort to digest it. It overworks the eliminating organs which must dispose of the surplus nutriment. The heart is overworked in forcing excess nutriment through the body. The glands of the body are overworked in trying to make secretion equal the demands made upon them by the excess food.

That man or woman who habitually eats beyond digestive capacity sooner or later wrecks his or her digestion and is poisoned by the many powerful toxins that form in the digestive tract from the fermenting, putrefying mass of undigested food. More people are killed by feasting than by famine.

People do not seem to be satisfied to supply the normal demands of their system for food. Rather, they resort to condiments and dressings of various kinds to stimulate their appetite and enable them to eat more. A soldier once wrote home from India of his fellow English soldiers stationed there: "They eat and drink, drink and eat, and they write home that it was the climate that killed them."

If you are not hungry it is a crime against your body to eat. It is a crime against your own best physical, mental, and moral interests for you to stimulate a false appetite by means of condiments, tasty dishes, etc. Alcohol, condiments, bitters, tonics, tasty dishes, etc., all conduce to overeating and they one and all retard digestion. Absolutely no good comes of their use. Indeed, their continued use deranges digestion, destroys the ability to relish plain foods and leads to troubles too numerous to mention. Those who desire real health, health that can be depended on in emergencies, will avoid all spurs to appetite and eat only when truly hungry. If one cannot enjoy good food without the addition of salt or pepper or some other equally harmful and equally worthless relish he should wait until he can, before eating.

Overclothing is a common means of weakening the body. Men are more prone to overclothe themselves than women. Present styles in women's clothes are far more sensible than men's. Particularly in winter do men overclothe themselves.

This business of bundling up like an eskimo begins in infancy. Fond parents weaken the reactive powers of their baby's skin by overclothing it. When the child grows older, his weakened powers of resistance cause him to feel the cold more than he normally should. He therefore keeps up the bad habit. The functional powers of the skin are weakened. It fails to do its full duty as an organ of elimination. It is unable to quickly and easily adjust the body to changes in temperature.

The failure of the skin as an organ of elimination throws more work upon the kidneys and mucous membranes of the body.

Dark clothing excludes the beneficial rays of the sun from the body and thus weakens, not only the skin, but the body as a whole. Sunlight is an absolutely essential factor-element in normal nutrition, as much so for the animal as for the plant. Man is, by nature, a nude animal and the nearer he approaches this ideal the more healthful will he become. Clothing should be light and porous in texture and made of light colors or of white. A free circulation of air about the body is essential at all times.

Indolence is also a weakening habit of mind and body. Muscular exercise or work is as esential to physical vigor, strength and development as air is to life. Those of light occupations who neglect to exercise become weak, delicate and sickly. By an irrevocable law, growth of mind and body is acquired through exercise. It is a mistake to think exercise builds muscle only. It trains the mind and develops the heart, lungs and other vital organs. Indolence is a crime against the body. It produces weakness in every tissue in the body.

Breathing impure air is a source of weakness and disease. Pure air is best for life. Air that has been breathed over and over again is poisonous. All the excretions of the body are, normally, more or less toxic, and they become more so as health is enfeebled. The character of the exhalations from men's lungs differs with the varying states and conditions of his health. In diseased states these exhalations are laden with toxins of various kinds. Some investigators have reported finding a toxin in expired air similar to the ptomaines.

Do not force yourself to breathe over and over again the air from your own or the lungs of some one else. Have your bed room, living room, office and workshop well ventilated at all times.

SEXUAL ABUSES.

Under this head I propose to treat of sex from a somewhat different point of view to the ones usually assumed in dealing with this subject. I hold that sex is governed by fixed laws of nature and that the sexual activities all fall under the realm of the laws already set forth in this book; but I propose to lay special stress on the *Law of Dual Effect*.

The sexual organs have at least two very important functions to perform— namely, (1) the development of the individual and (2) the propogation of the race. That it is the divine plan for perpetuating the race is patent to all. The sex glands supply an internal secretion which is necessary to the normal development and vigorous activity of almost every organ and tissue in the body. The sexual organs are not isolated and set apart from the rest of the body. They are integral parts of the body and are closely related to and correlated with every other part of it, as is shown by the results of castration and spaying, as well as by abuses of these organs.

I do not doubt that originally man was as perfect in his sex instincts and practices as the lion of the forest or the eagle of the air. He had no sex problems. But we do not find him in this condition now. Indeed, as he is at present, he is the victim of a great variety of forms of sexual perversion, some of which will be briefly discussed in another chapter. Only brief references can be made to these here.

Cases occur in which, from the perversion of the instincts of sex, women are hated by men instead of being desired and loved. This is especially likely to happen in the case of masturbators and sodomists, to whom the opposite sex has no attraction, and who think self-abuse or gratification by members of their own sex preferable to coition. This perversion is apparently much more frequent in man than in woman, although there are many women who abhor the legitimate method. Cases are on record of men masturbators who, though married, could not endure normal sexual relations and who so much prefered masturbation as to abuse themselves while lying beside their wives.

Between sexual aneasthesia (a condition in which there is lacking all sexual desire, perhaps an abhorrence of sex) on the one hand, and nymphomania and satyriasis on the other there exists all shades and colors of abnormal sexual conditions or perversions. Sexual anaesthesia is as much a perversion of sex as is nyphomania or satyriasis, and is found chiefly in women, although, often met with in men who have taken considerable quantities of nervines and nerve depressants. Nyphomania and satyriasis which represent identical conditions, are more common. Few people, if any, of today are normally sexed. For this reason we have a perpetual battle between the *idealists*, on the one hand, who would exact a perfect sex morality of a diseased race; and the *expressionists*, on the other hand, who would forever fasten the desires and promptings of a diseased humanity upon the race as a standard of conduct. Neither class bothers itself with the causes of the present condition.

The civilized and semi-civilized portions of the earth are given to sexual indulgences. Prof. O. S. Fowler wrote: "Every human function is perfect when exercised in harmony with its primitive constitution, but, when perverted, occasions suffering proportionate to the happiness its right exercise confers." The following words of Sylvester Graham presents us with the same thought: "So true is it that an infinitely wise and benevolent God has created us with such a nature, and established in our nature such constitutional relations to external things, that, while we have high and healthful enjoyment in the proper exercise of all our faculties and powers, we cannot make the gratification of any of our senses a source of enjoyment beyond the fulfillment of the constitutional purposes for which those senses were instituted, without jeopardizing all the interests of our nature, and finding disease and suffering in our pursuit of happiness."

With these words of Fowler and Graham the writer agrees in toto, and he is fully convinced that this principle is applicable to every department of life. There is pleasure associated with eating. But pleasure is not its end or object. It is merely an incident therein. So when one indulges his appetite and taste only for the pleasure and enjoyment he thus gains, giving no attention to the actual food requirements of his body, disease and even death results from his pursuit of pleasure.

In sex, the same rule applies. The procreative act should not be indulged for the sake of pleasure, for "relief" or "gratification," etc. Sex is the divine plan for the perpetuation of the race, and the pleasure associated therewith is only an incident, and not the end sought. The pursuit of happiness through sexual indulgence brings one to sorrow and pain.

Among those animals that are led by their unperverted instincts, sexual intercourse is never indulged in except for procreation. There is no foolish idea that such indulgence is essential to the perpetuation and increase of love. This is equally true among monogamous animals as among the polygamous kind. And in man we do not find such indulgence essential to the continuance and increase of love before marriage. On the contrary, it destroys love. In marriage, too, it destroys respect and love. "Incompatibility of temperament" is too often the outgrowth of sexual excesses.

In man as in the lower animals nature gives a sure and unmistakable answer to our query, "what is Nature's intent in the matter?" We have but to put the question frankly and fairly up to her, using no contraceptives or means to thwart her, and a few months later she presents her answer. "Here's my purpose," she says, as the new-born baby is ushered into the world. Her answer is final. No sophistry of the "communists" can appeal this decision.

The doctrine of sexual necessity has no foundation in fact. The sexual appetite bears no such relation to the individual welfare as the desire for food. Food is an actual physiological necessity, without which, the body would soon perish. Growth and repair of tissues, and the performance of physiological functions require food. Without food death must follow. The instinct of hunger is consequently a necessary provision. It forces the animal to seek for food. Food is a physiological necessity. Hunger is the instinct that causes the animal to seek food. If food is permanently witheld from the plant or animal death results.

The sex instinct bears no such demonstratable relation to the welfare of the individual. Rather, it was established for the benefit of the race. It is a biological necessity, without which the race would soon perish. Reproduction is an absolute necessity to the propogation of a species. Herein lies the true explanation for a strong driving force, such as the sex-instinct as we can readily understand how, without such a force, the bi-sexual animals would not reproduce their kind. But the natural history of reproduction gives no evidence that it bears any relation to the individual welfare, except that it represents a sacrifice.

There is no more necessity for coition inside than outside the pale of marriage. The physiological necessitites of man do not change with the marriage ceremony. Onanism is no more an essential to the welfare of the married than is masturbation, harlotry, or sodomy essential to the unmarried. The evil effects of sexual excesses in married life are the same—if we exclude any possible infectious diseases which may be acquired by certain extra-marital practices—as those produced by an equal amount of excesses in the unmarried.

. Marriage as an institution of Nature is not a thing to set aside the natural rules of conduct, but it furnishes the need of companionship on the intimate and personal side of life, and provides for the care and protection of the offspring.

In a state of unadulterated, unperverted, nature, the desires of the female is the law. And this is necessarily so. The female is not ready for intercourse except at certain periods, while the normal male is ready at all times.

We know that procreation is the natural outcome of complete intercourse where no contraceptive is used. This is the indisputable intention of nature in sex. Any use of sex for any other purpose is a perversion of it. The proper exercise of the sex function is for procreation. When so used it is exercised in harmony with its primitive constitution and it is only when so used that we get high and healthful enjoyment from its exercise.

I realize that everyone who reads these lines can think of a whole host of "authorities" who dispute this, who spin beautiful theories about superman, exchange of magnetism, sex communism, Dianism, Zugassents Discovery, etc., and who indulge in a lot of sophistry to prove their contentions. But, gentle reader, there is no authority but truth. If you fall into the bad habit of accepting authority for truth, rather than truth for authority, you will be led astray many times before death finally puts a period to your existence. Nature, not the "authorities," will speak to you in no uncertain tones if you but ask her what is the proper exercise of sex. Nature is our only authority.

Not the least among the evils that follow the excessive indulgence of the sexual powers is its tendency to develop every form of disease to which the victim may be predisposed. By producing enervation and by exciting the nervous system it readily brings out the weak points in one's constitution.

Many sufferers from epilepsy are certain of an "attack" whenever they indulge in venery. Other cases of epilepsy do not develop until after marriage. Asthmatic "attacks" are also frequently brought on by sexual indulgence. St. Vitus' dance is often perpetuated by sexual excesses; often by self-abuse. Indeed it contributes to the production of all disease in that it is a most potent cause of enervation. It is a mistake to look for some special or specific disease which is caused by sexual excess and by no other cause. These excesses produce enervation, enervation impairs organic function, toxemia develops and then, the resulting disease is the evolution of the individuals diathesis.

The genital organs are not the only sufferers. The constant excitement to which they are subject, and the trend of the mind to dwell on sex continuosly, keeps these organs filled with blood, and their glands over stimulated, so that a touch or even a lascivious thought or suggestion may result in a discharge of semen. Nocturnal emissions are frequent, almost habitual. Pains shoot and dart around or through the genitals and often their glands and even the penis itself atrophy. But these organs do not suffer alone. The nervous system is depleted, palpitation of the heart upon the slightest excitement often occurs. Pain in the back and spine is common.

Anything which over-stimulates the sexual centers finally exhausts them. Alcohol, for instance, if not used in sufficient quantity to make sex relations impossible, both increases the sexual appetite and diminishes the capacity for its satisfaction. Few things are more destructive, ultimately, to the reproductive powers. Strychnine, frequently used as an aphrodisiac, ultimately destroys potency. Small doses of morphine and cocaine, thought by many to arouse sexual desires, if habitually employed, result in impotency. Frequent and long continued petting, or eroticism, weakens the sexual powers. The young man who has indulged in these for sometime before marriage often finds himself suffering from prematurity or impotency upon getting married.

When the sexual organs of either sex are stimulated either from within or without, they become surcharged with blood, erect, and eventually relieve themselves by a flow, in man of semen, in woman of mucous. In common with every other passion, when the paroxysm is ended, a sensation of weakness, perhaps also of sleepiness, ensues. This weakness is due to the large amount of nervous energy that is consumed in the act, and not to the loss of fluid. The semen, for all practical purposes, is already out of the body when it is stored in the seminal vesicles.

Coition excites, in a degree proportionate to its intensity, all or nearly all of the functions of mind and body. Probably no other function does this to the same degree. Heart action is accelerated, perspiration is increased, respiration is increased, the man often literally panting for breath sufficient to supply the increased and increasing demand for oxygen. The whole muscular system is involved in the act and the tax upon this is not light. Blood pressure is increased and mental activities are accelerated. Some writers tell of seeing visions while in the act. During the act of coition nearly all the powers of mind and body are stimulated to the highest degree.

Of course, a corresponding reaction must necessarily follow such an act. It is impossible that such intense vital actions and emotions should occur without an immense expenditure of nervous or vital energy and a corresponding lessening of the funds of life. In point of fact no act or function is so exhausting to the whole system as this. If excessively indulged in, no practice can possibly be so enervating. J. Bradford Sax probably overestimated the amount of energy consumed in coition when he said (Organic Laws): "Probably more of the nervous fluid or influences is expended in a single sexual crisis than would suffice to carry on all the vital operations, perhaps for a day." At any rate the energy expended is very considerable and if the act is indulged in daily, or even weekly, the indulgent individual need not hope for health and strength.

Sexual excesses constitute a very common and very prolific source of disease, degeneracy and death. These may take any form from self-abuse to sodomy and other perversions. They may be practiced either within or without the pale of marriage and by both young and old alike. Both sexes, but particularly the male sex, are prone to these excesses.

What constitutes excess? The reply has been given: Anything is excess when procreation is not the end. Is this answer correct? It is true that in a state of pure, unperverted nature this is the invariable rule. Is it excess when used for other purposes? Yes, if our definition of excess is a correct one.

This answer would limit sex relations to the married and confine them to but few relations during life. I do not expect this answer to be regarded seriously by my readers. They will not be so restricted. Every animal possesses a sexual reserve for emergencies. It will not produce harm if this reserve is not over stepped. But this same is true of the unperverted animals and they all conform to the rule of intercourse for procreation only.

Prof. Fowler declared it to be a "law of things that the product of any given function is more or less perfect in proportion to the perfection of the function itself," and that "every function becomes diseased" or abnormal "when its organ is diseased" and this "accruing in the organs of the mind, produces, and even constitutes depravity." Disease of the sex organs usually arises as a result of the abuse of them and like all other abuses of the body, after the abuse has become habitual there is a morbid craving for the abuse. It is indeed true that the more the sex organs are abused the more abuse they demand, even after they have been reduced to a state in which they are no longer capable of normal response. The Talmud truly declares: "There is a small organ in the body of a man which is always hungry if one is trying to satisfy it; and is always satisfied if one starves it."

The frequent and habitual indulgence of the sex appetite quickly produces enervation showing itself in languor, lack of endurance, fatigue, lack of appetite, deranged digestion, impaired vision and hearing, palpitation of the heart, lack of mental concentration, "nervousness," and, as it continues, worse disorders.

In most cases excessive venery metes out a fitting punishment. It destroys the love existing between man and wife. Satiety results in disgust and so-called "sex-antagonism." Repulsion and resentment make peaceful companionship impossible. The couple reproach each other that they were quite "different before marriage." The man becomes as grouchy and irritable as an old bear. The meekest girls often become vicious, the most equable turn into tear fountains. Perhaps they quarrel so violently that they separate or seek a divorce. But after a time apart they feel that there is nothing wrong with themselves and return to each other and find their old sentiments revived. Others, after a stormy season, cool off after the passionate indulgences of the honeymoon, and, as they commit less excesses, get along together much better. Outraged sexuality breeds a degree of hatred and antognism between a man and woman commensurate with the former intensity of their love for each other.

These things may be appropriately defined as "sub-conscious" nature defending herself. Who does not know the ardor of the passionate man or woman in love making? A young lady once said: "I like to get men passionate, for then they make such ardent lovers." One woman writer, speaking of sexual intercourse declares: "and not uncommonly visions of a transcendent life are seen and consciousness of new powers experienced." For the man the ugliest of women, becomes temporarily, beautiful and lovely. These things are but parts of the primary effect of sexual excitement. The secondary effect is the exact opposite of this. One writer thus describes its effects upon the parties concerned:—

"The abuse of the sex function brings about a peculiar state of affairs between husband and wife. The desire to marry her arises, in the first place, out of the strong physical attraction she has for him, so that he desires her as a companion for life; not primarily to satisfy his sex appetite; this, however, is regarded as a legitimate function of the married state so he proceeds to do so without thinking much about it, subconsciously regarding it as much a part of marriage as taking his meals, but through this very indulgence, his wife loses the attraction that first drew him to her. Having satisfied his appetite he does not want to see her for a time, even her touch irritates him. That such cases are not exceptional has been proven over and over again, many young husbands have admitted it to their intimate friends, wondering at themselves and uneasy at what seems to them the begining of an actual dislike for the wife whom they married because they loved her. The following statement of a husband seems to express the consensus of opinion. 'It is the plan of nature that the two sexes should meet and then ignore each other for a time. I know I do not want to see or hear my wife for several hours, and I am greatly bothered when she speaks to me. She says I am at one time a very affectionate man, and then cross as a bear. This is Nature.'"—*Sex Force.*

Many examples of the workings of the *Law of Dual Effect* in the realm of sex might be given. The practice of masturbation supplies us with some. By repeated irritation over a long period of time, the penis has been known to become tolerant to all ordinary impressions so that the usual methods of exciting it produce no pleasurable sensations at all. But the tyrant of desire and perverted instinct calls loudly for gratification. The tortured victim of such desires connected with such impotency resorts to all manners of expedients to secure the desired gratification. Cases are on record in which the palsied nerves were so near dead that only by cutting the penis with a knife or other sharp instrument could any sensations be produced, and these, instead of being painful, were pleasurable.

Excitement follows the laws of stimulation and dual effect. If we are to secure the same internal effect, the same feeling, greater and stronger and new stimuli are required. Sensual pleasures do not last beyond the period of gratification. Whether we gratify sexual desire or the gustatory sense, the pleasure goes at once. It is momentary and fleeting. Often, very often, it is followed by a positive repulsion for sex or for food.

We get used to a thing by repetition and this both removes the pain from hurt and the novelty from joy. This causes us to search for new and more novel forms of excitement and gratification. Bitter foods give pleasure to the jaded appetite because the disagreeable element is just enough to excite pleasureable sensations in the palsied gastro-intestinal tract. The more jaded one is, that is, the more used to excitement he is, the greater the excitement needed to produce the desired feelings and sensations. Thus, the more such people seek excitement in what are, ordinarily or normally, disagreeable and even painful practices. To such jaded people, pain in a slight degree is exciting. Dr. Jennings tells of pulling a man's tooth, and of the man experiencing pleasure and not pain from the operation. He explained that the nerves were so near dead that the operation was able to excite them only enough to produce a pleasurable sensation. In the sexual sphere pain is often sought, by women and by the roue, as a means of increasing sexual pleasure.

The more often coition is indulged in, the longer time and more irritation is required to bring about the orgasm, and the less is the pleasurable sensation connected therewith. Sometimes hours are required and sometimes the crisis is never reached. The excessive exercise of the sex function produces impotency, nature thus protecting herself from complete exhaustion.

Impotency is of two kinds: (1) Those cases in which there is inability to have an erection, and (2) Those cases were there is constant erection (priapism), the victim of which imagines himself to be a veritable satyr in strength. Of this latter class Dr. Tilden observes:—

"I have been consulted by libertines who have acknowledged to continuous friction in intercourse, of hours duration. On my expressing surprise that a woman could be found who would stand for such treatment, I was told: 'She loves me, and is so anxious to satisfy me that she would not protest if I should be with her all night.' Such fiends have boasted that, if it were not for beccoming raw or excoriated, they could continue the sex act indefinitely. This statement being made to prove that they were very powerful sexually, but which proved to anyone who knows that they were badly enervated and in reality sexually impotent."

Sex is not a plaything for idle hours and should not be indulged merely for "pleasure" or "relief" or as an "indulgence" or as a "gratification" but should be restricted to its legitimate function. "Restriction, however, is not appropriate," as Prof. Fowler declared. "We are not restricted from eating stones, or swallowing poison. To follow the ordinances of nature is neither restriction no self-sacrifice; but our own highest happiness."

"We are told, on the most undoubted authority, that two of the most celebrated scholars that ever lived, Locke and Newton, passed through life without ever having intercourse or voluntarily gratifying that organ, and yet see the immense results which they attained."—*Philosophy of Generation*, John B. Newman, M.D., published by Fowler and Wells, 1892.

The intensest pleasures are the costliest. The more intense the pleasure the greater the expenditure of power. The more often they are repeated the less pleasure they give. The more frequently sex is indulged the less intense the pleasure and the longer the time required to complete the act. Man should resist being tyrannized over by *pleasure*. Plato, Spinoza, Descartes, Leibnitz, Kant, Berkeley, Hume Hobbes, Spencer, Newton are but a few of the great thinkers who flourished on a Shaker system. And look at the ages of them! On the other side, as early victims of the "standard of pleasure" are Burns, Byron, Maupassant, Murger, Mirabeau and others. Epicurus advised men to eat moderately, excercise much and have nothing to do with women. It is suggested that his advice to women would probably have been the same.

It is true that super-normal desire is the rule among men while sub-normal desire is almost the rule among women. No man save the impotent fails to secure pleasure from coition. Thousands of women spend their whole married lives without ever once experiencing the least pleasure in any way from the act. In many cases they receive pain from every indulgence. Such a condition is by no means normal and is often associated with a very ardent affectional nature. Woe is that man whose wife has no sexual desire but craves and demands constant affection. Life becomes a constant petting party which rapidly saps his energies but leaves her uneffected. In self-defense he is forced to avoid such parties as often as possible and is then daily accused of having ceased to love his wife.

Petting parties are intended by nature to culminate in intercourse and they quite naturally arouse desire, often almost uncontrolable desire. Gratified or not, if this is frequently and habitually indulged in, weakness, loss of virility, and even sterility and impotence may result.

"Very shortly ofter the fertilizing act," says Dr. E. Rosch, "there may still remain in the sexual organs of the female animal so much responsiveness, that she does not resist the second or third coupling. But after a few days nature takes another direction, or we might say, the other direction." The female has lost the capacity for sexual enjoyment until she has given birth to and ceased to suckle her young.

Among the lower animals the desires of the female is the law. She will receive the male only at certain times and this results in pregnancy. During pregnancy and the early part of lactation she will attack to kill any male who would attempt to approach her, a thing that rarely occurs. But man demands of woman gratification during pregnancy and lactation, and often during menstruation and while ill. He has even had woman's "duty" to minister to his desires incorporated into law as her "marital duties."

By what right does man claim to be an exception to the uniformities and regularities of nature? How did he ever secure exemption from the operation of these uniformities? No stock raiser would permit the males to tease and annoy his pregnant females. Why shall a pregnant woman not be given as much consideration? Normally she is averse to coition during pregnancy and lactation and finds it painful for some time after parturition. Intercourse during this time is frequently responsible for morning sickness, irritableness, hysteria, miscarriage, etc. It increases the pains of parturition and prepares the soil for post-partum fever, etc.

There is a whole school of writers and lecturers who, have somehow acquired the idea that by suppressing the orgasm, coition may be indulged in as frequently and as long as desirable without harm. This practice which is both destructive and habit forming, is called by many names. It tends to make sex gluttens out of those who practice it. It makes them irritable, weak, nervous, and impotent. I do not doubt that it contributes largely to the production of cancer of the sex organs due to the fact that it leaves them in an almost continuously congested state. Eroticism and perpetual petting must do the same thing.

It was long ago discovered that the longer the duration of the venereal paroxysm, the greater is the prostration and consequent injury. In normal sexual intercourse, the act, by its very nature, cannot last long, and everything hastens its completion, but when performed in an unnatural or modified way, whether by masturbation, onanism, etc., or by "communion," "coitus reservatus" or by similar practices, the party is desirous of prolonging the feeling and thus retards the *denoument*, and thereby makes his frequent gratification a greater source of weakness.

If desire has been aroused to the extent of demanding coition, and this has been entered into, it should be completed in a natural manner. The suppression of the orgasm, as advocated by some, is probably more vicious than any other form of excess.

Man is sexually perverted. He is the only animal that has his "social problem," the only animal that supports prostitution, the only animal that practices self-abuse; the only animal that is demoralized by all forms of sexual perversion, the only animal whose male will attack the females, the only animal where the desire of the female is not the law, the only one that does not exercise his sexual powers in harmony with their primitive constitution. This animal is driven by his perversions in all his sexual relations.

Even his and her so-called love life is based upon sexual perversion. "Making Love," or as it now commonly called, "petting," is simply a means of arousing the sexual powers and passions. The petting, fondling, hugging, kissing, etc., that accompanies this orgy of animalism cheapens love, renders love almost impossible and keeps the purely animal powers ever active. The cultivation of sex thrills for their own sake, even when no sexual relations follow, constitutes a terrible drain upon the powers of life. It matters not whether this is indulged in within or without the pale of marriage.

In these days of promiscuous and unrestrained petting, it is no longer a secret that both sexes frequently reach a sexual orgasm through petting alone. This is one reason for the great popularity of this form of masturbation.

"Petting," "spooning," "sparking" or "love making" as we call this manifestation is natural and serves a definite end. It is common to man and animals alike and in both serves the definite purpose of arousing the sexual energies and desires, and preparing the sexes for the function of procreation. It is this fact that makes it dangerous for young people who are frequently swept, by the almost uncontrollable desires thus aroused, into greater mistakes.

Custom sanctifies (?) petting orgies in married life but this does not deprive it of its enervating effects. Young men and women today openly indulge in this form of self-abuse and honest and sincere men and women defend the practice. It is unfortunate that a man may be both honest and sincere and at the same time be as ignorant as a child. When petting is not to serve its primitive purpose it should be avoided. This, the pervert, man (both sexes), will not do, however. And in most cases, to caution moderation is simply waste of time. This habit, like all other habits grows on one and holds one in its vice-like grip.

Ardent love-making, if frequently repeated, will injure one in more ways than one. There is the injury to the emotions due to ungratified sexual excitement. Then there is the weakening effect upon the sex organs themselves caused by the congestion and later inflammation in these due to arousing the passions and leaving them ungratified.

Ardent love-making prior to marriage is often followed by serious consequences. A lover's kiss accompanied with an ardent embrace is sure to arouse the sex passions and often they are aroused to great intensity. Love making of this kind, if frequently engaged in, is productive of great physical harm. Too free and ardent love making prior to marriage also carries with it the danger that the young couple will be carried beyond their abilities to control themselves; when the impulses aroused by intimate contact will be irresistible. Too much spooning is therefore dangerous as well as unhealthful. In addition to this, the force of physical attraction may cause one to make a serious blunder in choosing a husband or wife. The social policy enforced among certain Indian tribes, of "hands off," would mean better health and fewer mistakes. Bodily contact and too intimate association between the sexes, when carried too far, is certainly among the most weakening of the sexual errors. The young man who fondles a woman's body, holds her on his lap, embraces and kisses her, has his seed to run from him and soil his pants. An analogous thing occurs in the woman. If the desires thus aroused are not gratified, the over-stimulated sex glands and over-distended seminal vesicles, of the man, will be relieved in a nocturnal emission accompanied by a lascivious dream.

Petting parties cause enervation, lessen strength, and endurance, cheapen love, produce disgust and a whole train of mental and physical ills.

Sexual desire in girls frequently does not develop before twenty to twenty-five, although there is a small class of girls of much younger age in whom passion is often very strong, even uncontrolable. These cases, however, where they are not due to disease of the sex organs, or of the mind, are the result of artificial stimulation. Eroticism has been aroused in them by salacious reading or by pornographic plays or by the stories they hear from their newly married sisters or friends.

Contact with the opposite sex may easily excite the affectional nature into activity and this in turn may arouse the sexual organs into activity. The exercise of the affections may lead to satiety and exhaustion as quickly as coition. Strangely enough men and women are accustomed to thinking that sexual activity begins and ends with coition. The culmination or climax of sexual activities is considered to be the whole act and its antecedents are looked upon as of no consequence. Yet the stimulation of sex through sight, smell, hearing, feeling and even taste, by caresses, etc., which arouses desire and produces the turgescence of the sex organs are the most important parts of the chain of sexual manifestations. The amorous caress, be it of thought, look, or touch, as in hugging, kissing, fondling, etc., is the beginning of the sex act. There is great danger in the frequent and habitual stimulation of the sexual centers, in these ways, "without the safety-valve of physical and nervous relief which follows as a natural sequence in the ordinary sexual relation." Dr. Talmey correctly says:—

"Worse than mental erethism is tactile eroticism. By tactile eroticism is understood, keeping the genital organism constantly irritated by dalliance with individuals of the other sex, stopping short of the act of copulation. On a walk through the city parks, any summer evening, or on a trip on the Sunday excursion boats, young men and women may be observed lying in each other's arms in a continual caress, kissing, hugging, and fondling each other for hours, scarcely confining themselves to the limit of decency. These couples are acutally exercising the sexual act, although they do not obtain sexual congress. These tremors and ecstacies, these amorous ardors and intoxications, these sensual joys which stimulate with rapture the higher centers and infuse the mind with sexual gratification, all these are a part of the sexual act. The interruption of this chain of impulses short of copulation may satisfy the moral conscience of the young people, but it does not make such excesses less injurious. On the contrary, the genetive organism is deprived of the relief which complete coition lends to the sexual organism. ****The normal outlet of sex-activity has been cut off by a special process of repression."

"If these frustrate stimulations are frequently repeated, they perpetuate the genital congestion, and through the retention of the secretions, a catarrh of the genital organs ensues, just as inflammations often originate in the mammary glands through the accumulation of the milk after weaning the child. These perennial congestions are the cause of prostatic inflammations not seldom met with in young men. The ulcerations of the cervix so often found in young girls, may be attributed to no other cause than to frustrate eroticism. The cervix is damaged in the same way as the soil, burned by the sun, in the absence of a beneficient rain, cracks and slits. The frequently repeated engorgements of the blood-vessels which do not receive the normal physiological relief, provoke in both parties an exaggerated sex-sense and provoke the emotions known as satyriasis in men, and nymphomania in women. The exaggeration is followed later on by exhaustion of the libidinous impulses, and the men become hypochondriacs, and the women neurotic and sallow."

Keep watch over your emotions, avoid prurient or pornographic literature and "art" and put away thoughts of sex as well as sexual acts. Nine-tenths of all the sexual errors and evils and ungovernable passions are of a mental origin. Overt sins usually begin as covert sins. Eroticism of thought and imagination becomes habitual and finally the sexual passion absorbs and dominates the waking hours and one's very dreams as well. These libidinous fancies may be kept up in the mind there to burrow and fester, or they may find vent in vices of various forms. In either event they are evil and damaging.

Dr. Dio Lewis tells of a young clergyman of fine culture and morals who came to him with nervous symptoms which he immediately suspected of having their origin in some abuse of the sex organs. The man denied ever having practiced masturbation, or ever having had intercourse with a woman and had never had a nocturnal emission, to his knowledge. Upon questioning the man more closely Dr. Lewis learned that he was engaged to a young lady whom he visited every Thursday evening. He caressed her and permitted his mind to dwell on sexual fancies. He admitted that Friday was always a wretched day with him and that he had wondered why. The doctor relates another case as follows:—

"A gentleman of some intelligence had lived a chaste life up to the age of thirty-nine. A successful manufacturer, he had acquired wealth and kept up a hospitable home, but had never married. In point of personal purity he was regarded as a very Joseph by his friends, among whom I had the honor to enjoy a place. What was my surprise when he consulted me with reference to seminal weakness! I made careful inquiries about his habits. Had he practiced masturbation? 'Never?' Had he indulged in familiarities with some woman? 'Never?' And yet here was a case of frequent nocturnal emissions, with all the usual symptoms of exhaustion.

"I said, 'there is but one explanation, and that is, that you have morbid imaginations!'

"He owned it. 'If that is important, I am free to confess that I am rarely alone a moment without being occupied with erotic fancies. And my dreams, too, are full of them!'"

This man made a quick recovery after he was instructed how to control his fancies. Dr. Lewis relates another case of a young man of Boston who visited the East Indies, twice a year in control of a sailing vessel. In India he maintained a native mistress but "never indulged himself excessively." He denied ever having practiced masturbation more than five times in his life. Then upon being asked if there was anything about his sexual life which he had concealed he replied:—

"Nothing that I know of, except that I indulge in thoughts about women. During my long voyages I have given myself a good deal to such things. I have taken with me a score of French novels, in which sex has been treated in a very fascinating way. Certain passages in these books, I have read over and over, and then I have indulged for hours and days in thoughts to which such reading naturally gives rise."

"Have you observed," asked Dr. Lewis, that "after several hours abandonment to such fancies that your nervous system was greatly exhausted?"

"I have constantly observed it," was the reply "I have noticed that intercourse with my Indian woman did not exhaust me half so much. But sir, it is impossible to control my thoughts. Such fancies will haunt me and it is impossible to get rid of them."

He was then instructed how to control his thoughts and on his return from his next voyage with greatly improved health he said to the doctor: "Cleaned out, sir! I wouldn't go back again to wallow in the mire for my life."

Ungratified desires have a weakening effect upon both body and mind. An occasional arousing of the passions without gratification will have little effect upon a vigorous man or woman but it is the height of folly to habitually arouse these forces when they cannot be gratified in a normal manner. Close personal intimacy between the sexes, with fondling, caressing, kissing, spooning and other personal liberties cannot be but injurious to both parties.

There is an excess of blood sent to the sex organs and the glands are stimulated to increased action. If this is frequently repeated they are over stimulated. The man loses, more or less semen, often reaching a climax and having a full discharge, the woman has a quantity of "mucous" to run from her and soil her clothes. A very ardent woman may even reach an orgasm in spooning.

The evils that are, in many quarters, charged to continence, are usually, if not always, caused by this form of dalliance. Dalliance is not continence. Passions that cannot be gratified should not be aroused. Sexual stimulation should be avoided if one desires to avoid sexual indulgence. Physical intimacies should be abstained from. Erotic thinking, is, however, equally as harmful, and, after the habit of stimulating the sexual centers in this way is once established it is very apt to be persistent and insiduous in its influence.

Within recent years there has grown up a crop of writers on sex who have visited the reservations and brought back with them all the perverse forms of sexual relations they have found there, and through their books and lectures, have introduced these into society, some of them even are advocating their use among the unmarried. This class of writers parade their filth under the proud banner of pretended science. They do not seem to be content with the amount of sexual perversion that already exists, and are bent on producing far more. An ally of theirs, in this corrupting work is psychoanalysis and pretended psychology.

The claim frequently made by pretended psychologists that nervous diseases are due to sexual repression and that these may be cured by destroying the morals of the man or woman is unsound in principle and dangerous in practice. Those cases of nervousness that are claimed to be due to repression are due to dalliance, to eroticism of thought and act without the normal relief in intercourse. But the remedy is to remove the eroticism not to convert them into concubines and libertines.

SELF-INDULGENCE.

The sensuous and voluptuous usually keep up their bad habits until a collapse of function forces a halt. Anorexia and nausea, perhaps vomiting, force them to eat less. Repugnance to smoke and drink forces them to cut down on these for a time. A breakdown forces them to rest. Functional collapse is due to enervation brought on by the HABITS that KILL.

Once these sufferers are able to be up and around and they return to their bad habits. Repeated functional collapses do not teach them the way or life and health and, finally, chronic disease becomes their portion. They then seek for "cures" that will restore them to health without restoring them to sane living. Graham says:—

"The grand experiment of the whole human family seems ever to have been to ascertain how far they can go in indulgence, how near they can approach the brink of death, and yet not die so suddenly and violently as to be compelled to know that they have destroyed themselves."—*Science of Human Life*, p. 350.

These people do not desire to reform their modes of living. They do not care to discipline themselves. They are slaves to their habits. Almost anyone can give up habits for a few days or even for a few weeks, but to continue to live correctly for years is beyond the powers of the average individual. So enslaved are they by their habits that they declare they cannot see what one gains by abastaining from "all the good things of life" even if it does enable him to live a few years longer. Now if these

161

bad habits really constituted "*good things of life,*" nothing would be gained, not even increased length of life, by abstaining from them. We do not ask you to deny your-self a single one of the good things of life. We only ask you to abstain from the harmful practices and harmful excesses that enslave you. This will entail no hardship upon you. But there is another and even brighter side to this picture. To cease abusing your body and mind will not only add years to your life but life to your years. Instead of weakness, misery, aches, pains, disease, and suffering; health, strength, joy and happiness will be yours. The highest and greatest joys of life are based on health.

There is a heedless class who declare they are strong. They are masters of them-selves They harbor the delusion that they shall always be as able to control them-selves, that they shall be free to choose their course after frequent departures from the path of virtue as they feel while they are yet only in contemplation. They vainly imagine that when they will they can take their stand in unbroken strength of soul upon the fartherest verge of harmful indulgence and say to the surging torrent of undisciplined passions and desires: "Thus far shalt thou go and no farther and here shall thy proud waves be stayed."

These people are not conscious of the growth of their habits. They forget that habit is bondage. They cannot see the end of their strength and foolishly conclude it has no end. From master they are soon reduced to slave. Heedless of the warning voice of wisdom and experience they go recklessly on in their mad pursuit of false pleasures.

There is another class who can be good for a brief period and then must break over the traces and return to their idols. "Just this once won't hurt me," they say. And yet there is a first step in every career of excess and dissipation. The Chinese proverb truly says: "The thousand mile journey begins with the first step."

Once a man or woman yields to the temptation to do a thing resistance is weakened—and it becomes all the easier to yield next time. One's powers of re-sistance can be strengthened only by using them. "Just this once" all too often grows more and more frequent until a formidable habit is forged and the victim of his own folly becomes bound to a practice he did not intend to engage in. That "abstinence is easier than temperance" is an old and true saying.

Bad habits are always bad. The repeated use or application of any substance which is pernicious soon reconciles us to it. That which is at first disagreeable and manifestly injurious, may become apparently neutral or even apparently salutary. Such is the blinding influence of habit by which the vital instincts are rendered insensible to constant irritation, if it possesses only a moderate degree of force, so that, eventually, a craving or appetite is formed for a substance or practice that is harmful and foreign to the needs of the body.

Under the constant sway of such influences the body is perverted and its functions subverted. The effects ultimately produced must be commensurate with the magnitude and duration of the harmful habit. In the end, weakness, suffering and premature death must result. The combined and cumulative effects of the many harmful practices to which the human race is addicted are weighing down upon the health and lives of the race and gradually crushing it.

It is the constant falling of the little drops of water that wears away the granite boulder. It is the constant falling of the little flakes of snow that stops powerful locomotives and ties up the nation's commerce. So, it is the habitual repetition of injurious practices, however slight the injury resulting from one act may be, that wrecks health and life No man or woman exists who has only one bad habit. We all have a collection of them. As the combined effects of this collection of bad habits accumulates weakness, disease, premature old age and an untimely death result. As Graham declares:—

"They who make sensual enjoyment the chief end of their existence, and live in the continual violation of the laws of their nature, must of necessity either perish untimely by violent disease or sink into that melancholy and shocking decay which is so common to old age."

The nervous system may be said to possess two vital endowments, the motive and the sensorial power. The motive power is employed in those important vital operations which are concerned in the growth and sustenance of the body, and in the actions and functions of its various organs. The sensorial power is employed in the functions of sensation, perception, reflection, volition. These two properties of the nervous system, though somewhat different from each other, are yet so intimately related, that they both equally depend on the most healthy and perfect state of the nervous system for their highest and best condition; so that whatever in any measure deteriorates the nervous structure, or impairs its vital properties, always necessarily diminishes both the motive and sensorial powers of the system. And it is an invariable law that all excessive exercise or expenditure of the one, always diminishes the functional energy of the other; all excessive exercise of the passions and of the mind always necessarily diminishes the functional power of the stomach and all other organs concerned in the growth and sustenance of the body and which depend on the nervous power of the system; and on the other hand, everything that increases the demand for the concentration of the nervous power in the stomach and other organs, for the performance of their functions, beyond what is indispensibly necessary for the healthy operations and results of the vital economy, always necessarily diminishes the sensorial power of the system.

All men are so intent on present enjoyment, that they are little inclined to practice present self-denial for the sake of a future good which they consider in any possible degree contingent; and will only consent to reform their modes of living when compelled by necessity, or when they find it the only means of shunning imminent destruction, or of escaping from intolerable evils. Hence, so long as a man is favored with even a moderate degree of health, he rushes headlong into the eagerly desired excitements of his various pursuits, pleasures and indulgencies, and nothing seems to him more visionary and ridiculous, than precepts and regulations and admonitions concerning the preservation of health. While he possesses apparent health, he will not believe that he is in any danger of losing it; or if he is, nothing in his habits or practices can have any effect, either in destroying or preserving it. Nor can he be divorced from the universal delusion that, if he enjoys health, he has within himself the constant demonstration that his habits and practices are conformable to the laws of health, at least in his own constitution. He will not, therefore, consent to be benefitted, contrarily to what he regards as necessary to his present enjoyment, either by the experience or by the learning of others.

The consequence is—as a general fact—that, while in health, mankind prodigally waste the resources of their constitution, as if the energies of life were inexhaustible; and when, by the violence or by the continuance of their excesses, they have brought on acute or chronic disease, which interrupts their pursuits and destroys their comforts, they fly to the physician, not to learn from him by what violations of the laws of life and health they have drawn the evil upon themselves, and by what means they can in future avoid the same and similar difficulties; but, considering themselves as unfortunate beings, visited with afflictions which they have in no manner been concerned in causing, they require the exercise of the physician's skill in the application of remedies, by which their sufferings may be alleviated and their disease removed.

Popularly and professionally, if a man appears well and feels well, this is enough. No matter if he is on the brink of the grave, his most vital organs so impaired and deficient in vital power that as soon as they begin to falter the whole system is broken up and life becomes extinct.

So long as they possess a modicum of health, they cannot be persuaded to observe the laws of life. Why should they "diet"? Are they not healthy? Why should they bother themselves about health rules and regulations? Is not their health sufficient evidence of the healthfulness of their manner of living? When they are well, is this not proof that their haphazzard course of living agrees with them? Why then, should they deny themselves the pleasures of the palate and the sensuous enjoyment that comes of doing as one pleases? This is the way men reason. How deceitful this reasoning may be!

Present health is no guarantee of future health.

There are no iron constitutions. A strong constitution will stand a lot of abuses before their effects finally make themselves apparent, but the strongest constitution that ever existed must ultimately succumb to repeated violations of the laws of our being.

Dr. Chas. E. Page, represents the matter thus:—

" 'Nothing hurts me—I eat everything!' (Next year:) 'Nothing agrees with my stomach—I can't eat anything!' Thus the dyspeptic's ranks are kept full with recruits from those who don't want any advice about diet."

Dr. Page has not overdrawn the picture one bit. There is hardly an invalid, semi-invalid, and has-been-perfect-physically man or woman, in America today, that did not, at one time, say: "Nothing hurts me—I eat everything." All those who will recuit the great army of invalids as the present ones die off, are, today, following this same delusive idea. They are laughing at the idea of dieting, and are following no regular health rules. There are no copper lined stomachs. You may be able to digest pig-iron as you say, but *you are a fool if you try it.*

What is true of diet, is equally true of the other factors of life. Every day, the physician is forced to listen to the tale of woe of the has-beens in the great army of haphazzard livers, and it always runs something like this: "Doctor, I cannot do the things I once did. Once I could digest nails, now I have to eat baby foods; once I could go all day and night without fatigue, but now I tire in a few minutes or hours. I cannot indulge as I once did without suffering." They thought they had cast iron constitutions and copper-lined stomachs. They found they were made of flesh and blood and bones. THEY TRIED TO SEE HOW MUCH THEY COULD GET AWAY WITH INSTEAD OF TRYING TO LIVE IN THE HIGHEST SENSE. THEY ONLY GOT AWAY WITH THEIR HEALTH, STRENGHT, USEFUL-NESS AND LIFE.

I wish here to state a proposition that is of greatest importance to the human family. Present health is not a conclusive proof that the dietetic and other habits of the individual are most favorable to health, nor does the continuance of apparent health prove that those habits are most conductive to long life. Millions of human beings perish by disease, in all periods of life, from excessive alimentation and other causes, where one man is enabled to maintain health under the action of such causes, till he dies from the exhaustion of his vital powers. Says Graham:—

"This fact, however, does not in any degree militate against the general conclusion established by anatomical and physiological evidence; for, it should ever be remembered as one of the most important and invariable laws of our nature, that we may maintain health at the expense of life.**** Or, to state the proposition with more exactness and accuracy, we may, by virtue of a sound and vigorous constitution, and by the help of many circumstances and habits favorable to health, strength, and longevity, maintain comparative health and vigor, until we attain to what in modern times is ordinarily considered old age, in spite of some circumstances and habits which are unfriendly to the highest physiological interests of our bodies, and which necessarily hasten the consumption of life, and consequently shorten the period of our human existence. For as I have stated nothing is more true than that *intensive* and *extensive* life are incompatible with each other, and it is universally admitted that flesh meat always causes more vital intensiveness than pure and proper vegetable food does. High-toned and vigorous health, therefore, is not a conclusive proof that our dietetic habits are most favorable to health, nor is the long continuation of such health a proof that our dietetic habits are most conductive to longevity. The truth of this important proposition is often strikingly demonstrated by individual experience. I will present a single illustration. (At this point it may be well to caution the reader against the idea that Mr. Graham held that true health shortens life. This mistake is likely to occur here because he has not sufficiently emphasized the difference between true and apparent health. Although, anyone who will take the trouble to carefully study the example he gave—see it below—can see that the gentleman referred to did not possess true health. It was only apparent. Author's note.)

"At the close of my introductory lecture, in one of the beautiful villages of New England, I was addressed by a professional gentleman of very considerable intelligence, who was not far from seventy years of age, of portly appearance, and seemingly in what is commonly considered good health. He had a large frame, well clothed with flesh, and a somewhat florid complexion. Yet he was strictly temperate in regard to alcoholic liquors. 'I am glad to see you,' said he, 'and rejoice that you have consented to come and give a course of your lectures to our people. I think there is great need of such instructions at this present day. In our land of over-flowing abundance, everybody is in danger of excess, and I lament to see our young people so much devoted to the indulgencies of luxury. I shall certainly attend your lectures, and doubt not that I shall listen to them with great interest, although I do not expect to be benefitted by them in my own person. I am now too far advanced in life to make any changes in my habits with the hope of being benefitted, even though some of my practices might be considered a little exceptionable. Yet I have by no means been inattentive to these things; and I think I have the best evidence in the world that my habits have been very salutary; for I am now an old man, in the enjoyment of uncommon health and vigor for one of my age; and during my whole life, since my remembrance, I have not been so much indisposed as to able to keep my house for a single day.' 'Indeed, sir!' I replied, 'that may be very greatly your misfortune.' 'Misfortune!' he reiterated with much emphasis and surprise, 'How can it be a misfortune to enjoy uninterrupted health for seventy years?' 'Because, sir,' I answered, 'judging from the original soundness and vigor of your constitution, you are now but little past the meridian of your natural life; and the continued health of which you boast, may only have served to blind you to your dietetic and other errors relative to the laws of life, and to give you full confidence in the correctness of those habits which may in the end prove to have robbed you of nearly half of your natural existence. It should be remembered that not one human being in a million dies a natural death. If a man is shot or stabbed or poisoned or killed by a fall, or some other means of this kind, we say he dies a violent death; but if he is taken sick and is laid upon his bed, and is attended by physicians and friends, and waxes worse, and finally dies, perhaps with dreadful agonies and anguish, we say he dies a natural death. But this is wholly an abuse of language, a misstatement of fact; the death in this latter case is as truly a violent death as if the individual had been shot or stabbed or poisoned. Whether a man takes a dose of arsenic and kills himself at once, or takes small doses which more gradually and by imperceptible degree destroys his life, he equally dies a violent death, though the convulsive agonies which attend his dissolution may be less violent in the latter, than in the former case. And whether he gradually destroys his life with arsenic, or any other means however common, he equally dies a violent death. He only dies a natural death, who, during his whole existence, so perfectly obeys the laws of constitution and relation established in his nature, as neither by irritation nor intensity to waste his vital energies, but naturally and slowly passes through the progressive changes of his system from childhood to old age, and finally, in the sheer exhaustion of his vital powers, lies down and falls asleep in death without a struggle or a groan.

"The worthy gentleman, if not entirely convinced, was at least made thoughtful by my remarks; and so we parted. At my next lecture I observed he was not present. The third and fourth were given, and he was still absent. This excited my curiosity to make inquiries after him, and I was surprised to learn that he was very ill. A few days more elapsed, and I was informed that his physician considered him dangerously sick; that his disease had thus far baffled the physician's skill; and his symptoms had from the first continued to become more and more violent, in spite of all the means which had been used to subdue them. I now called to see him, and was exceedingly astonished to behold how great a change had taken place in his appearance in so short a time. A few days after this, he died. (That this man still possessed much vitality is evident from the continued increase in symptoms in spite of all efforts to suppress them. He would probably have recovered except for the suppressive treatment. Author's note). I however, visited him frequently before his death; and at each interview, scarcely had I entered his room before he began to exhort me with much earnestness and pathos to be faithful to my public labors, and warn the rising generation of the dangers of the table, and to entreat parents not to destroy their children by multiplying and pampering their appetites in early life, till they had become such perfect slaves to them as not to be able to deny themselves, but were led captives by their lusts to their destruction. Before he died, he requested that his body might be opened and examined after his demise. I was politely invited to attend this post mortem examination. And though I have seen many diseased bodies opened after death, yet never in any instance have I found disease so extensive as in this case The entire stomach and intestinal canal and other portions of the abdominal contents presented one general mass of deep and irremedial disease which clearly indicated a progress of several years, and which was of a character that fully evinced that it was not produced by any sudden or violent cause, but that it was the result of causes which had been gradually operating and by imperceptible degrees developing their effects, probably through the whole course of life."—*Science of Human Life,* pp. 492-93-94.

Protracted impunity tempts sinners to believe in the innocence of their habits. Because they are not knocked down avery time they do a thing they refuse to believe that it harms them.

Graham declares:—

"Indeed it seems as if the grand experiment of mankind had ever been to ascertain how far they can transgress the laws of life, how near they can approach to the very point of death, and yet not die, at least so suddenly and violently as to be compelled to know that they have destroyed themselves."

For years the infinite patience of nature labors every night to repair the waste and undo the mischief of every day, and before morning the wasted organs again report ready for duty. But by habitually working beyond the recuperative capacities of the body, or by keeping the body lashed with stimulation, or by the habitual failure to secure sufficient rest and sleep for recuperation, the powers of life are depleted and exhausted. All form of activity--mental, physical and physiological—require the exertion and expenditure of power, and so long as the sources of power that lie back in the nervous centers, are adequate to a good supply of motive force there will be none of those developments which we know as disease.

By reason of the "isolated" state of the different nervous centers, which are the immediate sources of organic power, we often see local derangements due to the exhaustion of one or more nerve centers. One set of organs may be reduced to the necessity of perceptibly faltering in their functions, while others are still able apparently to maintain their usual standard of healthy action.

Only those who can see in wrong living the cause for man's discomforts and misery, and in correction of his mode of life the proper remedy for these things, are in line for a rational solution of the problems of health and disease.

IMPAIRMENT OF ORGANIC FUNCTION.

All the functions of the body are controlled by the nervous system—the nervous function being the only exception. It is a self-evident fact that these functions are efficient or not depending on the power or weakness of the nervous system. With a full tide of nervous energy every function of the body will be vigorous and efficient. With nerve force inadequate, function lags—it becomes weak and impaired.

With impaired function—due to lowered nerve force, ENERVATION—the processes of nutrition and drainage are not conducted normally and, as a consequence, the slow, gradual starvation and poisoning of the cells begins. The functional and structural integrity of the body suffers and the process of dying commences. How long it will require for dying to culminate in somatic death—that is death of the body as distinguished from death of the cells--matters little.

Nerve energy is a fluctuating quantity. It rises and falls from day to day, from hour to hour and from minute to minute depending on the nature and degree of our activities and the nature of our environment. With every rise and fall of our nervous energies there is a corresponding rise and fall in functional efficiency. Those organs which, through heredity or abuse, are the weakest will suffer the greatest impairment of function when the nervous power is lowered. The degree of functional impairment may range from an imperceptible impairment to an almost if not total suspension of function as is frequently seen in shock.

Digestive powers are lowered. Secretion is not adequate to meet the needs of the food intake. Indigestion—or bacterial decomposition of the food—with the formation of a whole series of toxins, some of which are absorbed into the body, occurs.

Bowel action is weakened resulting in constipation. Kidney action is impaired. Excretion and elimination through this channel lags. The liver and lymph glands are impaired. Their power to detoxify, through chemicalization, the waste and toxins in the body is weakened. The functions of the liver, pancreas and other glands of the body in preparing food for use by the cells lag. Elimination through the skin and lungs is impaired. All this results in the slow, gradual accumulation, in the blood, lymph, secretions and cells of various toxins or poisons, "arrears of expurgation," as Dr. Jennings called them, and also in the slow, gradual starvation of the cells. Enervation impairs organic function and impaired function permits the slow, gradual starvation and poisoning of the cells. The process of dying which then begins is slow and gradual and may be prolonged over many years.

Poisons, irritants, excitants, "stimulants," "tonics" inflict a wound on the texture or substance of the organ, for by their *goading, pricking and wounding* processes they irritate and excite to action, and lay the foundation for disease. Poisoning and severe injuries produce in this or that organ all the phenomena which are exhibited in the various forms of disease. They produce them in the greatest simplicity, often, for the reason that the injured or poisoned person was previously in an excellent state of health. Diseases manifest all the phenomena of poisoning and injury for the reason that they are cases of poisoning and injury only developed over a longer period of time.

Much and long-continued abuse is necessary to weaken the organs, of the body sufficiently to subject them to disease, if they are normal at birth. Nature places a strong safeguard over the functions of every organ and makes every organ much stronger than the needs of a normal life demand, so that disease can develop only after this safeguard is broken down.

"For, it ought to be well understood," says Graham, "that disease is never the legitimate result of the normal operations of any of our organs. The natural and legitimate result of all the normal operations of our vital economy is always health, and only health: and if disease is induced, it is always by causes which disturb those operations."

Diseases of all kinds give every evidence of being caused by poisons. Trall declared: "There are aside from accidents—mechanical injuries—but two sources of disease in the world, viz, poisons or impurities taken into the system from without, and effete or waste matters retained." All the causes of disease, he said, "may be summed up under the heads of impure or obstructing materials (toxemia), and exhausted nervous power" (enervation), due to "unphysiological voluntary habits." Let us then turn our attention to the sources of these toxins.

TOXEMIA: We define this to mean the presence in the blood, lymph, secretions and cells, of any substance, from any source, which is inimical to health and which, in sufficient quantity, will impair organic functioning. Recently Dr. Tilden insisted on limiting the use of the term to retained and accumulated end-products of cellular activities. This seems to us to be narrowing the term down more than ·its etymology permits. To toxemia, derived from such a source, we would prefer to use the term AUTOTOXEMIA or endogenuous toxemia.

Enervation must always lower physiological efficiency. Among its other results is the checking of elimination. Elimination, which is one of the fundamental functions of life, must be maintained at its highest degree of perfection if health is to be preserved.

Wherever the processes of life are being performed toxins are found, for they are being constantly formed in every cell and tissue of the body. The tremendous importance of elimination by which these toxins are removed from the body will be realized when one considers that if the urine is suppressed for fifty-two hours death results; if the skin is varnished so that elimination through this channel is suspended, death comes in a few hours; the carbon dioxide exhaled in one day would kill many times over if retained. If a wound is pent up so that drainage is stopped, septicemia and probably death results. If the bowels, skin, lungs, liver and kidneys fail in their functions the accumulation of autogenic poisons takes place. This condition we shall call *primary* or *retention* toxemia. The body is poisoned by the retention and gradual accumulation of those same wastes and poisons that are thrown off by the healthy body every minute of life, asleep or awake, from birth to death.

Primary toxemia forms the immediate basic cause of all forms of disease. It is the only form of toxemia that is constant—that is, ever present. It is doubtful if most of the other toxemias would or could ever develop without the presence of this *endogenuous toxemia.*

Toxemia tends towards the further production of toxemia. The more the body is loaded with toxins the less able it is to function properly. Just in proportion to the extent to which the body is free from incumbering material is it capable of receiving and manifesting energy. Thus, toxemia itself becomes an inhibitor of elimination.

INTESTINAL TOXEMIA: This is, as Tilden declares, an infection and is not an autotoxemia. It develops in the stomach and intestines, that is, outside the body, and is, therefore, of an exogenuous origin.

Enervation checks secretion and lowers digestive power. With the powers of digestion impaired the food eaten is slowly and improperly digested, if at all. Fermentation and putrefaction set up in the food eaten, resulting in the formation of a whole series of toxins, a part of which are absorbed into the body, thus adding to the primary toxemia already present.

Whether foods decompose in the ice box or within the digestive tract, they give rise to poisons of varying degrees of virulence, depending on their chemistry. Intestinal toxemia is a ptomaine poisoning coming as a result of indigestion. It never develops, at least not sufficiently to cause any trouble in those who are not already autotoxemic. It must be absorbed before it can cause any trouble, and absorption will not take place until resistance has been broken down. Before resistance is reduced, the decomposing food is washed out of the body by means of a diarrhea.

ORGANIC TOXEMIA: This term we apply to those toxins arising within the body as the result of destructive processes going on in some one or more of its organs. An abscessed tooth or tonsil, a pent up wound, a tumor that is breaking down, suppurating ovaries or appendix, or other organs, give rise to septic matter chiefly in the form of pus which, when absorbed, as it often is, causes severe troubles. This absorption will not occur in those who are not already autotoxemic, unless forced. As Dr. Tilden declares:—

"A suppurating wound, ulcer, or chancre, is on the outside of the body, and if it causes septic (blood) poisoning, it will be because the waste products are not allowed to drain—to escape. The discharge being obstructed, it becomes septic, and its forced absorption poisons the blood. Even vaccina fails to produce septic poisoning because its poison is discharged on the surface—on the outside of the body. Occasionally the waste products are forced to enter the blood because of faulty dressings; then septic poisoning with death follows."—*Toxemia Explained,* p. 50.

CHEMICAL TOXEMIA: I have employed this term for the want of a better one. By this I mean poisoning by drugs, chemicals, dyes, food adulterants, bleeches, serums, vaccines, so-called anti-toxins, etc. The sources of these are innumerable, but the greatest source is in the use of so-called medicines. Every drug, vaccine and serum in use is a cause of disease. They are all poisonous and destructive. They are sent into the body through the lungs by inhalation; through the skin by absorption and by injection; through the mouth by swallowing, and by being injected into the eyes, ears, colon, vagina, womb, urethra and bladder.

Intestinal toxemia and organic toxemia we call secondary toxemia, while these together with the drug and serum poisoning we call ABSORPTIVE TOXEMIA— or Exogenuous Toxemia. It should be well kept in mind that these toxemias exist together, each of them contributing more or less to the production of each and every so-called disease.

Toxemia forms the immediate cause of every so-called disease. Exposure to cold or dampness, or becoming overheated or fatigued, etc., act as *exciting causes,* and would never bring on a crisis if no toxemia were present. These things are normal elements in man's environment and would occasion no trouble were he always to maintain his resistance at the normal standard. These factors are not primary causes of disease, but may serve to induce a crisis after the body is already greatly ENERVATED and TOXEMIC. No doubt every one of my readers can recall a time when he or she was exposed to severe cold without resulting in anything more than a feeling of chilliness, and can recall another time when upon slight exposure a very severe cold or rheumatism, or perhaps a pneumonia developed. The developments depend on the state of the system.

Toxemia is a chronic state with most people, due to the present mode of life. The body learns to tolerate these toxins just as it learns to tolerate tobacco or alcohol. After toleration is established, crises, or acute diseases develop only when the toxins rise above the toleration point, and subside when they have reduced the toxins to this point or slightly below.

As repeated crises develop and repeated reaccumulations of toxins follow, the irritations, congestions and inflammations produced by the toxins bring about more or less destruction of the tissues of the body, resulting finally in organic disease.

What we call disease is a culmination or summing up of a long series of causes and conditions that followed each other in orderly fashion. Wrong living lowers nervous power, producing enervation. Enervation lessens, functional vigor and efficiency, resulting in impaired secretion and excretion. These latter result in the retention and gradual accumulation within the body of the toxins that are normally eliminated from the body every moment of life from before birth to the instant of death. The toxins set up irritations and these cause congestions, inflammations and functional derangements. As the toxins increase and inflammation progresses, and as functional disturbances continue, structural changes occur in the body. These latter may progress to an incurable stage, or the sufferer may learn how to live in time to stay the progress of degeneracy and place the process of regeneration in the ascendancy and thus gradually return to health.

He does not usually do this. It is the custom to continue the wrong living on the theory that germs cause disease, and to resort to drugs, serums, vaccines, and surgical operations to accomplish a cure. True cure is a reverse process to the process of building disease. It can reach fruition in good health only after the disease building factors and influences are corrected and their places filled by health building influences and conditions. If extensive degeneration of structure has taken place, complete regeneration will not occur, although improvement and partial regeneration may be brought about. The rule of curability in any disease may be stated thus: If the functions of an organ are deranged, cure is probable by proper living; but if the structure of the organ is deranged, a complete cure is improbable, if not impossible. However, in most cases comfort and a high degree of health and vigor may be attained.

The fundamental cause of disease is the same whether it is located in the big toe on the right foot or the little finger on the left hand. In other words, whether it is one organ or another that is the SEAT of the trouble, the underlying cause is the same. Real and permanent cure of such conditions results only when their causes are corrected. The mode of life must be reformed to the end that ENERVATION may be overcome and TOXEMIA eradicated.

INFECTION: Infection is the introduction of decomposing organic matter into the living organism. It requires positive contact with, and absorption of septic or putrescent matter to result in infection. Medical men define infection as the invasion of the body by disease germs. But, as Tilden declares: "It should not be forgotten that unobstructed free drainage from wounds, ulcers, canals, ducts, keep them aseptic (non-poisonous). The *deadly germ* on the hands, lips, drinking cups, hanging straps of street cars—in fact, found anywhere and everywhere—is not deadly until it gets mixed up with man's deadly dirty, filthy physical and mental habits." Germs do not become toxic until they get into a toxic environment.

Infections, thought Jennings, are the products of impaired or vitiated secretory actions, or of the decomposition of vegetable and animal substances, and indirectly occasion derangement in the human system by directly wasting itself in damaging the structures and substances of the body and thus calling for an extra outlay of effort, in renovating the body and are acted upon by the body in the same way as drugs and serums. Two conditions were thought to be essential to the effective operation of infection—(1) A "sufficiently concentrated and virulent" infection, and (2) A "state of susceptibility to its action" in the subject of infection. "These conditions admit of extensive circumstantial range; the contagion, from various causes, may be more or less active, and the subject too may be more or less predisposed to its action. ****The contagion will do its utmost to impair and destroy life, and the organs on which it has expended its force will fall in their action and structural condition just as low as a sufficiency of sustaining energy compels them to and not one jot lower, for when they have found the level of their conjoint ability to arrest retrograde action, however short this may be of annihilation, they take their stand upon it and maintain it, until their strength is sufficiently recruited to enable them to commence and prosecute their upward and renovating march."—*Philosophy of Human Life,* p. 126.

The idea of specific infection has no place in a rational philosophy of cause. So-called specific infection is septic infection. Sepsis is the only inflecting agent in all the so-called specific diseases. Sepsis arises from decomposition. All secretions, excretions and exudations are non-toxic until they decompose, whereupon they become toxic.

There is no apparent difference in the effects of infection, whether that infection comes from an infected wound, a wound of the womb in childbirth, or abortion, ulceration, an ulcer in typhoid, etc. The only apparent differences are those of degree, and this depends on the condition of the patient, and the amount of septic matter absorbed. Whatever the part that may be played by germs, the constitutional effect is always the same.

The supposition that there are specific diseases caused by specific infection arises from the fact that every organ or tissue in the body lends its own individuality to disease processes. We do not expect to find identical symptoms in disease of two totally different parts of the organism. Disease of the lungs would present symptoms which differ from some of the symptoms of disease of the liver or bowels. However, inflammation is always the same in whatever organ or part it is located. And any inflammation in any part of the organism will, if great enough, occasion systemic sympathy—fever and general nutritive disturbances.

So-called specific infections are limited in their operations to particular parts of the body, and when these parts are barred against their action, there is no development of the supposed specific disease. Where the parts are susceptible to the action of the infectious matter, the effect or injury that will be produced by a given amount of virus of a definite virulence or toxicity, will depend on the vitality of the parts, and the circumstances under which it acts. Some men are naturally and habitually invulnerable to infection, while others are proof against its action at one time and liable to be affected by it at another. Resistance depends on an abundance of nerve force and normal secretions.

A simple infection arises from any injury or non-toxic irritation. These quickly heal, if the cause is removed. However, such an infection can easily be forced to take on sepsis if the cause is not removed and strict cleanliness observed. A thickening of the mucous membrane and ulceration will result. After this has taken place, if the exudate cannot drain away fully and freely, it will undergo decomposition, resulting in local septic infection. If drainage is not established there is then a possibility of systemic septicemia.

Infection or sepsis is generated by the decomposition—fermentation and putrefaction—of dead animal and vegetable substances and secretions. We hold to the theory of the UNITY OF INFECTION. Infection is due to the absorption of decaying animal or vegetable matter and is always the same in whatever part of the body it takes place. A specific infection is not more nor less than a septic infection. Contact with putrescent discharge is essential. This is primarily a skin infection and does not menace life. However, should blood infection be forced, then life is endangered.

The differences in the various septic substances, that is the differing degrees of toxicity, are derived from the chemistry of the substances from which they are derived and the stages of decomposition in which they are found. As an example of the unity of infection, smallpox vaccination serves admirably. It is sterilized pus, that is pus which has had all germ life therein destroyed, yet it is admitted by its advocates to be frequently responsible for generalized vaccina, cellulitis, septicemia, urticaria, erysipelas, so-called syphilis, tuberculosis, lock-jaw, menengitis, sleeping sickness, and many other conditions. Yet it is always septic pus from a cow.

So-called syphilitic infection, which is a skin infection and spends itself on the skin unless forced deeper, serves to illustrate the same fact. It is putrescent matter and when inoculated into the skin may end as the primary ulcer or may give rise to a wide variety of skin infections. So greatly does it resemble skin diseases of various "kinds" that syphiologists declare that it is not worthwhile to attempt to distinguish it from other skin diseases.

Sepsis in the intestines may give rise to cholera infantum, typhoid fever, pneumonia, diphtheria, menengitis, inflammation of the brain, peritonitis, appendicitis, or other infections, all depending on the virulence (chemistry) of the toxins present and the systemic and organic resistance offered to it. Intestinal toxemia is correctly considered as an infection. So, also, in organic toxemia and vaccine and serum poisoning. The phenomena of *anaphylaxis*, which follows serum injections may manifest in a very extensive variety of diseases, ranging from aching in the joints with slight fever, to tetanus, convulsions and immediate death. Usually several forms of disease are present together as a result of serum inoculation.

The consevative power of the body limits all infections, as long as possible, to the lymphatic glands. These glands possess more immunizing power than ordinary tissue. The spread of all infections is along the lymphatic channels, but where lymphatic restraint is broken or overwhelmed, all the fluids of the body become infected and death may follow quickly. The lymph nodes in the groin, for instance, arrest so-called venereal infection and hold it up long enough to neutralize and destroy it. If the amount of infection is great and the immunizing power of the glands is inadequate, suppuration follows and a heavy pus discharge carries the infection out of the body. If toxin infection in the lungs is great enough to cause suppuration of the lymphatic glands in these, the resulting disease is called tuberculosis. Before a morbid process can evolve, the power of the part or of the body as a whole to generate its own immunizing agents must be broken down or overwhelmed. The reason two people similarly infected do not suffer alike, is that the one is more enervated and toxemic than the other and hence has less resistance; less self-immunizing power. Immunizing power has nothing to do with muscular strength.

One patient has a mass of putrefying food stuff in his intestine and has diarrhea Another has a similar mass and develops typhoid. In the first, the powers of resistance were sufficient to resist infection, and the decaying matter was expelled. In the second, there was low resistance which permitted infection.

Sepsis is often generated in the intestine, in the uterus, under a tight prepuce, etc. Lack of drainage, uncleanliness, etc., account for this. The disease resulting therefrom will depend upon the structures involved. Its severity will depend on the amount of septic matter absorbed, the condition of the patient and the aid or interference that the organism is given.

In septic infection, if proper drainage is established and the exudate washed away—this is, if cleanliness is observed—the primary infection will end within a few days. However, if drainage and cleanliness are neglected, reinfection will take place. General septic infection may follow.

The healthy individual, and by this we mean one who possesses real health, not merely one who conforms to the conventional health standard, easily resists infection where it is not so great as to completely overpower the organism at once. One individual may handle the poison ivy freely and not be affected, while another handles it but slightly and is poisoned by it. Again, the same individual may handle it at one time and not be infected, and at another time he may handle it and be infected. Infection is powerless against the healthy organism.

TOXIC DEPOSITS: We hold to the theory that the body deposits at various places in the tissues much of the uneliminated toxins and renders them as harmless as possible. So far as we have been able to trace this theory it originated with Sylvester Graham, who wrote:—

"I have known persons who have been greatly addicted to chewing, smoking or snuffing tobacco, and who, after an entire abstinence from it in every form for several months, on coming from a vapor bath which had caused profuse perspiration, emit a powerful tobacco odor from their whole surface. Indeed, I once saw a young person made sick at the stomach by rubbing the body of such an individual when he came from the bath. The individual was a friend of mine whom I had taken to the bath on purpose to try the experiment, and he assured me that he had not used a particle of tobacco in any form for four months. The Keeper of the bath informed me that he had observed the same fact in many instances; and that some invalids who had boarded and been under his care, taking the bath three times a week, had continued to emit the tobacco odor on coming from the bath, for several weeks in succession, when not a particle of tobacco had been used by the individuals for months. The same thing he had also observed in persons who had previously been much addicted to drinking alcoholic liquor, and others who had taken much medicine of certain kinds.

"These facts, which may be relied on with entire confidence, clearly prove that the vital economy has some depository out of the general circulation, and at the greatest remove from the most important vital properties and functions of the system, where it disposes of those deleterious and other offensive and superabundant substances which, from any cause, it is unable wholly to eliminate from the vital domain; and this, as we have seen, is none other than the adipose tissue. And hence it is evident that when, from poisonous or unwholesome food, or from any other cause, morbid and deleterious deposits take place in the animal system, the general receptacle is that portion of the cellular tissue which contains the adipose matter; and there is the strongest reason to believe that those substances become closely associated with the fat."—*Science of Human Life,* p. 500.

"The cellular tissue, we have seen, is the lowest order of animal structure; the lowest in vital endowment and functional character; and of all the forms of this general structure, that in which adipose matter is deposited is the lowest species. In the cells of this loose tissue, which is simply employed as a kind of web to connect other and more important tissues and parts, the vital economy, therefore, may, with greatest safety, in its particular emergencies, deposit for a time whatever substances it is obliged to dispose of in the most expeditious and convenient manner, and which it is not able to eliminate from the vital domain for—in these cells, such substances are at the greatest remove from any important vital power or function that they can be within the vital domain, and hence it is that such substances are deposited here and, in some cases retained for years, are of the most deleterious character, as we shall see hereafter."
—*Science of Life.*

We have an excellent example of this in the dropsy that forms in nephritis, due to impaired or suppressed kidney function. The waste matters normally eliminated by the kidneys cannot be permitted to circulate in the blood and lymph. These are deposited in various cavities and in the tissues under the skin, as dropsy, where they remain, in solution, until kidney function is restored, after which they are gradually reabsorbed, this taking place as rapidly as consistent with vital integrity, and eliminated. The amount of dropsy that develops under such conditions will depend on the amount of uneliminated salts or ashes that must be held in dilute solution.

Rabagliati holds that the "connective tissue is the first great place or part in the body where the products of an excess of food materials, finding their way into the blood, are primarily deposited." He called the connective tissue the "great dumping ground of the blood, the place which was, so to say, chosen by the blood as the least hurtful place or site in which to lay down any excess of material which it might be carrying, and for which it has no use."

A few years after Graham, Rausse of Germany presented a similar theory concerning drugs and he was followed a few years thereafter by Louis Kuhne who worked out an elaborate system of diagnosing disease by carefully observing the size, location, etc., of these deposits, which he called *Facial Diagnosis.* As a method of diagnosis, it is worthless and the careful observer will note that the deposits he pictures are accumulations of fat. Perhaps without knowing it, Kuhne agreed with Graham that the deposit of toxins was made in the fat, or in the least vital and most dispensable elements of the body.

It is evident that as the accumulation and deposition of these toxins continue and, as the cells of the body grow weaker and offer increasingly less resistance to the toxins, they are deposited more or less in all the cells and tissues.

172

If this is true, then the real cure of disease must begin in the cell. The real process of elimination must begin in the cell. The cell must disgorge itself of its accumulated toxins—must throw these into the general circulation to be carried away by the blood and lymph and eliminated by the various emuctories. Merely to force the bowels, skin and kidneys to increase their activities is not enough. This will not affect the deposited toxins in the body. It only weakens the organs so stimulated.

To force the deposits into the general circulation by any means that does not increase the body's powers of elimination or its ability or readiness for the absorption of these toxins from the tissues is only to increase the amount of toxins in the blood and lymph and cause trouble. This trouble may be labeled a *healing crisis*, but it is none the less true that the patient is harmed by this kind of treatment. If deposits are causing trouble in one part of the body and these are, by treatment, forced into another part where they set up trouble to which a different name is given, it is no true healing crisis. The crisis is being worked overtime by ignorant pretenders as a cloak for their ignorance and to hide their mal-practice.

True cure is found in natural living. This will gradually build up the body and purify the blood and lymph and enable the increasing strength of the cells to throw out the toxins. Often in the course of such a process, acute reactions (crises) arise and much of the toxins are cast out in the course of a few days. After each of these crises the general health and strength of the individual is seen to be improved Thus proving their beneficial and renovating character.

HEREDITY.

One-celled beings like the amoeba multiply by a process of division. It is not a new being springing from an old one, but the old one becoming two. "Their growth has no termination," as Weismann puts it, "which is comparable with death. The origin of new individuals is not connected with the death of the old."

There is something very similar to this in what we call the process of "reproduction" in higher animals. The birth of new beings also takes place by cell division, but every cell does not possess the power of producing the whole organism. We have two general classes of cells—somatic (body) cells and germ ("reproductive") cells—ova and spermatozoa. The "immortality" we see in unicellular organisms belongs not to the somatic, but to the germ cells. The *essential* "reproductive" part of the germ-cell is referred to as germ plasm. A portion of this germ plasm, when united with a portion from the other sex—the union of spermatozoa and ovum—will, under proper conditions develop into a new being like those from which the germ-plasm was received.

Only a portion of the germ-plasm is used up in the production of the new individual, the rest is stored away in the germ-cells in the sex glands of the new organism for further reproduction. In a strict sense the germ-cells are not a part of the body. The body simply acts as a repository, a safety vault in which they are stored. The body simply supplies the germ-plasm with room and board. There is, then, an unbroken stream of germ-plasm beginning in the misty ages of the past which has gone on dividing and re-dividing down the ages to the present and which will go on dividing and re-dividing for ages to come. This is called the "continuity of the Germ-plasm."

The germ-cells of Smith are not derived from his body but are the offspring of the germ-plasm from which his body evolved. The line of descent of from germ-cell to germ-cell—the body cells of each generation being offshoots. They serve no function in the work of "reproduction" beyond guarding and nourishing the germ-cells. Thus the characteristics of the son are not derived from the father but from the same germ-plasm from which the father derived his.

The child is not the offspring of the parent, but they are both the offspring of the same germ-plasm. A mother and her daughter are sisters and a father and his son are brothers in the biological sense. There is no *reproduction*. There is only *successive production*.

A child resembles his parent because he is derived from the same line of germ-plasm. He does not exactly resemble his parent for three reasons—(1) He is derived from a mixture of two lines of germ-plasm, the one derived from the father, the other from the mother; and, (2) Each of these lines of germ-plasm are themselves, the

173

results of past mixings so that many possibilities are potential in them; and, (3) They are not subjected to identically the same influences in developing the soma.

HEREDITY may be properly defined as "the *continuity from generation to generation of certain elements of germinal organization.*"

It is not intended, here, to go through all the maze of materials, symbols and merely mechanical explanations of heredity that exist. This would require several volumes and we cannot devote so much space to this subject in this one volume. A few practical points require to be noticed.

Above it was pointed out that the differences in a man and his son are due to causes inherent in the germ-plasm and to causes extrinsic to these. The same is true with regard to the differences between two brothers. However, experience has shown that the differences intrinsic in the germ-plasm are the predominating causes of differences in the offspring. In the same environment one egg becomes a duck another a chicken and another a snake, etc. The same pair of guinea pigs give rise to white and black pigs in the same litter. The germ-plasm, not the environment is specific. This fact was formerly expressed in the law that *like produces like.* This law in its true sense means that chickens produce chickens, dogs produce dogs, apes produce apes, men produce men, etc. It never did mean, and never can mean, that the offspring will be exactly like the "parent body" in every particular. Variation around a common center and with limits prescribed by law as fixed as the law of gravitation, is certain. In the strict sense there is *absolute uniformity.* Variation is greater where the parents are not related or are but distantly related, and less as the parents become more closely related—that is, variation is in proportion to the differences in the germ-plasm.

What we inherit is organization. "Heritage is the sum of all those qualities which are determined or caused by this germinal organization." A narrow chest is a question of organization and it is often a heritage, but whether or not it takes on consumption will depend on environment. Blue-eyed parents have blue-eyed children, for blue eyes is a matter or germinal organization. But one armed persons have two armed children, because the loss of an arm is a somatic loss.

Now organization may be largely determined by the selection of parents, and animal breeders make use of this fact. However, they breed for commercial purposes to produce specialized types which, due to the disturbance of the correlation that exists between the various organs of the body, both in structure and function, often leads to biological disaster. Loss of size, delicacy of constitution, and general deterioration, result from too close in-and-in breeding, and similar breeding.

Full health of the whole, or full functional activity of the whole organism, subsists not in the development of some parts or of some organs alone, but solely in the full development of them all. In all organisms, there is normally a reciprocal balance of all the organs and parts of the respective species. The maintenance of this balance constitutes full physiological perfection; and, when any part or parts are wanting or reduced, this balance is impaired and an evil effect is wrought. Perhaps no better illustration of this can be given than those evils often wrought by close inter-breeding of animals and plants. Darwin says of pigeons: "The young of all highly improved fancy breeds are extremely liable to disease and death." He collected hundreds of instances showing that the further a special "desirable" (desirable from the breeder's point of view) character is pushed by selective breeding at the expense of other less desirable qualities, the greater was the decrease in fertility and the greater became the susceptibility to disease and early death. The greater the degree of divergence the less the ability to survive. On the other hand, he presented numerous other examples where close interbreeding had been carried on for generations with little or no harm, with no reduction in fertility and no increased susceptibility to disease. These cases were, without a single exception, confined to not "highly improved breeds;" that is, to breeds that were not greatly divergent—common instead of fancy stock. To complete the thought here it is necessary to mention that Darwin collected hundreds of facts showing that an occasional cross between varieties increased the fertility and lessened the liability to disease in the offspring; or, in other words, the positive characters possessed by two divergent varieties were mingled in the offspring, the offspring, thereby approaching nearer to the normal or primitive perfect type, and for this reason is better able to survive. The same is true of cases of reversion by which lost or, more properly, suppressed characters are restored or regained. Says Darwin: "With pigeons, the more distinct the breeds, the more productive are their mongrel offspring." This is due to the fact that the offspring of such a union gain more positive characters than do the offspring of breeds more nearly alike. By such a cross the characters suppressed in the distinct varieties are regained by the offspring, thus bringing them nearer to the primitive type and thereby restoring, in great measure, the proportionate development of all the chraacters of the species.

Thus, it will be seen that the breeder subordinates the health and fertility of the animal or plant to the special object in view and reduces or suppresses parts or characters in the organism and keeps them reduced or suppressed if he fancies that such characters are in no wise profitable to him. He never considers how profitable they may be to the animal or plant. The full proportionate development of all the parts which is so necessary to perfect physiological function and the normal balance that exists between correlated parts and organs is, thereby, destroyed. The whole animal or plant is sacrificed to one or two qualities or characters which, in the eyes of the breeder are desirable ones. For instance, in fowls, many breeds either lack entirely such characters as the following, or have them greatly reduced in size: the beak, spurs, comb, wattles, tail feathers, crest of feathers, hackles, wing feathers, head, neck, wings, feet, etc. Many are greatly reduced in size while in some a vertebrae or two is missing. On the other hand they may have one or more such characters pushed to the extreme point of development at the expense of the reduced ones. Many other such modifications of characters of both a positive and negative nature could be given, not alone among fowls, but among other animals and plants as well. Similar changes are observed to follow the early removal of the gonads of animals.

A few quotations from a more recent study of this subject may be advantageous at this point. More recent works are chosen, not because the facts have changed, but to show that the greater knowledge of heredity gained through Mendelism only confirms the old facts. These quotations are taken from a paper by D. F. Daurie, Australian Poultry Expert, and published by the Australian Government. He well says: "DeVries, the author of the modern theory of mutation, as opposed to Darwin's theory of natural selection, has now a large following who may forget that Darwin and his disciples wrote what can neither be forgotten nor disproved; and we must remember that much which is thought to be new is old." To show that the new is old, the following quotations are selected:—

"The main principle involved in this scheme of breeding is to concentrate the blood or strain, and by the knowledge gained of its breeding characteristics, gradually to eliminate undesirable features. Where crossing is resorted to promiscuously, no definite results can be forecasted."

"Experience long ago taught many of the most successful poultry breeders that the direct infusion of fresh blood—a raw outcross—was invariably attended with disaster" (he means here disaster in a commercial sense—that is, the "pure" breed by the cross has new and, to the breeder, undesirable characters introduced. As he had previously remarked: "Most breeders forget or, perhaps, never knew of, the truth of Darwin's remarks on the crossing of alien families, and thereby the tendency to revert to lost characteristics—not lost, however, in modern phraseology, only digressive or latent." Author's Note). Mr. Felch's method clearly shows how type, purity and other desired characteristics can be maintained without loss of vigor; a modification also permits of the introduction of fresh blood if deemed, through any circumstances, absolutely necessary. I am, of course, referring to the breeding of pure-bed poultry of undoubted pedigree; the mongrel is not worthy of consideration."

Such methods of selection are often disastrous to the breed. In order to offset this evil there often occurs reversions of various characters by which the fowls are enabled to at least partly overcome the disturbed physiological balance. For instance, he writes: "Breeders of many strains of these Leghorns find that continued selection is resulting in what is apparently reversion to the long-lost (suppressed) maternal instinct of a desire to incubate. Birds which under careful test produce from 220 to 270 eggs in a year occasionally act as if developing the characteristic 'broody fever.' In some strains this feature is apparently increasing, and endeavors are being made by some to eliminate the feature by discarding all females showing a tendency to become 'broody.' Others again look upon the short rest—when the birds are in this condition and not laying—as a period of recuperation." Another feature that may be only a means of recuperation is stated by him as follows: "Although observation and evidence upon this point are not complete, there seems to be strong probability that the high laying power of a hen will not be directly transmitted to her pullets, but to the grandchildren or pullets bred in the third generation."

Perhaps it will be doubted that any period of recuperation is essential. The following quotations will show that these doubts are not well founded, as well as showing some of the physiological evils that are brought about by breeding for greatest commercial returns rather than for the greatest physiological benefits to the poultry.

"There may be reason to think that, as regards egg production in certain highly developed strains of fowls, we are in a similar position to the trotting horse people. By careful breeding to a definite type a trotting horse of great speed has resulted, but his speed is of short duration, and the chief organs affected will be the heart and lungs; legs and feet may be assisted by specially prepared elastic tracks. The laying hen is, however, different; it is not merely a question of development of type and motor muscles. Here we are selecting for the development of the organs of reproduction, which are the most sensitive in the body. We cannot be certain, but personally I have strong suspicions that the induced activity of the ovaries is in excess of the capacity of the glands in the oviduct, and the shock due to continuous laying accounts for many abnormal features.

"To conclude, I am of the opinion that our most noted strains have almost reached the level of highest development for egg-production, and experience is proving that vigorous selection for hardiness and constitution are absolutely essential to ensure this high egg-production." It is highly probably that a return to those anatomical and physiological conditions necessary to hardiness and constitution will also result in a return to a more normal egg production. For this exeremely abnormal over-production of eggs is secured in the same way as the following characters are secured, and is desirable only from the commercial, not the physiological point of view.

"In the case of egg-production there is a strong tendency for selection for numbers of eggs only without having regard to the size of the eggs. Again, many novices consider the number of eggs produced by a hen to be the only utility point worth considering and often find that undesirable points have been so firmly established as to render the whole breeding scheme negative. Those who breed for exhibition at poultry shows only as a rule have little, if any, regard for egg-production; in consequence, no selection having been made for that point, it is generally poor. On the other hand, through disregard for type and breed characteristics, the utility breeder, with egg-production as his only end, very often builds up a laying strain of what appears to be unprepossessing mongrels."

That selection—whether natural or artificial—cannot be depended on to do more than preserve the status quo after the improvement (regeneration) has been made that can be made under favorable conditions is very obvious, when one considers all the facts that have been accumulated bearing on this point. The following quotation from "Scientific Breeding and Heredity with some Notes on Research in Mendelism" by D. F. Laurie, are to the ponit:—

"The chief point, from a commercial aspect, is whether a race of birds can be selected which can be depended upon to give as high an average as the selected birds at present, and whether by selection we can accomplish even greater records of laying. DeVries holds that natural selection of individual differences can never lead to definite and permanent distinctions. When one considers that some individual fowls of a pure breed will lay only 120 eggs a year, and others of the same breed 300 eggs a year, we may look on laying as coming under this heading. Lock refers to the sugarbeet industry, 'in which elaborate care is taken to select those roots which contain the highest percentage of sugar for the purpose of propagation. This process was followed at first by rapid improvement, but the rate at which the percentage of sugar increased soon fell off, until at the present day all that selection can effect is to keep up the standard of excellence already attained. From his own experiments DeVries has come to the conclusion that, when selection is really efficient, the full possible effect of this process is exhausted in quite a small number of generations, and that then the only further effect of selection is to keep up the standard already arrived at.' Again, Lock's remarks are noteworthy: 'We have seen that the theoretical conclusions of the biometricians are in agreement with the opinions here expressed, as long as selection is understood to be confined to the choosing out of parents which show a definite standard value of the character under consideration, this value being the same in each generation. Under these circumstances, Professor Pearson concludes that in the first two or three generations a marked advance in the desired direction will take place, but that further selection (in this sense) will have comparatively little effect."

It may be emphasized, then, that the highest physiological integrity and most vigorous organic function depend, primarily, upon full and proportionate development and normal condition of all the organs, tissues and substances of the body; and, secondarily, upon a perfect conformity to the laws of constitution and vital relation established in organic nature. Whatever influence tends to weaken and impair one organ or part and its functions, thereby cripples the efficiency of all the organs and parts of the body; for, so great is the interdependence of all parts of the body upon every other part and of one part upon the whole, that no part of it can be impaired without more or less damage resulting to the whole organism. Necessarily, some organs, such as heart, lungs, brain, etc., bear a more vital relation to the whole than some others, but this in no way invalidates the general proposition as stated.

The mere lack of spurs or feathers, or wattles or horns, or of maine or color, or of the beard, as in the eunuch, the shortening of the legs or of the snout or tail, etc., may not seem of any great importance, but they are evidences of a deep-seated, far-reaching and fundamental constitutional deficiency in the organism which manifests not only in the loss or partial loss of these characters, but, by sterility, loss of size, lessened resistance to disease, fatty degeneration, changes in muscles, bones, nerves and other organs, and by shortened life. The more positive and fewer negative characters possessed by any variety over that of another variety of the same species, the greater are its relative powers of life, and the greater its chances of survival. Certain conditions are needed for the full and proportionate development of all the characters of each species. The withdrawal of some of these conditions entails the reduction and suppression of some of these characters—of those characters to which such conditions are immediately correlated. Those conditions of environment, therefore, that favor the full and proportionate development of all the positive characters belonging to the species are the ones best calculated to preserve health and life. On the other hand, those conditions of environment that are so disadvantageous to life that only the fittest, or more properly, the least degenerated survive under, are the least calculated to preserve health and life. What is termed "natural selection" is, at best, only a struggle or a protest against degeneration under such adverse conditions.

The results of breeding show that an organization that predisposes to disease may be inherited, but that the disease does not develop until the producing causes are present. A hereditary predisposition to disease is intensified when it exists in both parents.

Thomas Shaw, Professor of Animal Husbandry at the University of Minnesota, in his *Animal Breeding*, p. 78, thus describes the organization in animals which predisposes to tuberculosis:--

"These indications are various. They include the following, viz: 1. A thin carcass and lacking in depth, a narrow chest and loin, flat ribs, large barrel depression and hollow flanks. 2. Extreme thinness and fineness of the head, neck and withers, want of fullness in the eyes, hollowness behind the ears, undue fullness under the jaws, and a small and narrow muzzle. 3. Much prominence of the bones in certain parts as at the joints, and a coarse and ungainly appearance. and 4. A hard, unyielding skin, thin and dry hair, and irregularity in changing the coat. A thin carcass, of course, means one lacking in width throughout its entire length. Narrowness of the chest, flatness of rib and smallness of muzzle are all associated with circumscribed respiration, and a low vitality. Want of width and depth in body are associated with a lack of digestive capacity. The low vitality and the lack of digestive capacity account for the lack of fullness in the eyes, behind the ear and in the flanks. They are the outcome of a weak nutrition, which in turn is the outcome of the causes named. The undue length of the limbs in such instances is probably a result of the law of correlation discussed in Chapter VIII. The undue prominence of the joints arises from perverted nutrition. The harsh, unyielding skin, and the characteristics of coat mentioned are the outcome of a feeble circulation, which in turn grows out of a feeble digestion. Animals thus formed fall an easy prey to tuberculous diseases, hence, to breed them would be very unwise."

But this organization is not tuberculosis nor its cause. It is one of the SEVERAL CAUSES of tuberculosis. Among the "predisposing causes of tuberculosis" in animals the professor lists—"digestive disorders, food deficient in quantity, and quality, impure water, confinement in dark, damp, filthy, unventilated apartments, and undue exposure to cold *or to any other influence that lowers the action of the vital powers.*" (Italics mine). These influences, he declares, are chiefly responsible for tuberculosis in animals, and we have found them to be so in man, and he adds: "Cattle reared on the ranges are but little subject to tuberculosis, notwithstanding that in many instances they are frequently subjected to privation because of short supplies of food." He tells us also that the disease may not develop for several generations, due to the "absence of the exciting causes" or "owing to favorable sanitary conditions."

It is *organization* and *environment* which are inherited. The germ-cells are set apart at a very early stage in embryological development and a strong safe-guard is thrown around them, so that they are not easily influenced by the causes of disease. Should they be too greatly influenced by these they are unable to evolve into a new being. It is highly improbably that either the ovum or spermatozoa could carry enough infection to result in disease in the embryo. They would be more likely to be destroyed before any development took place. But this does not preclude the possibility of inter-uterine infection, although in most cases the membrane separating the embryo from the mother is a sufficient barrier against infection. Infection may also occur in the vagina in birth.

Children are said often to be born with venereal disease. This may be true, but such children were infected after conception. Inter-uterine infection is in no sense, heredity. We must keep our meanings clear. One inherits only that which is inherent in the germ-plasm.

When, in normal intercourse, thousands of spermatozoa are thrown into the womb and vagina of a woman, only one of which can ever survive, and all of which are struggling with might and main to be that one, there is a "struggle for existence" which eliminates the weaklings and unfit and assures the survival of the fittest. The accident of position may prevent the most fit from surviving but we may be reasonably sure that the least fit perish in the race. Infected spermatoza could hardly be expected to reach the ovum, or, should they do so, they must be unable to result in development.

Dr. Jennings declared:—

"Predisposition to disease—and I now use this term in its common acceptation for convenience sake, as my meaning will be understood—is constitutional and hereditary to a greater or less extent in all families, and every individual, derived by a law of descent; and this hereditary predisposition often manifests itself in great inequality of structure and functional vigor, in consequence of which some families are especially subject to lung consumptions; others to gouty or rheumatic diseases; and others again to sick-headache, or some particular affection, which is more common to those families respectively than to others; and this liability is traceable in such families from one generation to another, and in some instances in a long line."— *Philosophy of Human Life*, p. 112.

Many begin life with a *bias* or *predisposition* towards a sick-headache, or indigestion or rheumastim, due to an inherited or congenital defect of the local tissues, an "ancestral legacy," as Dewey called such conditions, so that a less amount of impairing causes are necessary to reduce these tissues to an uncomfortable and painful state, than is requisite to produce a similar state in the same set of tissues or organs in most other individuals. Those parts of the body that are constitutionally the most defective, or have been made so by accidental injury or abuse or otherwise, suffer soonest and most upon a general declension of the powers of life. If such people will learn to lead a reasonable course of life, conform to a proper dietetic regimen, take more exercise in the open air, etc., they may escape suffering. It should be generally known that a strict conformity to the laws of life is not only the best preventive of the common ills of life but is also the only reliable defense against epidemic influences.

But there are causes which acting upon the body, extend their influences to the germ-plasm and weaken this in consequence of which children are born with such weaknesses. In the chapter on sun baths we have recounted a series of experiments which show this to be true of a lack of sunlight. It is generally known that plants grown in poor soil are smaller and generally produce smaller seeds than do those grown in good soil. Experiments have shown that such seeds, even when planted in good soil give rise to smaller plants and seeds than those of the normal seed. Cold, alcohol, etc., have analagous effects on plants and animals. Fortunately these changes, being quantitative and never qualitative do not change the hereditary constitution, and, if their causes are removed, disappear in one or two generations. Indeed, Nageli found that plants which have acquired certain adaptive modifications by living on the Alpine heights since the "ice age," "lose these characters perfectly during their first summer in the low lands."

Defective nutrition, particularly in childhood and youth, not only cause defects and troubles that persist throughout life, but affect also the offspring of the child after he or she has grown up. Upon this point Dr. Taliaferro Clark, expert in child feeding for the United States Public Health Service says:—

"Underfeeding in certain essential food elements to a degree not necessarily accompanied by evidences of ill health or the production of pathological change, when continued from generation to generation will cause marked changes in hereditary characteristics."

Dr. Clark quotes definite experimental proof showing that rats when fed for several generations on a slightly deficient diet, produce offspring that, even when fed a complete diet, do not thrive as well as rats that possess well fed ancestors. In addition to this he gives evidences from observation on human beings that reveal the same thing. It is evident that a defective diet impairs the germ-plasm to some extent and thus injures the offspring. It is obvius, of course, that a defective diet eaten by the pregnant mother will injure the offspring. Proper feeding should begin, then with our great-great-grand parents—or, to put it the other way around, if "civilized" peoples continue to eat denatured foods each succeeding generation of our posterity will be more defective and ailing and shorter lived.

Alcohol is also known to weaken the germ-plasm. It is probable that many other drugs and poisons do likewise. As Trall declared, *Mother's Hygienic Handbook*: "It is a very prevalent error that persons may impair the functions of individual life without materially affecting the integrity of the reproductive organs. Many persons will eat and drink pernicious things, use liquor and tobacco, indulge in the most violent passions, etc., with little or no thought that such practices and habits deprave and enfeeble their sexual powers.**** This is why so many persons of vigorous constitution are the parents of feeble and sickly children."

But as Prof. Conklin says, *Heredity and Environment*, page 247, "probably such cases are not instances of true inheritance; they do not signify a change in the hereditary constitution but an influence on the germ-cells of a nutritive and chemical sort." Such cause must act through more than one generation to sufficiently deteriorate a hardy strain of germ-plasm to result in disease or a predisposition to disease.

"No doubt," says Jennings, "it required ages of the continuous action of appropriate causes on definite tissues or sets of organs, to prepare them for the first exhibition of the phenomena—and these mild at first—of smallpox, measles, and other forms of disease that are denominated specifically contagious. And they who have the misfortune to possess a cachectic or scrofulous habit of body, in consequence of which they are ever liable to serious maladies from slight causes, have not fallen into this dire condition accidentally, or suddenly. If their pedigree could be traced back to a strong healthy race or stock, and all the impairing causes that have been instrumental in reducing them to their unenviable inheritance could be correctly computed and presented, it would exhibit an appalling spectacle."—*Philosophy of Human Life*, p. 100.

PREDISPOSITION TO DISEASE.

"Medical books," wrote Trall, "are full of amusing specimens of thoughtless statements on this prolific subject. Thus Hooper in his 'Physicians Vade-Mecum, with Improvements by Guy and Stewart,' gives us the predisposing causes of inflammatory fever in the following words: 'Plethoric habit of body, with a *strong muscular system;*

a good and unimpaired constitution.' If muscular strength and a good constitution predispose us to disease, it is certainly very dangerous to have good health! The same author gives us as among the predisposing causes of yellow fever, the 'male sex,' and among those of miliary fever, 'the female sex.' It is of such stuff that many medical books are made. I only marvel that some transcendent genius has not recorded *human nature* as a predisposing cause of disease!"—*Hydropathic Enc.*, Vol. 2, p. 74.

Anyone who will take the trouble to examine the very latest books of today on the practice of medicine will find that the "male sex" and the "female sex," "pregnancy" and other perfectly normal healthful conditions of human life are still listed as predisposing causes of disease. These apparent predispositions in males or in females, etc., we hold to be due not to greater susceptibility of one sex over the other to disease of one kind or another but to differences in their mode of living and in the conditions under which they live.

The human organism is a complex of varied organs and tissues each of which is designed to serve various functions. There is not one superfluous organ in the whole body, nor one too few. Every organ of the body is essential to wholeness of life. Some are of relatively more importance than others, but none can be dispensed with without disturbing more or less that nicety of physiological equilibrium which is necessary to normal function of the whole body. It is not the mere possession of organs, but their functioning that determines health. A corpse has all the organs of a living body, but it lacks the power to function.

Normal function is the basis of an enduring health. This is dependent upon two general factors—namely, the structural integrity of all the organs of the body and sufficient functional power to carry on the functions of life. If there is no power in the power-house, the motors do not run. Similarly, the organs of the body, however perfect may be their structure, function vigorously or not, depending upon the amount of power that reaches them.

Constitution: is the sum total of the comparative development and soundness of all the organs of the body at any given time. It is susceptible of improvement or impairment.

The best constitutions among modern civilized man are more or less organically defective, these defects resulting either from heredity, defective nutrition, injury or abuse, and have tendencies toward functional disturbances in different directions, and in different degrees. One may be safe in saying that whatever his organization may be, no man in civilized life enjoys, at any time, a perfect equilibrium of functional action throughout his whole organism, nor enjoys it to the same extent at all times.

Few, if any, of us possess perfect organisms. Almost every one of us has one or more congenital or acquired structural defects—some anatomical weakness or deficiency that cripples life more or less. Dr. Dewey called these *"ancestral legacies,"* and regarded them as *"constitutional tendencies to disease."* Dr. Jennings referred this *"bias"* or *"Predisposition to disease"* to an "inherited constitutional defect of the tissues of the organs concerned."

However, in most of us these anatomical defects do not make themselves felt so long as we are possessed of sufficient nerve force to maintain normal function. Once the powers run low from whatever cause, these weaker parts take on disease. With a lessening of the powers of life, these weaker structures fail in their function more than do the better constituted organs and, as toxemia develops, due to lessened functional vigor, they offer least resistance to the destructive effects of the toxins. It does not matter whether these toxins arise within the body as a normal result of the functions of life, or are taken into the body from without as in gastro-intestinal putrefaction and fermentation, or, as in the use of drugs and serums, those organs whose structural integrity is least perfect suffer most. These are the organs too that break down first when the body is subjected to over-stimulating or to depressing influences.

Dr. Dewey observed: "By whatever means brain power is lessened abnormality is incited in the weak parts; hence gradually from the original weakness there is a summing up, as . . . acute or chronic, local or general diseases." By brain power, Dr. Dewey meant the same thing that we mean by nerve power.

Dr. Jennings well said:

"The recuperative or renovating work never begins but once, with the beginning of life, and only closes when that closes. And the only difference between the renovating work in health and in disease is this: In health there are vital forces enough to sustain all the departments of labor, synthetical and analytical. In disease there is lack of sustaining energy for all purposes, and this deficiency of power or disproportion between ability to do and work to be done, or between supply and demand, constitutes the whole of the proximate or fundamental reason of disease in all cases."

In an organism, which, starting as a single cell, has built itself up step by step, evolving its various organs and parts, manufacturing them from material supplied by the mother, and linking all these organs and parts together by means of the nervous system, glandular system and the blood and lymph systems, and making each part dependent on the whole and the whole dependent on each of its parts, there exists such a close harmony and inseparable unity that no organ can act as an independent isonomy. If an organ is weak it is not permitted to become sick (diseased) so long as the general economy is able to sustain it. Not until there is a lowering of the general health standard, due to enervation and toxemia can an organ which is below the general standard of excellence become the center of an affection. When enervation is brought on, and because of this secretion and excretion are impaired, and toxins resulting from faulty digestion are added to the retained cell-waste, the weaker organs or systems of the body become diseased.

Predisposition is nothing more nor less than weakness or "inverse resistance," as Rabagliati called it. Resistance is a quality of organized matter, and if organization is weak resistance must be weak. If organization is inherited, as we claim, then predisposition to disease, or a less amount of resistance than usual to the causes of disease is hereditary, providing this weakness is inherent in the germ plasm and is not merely somatic in character and having its origin in defective development from causes acting upon the soma from without.

Some parts of the body are weaker than others. This weakness may be hereditary, congenital or the results of abuse and defective development from one or more causes. Some of the circumstances and habits of life bear more heavily upon some organs than upon others. A character is the product of nature (heredity) and nurture (environment).

When energies are low hereditary and acquired tendencies (weaknesses) are most troublesome. They are unable to keep up their end of the game. If the energies of the body are just sufficient to maintain comfortable action under favorable circumstances, a little additional strain placed upon them will produce discomfort, pain, faltering of functions and other evidences of weakness and disease. If these changes in external conditions that put a tax upon the body are sudden or great, this makes it more difficult for the enfeebled organs to keep up comfortable action. Any change that necessitates a little additional expenditure of power to maintain the usual functional standard, when the extreme of forbearance has been reached, will cause a faltering of organic function with an added check thrown upon elimination. Those who are strongly predisposed to diseases of the lungs, for instance, require only to be subjected to sufficient enervating causes to break down resistance and then the lungs become diseased.

Diathesis means a constitutional (usually inherited) tendency to develop a particular form of disease. It is really the sum of nature and nurture; largely a defective anatomism—hereditary, congenital or acquired—which acts as the localizing agency. Sometimes it is a defective function where no anatomical defect is discoverable. Diatheses are divided into general and special.

General diatheses are the gouty, (arthritic, lithic, rheumatic, uric acid), neurotic, tubercular or scrofulous, strumous, cancerous, furucular, etc. A scrofulous diathesis is a defective structural development of the lymphatic system which favors the development of tuberculosis. It is accompanied with other defects in the organization—in the size and shape of the head, chest, bones, texture and color of the skin and hair, and other defects. The neurotic diathesis predisposes to nervous diseases.

Special diatheses are defective anatomisms of the various organs of the body. Special or organic diathesis is the only explanation of why people develop different organic diseases—why one develops a heart, another a liver, another a kidney, etc., affection—from the same causes.

181

Two men acquire the drink habit. Shortly thereafter one develops hyperemia of the liver which goes on to the production of cirrhosis, ascites and death. The other develops neuritis, and, if he continues to drink, graver forms of nervous degeneration. One man may drink large quantities of alcohol and yet live to old age. Another may die in early life from but a few years of drinking. It must be evident that when alcohol produces liver disease in one man and nervous disease in another the difference is in the vulnerability of the respective organs of these men and not in the alcohol. When comparatively moderate drinking kills one man at an early age while another who drinks heavily lives to an advanced age this must be due to the relative resistance of the two men and not to a difference in the alcohol used.

A diathesis is not disease. It is only a constitutional peculiarity or defect which determines the type of disease that will develop when sufficient impairing causes are brought to bear upon the organism. It is not a cause of disease except in that it is a weak point, a vulnerable point, in the fortifications of the body. The producing causes of disease lie elsewhere and the diathesis must always lay dormant unless these are present.

Page truly declared that, "the gouty, the rheumatic, the strumous, the 'colds,' and all other diatheses, are practically unimportant distinctions. The technical difference is, of course, well understood and admitted. In any event, it is certain that the course of living best suited to prevent one, is also best adapted to prevent or remove all. For all practical purposes, however, they may be all classed together; and whoever desire, either for themselves or their children, exemption from, or the alleviation of suffering, have only to adopt a pure mode of living in order to escape, or emerge from, the disease diathesis."—*The Natural Cure*, p. 132.

EPIDEMICS

Epidemics are due to germs. But germs are ubiquitous. They are always with us and "carriers" are always present. If germs produce an epidemic, how do they do it and why do they only produce an epidemic at certain times, and not at all times?

Orthopaths have always assumed that what they prefer to call *epidemic influence* is of an atmospheric nature, some advancing the theory that certain "electro-magnetic" influences favor decomposition and the development of disease, or of disease of a particular type. Even if we grant germs a place in this epidemic influence, we are forced again to relegate them to their usual subordinate position. Only those of poor constitutions, feeble vitality and toxemic bodies are overtaxed and crushed by epidemic influences.

Jennings explained the matter thus:

"By reason of debilitating or health-destroying agencies on the one hand, and the rotary renovating operations of nature on the other, that are in ceaseless progress in most constitutions, the members of communities always stand in different and constantly varying attitudes in relation to all great and general causes of physical derangement, to which they are equally exposed; and when such causes sweep over them, they learn who of them at those times possess similar local infirmities, so far as those cases can make the revelation. It is on this account and in this manner that the great periodic atmospheric revolutions prove such mighty revealers of secrets; that they disclose the weakest parts of men, and make 'violated law speak out its thunder' in such terrific accents."—*Philosophy of Human Life*, p. 123.

Whatever all the causes of an epidemic may be, it is absolutely certain that only those who are ready for the development of the disease will develop it. In all the epidemics, endemics and pandemics that have occured in the world or parts of it, in any and all ages, "some constitutions have been," as Jennings says, "able to stand erect amid all the disturbing elements that have prevailed around them."

Again:

"Atmospheric revolutions, the vicissitudes of the seasons and sudden and considerable changes of the weather, affect persons with different predispositions, or that possess different structural proportions and endowments, differently;" but "a man with an iron constitution may fix his abode where he pleases and health will be his portion." —*Philosophy of Human Life*, p. 122.

The vicissitudes of the seasons and weather are not, on the whole, prejudicial to health in sound, vigorous constitutions. Rabbits may sit all day in the snow and do this day after day without developing colds, pneumonia, influenzas. Young kittens may be well frozen and then if warmed, will revive and develop no disease as a result. Years ago, when ranchmen took less care of their stock than now it was no uncommon occurrence for a man to lose forty per cent of his herd in a Texas blizzard. Yet those cows that did not freeze to death developed no disease as a result of exposure. Men can withstand all kinds of climates, hot and cold, dry and damp, high and low altitudes, and withstand sudden changes in temperature or work day after day in water without developing disease if they are sound and vigorous. But those who are weak, who are of weakened constitutions, feeble vitality and who are heavily toxemic fall victims to such influences. Jennings truly declared:—

"Those persons whose capital stock is not equal to the emergency, are prostrated more or less, according to the amount of sustaining energy which they have in store at the time. Those individuals who are the nearest to bankruptcy in this essential article, fall first and fatally, others hold out longer, some recovering and others dropping off. Here too is to be found the reason why a much larger proportion of the cases that occur in the first stage of an epidemic prove fatal, than in the later stages."—*Philosophy of Human Life,* p. 115.

Those who are weakest and who are the most heavily toxemic fall first and have less recuperative power. Of these Tilden says:

"All they need is a fulminant—in disease a sudden drop of ten or more degrees in temperature, a slight indigestion, a mental shock, fear, etc. A long warm season followed by cold, a long dry season followed by wet weather, bring many to such a state of enervation that the change becomes the fulminant—the last straw—that starts an epidemic."—*Philosophy of Health,* April, 1923.

Every epidemic stops somewhere. They always did this all down the ages. As soon as all the "susceptible" have had the disease the epidemic ends. Only a small percentage of people in any community are "susceptible" to any epidemic influence. This allows the "guardians of the public health" to show how wonderfully they stayed the ravages of the deadly epidemic and saved the lives of the community. They trade upon the natural immunity of man and an ignorant public worship at their feet. They first create frenzy and panic by every avenue of propaganda and follow this by saving the precious lives of the dear people. It is a great game when it is skilfully worked and it nets the doctors and vaccine and serum manufacturers many thousands of dollars.

That atmospheric conditions have something to do with the occurrence of epidemics seems certain. Take the great plague of London, as an example. This came in one of the hottest and driest summers in London's history. This followed immediately upon a dry winter. It was a year of comets and these were looked upon as responsible and regarded with awe, dread, apprehension and fear.

There was but little water for drinking or cleanliness, and this was more or less stagnant.

The plague perceptibly abated when the first rain fell and almost died down when winter again arrived.

Humidity, damp cellars, damp houses, damp weather, etc., favor the development of diphtheria.

In 1925 London suffered an epidemic of tonsilitis. It was an unusually hot and dry summer. But there was plenty of good water and the filthy, crowded slum-like conditions of the middle ages were lacking. No plague would or could develop in the London of today.

Most epidemic outbreaks have held a more or less intimate relationship with decomposing organic matter. Defective drainage, and sewerage, cess pools, open sewers, over crowding, and, in the country, cow lots, etc., have all contributed to the production of epidemics.

"When we do away with organic filth, banish corruption from the haunts of men, we shall put an end to epidemics of putrid diseases. Thorough sanitation is the one thing needed, first, last, and all the time."—Dodds, *Drugless Medicine,* p. 455.

We do not favor the view that disease is transmitted from one person to another and thus an epidemic rages. The first case of smallpox must have been produced without infection from a previous case, and many cases since must have so originated and

183

must so develop yet. The first case of measles or of scarlet fever or of bubonic plague must have developed without contact with a prior case and many cases must have so developed since. The law of parsimony demands that no more causes be admitted than are necessary to the production of any given effect.

A cause, or combination of causes, which is sufficient to produce a given effect once may do so again and again millions upon millions of times. The author's own children have been repeatedly "exposed" to so-called contagious diseases without contracting a single one of them as a result. The author has been through unnumbered such experiences.

If one's physical condition is ripe for the development of a disease he will develop it, even though there is not another case on earth—that is the way the first case developed. If one's condition is not ripe for its development he will not develop the disease even though there is a case in the same bed with him—there are millions of instances like this.

"Only those individuals in the peculiar physical condition causing the outcome of bubonic symptoms," says Dr. Page, "will have the disease; when the last one of these is down the so-called plague is 'controlled.'"

The disease is individual. By this I mean the state of the individual and his body chemistry determines his disease. No so-called epidemic disease ever comes alone. There are plenty of "other" diseases but they are not made head-liners. Indeed these "other" diseases are frequently, it is almost correct to say commonly, diagnosed as the epidemic disease. You are only asked to keep your eye on the head-liner. Scarlet fever and diphtheria are often epidemic together, sometimes, though rarely, coexisting in the same individual. The so-called influenza-pneumonia pandemic of 1918-19 was really a whole group of symptom-complexes—"diseases." Pneumonia, pleurisy and bronchitis were frequently diagnosed as pulmonic influenza. Typhoid fever, appendicitis and other bowel diseases were frequently diagnosed as intestinal influenza. Sleeping sickness, menengitis, etc., frequently were diagnosed as nervous influenza. The epidemic was a state of mind or a method of diagnosis, a panic. In the training camp where the writer was stationed hundreds of cases of mumps developed during the "influenza" pandemic.

An epidemic is an increase in the amount of disease in a community and whether it is one epidemic or another will depend very largely upon the diagnosis. Chicken pox, cuban itch, Philippine itch, varioloid-varicella, amaas, kaffir milk-pox, sanaga smallpox, West Indian modified smallpox, Weisse pocken, indigestion, influenza and ivy poisoning are all frequently diagnosed as smallpox.

The 1918-19 pandemic followed upon the heels of the war. Years of fighting, coupled with fears, dreads, anxieties, griefs, sacrifices, deprivations, etc., had so prostrated the world—had produced so much enervation and toxemia—that there was simply an increase in the "diseases" that are always prevalent at that period of the year. When the Spartans besieged Athens during the reign of Pericles, an epidemic broke out in Athens. The city was overcrowded, the people from the outlying districts having retreated, with their cattle, within the walls of the city. Water was scarce, food was scarce, the city became filthy; the stress and strain of war enervated the people and sickness developed. Such a plague was undoubtedly composed of many different forms of disease.

Whether germs, fleas, white ants, rats, ground squirrels, etc., have anything to do with the production of epidemics or not, these other conditions are the primary causes of the epidemic. If we avoid filthy surroundings, enervation and toxemia there can be no epidemic.

ANIMAL AND VEGETABLE PARASITES.

There exist many parasites that find a habitat in and on the human body and, under certain conditions these are capable of causing much trouble. Under these conditions these parasites multiply very rapidly, whereas, under other conditions they multiply slowly, if at all, and appear to do no harm.

Agriculturists and horticulturists know that when plants and trees are deprived of some of the elements of normal nutrition, they become victims of parasites. They can control these to a limited extent by spraying the plants and trees but their attack will continue until the plants and trees are destroyed unless the lacking elements of normal plant nutrition are supplied, after which the plants are able to defend themselves.

This same is true among animals including man. Those of lowered resistance are not able to prevent parasitic invasion. However, as soon as normal resistance is restored the parasites disappear.

Dr. Shew tells us:

"The children of the Indians were never known to be troubled with worms; so that, we have reason to believe, that if a hardy course of training and diet were pursued with civilized offspring, such would uniformly be the result in their case as well. Worms are an evidence of debility. They cannot generate in the living body if it is preserved in a truly healthful and vigorous state."—*The Hydropathic Family Physician*, p. 21.

Tilden declares:

"It should not be forgotten that parasites will not find lodgment in the intentinal tract of normally healthy people. To find anyone troubled with any kind of parasitic disease is proof positive that his nerve energies have been broken down, and as a consequence, his digestive power is below normal; hence everything must be done to restore his resistance." "It is impossible for parasites to develop in the intestines of a child or adult unless the digestive secretions are weakened to such an extent that they have no destructive influence on the ova, or eggs of the parasites taken in with the food."

Jennings declared that only a "depravation" of the secretions of these organs gives the parasites a "title" to a "residence" therein.

Not all whose resistance is impaired are troubled with parasites, but some are. Particularly the poor and those who live in unhygienic, unsanitary surroundings and eat poor or unclean food and drink polluted water are affected by parasitic diseases. Filthy houses, dirty beds, lack of body cleanliness, etc., favor the acquisition and development of parasites. The kind of parasite that one will acquire will depend upon what parasites are indigenous to his locality and climate, as well as to the season of the year. Or, one may receive an imported variety from some one else who is infested with them.

It is true that parasitic diseases are sometimes, though rarely found in the well-to-do, who live conventionally clean lives. These people have broken down their resistance to parasitic invasion by an unwholesome mode of life and have, through some channel, come in contact with the parasites.

Some parasites are found chiefly in the skin. Before most parasites can gain a foot hold in the skin and thrive therein, there must be a lowering of the powers of life. Nutrition must be abnormal and renewal of tissue slow and imperfect. The skin must be weakened and debilitated and ready to undergo degeneration. In such a condition, the normal scaling of the skin takes place prematurely and the skin does not renew itself promptly and perfectly. This gives opportunity for parasitic invasion. That this is true is proven by the fact that the improvement of the skin by sun-bathing soon ends most parasitic skin diseases.

Because of a lack of some of the elements and conditions necessary to the production of high-grade tissue, retrogression takes place and parasites find a ready entrance into the skin. It should be easy to comprehend that any influence that impairs the powers of life, and thus impairs and disturbs nutrition, will build a systemic condition favorable to the invading parasitic hosts. It will also be readily seen that in order to bring about a complete and permanent cure of parasitic diseases it is necessry to build up the general health and correct all environmental factors that are impairing health.

Parasites are supposed to be conveyed from one person to another in a wide variety of ways—the use of common hair brushes, combs, towels, caps, wearing apparel, sleeping in the same bed or coming in contact in any way with the body or clothing of the infested individual. Some parasites are supposed to be carried by dogs, cats, birds, etc., and spread among men through these agencies. Many find their way into the body in food and drink, usually in the form of eggs. Others like fleas, bed bugs, lice, etc., when they get into a house find many hiding places from which they sally forth and bother almost every one that stops for a time in the house. Some, however, seem to be immune to attack by bedbugs, although the room may be full of them and other occupants of the room are much annoyed by them. Some are never annoyed by mosquitoes. This peculiarity is, by some, thought to be hereditary. Skin parasites live upon the skin. They feed upon its tissues and fluids and produce their young in its layers. They thus form a constant source of irritation which causes itching, inflammation and various efforts of the skin to protect itself. These efforts on the part of the skin, at self-defense constitute the symptoms of the disease or diseases caused by the particular parasite. The excretions of the parasites are, of course, poisonous and form part of the cause of the skin disease.

Intestinal parasites live upon the food in these organs. Where they get into the body they may find lodgment in the liver, kidneys, lungs, heart or elsewhere, where they live upon the blood and tissues of their host.

GERMS

Chapter 17

OFTEN things are asserted to be scientifically proven when they have only been accepted by self-constituted authority, and "authority" allows no contradiction. They merely rest upon the teachings of a certain school of thought and hold their field only so long as that particular school is able to maintain its ground. With the passing of one school of "science" another school of "science" arises with new theories, new doctrines, new dogmas, but the same pedantry, arrogance and bigotry.

Just now the germ theory of etiology is a reigning dogma of "science." There are, however, signs that the theory is beginning to wane. It is regrettable that the various drugless schools are beginning to accept more and more of the germ theory at a time when there is evidence of a distinct medical trend away from it.

Medicine is now claimed to be a science. Before the discoveries and pseudo-discoveries of Pasteur it was "a medley of diversified diseases and imaginary causes, treated symptomatically and empirically." Up to this time the evolution of medical thought was but a slow transition from superstition. The profession groped blindly about in search of a tangible basis upon which to base their theories and practices. Pasteur, while exploiting the work of Beaucham, and other scientists of that period, gave the profession the germ. Here, at last, was a tangible and basic theory which could be developed without limit. The microscope made it possible to visualize, differentiate and classify the organisms. With a frenzied and hysterical outburst of enthusiasm the medical profession seized upon this new theory since which time practically all medical investigation has been carried on with the germ theory of disease as its basis.

From that day to this they have labored and suffered in an effort to fit a special germ to the pre-Pasteurian nomenclature—to find a specific germ to cause each disease they brought with them from the old order. The unity of disease is not understood and each symptom-complex must have a special germ as its cause.

The Boston Medical and Surgical Journal, March 12. 1924, in an editorial entitled "New Conceptions of Disease and Treatment," discusses the trend away from bacteriology, the laboratory specialist and toward bio-chemistry and a return to clinical methods and says:

"The reason, therefore, of an eclipse or partial eclipse of bacteriology may be found in the belief that this branch of medicine, if it has not come exactly to a blind alley, has at least come to a halt*** There are signs, more or less vague as yet, that new conceptions of disease are arising, although such views are themselves nebulous. It is thought by some that there is more or less fundamental unity of disease, and that many of the nosological labels attached to them are superfluous and confusing."

There is hope, then, that medicine may yet come to the orthopathic conception of the unity of disease and perhaps we may dare to hope that they will also come to see its beneficent nature. Then will the present vagueness and nebulosity pass away. It will then be seen to be as inaccurate to say "a disease" as to speak of "a health." Let us hope that the drugless schools will also see the light.

Bacteriologists divide germs into two general classes—namely: Saprophytic, or those which live off of dead organic matter, and Parasitic, which live off a living host.

The saprophytic form the largest class, constituting omnipresent scavengers and are ever busy in Nature's great laboratory, the soil, in breaking down and working over dead organic materials into forms appropriate to the nourishment of growing vegetation. They are ferments and their work is to break down dead matter and reduce it to simple forms to be again used by plants. In the septic tank, sewerage is reduced by them until it finally passes out pure water in which fish may live. They are essential nitrifying elements in the soil. Without them neither plants nor animals could long exist and the earth would rapidly become encumbered with dead bodies. From both the esthetic and economic viewpoint they are benefactors. They are the best friends of life that we know. We live in a balanced and interdependent world which is too complex for man ever to fully understand, but his dependence upon germ life is, at least partly, understood.

The parasitic group, which constitute only about two per cent of germ life, are said to live always off a living host and to produce poisons, are also called pathogenic, or disease producing. They do not differ in any respect from the innocent varieties except in their ability to live off other forms and "cause disease." "The essential difference between the disease producing and the innocent bacterial species is that the former possess as their most striking physiological peculiarity the power of elaborating poisons, toxins, technically speaking, that they have a direct destructive action upon the tissues of their host."

The *Ency. Britannica*, Vol. 3, p. 172, has the following to say in the article under "Bacteriology":

"As our knowledge has advanced it has become abundantly evident that the so-called pathogenic bacteria are not organisms with special features, but that each is a member of a group of organisms possessing closely allied characters. From the point of view of evolution we may suppose that certain races of a group of bacteria have gradually acquired the power of invading the tissues of the body and producing disease. In the acquisition of pathogenic properties some of their original characters have been changed, but in many instances this has taken place only to a slight degree, and furthermore, some of these changes are not of a permanent character. It is to be noted that in the case of bacteria we can only judge of organisms being of different species by the stability of the characters which distinguish them and numerous examples might be given where their characters become modified by comparatively slight changes in their environment. The cultural as well as the microscopic characters of a pathogenic organism may be closely similar to other non-pathogenic members of the same group, and it thus becomes a matter of extreme difficulty in certain cases*** in differentiating varieties."

Was ever such a muddle presented? By far the greater number of "varieties" of bacteria are non-pathogenic. The pathogenic bacteria cannot be distinguished from the non-pathogenic except by their power to produce toxins. Their cultural and microscopic characters are so similar that it is extremely difficult to distinguish one from the other. Pathogenic bacteria are not organisms with special features but belong to a group of bacteria possessing similar characters, and have "we may suppose" evolved their power to invade living tissues and produce disease. Yet they have acquired their pathogenic properties "in many instances" to a very light degree and some of these characters are not permanent. They are judged to be of one species or another only by the stability of their characters but such characters are so unstable that they become modified by comparatively slight changes in their environment. Where are they going? Probably non-toxic bacteria become toxic bacteria in a septic environment.

Sir Richard Douglas Powell, a leading English bacteriologist, admitted a few years ago that if tetanus and gas gangrene germs are washed clean and freed from their environment, they are quite harmless. It would seem that they depend for their toxicity and supposed specificity upon a toxic environment, and if this is so, the chemistry of their environment really determines toxicity. The same is true of all germs.

Organized ferments (germs) are as necessary to life as unorganized ferments (enzymes) and become dangerous only when their environment is toxic. For instance, in wounds germs must be pent up before they can set up their peculiar fermentation in the surplus material that has been sent there. Unless they are able to produce a specific disease without the aid of an unnatural environment they cannot be rightly regarded as *the cause* of disease, although they may be regarded as *a cause,* just as any beneficial influence may help to produce disease when it is perverted.

Germ theorists estimate that an average of 14,000 germs pass into the nose in an hour's breathing. On the subway and in a crowded building, we probably get this many into our noses in a few minutes. Many more are taken in in food and drink. Prof. Haas, of Leipsig, the renouned German physicist, who calculated the number of electrons in the universe, said:

"It is well known that bacteria are peculiar in that they propogate by a process of division of the individuals. From one bacterium in the course of an hour, there results two bacteria by this splitting process, and after an interval of two hours there are four and so on. Let us suppose we have a single bacterium in a glass of water. We shall further assume that in some way or other sufficient nourishment can be supplied to insure that reproduction is not adversely affected by lack of food. In such circumstances there would be present some 16,000,000 of bacteria after one day of twenty-four hours; and at the end of the second day there would be 3,000,000,000,-000; and after three days 5,000,000,000,000, which would already correspond to a weight of thousands of tons. In the course of the sixth day the mass of the bacteria would exceed the weight of the earth; in the course of the seventh day the mass of the sun; in the course of the tenth day the weight of all the bacteria would attain the total weight of the universe; and, finally, in the course of the eleventh day the number of all the bacteria would be as large as the total number of electrons in the universe."

Imagine taking a few millions of germs into your body in your food and drink and have them start multiplying at such a rate as that! Remember the above figures represent what one bacterium would amount to in the times stated, if not prevented from multiplying at their normal rate by adverse influences. If you take a few millions of germs into your body in meat or milk, you have not one bacterium to start multiplying, but millions. You will readily perceive that we must be germ-proof, or we perish.

Let us go away to the forest. It is a beautiful summer day and we take a stroll along through the shade of the trees. There before us we see a beautiful deer. He does not know what it is to be sick. He has never been sick. From birth he has enjoyed uninterrupted good health.

Suddenly the crack of a rifle sounds on the air and the deer drops in his tracks. Life is gone. All the functions of life cease and that beautiful and once vigorous organism lies stilled in death. A few hours pass and it begins to smell bad. A few hours more and it is a corrupt mass of putrid flesh. It is literally swarming with bacteria. They are at work destroying the body of the deer. They are multiplying rapidly. In a few days they complete their work and what was once quickened flesh is now dead and inorganic matter—returned to the dust of which it was made. Germs have destroyed that flesh. They have consumed it and returned it to its primitive elements.

Why did not they do this while the deer was still alive? Why were they unable to destroy the living, healthy flesh? How was that deer able to maintain such a high degree of health and vigor in a world swarming with germs of all kinds? If germs are the enemies of life, if they attack and devour living flesh, where they can, is it not obvious that the body of the living animal possesses some very adequate defenses against their encroachment? It is not proven that germs ever attack living matter, but assuming that they do, and seeing that we cannot destroy all the germs on the earth, does it not appear that nature's own defenses are adequate so long as by proper living, they are maintained at their normal standard? So long as they are not broken down by a mode of life that saps the powers of life and weakens its functions, germs, if they are the foes of life (which they are not), are powerless against the body.

The Medical Journal and Record, for March 17, 1926, says editorially, that:

"Many acute and semi-acute diseases originate in the mouth, nose or throat by inhalation of microbes or germs there present which are excited into activity by causes as yet unknown. . . . This seems to be the theory that is gaining in favor, that some unknown cause activates latent germs into activity."

The medical profession is hard pressed for a means of saving the tottering germ theory. They first assumed that germs caused disease. But since their presence does not cause disease, they have to have an *unknown cause* to cause the germs to cause disease. This helps them out of their dilemma. There are many unknown causes in what is known as *Modern Medical Science.* It is a strange "science" that is based on the unknown.

Warmth, moisture, food,—these are the causes that activate latent germs and arouse them to activity. They exist, all except the food, in the mouth, nose and throat at all times. The food is thrown out into these, as excretions, in disease. The germs feed on the excretions. They are scavengers. They were never anything else and will never be anything else. They break up and consume the discharge from the tissues. This is the function ascribed to germs everywhere in nature outside the body and is their real and only function in disease. They are purifying and beneficial agents. The medical profession has Coued itself into hysteria over the germ theory and is using it to exploit an all too credulous public.

Germs are ubiquitous. They are in the air we breathe, the food we eat, the water we drink. We cannot escape them. We can destroy them only to a limited extent. It is folly to attempt to escape disease by attempting to destroy or escape germs. Once they are in the body the physician has no means of destroying them that will not, at the same time, destroy the patient. We cannot avoid germs. We must be proof against them. We have to accept them as one of the joys of life, and if they are really causes of disease, we can avoid disease only by keeping ourselves in such a high state of health that they are powerless against us just as they were powerless against the deer.

It is not yet definitely proven that germs are essential elements in the production of any disease. It seems probable that they are only incidental and perhaps beneficial factors. However, this much is certain; whatever part they perform in the production of disease, germs alone can no more produce disease than a seed alone can produce a tree. Just as a seed must have fertile soil, moisture, warmth, air and sunlight, if it is to grow into a tree, so the germ, if it is to produce disease, must find certain essential conditions existing in the bodies of those it enters before it can do the slightest harm. If the body is normal, if it has an abundance of nerve force, if its blood stream is pure, if there is prompt and vigorous action of all its essential organs, no germs coming in contact with it can grow and multiply. Good health is proof against germs of all kinds.

There is a class of individuals to which the medical profession and the bacteriologists have fastened the term "carrier." This is an individual who carries around on or in his person the germs of some disease. Every epidemic, we are told, develops a number of such cases. But these people, while they are accused of harboring so many of the deadly germs and of spreading the disease wherever they go, themselves do not have the disease. "Typhoid Mary" is still fresh in the memory of many of us. These "carriers" when found, are isolated, quarantined, kept away from family, friends and work and forced to undergo many hardships. Why do not these people develop the disease they are said to be spreading among others, if the mucous membranes are especially susceptible to such germs? Why if not for the reason that these membranes are susceptible to bacterial invasion only under certain conditions? Medical men say they are immune but upon what does this immunity depend?

All the standard works on bacteriology state that a person may have germs of diphtheria, typhoid fever, tuberculosis, pneumonia or any other disease within his body, that is, in his mouth, throat, air passages, stomach and intestines, without having the disease these germs are supposed to cause. Why do not these germs produce disease? Isn't it obvious, that, whatever their part in the production of disease, they alone cannot produce disease?

Medical men and bacteriologists are practically a unit in declaring that germs cannot secure a foothold in a healthy body, but that a "nidus" or "suitable soil" is essential to their genesis. They do no harm in a body that is in a normally healthy condition. If germs cause disease why don't they produce disease in a healthy body? Why must the body already be diseased and its resistance low before they can produce disease?

If there is a natural immunity to germs as the above facts and many more easily show, if germs are powerless against a healthy body, then, is not the logical preventive procedure that of finding out the factors upon which immunizing health depends and cultivate these? The cultivation of health as a defense against disease is far more sensible than the mad-house effort to immunize everyone with serums and vaccines.

The natural antiseptics of the body are found within the body itself when it is not impaired, and it is maintained in a normal state by the proper use of those eternal elements of hygiene—sun, air, water, proper food, muscular exercise, etc.

Investigations in the bacteriological laboratory throw no light on the conditions in the body which permit the germs to grow or which prevent them from growing. They tell us of a few germs which, it is claimed, are the active agents in disease but they tell us nothing of the conditions which permit these agents to become active. They grow in those conditions and only in those conditions of life which give rise to such complaints as indigestion, catarrh, etc.

The view I would put before the reader is that disease is caused, not by the germ, but by the state of the body that allows the germ to flourish. And this condition of the organism or any part of it which renders possible the growth of the germ therein is the much sought for "filterable virus." It is the outgrowth of violations of the laws of life and is no chance or haphazard condition. We also favor the view so long stressed by Dr. Tilden, and now made feasible by the knowledge of the transmutability of the "various" forms of germs, that the disease condition present determines the morphology of the germ and not vice versa. The germ takes on a form and character in keeping with its environment—environment does not change to conform to the germ.

It is admitted that the body is built to offer very powerful resistance to the entrance of germs. The skin is, if unbroken, impermeable by them. The internal skin, or mucous membrane lining all the cavities of the body which communicate either directly or indirectly with the outside world, if unbroken, is invulnerable to them. The normal secretions of these membranes are germicidal. There is no susceptibility on the part of any healthy organ, to bacterial injury. It is obvious that, living in a world swarming with microbes, if these cause disease, man must have powerful resistance to them, else he would have perished long ago.

In *Physical Culture* for May 1919 is an article by John B. Fraser, M.D., C.M., entitled "Do Germs Cause Disease?" giving an account of some experiments in this connection carried out in Toronto during the period between 1911 and 1918. He says:

"In an earnest endeavor to determine whether germs are dangerous, Toronto has taken an honorable part. In solving this question the first three years, 1911-12-13, was spent in studying a single point, viz. 'When does the germ appear?' The verdict was 'after' the onset of disease; and this fact led to the supposition that germs were simply a by-product of disease, and possibly harmless.

"In 1914 a small group of citizens undertook to prove the latter point by adopting Hunter's method of direct action, viz., incorporating fresh vigorous germs in food and drink and then using that food in the ordinary way.

"This proposal was vigorously opposed by friends and acquaintances who pointed out the danger and said it was tempting Providence but experience showed there was no danger, and that one could tempt Providence in that line (taking germs) with impunity.

"The first experiment made was taking fifty thousand diphtheria germs in water, and after a few days suspense and no sign of the disease it was considered that the danger had passed. The reason for choosing diphtheria germs for the first experiment was that in aconite, we had an especially reliable remedy for aborting the disease, providing it showed signs of developing.

"In the second experiment one hundred and fifty thousand diphtheria germs were used in milk, and again no signs of diphtheria appeared.

"In the third experiment over one million diphtheria germs were used in food without producing any sign of the disease.

"In the fourth experiment millions of diphtheria germs were swabbed over the tonsils and soft palate, under the tongue, and in the nostrils and still no evidence of the disease was discernable. As these results were very satisfactory it was decided to test out some other kinds of germs. A series of tests were made with pneumonia germs in which millions of germs were used in milk, water, bread, potatoes, meat, etc., and although persistent efforts were made to coax them to develop absolutely no sign of the disease appeared.

"Another series of experiments were carried out with typhoid germs, especial care being taken to infect distilled water, natural milk (not pasturized); bread, meat, fish, potatoes, etc., etc., with millions of the most vigorous germs that could be incubated, and but for the knowledge that they had been taken, one would have known nothing about it.

"Another series of tests were made with the dreaded meningitis germs, and as the germs are believed to develop mainly in the mucous membranes of the nostrils, especial pains were taken to swab millions of the germs over the floor and sides of the nostrils, into the turbinated sinuses, over the tonsils, under the tongue, and back of the throat. In addition to these tests other tests were made in food and drink—millions of germs in each case, and yet no trace of the disease appeared.

"The experiments with the tuberculosis germs were carried out in a different way

—more time was given between the experiments so as to allow the germs to develop; for clinical evidence has shown that this disease may remain latent, or imperfectly developed for months. Consequently it meant months of watching and waiting before one could be positive that the germs would not develop.

"Here again millions of germs were used in water, milk, and food of various kinds; every facility was given for the germs to develop as far as time and virility, numbers, and variety of food and drink was concerned; and as almost five years have elapsed since the experiment with T. B. began and no evidence of the disease has appeared I think we are justified in the belief that the germs are harmless. In addition to those experiments combinations of germs were used, such as typhoid and pneumonia, meningitis and typhoid, pneumonia and diphtheria, etc., etc., but no evidence of disease followed.

"During the years 1914-15-16-17-18 over one hundred and fifty experiments were carried out carefully and scientifically and yet absolutely no signs of disease followed."

The London Lancet Medical Journal of Canada (June, 1916) records some of the same or similar experiments by a medical man and six others which covered a period of two and one-half years, and, in which cultures of the germs of various diseases, particularly those of diphtheria, pneumonia and typhoid were used in all kinds of foods and under the most favorable circumstances. The germs were administered in doses ranging from fifty thousand to one million and five hundred thousand without producing a single evidence of disease.

Surely such results or lack of results do not speak well for the germ theory in general nor for the idea in particular that the mucous membranes of lungs, intestines, etc., are particularly susceptible to germ invasion. Rather, we would say, they completely negative the whole theory. They show, at least, that germs alone cannot cause the diseases which they are supposed to cause.

A celebrated physician and professor of the University of Vienna, Dr. Pettenkofer, came to the conclusion that germs alone do not cause disease and for many years defended his position from the lecture platform and in his writings. On one occasion, while instructing his class in the bacteriological laboratory at the University he startled his students by picking up a glass containing millions of living cholera bacilli and swallowed the entire contents of the glass before the astonished students. Dangerous as this experiment appeared, it resulted only in a slight nausea.

Dr. Thomas Powell, who died a few years ago in California in his eightieth year, is thought to have taken more germs than any other man. Years ago he challenged his medical colleagues to produce a single disease in him by germ innoculation. For years many of the germ theorists did their best to silence this discordant note. Cholera germs, bubonic plague germs and germs of every description were innoculated into his body and fed to him in every kind of food. Again and again they scraped his throat raw and painted it with diphtheria germs. But in all these many efforts, not once did they succeed in producing a single disease in him.

There was the celebrated attempt of Dr. Waite to kill Colonel Peck. Waite fed his victim cultures of all the supposed disease producing germs, that he could secure, both home grown and imported. These cultures included cultures of the germs of the most "deadly" disease known but Colonel Peck seemed to thrive on them. Waite was finally forced to resort to chloroform and a pillow to get his victim out of the way.

A number of experiments were made in the Naval Detention camps during the influenza epidemic of 1918-19 to transmit the disease from the sick to the well. Several such experiments were made on sixty-eight volunteers from the U. S. Naval Detention Training Camp on Deer Island.

Several groups of volunteers were innoculated with pure cultures of Pfeiffer's bacillus; with the secretions of the upper respiratory passages, and with blood taken from typical influenza cases. About thirty of the men had the germs sprayed and swabbed in the nose and throat. The Public Health Report sums up the results in these words: "In no instance was an attack of influenza produced in any one of the subjects."

Ten other men were carried to the bedside of ten new cases of influenza and spent forty-five minutes with them. Each well man had ten sick men to cough in his face.

With what results? "None of these volunteers developed any symptoms of influenza following the experiment."

Some similar experiments conducted in San Francisco are described in another article. Here one group of ten men were given emulsifying cultures of Pfeiffer's bacillus with no results during seven days of observation. Other groups of men, in all forty, were given emulsions of the secretions from the upper respiratory passages of patients in the active stages of influenza. These emulsions were sent into the nose by a medicine dropper and by an atomizer. The results are described in these words: "In every case the results were negative, so far as the reproduction of influenza is concerned. The men were all observed for seven days after innoculation."

Similar experiments with the same negative results were carried out in Philadelphia.

In *The American Journal for the Medical Sciences*, June 1923, is an article by A. C. Abbott, Director School of Hygiene, Public Health, University of Pennsylvania, entitled "Is Our Knowledge of Pneumonia Sufficient to Explain Its Endemicity and Occasional Epidemicity?", in which he says:

"It would be superfluous to detain you with a recital of the prevailing view of the relationship between lobar pneumonia and one or another of the several varieties of pneumococus always present in the diseased lung. Because of this regular association, the opinion is very general that pneumococus is the one and only vital factor concerned in true lobar pneumonia. This view, is fixed in the minds of many as was at one time the view that the so-called hog cholera bacillus, always present in the characteristic lesions of that disease, was the cause of hog cholera—yet time has shown that through-out all the careful experimental work on hog cholera we were, for the most part, unconsciously dealing with at least two exciting factors: one, quite obvious, easily recognizable, and readily lending itself to experimental study, the hog cholera bacillus—the other, obscure, evasive, invisible, but apparently ever present, filterable or ultra virus The one, the latter, the real cause of the disease; the other, the former, only a regular accompaniment. As a result, years of labor and reams of publications upon hog cholera are today of but historic interest."

Hog cholera is not due to the demonstratable germ which is a "regular accompaniment," but to an ultra-germ that cannot be demonstrated but which must be assumed, if the germ theory is not to be scrapped altogether. Dr. Abbott seems to look upon pneumonia as also being due to some undiscovered and, at present, undiscoverable germ. Smallpox has long since been decided to be due to a germ which is so small it cannot be seen with the aid of the highest power microscope now in use. Other forms of disease for which germs have not been discovered also fall into this class.

Among those "diseases" for which germs have been "discovered" there are often several forms of germs that are thought to be capable of producing them. For instance, penumonia is thought to be caused by several forms of germs. It is thought that one may be immune to one or more forms and be vulnerable to one of the others. Meningitis is declared to be caused by several different germs. What was once typhoid fever has been broken up into three diseases, each presenting identically the same clinical picture, but each "disease" is said to be due to a different and distinct germ.

Diphtheria may be used as an example of another class of "disease" which refuses to run true to type. The patient may present a perfect clinical picture of this disease and yet no diphtheria bacillus be present. A case of this kind was investigated by the Department of Health of New York, two years ago, and it was finally decided that the disease was *Vincent's Angina*, because "Vincent's organisms" were found, but also because the child had previously been "immunized" with three dozes of toxin-antitoxin and because antitoxin failed to "cure the disease."

On the other hand, one may have a slight sore throat, and the supposed diphtheria germs and it will be declared to be diphtheria.

Walter R. Hadwen, M.D., M.R. C.S., of England, in a lecture at a public meeting in Los Angeles, Cal., June 16, 1921, quoted Dr. Muthu of the Mendip Hill Sanatorium, who he said is "perhaps one of the most experienced men in tuberculosis" in England, as saying, "In fifty per cent of his cases he could not find tubercle bacilli at all." Dr. Hadwen himself declared: "Nobody has ever found a tubercle bacillus in the earliest stages of tuberculosis!"

Dr. Paul Carton, long head of one of the largest sanitoria in France, for tubercular patients, declares in his *Consumption Doomed*, p. 19:

"In tuberculosis the soil is practically everything,*** one becomes tuberculous by enfeebling one's organism, and the only means of getting rid of the bacillus, once it is fairly engrafted, is the heightening of the spontaneous resisting power. In a word Koch's bacillus is not much more than a saprophyte, a moss, a parasite which fastens upon failing organisms and seals the fate of those already falling into ruin."

It is often asked in drugless circles, if it is not possible that germs are the factors that give individuality and localization to disease. In other words, it is admitted that toxemia is back of both typhoid and pneumonia, but it is asked: Why did toxemia cause typhoid in one and pneumonia in another? It is admitted that toxemia is back of both tonsilitis and diphtheria, but, it is asked: Why is diphtheria more virulent than tonsilitis? May these things not be determined by germs?

The answer to the first question, that is, Why does toxemia cause pneumonia in one and typhoid in another, will have to be found in the laws of heredity, nutrition and environment. It is certain that germs cannot answer this question. Those tissues offering least resistance to the toxins are the first affected.

The answer to the second question must be found in the nature and source of the toxins causing the trouble. Wood alcohol and grain alcohol are both products of fermentation—bacterial decomposition. The greater virulence of wood alcohol is not due to any difference in the yeast germs but to the differences in the substances from which the two forms of alcohol are made. Toxins resulting from protein decomposition are more virulent than those resulting from carbohydrate fermentation. Animal (meat and egg) proteins, when they decompose, produce more virulent toxins than plant proteins. Decomposing milk proteins produce less virulent toxins than some plant proteins. Some forms of flesh foods, when they putrefy, give rise to more virulent toxins than other flesh foods when they putrefy. There is also a difference in the virulence of the poisons formed by the decomposition of various vegetable proteins. This difference in virulence exists potentially in the animal or plant food—not in the germ. The difference in virulence depends upon the composition of the protein, not upon the germ decomposing it.

Tonsilitis, we believe, is the result of the less virulent plant toxins, while diphtheria results from the more virulent animal toxins. In both these diseases there is decomposition going on in the gastro-intestinal tract. This decomposition does not always result in tonsilitis or diphtheria. It may cause pneumonia or meningitis or typhoid or typhus or acute nephritis or some form of eruptive fever, as indicated in our answer to the first question.

We do admit the office of the germ in decomposition. Fermentation and putrefaction are the result of germ action under favorable conditions. In the gastro-intestinal tract these favorable conditions are, impaired secretion, plus eating beyond digestive capacity. Back of impaired secretion is wrong living. So, it will be seen that whatever place may be accorded to germs in the production of disease, that place is necessarily a subordinate and secondary or tertiary place. They are not and can never be primary causes. If they were primary causes, there would be no plant and animal life on the earth.

Putrescence, or the toxin resulting from decomposition, is not potential in the ferment, but in the fermenting or putrefying substance. The organized ferment (germ) takes on an individuality and personality in keeping with the chemical medium resulting from the disease process or the fermenting activities.

If more food is eaten than can be prepared for absorption the ever present organized ferments (germs) set up fermentation. Fermentation, irritation, catarrh, inflammation of the mucous membrane, gastritis, etc., develop. If great quantities of sugar and starch are eaten by children, gastritis, pharyngitis, tonsilitis, enlarged tonsils, adenoids, constipation, polyuria and nervousness result. In adults, rheumatism, flatulency, headaches, catarrh, constipation, glycosuria, diabetes, eczema, heart palpitation, nervousness, visceroptosis, colitis, piles, etc.

The materials out of which false membranes are made is a fibrogenic exudate, the same as is thrown out on any abraded surface, or into solutions of continuity in any

194

and all wounds. The quantity thrown out is always abundant, but the amounts are always greater where the local irritation is great.

Diphtheroid gangrene, supposed to be due to microbic infection, is the result of a toxin of sufficient virulence to produce death in the tissues involved in the inflammation. Before this can take place there must be profound enervation, lost immunization and putrescence of sufficient virulence to destroy tissues.

A ferment and a protein result in decomposition, if conditions do not inhibit bacterial action. The chemistry of the protein does the rest. Chemistry is the determining factor.

When excess of proteins are consumed a more severe type of disease will be developed. In children scarlet fever or diphtheria are likely to develop. If the patient is plethoric and the digestive tract is kept full of food, the fermention and puterfaction will continue. If the food is of a protein character, particularly animal proteins, fevers will take on typhoid or sepsis. Wounds and puerperal derangement will take on septicemia. The difference in toxicity between vegetable and flesh foods is colossal.

In the previous chapter we emphasized the fact that every form of disease is an evolution out of a great number of correlated factors which collectively constitute cause, and that no form of disease admits of a unitary cause. This holds true, even if germs are granted a place in causation. Germs alone can no more produce a disease than a seed alone can produce a tree. Just as the seed must have fertile soil, moisture, warmth, air and sunlight before it can become a tree, so the germ must find certain essential conditions existing in the bodies it enters before it can do the slightest harm.

A ready example is furnished us by what we know of digestion and indigestion. The individual with normal digestive powers consuming an ordinary meal and pursuing the even tenor of his ways, digests his food with ease. No fermentation and putrefaction takes place because the normal secretions of the digestive tract are able to prevent bacterial action.

But if the individual is enervated, his digestive powers impaired, the secretions deficient and of poor quality; or, if he is subjected, after eating, to mental and physical influences that inhibit secretion and digestion, then his food, instead of being digested, will undergo fermentation and putrefaction.

Under such conditions, the poisonous products of bacterial decomposition are absorbed into the blood and lymph, and if other conditions are right, disease develops. If the enervation is not great, if elimination is not markedly impaired, the toxins are quickly thrown off and no disease develops.

There are many factors entering into the production of disease from *intestinal toxemia*. There are first, the factors and influences that bring on enervation. Then follow in order enervation, impairment of organic function, and of secretion and excretion, fermentation and putrefaction, absorption, and constitutional defects which determine where the trouble will develop. Back of the constitutional defects are their causes. The virulence of the absorbed putrescence will depend on the chemistry of the food eaten. With so many factors involved in the unfolding "disease" it is hardly fair to pick on the germ as the cause of whatever form of disease that develops.

Some supposed disease germs are said to produce immunity when one has them once. How they are barred out by one operation has not been satisfactorily explained. That all supposed germ diseases operate this way is not claimed. That many do have those for which the claim is made, two, three, or more times is admitted. Such cases are far more frequent than is commonly supposed.

On the theory that immunity to infection is established by once being infected, and that this immunity can be transferred to another, the vaccine and serum practice is based. The practice is worse than a failure, it is a calamity. It should be prohibited by law.

It will be appropriate to close this chapter with the following by Dr. Page:

KISSING AND THE GERM THEORY
You may make a wound and poison it—
That is, vaccinate my child;
But kiss him! The very thought of it
Is enough to drive me wild.

195

Implant the seeds of Lock-jaw,
Consumption and decline
By any means save kissing him—
It's there we draw the line.

—*The Open Door*, Jan. 1918.

PERVERSIONS

Chapter XVIII

PERVERSION is derived from the Latin, *Perversus*, meaning, turned the wrong way. In pathology it is employed to designate an abnormal or wrong use of certain instincts and voluntary functions. The functions and instincts, by education or otherwise, have suffered inversion, that is they have been turned from their right purpose or use to another and different and wrong use.

Every power, faculty and instinct of man is good. So long as it is exercised in harmony with its primitive constitution its results are good. It is only when it is turned aside from this primitive purpose and inverted to another use, that is corrupted and abused, that its results are evil and harmful.

Man should possess in perfectly symmetrical combination, in his personality, all the superior, lovely and desirable traits of character, that have distinguished individuals in all ages and localities of the world, very largely amplified and embellished.

Throughout all nature we find every creature provided from the start with just so much of instinct and impulse as is needed to direct and propel it to the order and degree of development of which its organism is capable, leading it with unfailing regularity to the fulfillment of the law of its own being, and to the successful performance of its functions in the world. If the *unity of nature* means anything the higher as well as the lower gifts of man's nature must have been intended to lead straight and unerringly to the highest and loftiest development of which he is constitutionally capable, just as the dispositions and instincts of other creatures lead them to the perfect discharge of their functions in the *order of nature*.

There is no known creature, however terrible or loathsome it may appear to us, which does not pass through all the stages of its development, with perfect accuracy, or that fails to exhibit a corresponding harmony between its propensities and powers. Order and adjustment of the most perfect kind are seen to prevail throughout the whole organic world. Exceptions to this rule are found only among men and those animals that are controlled by men, and among men more than among his domestic beasts.

All animal beings, man included, are constituted upon certain physiological principles, out of which grow certain physiological wants; and upon which are established certain faculties of instinct which relate them to the forces and substances required for their maintenance. Animal bodies possess organic powers and physiological abilities to convert these external forces and substances to their own natures. The instincts in man, as in the lower animals, are determinate in their functional characters and in their final causes, and so long as they are preserved in their integrity, are a law of truth to all, but it was no more intended that man should find enjoyment in the exercise of his instincts and powers, beyond the legitimate fulfilment of their normal functions, than that the lower animals should do so. Man is not constituted with any more capability of doing this without injury to himself than are the lower orders. For the maintenance of healthy function certain conditions are known to be necessary, and if these be materially modified in the whole or in any part of the body, disease and death may be the result. Instinct relates the animals to these conditions in so far as they are external to him, and under his voluntary control.

Animals almost unerringly obey the laws of their being and fulfill the functions of their order. Man, man alone, is the victim of practices which cannot be properly fitted into the *unities of nature*. Well did the Duke of Argyle say, *Unity of Nature*:

"Man has been, and still is, a constant prey to appetites which are morbid—to opinions which are irrational—to imaginations which are horrible,—to practices which are destructive. The prevalence and the power of these in a great variety of forms and of degrees is a fact with which we are familiar—so familiar, indeed, that we fail to be duly impressed with the strangeness and the mystery which really belong to it. All savage races are bent and bowed under the yoke of their own perverted instincts—instincts which generally in their root and origin have an obvious utility, but which in their actual development are the source of miseries without number and without end. Some of the most horrible perversions which are prevalent among savages have no counterpart among any other created beings, and when judged by the barest standards of utility, place man immeasurably below the level of the Beasts. We are accustomed to say of many of the habits of savage life that they are 'brutal.' But this is entirely to misrepresent the place which they really occupy in the system of nature. None of the Brutes have any such perverted dispositions; none of them are ever subject to the destructive operation of such habits as are common among men. And this contrast is all the more remarkable when we consider that the very worst of these habits affect conditions of life which the lower animals share with us, and in which any departure from those natural laws which they universally obey, must necessarily produce, and do actually produce, consequences so destructive as to endanger the very existence of the race such are all those conditions of life affecting the relation of the sexes which are common to all creatures, and in which man alone exhibits the widest and most hopeless divergence from the Order of Nature."*** "It is, indeed, impossible to look abroad either upon the past history or the existing condition of Mankind, whether savage or civilized, without seeing that it presents phenomena which are strange and monstrous—incapable of being reduced within the harmony of things, or reconciled with the Unity of Nature. The contrast which it presents to the general laws and course of Nature cannot be stated too broadly. There is nothing like it in the World. It is an element of confusion amidst universal order. Powers exceptionally high spending themselves in activities exceptionally base; the desire and the faculty of acquiring knowledge coupled with the desire and the faculty of turning it to the worst account; instincts immeasurably superior to those of other creatures, alongside of conduct and of habits very much below the level of the Beast—such are the combinations with which we have to deal as unquestionable facts when we contemplate the actual condition of mankind. And they are combinations in the highest degree unnatural; there is nothing to account for, or to explain them in any apparent natural necessity." "But the idea of civilization is in itself separate from the idea of Virtue. Men of great refinement of manners may be, and often are, exceedingly corrupt. And what is of true of individuals is true of communities. The highest civilizations of the heathen world were marked by a very low code of morals, and by practice even lower than their code. But the intellect was thoroughly cultivated. Knowledge of the useful arts, taste in the fine arts, and elaborate systems both of civil polity and of military organization, combined to make, first Greek and then Roman, civilization, in such matters the basis of our own."

The only exceptional fact about man is not the possession of higher faculties than those possessed by other creatures, nor that these faculties are susceptible of a corresponding kind and degree of development, but that man alone manifests a persistent tendency to pursue a wrong direction, that is, one leading away from rather than towards the perfecting of his powers. Mankind, "savage" and "civilized" are a prey to habits, practices and dispositions which, measured by natural law, the unity and order of nature, and by their results, are monstrous and unnatural. They are not found among the lower animals "in those spheres of impulse and of action in which they have a common nature with our own." These practices, habits and dispositions are always directly injurious and often even fatal to the race. Such practices cannot be referred to the *order of nature*, but are evident departures from it. "The nature of Man," says the Duke of Argyle, "is seen to be corrupt not merely as compared with some imaginary standard which is supposed to have existed at some former time, but as compared with a standard which prevails in every other department of Nature at the present day."

It is as if weapons have been placed in man's hands which he has not the strength, knowledge, nor rectitude of will to rightly wield. In this he stands in marked contrast to the world around him.

The rule throughout the rest of nature is that every creature can and does handle the powers with which it is endowed with a skill which is as wonderful as it is complete, for the highest purposes of its own being and for the fulfilment of its functions in the *unity of nature*.

Man alone is out of adjustment. He alone is in constant antagonism to that wonderful order and unity of nature from which harmony and certainty result. He is in continual conflict with the laws of his being. As we shall later see, the analogies of nature are contrary to the supposition that this condition of things was mankind's original condition.

The laws of life have not changed and are not changeable. None of them have ever been modified, and amended or repealed. They are eternal, always in full force and cannot be beaten in any manner. They must be obeyed or we must pay the inevitable penalty.

From every side, one hears the cry, no man can perfectly obey all the laws of his being. Probably not, in our hyper-civilization, but in a truly natural state this complaint involves a monstrous absurdity. For it assumes that God or nature has constituted man with certain relations to external things and endowed him with corresponding instincts,—without equipping him with the necessary mental and voluntary powers to fulfill perfectly his relations to the external world; that man has been created with certain constitutional powers and capacities, but without the necessary abilities to control these powers and capacities. Such an assumption makes of God or nature a fraud and a cheat.

The trouble is not with man as he is constituted, nor with the natural order of things, but with the unnatural order of things with which he has surrounded himself. In spite of the perversity that we see around us and in us, we will not admit that man is totally depraved, or that he is not capable of improving himself and attaining to a higher degree of perfection. Man is inherently capable of fulfilling the functions of his being in perfect harmony with their laws.

One theory, which attempts to account for the vicious and destructive habits of man, holds that they are not aberrant phenomena at all, but are original conditions of human nature—hangovers or relics of a primitive condition. This theory holds that man, having come up from a lower form of animal life, still retains within his constitution vestigal characters of his pre-human self, and that the very worst of these evils have been primitive and universal, so that the lowest and most debased forms of savage life are the nearest representatives of the primeval condition of mankind.

This theory, it seems, is based on a failure to recognize clearly in what the real difficulty consists. The evils are not in those things in which man most resembles the brute but in those things in which he falls farthest below any known beast. If such a theory were correct, it would represent the contrast between man's instincts and those of the beasts as greatest and widest, at the very time when he first appeared among and sprang from these creatures. The beasts with regard to these instincts are higher, not lower than man. Such a supposition does not explain man's perversions—rather it presents another and greater difficulty, that of accounting for the fact that he was "far beastlier than any beast" at the time of his emergence from them.

"If man was, indeed, born with an innate propensity to maltreat his women, to murder his children, to kill and eat his fellow, to turn the physical functions of his nature into uses which are destructive to his race, then, indeed, it would be true," says the Duke of Argyle, "that

> Dragons of the prime,
> That tear each other in their slime,
> Were mellow music matched with him.

"If evolution is the law of life, as this theroy demands, it does not necessarily follow that primeval man stood on a level far lower than that of the lowest existing "savage." Such an assumption might be real if it were true," as the Duke of Argyle says, "that during some long series of ages Development had not only been always working, but had always been working upwards. But if it be capable of working and if it has been actually working, also in the opposite direction, then the element of time in its bearing upon conditions of modern savagery must have had a very different operation. For here it is to be remembered that the savage of the present day is as far removed in time from the common origin of our race as the man who now exhibits the highest type of moral and intellectual culture. Whether that time is represented by six thousand, or ten thousand, or a hundred thousand years, it is the same for both. If therefore the number of years since the origin of man be taken as a multiplier in the processes of elevation, it must be taken equally as a multiplier in the processes of degradation*** All the ages which have been at work in the development of civilization have been equally at work in the development of savagery. It is not possible in the case of Savagery, any more than in the case of Civilization, that all those ages have been without effect. Nor is it possible that the changes they have wrought have been all in one direction. The conclusion is that neither Savagery nor Civilization, as we now see them, can represent the primeval condition of man. Both of them are the work of time. Both of them are the product of Evolution."

We can safely say with the Duke, that the nearer we "may suppose the origin of man may have been to the origin of the Brutes, the nearer also would his condition have been to the fulfillment of a law which is of universal application among them. Under the fulfillment of that law the higher gifts and powers with which man is endowed would have run smoothly their appointed course, would have unfolded as a bud unfolds to flower,—as a flower ripens into fruit,—and would have presented results absolutely different from those which are actually presented either by the savage, or by what is called the civilized, condition of Mankind."

Cruel treatment of the female sex is almost universal among savages, and this is entirely unknown among the lower animals. "In every part of the world," wrote Malthus, "one of the most general characteristics of the savage is to despise and degrade the female sex*** Their condition is so peculiarly grevious, that servitude is a name too mild to describe their wretched state. A wife is no better than a beast of burden. While the man passes his days in idleness or amusement, the woman is condemned to incessant toil. Tasks are imposed upon her without mercy, and services are received without complacence or gratitude. There are some districts*** where this state of degradation has been so severely felt that mothers have destroyed their female infants, to deliver them at once from a life in which they were doomed to such a miserable slavery."

If space permitted it could be shown that this miserable degradation of woman has existed in all parts of the world in all ages in *civilized* as well as in *savage* countries. Indeed it does now exist in certain *civilized* and "*Christian*" nations. The emancipation of woman is a thing of today—it only began a few years ago. But the Duke of Argyle was eternally right when he declared that "it is impossible to find for this most vicious tendency a place among the Unities of Nature. There is nothing like it among the Beasts. With them the equality of the sexes, as regards all the enjoyments as well as all the work of life, is the universal rule."

This is but one among many of that long, black catalogue of perversions in man's sex life and the relation of the sexes. Polyandry, Polygamy, infanticide, "communal marriage" child marriages and many other perversions which might be mentioned, are among those practices of man which are stamped by many separate considerations as corruptions and gross departures from primeval habits. All such customs are fatally injurious to the propagation of the race. Many, if not all of them may be traced to causes existing outside the nature and needs of man. These customs, taken together with the necessary and inevitable results of the maltreatment and degradation of woman, its effects upon the constitution, character and endurance of the children, (we see how grossly unnatural is this last), must tend to a greater and greater degradation of the race and make recovery from this downward road more and more difficult. "These hideous customs which are everywhere prevalent among savage men, and which often, in their ingenuity of evil, and in the sweep of their destructive force, leave it a wonder that the race survives at all."

But these vices, and the evils arising out of them are not peculiar to the savage state. Some of them, more or less changed and modified in form, attain a rank luxuriance in civilized communities. They corrupt the very bones and marrow of society and have brought more than one rich and powerful nation to decay and death.

Savage life and customs are not all bad. Indeed, there are many respects in which it transcends much that exists in civilized life and customs. Some of the worst and most revolting forms of sexual perversions are found almost exclusively among civilized peoples. The mere cataloguing of all the forms and directions which sexual perversion takes would be enough to astonish the uninformed reader. Some of these perversions are plainly the result of pathological conditions confined to the individual; others are individual cultivations, while still others arise from, or are at least predisposed to, by hereditary weaknesses.

Nymphomania (in woman) and satyrasis (in man) is an insatiable sexual desire, often associated with certain sensations of anguish. The effect of such desire is to direct the appetite toward any object that is capable of gratifying it. In the absence of the opposite sex, masturbation is generally resorted to. All mucous surfaces (anus, mouth, etc.) and inanimate objects may serve to satisfy these desires. Animals are frequently used to this end. Rape and incest are often its outcome. "Men much distinguished in other respects," says Forel, "may abandon themselves to the most foolish or abominable practices." Men visit prostitutes. They quickly become excited by the sight of any woman who is neither too old nor too repulsive. Women introduce all manner of objects into the vagina in an effort to satisfy the craving. Many of these individuals have their minds filled with erotic images which may become an obsession.

Sadism or the association of sexual desire with cruelty and violence is a strange perversion. Cruel voluptuousness of this kind usually manifests itself only after excesses have brought the individual to such a state that coitus will not give satisfaction. History is full of such men who "lie in wait for their victims like cats, pounce on them, revel in their terror, assassinate them by inches, and wallow voluptuously in their blood." The law courts are full of them. The newspapers almost daily carry accounts of the evils of these beings. Nero, Tiberus, Caligula, Valerie, Messalina, and Catherine de Medici are prominent historical examples. There can be little doubt that most, if not all, vivisectors and others who revel in cruelty to animals and to children are sadists.

Masochism is the converse of sadism. It is a form of sexual desire in which there is a submission to cruelty and violence. Rousseau is considered to have been a masochist. The religious ecstasy of fakirs and flagellants who flog themselves, or who have themselves flogged, is a form of masochism.

Fetichism is the production of voluptious sensations by sight of or contact with certain portions of the body or clothes of woman, of certain body odors, or perfumes worn by women.

Exhibitionism is the term given to the practice found in a class of individuals who masturbate in the presence of women. They lie in wait behind a wall or a bush and masturbate openly when women pass. These people may only reach an orgasm when seen by women. It is also seen among women.

Homosexual love is the term applied to those abnormal conditions when the whole sexual appetite and psychic irradiations are directed to the same sex as that of the perverted individual, and in which the pervert is horrified at the thought of sexual contact with the opposite sex. Both sexes are found in this condition—the sexual appetite and amourous ideals of the man being directed wholly and throughout life to other men; the woman's sex feelings all being directed to women.

Pederosis is sexual appetite for children.

Sodomy or Bestiality is the term now applied to the direction of the human sexual appetite towards animals. The original meaning of Sodomy (see Genesis Chapt. IX) was that of "coitus" between men now called pederasty.

Masturbation (self-pollution, self-abuse, onanism,) is the artificial excitation and gratification of the sex appetite by friction of an artificial nature. The hands some soft object, another man, or woman, an animal, or other means are employed. It is usually associated with erotic images of nude females, or female sexual organs, in the male. Both sexes are guilty of this practice.

There is a broad general sense in which all the aberrant practices above mentioned are forms of masturbation as is also, "coitus" with a prostitute.

Prostitution, Concubinage, Pornography, rape, the desire for change in marital partners, coitus during pregnancy, lactation, menstruation and disease are all forms of perversion of the sex instinct and are not discoverable among the lower animals. I have indeed seen one hyena, in a New York Zoo, masturbating himself and occasionally this vice is seen among domestic animals, but such cases are extremely rare. Forel declares:--

"Human sexuality has been unfortunately perverted and in part grossly altered by civilization, which has even developed it artificially in a pathological sense. The point has been reached of considering as normal, relations which are in reality absolutely abnormal   For example, it is maintained that prostitution produces normal coitus in man.   How can this term be seriously employed in speaking of connection with a prostitute who is absolutely indifferent to it, and who seeks only to excite her clients artificially and to get their money, without mentioning venereal diseases which she so often presents them with.   Forgetful of the natural aim of the sexual appetite, civilization has transformed it into artificial enjoyment, and has invented all possible means to increase and diversify it."

Art, literature, dress, luxury, alcohol, etc., are among the elements named by Forel when he declares "the artificial culture of the human sexual appetite has given rise to a veritable high school of debauchery."   And may we not, when viewing all these forms of perversion and contrasting them with the *uniformities of nature* as exemplified throughout the Animal Kingdom, justly conclude that "free love" or "Varietism," and sexual indulgence within marriage which is "FORGETFUL OF THE NATURAL AIM OF THE SEXUAL APPETITE," but which is indulged frequently merely for pleasure, and not for procreation, are also forms of perversion. And "petting" or "spooning," now so commonly and openly indulged in, which does not fulfil its natural end, but is engaged in for pleasure and thrills only, is a perversion of a natural instinct.

Cannibalism, deliberate cruelty, systematic slaughter connected with war-like passions and with religious customs, animal and human sacrifices, wife-beating, child-beating, hunting for sport, meat eating, and many other things might be added to the list of perversions, but we cannot hope to deal with all these things in the space allotted to this subject.   A few other perversions must consume the remainder of this chapter.

BULIMIA is a voracious appetite.   It may be due to cultivation, to disease, such as diabetes, or from a very irritable condition of the nerves of the stomach.   Shew recounts a case related by Dr. Mortimer, of a twelve year old boy in whom the craving for food was so strong that he would gnaw his own flesh when not supplied with food. When awake, he was constantly eating; being supplied with bread, meat, beer, milk, water, butter, cheese, sugar, treacle, puddings, pies, fruits, broths, potatoes, etc.   Of these he swallowed in six successive days, three hundred and eighty-four pounds and eight ounces, an average of sixty-four pounds a day.

The disease continued in this case for a year, the food being usually vomited soon after being swallowed.   This condition of the appetite is usually associated with vomiting of this nature.

There are all degrees of bulimia and most cases are due to habitual overeating. The condition is frequently met with in dyspeptics.   The supposed hunger is but a morbid craving.   To satisfy it can never benefit the victim of such perversion.   A complete fast until the craving ceases is the more sensible means of overcoming it.

In discussing typhus and typhoid fever, Shew says:—

"The *appetite* is usually altogether absent after the disease has fully set in. Ordinarily, when there is a considerable degree of pyrexia present, the stomach is wholly unable to perform its function.   In some cases individuals have gone two and even three weeks without any nutriment other than water, recovering in the end perfectly well   Yet there have been cases of fever in which the appetite was voracious. Dr. Satterly is quoted by Dr. Elliotson as giving a case of a boy who labored under typhus fever, attended by marked inflammation in the head, and in which the exacerbations of fevere were always attended with a voracious appetite; so that in the midst of the fever he would eat four meals a day, and each meal sufficient for a stout laborer. Besides those four meals of meat and vegetables, he daily ate many pounds of dry bread, biscuit and fruit   He had no sooner eaten a meal, than he denied that he had eaten anything, so that the more he ate the more he desired.   If he was not fed the moment he requested it he sucked the bed-clothes and bit his fingers like a child.   He discharged several very copious stools a day, which evidently saved his life, for he recovered perfectly "

This was plainly a case of nervous irritation, and not of appetite and no effort should have been wasted in fruitless attempts to gratify it.   This was an extreme case. We daily meet with similar cases of all degrees of *craving* in chronic disease.

ANOREXIA is loss of appetite. There are many conditions in which a temporary loss of desire for food is quite normal. Such, for instance, as after great fatigue, from mental emotions, as grief, anger, etc., in acute and, usually, chronic disease, and after eating. Hysteria and too often repeated fasting and certain mental states often give rise to a loss of appetite.

The appetite may be depraved to an almost indefinite extent, as is exemplified in the dietetic habits of the various nations of the earth. The taking of chalk, charcoal, acids, dirt, cinders, ordure, fire, spiders, lice, toads, serpents, leeches, snails, bits of wood, mushrooms, hair, candles, paper, leaden-bullet, glass, stone, pieces of money knives, marbles, etc., are but a few such perversions. Depraved appetite is sometimes the result of cultivation, sometimes the result of disease. In hysteria, chlorosis, pregnancy and some of the mental ailments, the appetite sometimes craves the most singular and disgusting articles. In the cases of chlorosis and pregnancy, at least, this craving arises out of food deficiency and is usually quickly overcome by proper feeding.

DIRT EATING, or AFRICAN CACHEXIA, is a form of depraved appetite that prevails among the colored population of hot climates and appears to belong to the colored race almost exclusively. The individual so depraved experiences an irresistible craving for substances of an indigestible and disgusting character. Clay, earth, mortar, dust, ashes, chalk, slate, bricks, and shells are often devoured in enormous quantities, while food is almost wholly rejected as disgusting and worthless. The appetite seems to be wholly depraved. The condition has long been known in tropical America and has been seen in the southern part of the United States.

Of a similar character to filth eating is that perversion of the sense of taste that manifests itself in salt-eating, condiment using, tobacco chewing, snuffing and smoking, pickle eating, drinking of alcoholic and soft drinks, and the use of other such substances. None of these things supply any need in the human body. None of them are essential to normal enjoyment of food. All of them are harmful. A *taste* for them must be cultivated before they can be *enjoyed*, after which they enslave their victims as truly as the coffee habit, tea drinking or morphine using.

What Jennings called a "good physical conscience" is the sum total of an individual's unimpaired, unperverted instincts and "reflexes." It may be well to impress the reader with the "importance of maintaining a clear physical conscience. He may do this by attending to a comparison between a temperate and an intemperate man. They possess natively similar constitutions. A. has been provident of his, has been temperate in all things; B. intemperate. Aside from the fact that B. is using up his energy faster than A. and must of necessity come to the end of life sooner, even if no sudden providence cut off either, B. is always in danger of terminating his existence by pushing the law of stimulation too far, and drawing, unwarned, the vital current below the point of recovery. On a hot summer day, they both go into the field and mow for a trial of their strength. On the first day, perhaps, B. gains a victory—holds out longer than A., and appears less fatigued. The cold water man is ridiculed. On the second day B. drops dead over his scythe, or beside the bucket. A. may feel weary and tired as he leaves the field, or distress himself by drinking too largely of cold water, but is in no danger of destroying life. His clear physical conscience, or healthy sensibility, will warn him of his danger long before he reduces the vital energies to a fatal point.

"The advantages of a good physical conscience are too obvious and too numerous to need or admit of a full notice here. The individual who is so fortunate as to possess one, is in much less danger of violating physical law than one who does not. If the former were to receive into his stomach but a small particle of black pepper, though intimately mixed with his food, unperceived by him at the time, it would inflict a pang on the tender, upright sensibility, that would be remembered a long time, and operate as a caution against further transgression. Another benefit derived from a good physical conscience, is that while it guards against the admission of noxious substances into the system, it also imparts a very high relish to those plain, simple substances, that are adapted to the wants of the body.

"Everybody knows how cold water is relished by a 'thirsty soul.' The wise man compares it to 'good news from a far country.' This relish arises from the adaptation of the water to the state of the body; it is a *natural* relish; the water just meets a pressing want. Just so it is with simple nutriment taken into a healthy stomach, where there is a demand for food—and no one should eat without the existence of such a demand; and with a good physical conscience, one is in much less danger of eating without, or beyond a seasonable and salutary call for food. Indeed, a stomach restrained to plain, simple diet, (a *sine qua non* for a pure sensibility,) would never relish food unless there was an actual necessity for this raw material in the body, any more than such a stomach would relish pure water when the fluids of the system were already sufficiently diluted;—and it is equally true that a vitiated stomach would not relish unstimulating food, without a good appetite, and be in still less danger of being unduly loaded with such material. How strange, then, that anyone who has his physical conscience somewhat purified, should be willing to have it seared again.

"I have heard of men, who, having abandoned the use of all excitants, and lived on plain vegetable diet for a considerable time, resumed their old mode of living, for the alleged reason, that, as they were obliged to be much from home, and were under the necessity 'when among Romans, of doing as Romans do,' they suffered much from stimulating diet with stomachs unaccustomed to it! But what would be thought of a man who should act thus in relation to his moral conscience? He found it so painful, with a keen moral sense, to utter an oath, but being much among profane swearers, he could not at all times well avoid it, therefore he chose to be in the habit of swearing, that he might avoid the lashings and goadings of a tender conscience!"—*Medical Reform*, pp. 64-5-6.

The parts on which irritants habitually act are put in a position of defense by a hardening and thickening of the irritated parts, just as the hands of the laborer harden from the use of tools. This lessens their sensibilities and protects them, but, at least in the case of the internal organs, also lessens their functional powers. The nerves are weakened and depraved so that they are no longer able to appreciate their normal stimuli and are incapable of discriminating between various kinds and classes of stimuli. They become so weakened and depraved that they are unable to respond or "react" except to powerful irritants, and, as they grow weaker, larger and stronger doses are required to elicit an apparently healthy sensation.

The true condition of the system is revealed when these things are withdrawn. The headache, lassitude, depression, and general discomfort show how weak and impaired the system really is. The pains suffered by the opium addict when coming from under the influence of his drug reveal his true condition. The outcries of his nerves may be silenced with another dose of the drug, but this makes his condition worse still.

The first drink of alcohol smarts and burns. The eyes water, the nose smarts. The mouth and throat burn. The stomach smarts and burns under it. There is coughing and sneezing. But when the tisues affected have thickened and hardened and the nervous sensibilities have been blunted by the repeated use of alcohol, large doses only produce a pleasurable sensation. The "physical conscience" has been seared.

The first use of tobacco in any form produces headache, nausea, vomiting, dizziness, lassitude, tremor, and even prostration, as a vital reaction against it. Tobacco does not appeal to the unperverted sense of taste. The hardening and thickening of the membranes of the mouth and depravation of the nerves of mouth and nose, as a result of the repeated use of tobacco and the perversion of the sense of taste calls for the regular and increasing use of the foul weed.

The first employment of pepper smarts and burns in the mouth, throat, stomach, and often, in the rectum when it is passed on the day following. But its habitual use results in a thickening and hardening of the membranes of the alimentary tract, and a blunting of its sensibilities, so that larger and larger doses are needed to secure the excitation essential to pleasurable sensation. It is no longer possible for the blunted sense of taste to sense and appreciate the fine delicate flavors of foods. Unseasoned food is not relished. The glands of the mouth, stomach and intestine also suffer in the deterioration thus occasioned.

The first dose of salts causes griping and diarrhea, provided it is not vomited first. Its continued use results in a thickening and hardening of the intestinal mucosa, and a weakening of the glands of these organs. Larger and larger doses are required to secure bowel action. More and more weakness is the result.

In the following quotations from Graham's *Lectures on the Science of Human Life,* he accurately describes the process of perverting human instincts and senses:—

"Thus, if a person with a pure system and undepraved olfactory nerves, comes into the vicinity of a large quantity of tobacco, he instantly perceives the loathsome odor, and at once detects its poisonous character, and finds himself urged by many distressing feelings to avoid the deadly narcotic; but, if, regardless of these admonitions, he thrusts some powerful tobacco into his nose, his olfactory nerve still perceives and appreciates the poisonous odor, and the trifacial nerve feels the poisonous character of the irritating substance, and gives the alarm to the domain of organic life, and violent sneezing soon ensues as the instinctive means of expelling the offending cause. If the offending cause is not removed by sneezing, the whole system soon becomes so much affected by the poison, that the most distressing dizziness, and muscular relaxation and tremor and sickness at the stomach, and cold sweat, and vomiting and convulsions, follow in rapid succession, in order both to expel the poison from the vital domain, and to cause us ever after more cautiously to avoid so deadly and so foul an enemy. But by commencing this career of depravity with cautiously measured steps at first, we may in time succeed in utterly destroying the integrity of this important sentinel, and so completely deprave both the olfactory nerve and the nasal portion of the trifacial, that neither of them can any longer detect the poisonous character of the tobacco, but both of them will become so adapted to its properties, as to delight in its stimulation, with an intensity of morbid enjoyment equal to the depth of depravity to which they are reduced. And thus the organ of smell, instead of guarding the vital domain like a true faithful sentinel, against the encroachments of every enemy which it is naturally qualified to detect, not only ceases to give alarm to that domain when those enemies are approaching, but even throws open its gate and earnestly entreats those enemies to enter, and embraces the foulest and deadliest of them all as the dearest and most valuable friend, and ushers it into the vital domain, proclaiming with inebriated energy the introduction of a generous and glorious conservative. And thus, by sensual depravity, we transform a guardian angel of light into a treacherous demon of darkness; and still confiding in its integrity and fidelity to the vital domain, we receive into the very citadel of life the enemy which poisons all our wells of vitality, and with perfect infatuation rejoice in his destructive influence, and regard his withering embraces as the source of our highest enjoyment, and perish in the full belief that our destroyer is our truest friend, and perhaps with our dying breath commend him to the confidence and kind regard of all around us. Such are the natural consequences of disregarding the holiest and most delicate admonitions of those undepraved sentinels which a benevolent Creator has, for the preservation of our highest welfare and happiness, placed on the outposts of the vital domain. There is indeed a sense in which it may be said that sneezing is the voice of God in our nature distinctly and unequivocally commanding us to avoid whatever causes us to sneeze. And let it be remembered, that although the constant application of snuff and other poisonous and pernicious substances to the living membrane of the cavities of the nose, may so deprave the tissues of that membrane, and so impair their delicate and peculiar sensibilities, that they can no longer detect the poisonous qualities of those substances, nor give the alarm of danger to the vital domain, by which sneezing and other instinctive efforts are called up to expel the offending cause, yet the real character of those substances, and their true relations to the vital powers and interests of our bodies, remain unaltered, and equally hostile to our life and health and happiness."

"****When the organ (of taste) is in this state of integrity, if natural substances pernicious to life, or those which are not adapted to the constitutional wants of the body, are received into the mouth, their offensive character is instantly detected, a loathing is soon felt, and mucus and salivary secretions are poured into the mouth to shield the parts acted upon, and to flood the offending cause from the porch of the vital domain. If the character of the offending substance be such as to render it

205

exceedingly dangerous to the vital interests, or such as is wholly unfitted for the highest and best condition of our nature, the loathing will be so intense as powerfully to urge us to expell it from the mouth; and if we do not promptly obey this admonition, the sympathetic alarm will be diffused over the whole system, by the same means and in the same manner as in the nose, and dreadful nausea and dizziness and muscular relaxation and tremor and cold sweat and violent vomiting will ensue, as the instinctive means of the vital economy to relieve itself of danger. But by habitually debauching the gustatory nerve and the other tissues of the mouth, with poisonous or improper substances, we soon destroy the power of the organ to discriminate between salutary and pernicious substances, and the power of the parts to give the necessary alarm and call up the necessary efforts of the system to protect itself from danger, and in a short time the tissues of the mouth become so deeply depraved, and so completely conformed to the qualities of these improper substances, that they learn to delight in their stimulation incomparably more than in that of healthful and proper substances; and thus, by destroying the integrity of this sentinel, we are given up to believe a lie. Improper substances are received into the vital domain with more or less repugnance of the instinctive powers at first, according to the character of the substances, and according to the caution or excess of our incipient transgressions, till the depravity is extended from the mouth through the whole of the alimentary canal; and the mouth and stomach not only become reconciled to, but exceedingly delight in, the character and influence of the most pernicious substances, which either with hasty ravages spread ruin over our whole vital domain, and violently precipitate us into the grave, or slowly and treacherously sap the foundations of our constitution, and fill us with disquietude and feebleness and disease, which terminate in untimely death; and still we, with the utmost confidence in the integrity of those organs, strenuously contend for the rectitude and safety of our course, on the ground that it is pleasant to the taste and agreeable to the stomach. Indeed, these organs may become so thoroughly depraved, that they will reject the most salutary substances as disgusting and pernicious, and receive the most pernicious substances as agreeable and salutary."

Again, he wrote:—

"It is important to remark, however, that in the earlier generations of the human species, when the constitutional powers were least impaired, and all the vital susceptibilities and sympathies of the system most delicate and vigorous, all disturbing causes would produce more powerful effects in the physiological operations and results of the vital economy, than when the system has become more deteriorated or depraved in all its properties. Thus, we have seen, when all the organs are pure and undepraved, the presence of the baneful odors will not only be perceived by the olfactory sense, but if their quality or power be such as to endanger the vital welfare of the system the alarm will be given through the medium of the vital sympathies to the whole domain of organic instinct, and every part will be called into vigorous and perhaps violent action, to protect the vital interests; and in the general array of all the vital powers against a common enemy, the particular functions of the several organs are necessarily more or less disturbed. So, when a state is invaded by a foreign foe, the husbandman, and artisan, and merchant, and other members of the commonwealth, roused by a common sympathy of patriotism, rush to the field of arms to protect the common interest of the state; and by these means, the particular functions of these several men, in agriculture, arts, and merchandise, upon which the very existence of the state depends, are necessarily more or less disturbed; and if these disturbances are too powerful, too frequent, or too long, famine and poverty and pestilence and general ruin must result.

"But when the vital sensibilities and sympathies of the organs have become depraved and generally impaired, the poisonous odors, though equally hostile to the vital interests of the system, are not perceived and appreciated by the olfactory sense, and consequently no alarm is given and no general effort is made to resist the encroachments of the enemy, but the whole system stupidly succumbs, and gradually sinks and perishes beneath its baneful influence, and the unhappy subject never perhaps suspects the cause of his destruction. Or if, from the potency of the disturbing cause, the particular organ upon which it more immediately acts is somewhat irritated, the vital

206

sympathies of the system are too much depraved to communicate the alarm with integrity, and all the physiological powers of the body are too much impaired to admit of a prompt and vigorous co-operation of the several parts to resist or expel the invading foe.

"In the same manner, when the system is in a perfectly healthy and pure state, if any substance unfriendly to the vital interests be taken into the gastric cavity, the organic sensibility of the stomach will instantly detect its pernicious character, and not only will the stomach itself be disturbed, but it will probably give the alarm through the medium of the healthy sympathies to the whole domain of organic instinct, and all the vital powers will at once be arrayed against the hostile invader, and act with an energy and violence proportionate to the real banefulness and power of the disturbing cause. And perhaps in the mighty conflict, life will be expelled, and the system relieved from its destructive influence. Yet in such a case, death would be more the result of exhaustion than of poison. But when the physiological powers of the system have become generally depraved and impaired, pernicious substances may be introduced into the stomach habitually, and that organ will not detect their poisonous character, nor spread the alarm over the domain of organic instinct; and while a morbid irritation injurious in its effects will be more or less extensively felt, there will be no array of the vital powers against the invader, but the poison will be permitted to extend its ruinous influence into every part and substance of the whole system; the functional results of every organ will be deteriorated, and the constitution slowly impaired, and life destroyed. And perhaps through the whole progress of the work of death— except in the agonies of the first debauch—the sensibilities and sympathies of the system will scarcely indicate a struggle of the vital powers to arrest the career of the destroyer:—so completely will they be stupefied and subdued by that destroyer's influence. In such a case, death is truely the result of poison. Or if the disturbing cause is very powerful, the morbid irritations of the organ immediately acted on will be extended over the system by unhealthy sympathies, and there will be a blind array and violent action of the vital powers, which, instead of relieving the system, will only increase its suffering and hasten its destruction; and in these terrible conflicts, such a system will exhaust its vitality, and death will result much sooner than in a healthy body. So, when a state is generally depraved by the universal selfishness and sensuality of the people, the constitutional interests of that state may be assailed and gradually destroyed, and none will have the courage nor the inclination to rise in the cause of freedom and of patriotism, but all will stupidly submit to the encroach- ments of usurpation, and suffer their liberties to be continually abridged, and themselves degraded to very slavery; and when oppression bears so heavily upon them as to be intolerable even to a slave, they will groan under it as under an incubus, which by the very principle that gives distress, deprives them of the ability to act. Or if they should be goaded on to action, it will only be in blind and violent convulsions, without direction, without aim; and their tumultuous struggles will only serve to exhaust and destroy themselves, or sink them in deeper miseries, without effecting any good for the cause of freedom and the rights of man.

"But when I say that in the early state of the human constitution, when its physiological powers were far less impaired, and all the vital susceptibilities and sympathies of the system far more delicate and vigorous, all disturbing causes would produce more powerful effects in the physiological operations and results of the vital economy than when the system had become, in all its properties, more deteriorated and depraved, I do not mean that in the most healthy and vigorous state of the human constitution, disturbing causes more readily and more easily induce disease and death, but that all the vital powers, according to the instinctive economy of organic life, more promptly and more powerfully and more determinately co-operate to resist the action of those causes which are unfriendly to the vital interests; and, therefore, disturbing causes acting on particular parts, more powerfully affect the physiological operations and results of parts not immediately acted upon by these causes, but sympathetically affected by them. Thus, if a piece of tobacco is taken into the mouth of one whose system is in perfect and vigorous health, and whose physiological properties and powers are perfectly undepraved and unimpaired, the poisonous character of the

207

tobacco will be instantly perceived by the vital sensibilities of the parts on which it acts, and the alarm will be promptly given to the whole domain of organic instinct, and the physiological operations and results of the stomach, the liver, the lungs, and every other organ in the body, will be more or less powerfully and extensively affected by the sympathetic irritations of the system, and by the general effort of the vital powers to resist the poisonous effects of the tobacco and to expel the enemy from the vital precincts. (From this it will be seen that the ability to indulge in large quantities of tobacco, alcohol, opium, etc., with apparently no immediate ill effect is a sure evidence of depravity and weakness, not of strength. This is contrary to popular opinion. Author's note.) But when the system has become depraved, and its physiological properties and powers impaired by the habitual use of tobacco, its poisonous character is not detected, no alarm is given to the domain of organic instinct, and while the vital interests are continually injured, and life itself jeoparded by the habitual presence of the poison, no general and energetic effort is made to resist its action, and consequently the physiological operations and results of the stomach and other organs of the body are not at any time so powerfully affected by the tobacco, though they are continually suffering, to some extent, from its deleterious influence.

"Hence, therefore, when the physiological properties and powers of the human system are in the most perfectly healthy and pure and vigorous state, the disturbances of one special economy of the system will most powerfully effect the physiological operations and results of another special economy. Moreover, in such a state of things, the extent to which the physiological operations of the system deviate from the normal results, under the action of disturbing causes, must always be proportionate to the force of the disturbing cause and the physiological power of the disturbed economy.

"It therefore clearly and necessarily follows that the greatest deviations from normal results in the reproducing economy of the human system could only be effected by the influence of disturbing causes, in the early generations of the human species, when the constitutional powers were little impaired, and all the vital susceptibilities and sympathies of the system still nicely delicately and vigorously active. Abortive and puny and deformed results are infinitely more numerous in the more degenerate state of the constitution; but great deviations from the regular results of the economy, and enormous monstrosities, are only to be expected from disturbances of the most vigorous physiological powers."

THE DEVELOPMENT OF DISEASE

Chapter IXX

AFTER disease has reached a more or less advanced stage, or after the patient is dead the condition of the body in such states has been thoroughly studied. Diagnosis is the art of discovering effects, and these cannot be discovered until after they have reached a certain stage—until after they have advanced far enough to produce a physical sign. In the *descending pathological transit* a certain series of changes must necessarily occur before the damage becomes great enough to manifest as signs and symptoms, and these changes require time. When a pathological condition becomes manifest so that a diagnosis, right or wrong, may be made, this is not its beginning. Indeed, its beginning may be, and often is years prior to this. Its development is invariably slow, gradual, insidious, causing little or no disturbance to the body and no visible sign of its presence.

What of these initial stages? What of the stages which precede the production of a physical sign? Cause is here at work for weeks, months or years and the pathological condition is gradually developing. The individual imagines he is healthy and refuses to believe that his mode of living is harming him. His physician may examine him and tell him that he is alright, that all of his organs are sound, and yet, the condition that is later to manifest itself by physical signs and symptoms is developing. From this class of "healthy" individuals gradually emerges the many cases of advanced organic disease. These "pre-clinical" stages are the most important stages in the development of such conditions as cancer, insanity, paralysis, paresis, locomotor ataxia, Bright's disease, diabetes, diseases of the heart and arteries, cirrhosis of the liver or kidneys, etc., etc. If these "pre-clinical" stages are prevented the advanced stages will not develop.

The "Modern" methods of dealing with such conditions are faulty in that they consider an individual to be healthy, however evil his mode of living, if no physical signs of "disease" are to be found. The causes that produce these signs are wholly ignored; perhaps unknown to medical men. Indeed there is still "more truth than poetry" in Trall's observation made in relation to the various schools of medicine of the past:—

"One source of error, however, pervaded all their observations, as it does post-mortem investigations at this day. It is this: Structural appearances after death denote the effects of disease; and these morbid changes were and are often mistaken for or confounded with the causes of disease."—*Hydropathic Encyclopedia*, Vol. 1, p. 31.

"Medical Science" still goes to the dead and dying in its search for cause. Critical studies and examinations of end-results are the means employed in searching for causes.

"Functional derangements," says Dr. Tilden, "are of the same nature and from the same universal cause that ends in all organic so-called diseases. All so-called diseases are, from beginning to end, the same evolutionary process. All symptom-complexes—diseases—from their initiation to their ending, are effects, and the most intense study of any phase or stage of their progress will not throw any light on the cause."—*Toxemia Explained*.

At a necropsy, the chest of a young man who had died of tuberculosis of the lungs was opened revealing an ugly abscess of one of the lobes of the lungs. "There," said one of the physicians present, "I don't want to look any further for the cause of death."

But he was looking at the end, not at the beginning of the young man's trouble. How come the abscess there? How come the liver diseased? How and why do congestions, inflammations, etc., develop? Such conditions as was revealed in opening this young man's chest do not come into existence full-blown, any more than trees or flowers do so. Diseases never come butt-end first and Jennings truly said: "The ground is first broken at the surface, and there is a regular gradation from the summit level of physical soundness to the stagnant fenny region of disorder. It takes a great while and an amazing amount of opposing, noxious influences to reduce a healthy vigorous human system to a diseased state, according to the common acceptation of that term."—*Philosophy of Human Life*, p. 100.

There is no organic disease without previous functional disease; and there can be no functional disease except under a deficiency of functional power. Post-mortem examinations and physical examinations by the physiacian reveal effects, results, end-products, not causes. Let us trace the development of pathology from its initial beginnings to its final endings.

In tracing this development, let us first get a general view of the processes of life. The nutritive functions of the body may be roughly divided in two classes, namely:—

I. Those by which food is prepared for use by the body, and distributed to all parts of the body, and finally, used by its cells and organs.

II. Those by which waste and injurious matter is broken down, prepared for excretion and carried to the excreting organs and, finally, eliminated.

By the joint operation of these two general functions, the body is built up and sustained, on the one hand, and kept clean and pure on the other. Its perfection in size, symmetry and form, depends upon the integrity and efficient activity—granted a proper supply of building material—of these two functions.

Under the most natural and healthful activities of the vital organism there is necessarily a constant wear and impair of organic substance, necessitating a constant process of repair to prevent the rapid wearing out of the organic machinery. While, therefore, the general nutritive functions are efficiently and vigorously sustained, no sooner does any substance in the body become unfit for further use than it is caught up by the lymph vessels and hurried along to the blood and to its final expulsion from the body, while its loss is immediately made good by fresh material brought there by the lymph.

By these two processes, a sound body, after attaining maturity, if the laws and conditions of life and health are complied with, will retain for a long period, its identity of size, form, weight and complexion, while, at the same time, undergoing constant change, its tissues and organs being daily and hourly in process of renewal.

The powers of the various organs of the body may be appropriately classified as *fundamental* and *special*. The processes of building a machine must always be distinguished from the processes of the machine after it is built. The processes by which the body is built, and the processes by which the body or any of its organs works after it is ready for function are different. The evolution of a kidney is one kind of a process. The production of urine by the completed kidney is another kind of process. Every organ and part of the body may, therefore, be said to possess two powers—namely: (1) Its power of self-repair and self-maintenance, which is its *fundamental* power; and, (2) Its functioning power, that is its power to work, which is its *special* power. These powers are inherent in the organs or in their cells, although in the body they are governed and controlled by the nervous system and while this is true of both powers, it is especially true of the *special* power

The *fundamental* power maintains the organ in repair and in readiness for work when supplied with motive power by the nerves. It heals its wounds, removes its worn out cells and replaces these with new ones and repairs its damaged structure. This work is largely dependent upon the blood and lymph for its success.

Jennings called this power the *recuperative function*, and pointed out that so long as there is sufficient power to maintain repairs no organic defects will or can develop in an organ for as rapidly as it sustains wear and tear this is repaired and structural soundness is maintained. It is only after the body has been abused and weakened so that its various parts are no longer fully capable of recuperating and repairing themselves as rapidly as they sustain wear and tear that the various organs of the body begin to take on change.

Let us for convenience break up the development of disease into three distinct stages or steps, keeping in mind, at the same time, however, that there are no distinct lines of demarcation between these stages. They are all of a piece and each shades gradually, imperceptibly into the other. In doing this we have:—

First: *Declension of power:* No portion of the living organism ever takes on disordered action, except where it suffers great violence, until its energies have been reduced to a point below that necessary to sustain it in normal function. The vital properties were made to act just as they do under the circumstances in which they act, and they possess neither disposition nor power to act in any other way. The highest possible good of the organism in general, and of its several organs in particular is the end always before the forces of life and toward this end they aim as steadily and unerringly as the needle to the pole. When all parts are well supplied with power, there is GOOD HEALTH, general and local. When there is a deficiency of functioning power, that is, less power than is required to sustain a healthy functional standard, the health of the part or parts is IMPAIRED, and impaired to the extent of its lack of power.

By virtue of the *law of life*, each organ of the body has a specific and distinct function to perform, which it must perform, or attempt to perform, while it has the power to act. The vigor and efficiency of any function, and the perfection of its work, is proportioned to the ability of the organ to labor—a due supply of appropriate material being understood.

As an example, the liver must secrete bile, and supply this just when, in the exact quantity and precise quality required, if there is power enough at the command of the vital economy to effect this. If there is not sufficient power to enable the liver to supply perfect bile as required, the liver must meet its obligations in this particular according to the power it possesses and not according to the power it does not have.

Second: *Impairment and derangement of function, functional disease*: When the energies of an organ or group of organs have been reduced to a point below that essential to the maintenance of healthy function, its functions are impaired or deranged. In a sound state of the body, when all the parts are sufficiently supplied with power, there may be a large temporary diminution of the power of one or more organs of the body, without any derangement of function, but when the general stock of energy is reduced to a supply barely adequate for ordinary use, any reduction below that level must be followed by derangement. When such a condition exists and the body is subjected to circumstances that require more energy to maintain its functions at the standard-level of comfortable health, than is required under the usual conditions of life then impairment of function must follow. Sudden and great changes in weather, exposure, fatigue, overeating, excitement, grief, shock, prostrate the greatly enervated, not the vigorous and strong.

Every organ and part of an organ is liable to functional impairment as a result of a reduction of its sustaining energy. The manifestations, or symptoms, which announce the defective state of the part or parts, will depend on the organ or parts of the organ affected, and the extent of the affection.

A change in the substance or structure of an organ, can only be reached through functional impairment and derangement and this can only take place through a pinching scantiness of functional power. There is, in all violations of the laws of life, an actual loss of power, but, as Jennings said, "We have no vitometer by which to graduate this defect; and it is only when power is reduced so low that action falters, or structure changes that we can begin to measure the damaged condition of the body; and from this point the symptoms become our guide, and our only guide to a knowledge of the quality or kind, seat and extent of disease—in the *common* use of the term."

Although the action of pathoferic substances is primarily and directly, upon the substances of the organs of the body, yet the injurious effect would be discovered first—if we had means of measuring the vitality of its parts—in a reduction of power. For even in a tolerable sound and vigorous body, there is power in reserve, over and above what is necessary for ordinary purposes. This capital stock of energy, over and above the usual expenditures, is held in store for an emergency, and while, therefore the draft upon this reserve is increased by every assault, the supply necessary for the work of maintaining functional action and structural integrity will be furnished till the reserve is exhausted. After this, if the demand for power to sustain functional soundness exceeds the income, the organ or organs must falter in their functions, and here commences FUNCTIONAL DISEASE.

Dr. Tilden admirably traces the development of functional diseases as follows:—
"The stomach is the most abused organ of the body. Almost immediately after birth the child is often enervated from fondling and overfeeding. Meddlesome midwifery, called modern medical science, enervates both mother and child, rendering the mother's milk, if there is any milk at all, unfit as food. Very soon after birth, symptoms

of indigestion appear in the child, and as often in the mother, which automatically starts a cinema of infant-feeding and care that competes in exquisite torture with the inventions of the fiends of hell. Here is laid the foundation for the universal gastro-intestinal catarrh that extends on and on, involving more or less all the mucous membranes of the body, becoming the father of all diseases *peculiar* to children—all the diseases recognized as catarrhal: colds, croup, tonsilitis, and others of the respiratory organs, all of which are reflex irritations of gastro-intestinal catarrh. And, as the skin is the mucous membrane without the body, the extension of the catarrh at times reaches the surface of the body, manifesting itself in one form or another of the exanthematous or eruptive gastro-intestinal catarrhal diseases, including smallpox. Respiratory diseases and eruptive diseases are interchangeable. (It was learned in the chapter on *Crises* that the suppression of the exanthemata most often results in respiratory and other mucous membrane complications and sequelae. Author's note).

"This brings us to the relationship of pneumonia and smallpox—the former an extension of grastro-intestinal catarrh to the lungs, and the latter an extension of gastro-intestinal catarrh to the surface of the body. Both these types of disease vary from a light, almost insignificant derangement to a malignancy that is fatal in almost every case. The cause of the great difference in severity, from almost nil to fatal malignancy, is the state of the body—it is a question of the degree of Toxemia. In pronounced enervation and Toxemia, with gastro-intestinal putrescence from an excessive intake of animal protein, infection from absorption of the intestinal decomposition, added to the existing Toxemia, often builds a fatal malady."—*Philosophy of Health*, Aug. 1924.

Third: *Structural impairment or change—organic disease*. Every part of the body is susceptible of change or impairment of its structure and substance, to a greater or less extent. This results from functional derangement which, in turn, results from enervation. When the *fundamental* or *recuperative* power of an organ is unable to repair itself as rapidly as it wears out or is damaged, a change in structure ensues. Every day happenings evidence the fact that wounds and broken bones heal without difficulty even under unfavorable external circumstances and that there are cases where neither cuts, bruises, or broken bones will heal under very favorable external circumstances. When power is low and the blood exceedingly foul the ability of an organ to repair and renew itself is greatly impaired. In toxic states of the body there is more or less destruction of the functioning cells of the body, and these, due to the ease with which they are destroyed by the toxins, instead of being replaced by others of their own kind are replaced by a functionless substitute of connective tissue or "scar tissue," which is better able to live under the circumstances. The damaged section of the organ is repaired by this tissue—the only tissue that may be used for repair under the circumstances. Thus, even cirrhosis or the hardening of an organ is a defensive measure, one designed to prolong life as long as possible. The forces of life always work for the preservation of life and when they cannot do as well as they would, they do as well as they may.

In functional derangements there is ordinarily more or less change of structure; but as this is only temporary, and the parts are soon restored to the natural state, it is not regarded as organic disease. It is only when functional derangement has persisted long enough that these changes have become extensive and permanent, that the condition is regarded as organic disease. Thus it will be seen that *functional* and *structural* diseases shade insensibly into each other. Structural disease does not always end in death, nor does functional derangement always result in organic change.

First, then, there must be exhaustion of power below a certain standard before there can be impairment or derangement of function. Impaired function must be impaired still more and prolonged before structural derangement can take place.

Want of power, then, the most *vital* kind of power, is the immediate cause of impaired, or what is called morbid or diseased action, for nothing constitutes good health, the highest degree of vigor, but a full and overflowing state of the vital treasury in every department of life. And not only should the fountain of supply abound and superabound, with vital energy, but every tissue and organ, and all the fluids and secretions of the body should be sound, and pure. Unfortunately, in the present state of mankind, there are no perfect constitutions, and but few that can be rightly clased as *sound* or *good*. One or more organs of the body are weak and faulty. They are more easily brought into a state of disease than the stronger more perfect ones, and take an organic change more readily when through oft repeated, protracted and aggravated violations of physical law, nature is unable, uninterruptedly, for any length of time, to maintain a nice balance between waste and repair.

The loss of power that must precede the development of disease is due to waste of power largely occasioned by the use of irritants and excitants—*stimulants*. Hence the egregious folly of the habitual employment of stimulants or tonics of various kinds, until the vital economy is forced to hang out its distress signals, and then employing the same means in larger amounts, or others of similar character and greater power, to remedy the damages of the habitual over-stimulation.

When over-stimulation has lashed an organ into impotency and organic change is taking place nature calls loudly for a let-up in activities. If this is granted the work of cure proceeds. The most rigid economy is exercised in the expenditure of power. Reinforcements are called in as far as can be done without incurring greater peril in some other organ, and every favoring circumstance is employed to avert, if possible, the ruin of a vital organ. Depleted energies hold out for a time, then lag behind for a brief period, then as if having gathered fresh strength, they rush forward in a greater effort and regain what they had previously lost. But if no change is made in the mode of living, and cause is not corrected, and as the treatment employed produces more enervation and more damage to the body the forces of life are worn down. The unequal contest finally balances against feeble vitality. The organs of elimination "fail to remove the cumulative mass of useless matter," as Jennings puts it, and wastes are no longer adequately repaired. Another stage in the *pathological descent* is reached— ORGANIC DISEASE.

The development of organic disease is never sudden and never without repeated warnings. Their earliest stages are purely functional and, as previously pointed out are evanescent. If causes are corrected they never become organic.

Let us assume that an infant begins life with semi-perfect health. He is fed too much and too often. He is bundled up too much, denied fresh air and sunshine, handled too much and subjected to too much noise. Colic develops. The baby cries. He is fed and drugged. Colds, constipation, punctuated with frequent diarrhea, skin rashes, tonsilitis, etc., develop. The stomach and bowels become sensitive. Indigestion becomes a "habit." Gastritis, bowel diseases, sore throat, the exanthemata, or erruptive diseases develop as crises. Chronic catarrh develops.

A sensitive stomach, enlarged tonsils, adenoids, impaired bowel action, glandular swellings and perhaps richets and other troubles follow the child through the next few years of white bread, potatoes, cakes, candies, pie, cereals with sugar, milk, eggs, meat, and repeated drugging. Frequent crises develop and these are palliated or suppressed. Puberty arrives and this may carry them by sheer force of developmental power through adolescence with but a part of their childhood troubles or with none of them.

After adulthood is reached there comes indigestion, nausea, vomiting, gastritis, sleeplessness, headaches and pains in various parts of the body.

In women painful menstruation develops, if indeed they have not had this from the first. They become morbid, and perhaps more or less hysterical.

The excesses and dissipations of this period from twenty to thirty-five, coupled with imprudent eating and frequent drugging—cathartics, headache remedies, bicarbonate of soda, etc.—and operations soon lay a secure foundation for shronic disease. Anemia, gastric ulcer, visceroptosis, chronic rheumatism, tuberculosis, etc. develop. At first these symptoms are only functional and periodic but as the causes are continued and intensified the affected organs undergo structural changes. From their *functional beginnings* in infancy to their organic endings in middle life these so-called diseases represent a continuous development out of ever increasing causes. Every chronic disease is of slow development and cannot exist without previous systemic impairment. Each toxemic crisis is palliated by drugs or treatment that produce greater enervation and build a greater toleration for toxemia. Chronic diseases are the legitimate outcomes of palliated acute troubles. Dr. Tilden well pictures the gradual evolution of disease in these words:

"When the organism is enervated from the thousand-and-one influences incident to life, and intoxication has brought on such a state of metabolism that the organism is overwhelmed by waste—excretory products—it is then that inherited diathesis takes on activity. If the diathesis is tubercular, gouty, neurotic, or of any of the special organs of the body, it is in keeping with the laws of health and life for the affection peculiar to the diathesis to spring up. If the causes are not removed, the affection will remain functional for a time; then organic change will take place. It is then that affections become diseases; it is then that irritation and an inflammation from indigestion become ulceration of the bowels or stomach, and the ulcer perforates, and death ensues from peritonitis caused by the perforation. The peritonitis was caused by the perforation; perforation was caused by ulceration; ulceration was caused by inflammation; inflammation (catarrh) was caused by irritation; irritation was caused by indigestion; indigestion was caused by fermentation; fermentation was caused by enervation; and enervation was caused by the thousand-and-one influences which build or destroy the body and mind of men, depending on whether they are wisely or unwisely applied."—*Impaired Health*, Vol. 1, p. 258.

Despite the evident looseness in the use of terms, the above description of the development of disease conditions is excellent. Each step is built on or out of the preceding one as a result of the continued operation and intensification of the same cause or causes. It were rank folly to regard disease in any other light.

Catarrh is a hypersecretion of the mucous membranes made necessary by plethora or a full habit—an overcrowded state of the blood-vessels—and by irritants and excitants. It is a conservative measure—a natural means of relieving the blood pressure and the engorged state of the mucous membranes. When this conservative measure is worked overtime there results a gradual impairment of function followed by inflammation of the mucous membrane. This passes into ulceration.

The poisons produced by carbohydrate fermentation give rise to the simple forms of inflammation such as are seen in colds, catarrh, etc.

If no more food is eaten than can be fitted for use by the body, secretions and excretions are closely enough balanced to maintain health. If the body is abused by excess of all kinds, by overclothing, living in overheated, poorly ventilated houses and by overeating, then passing from a hot room into the cold outdoors, or from a warm bed into a cold room will set up enough irritation of the exposed mucous membranes to bring on congestion—a cold, catarrh, hay fever, bronchitis, laryngitis, pharyngitis, etc.

Where enervation is pronounced, due to mental and physical habits that use up nerve force to excess, secretion and excretion are impaired. They fall below the level demanded by health. There is a consequent increase in the amount of waste matter circulating in the blood. If, as is usual, the accustomed amount of food is eaten, or if some unusual drain upon the nervous energies is sustained, digestion will not be perfect. Secretion will not be adequate to the work of digesting all the food eaten and there will be some left over which will fall to the bacteria, that are always present in the digestive tract, to be broken down. Fermentation and putrefaction will occur. A catarrhal inflammation of the stomach, intestine, or other part of the body will be set up. The catarrhal condition becomes general and forms the foundation for the development of many affections of the body.

Where the catarrh develops in the stomach and intestine, as in gastritis, it may easily spread to the common bile duct and from this to the gall-bladder and other bile ducts, even passing on into the liver itself.

Gastritis is the same condition in the stomach as a cold is in the nose and throat. Back of it are the same causes that produce a cold. Chronic catarrh of the stomach and intestine is the same thing as chronic catarrh of the nose and throat. Back of these conditions are the same causes. An acute catarrhal inflammation of the common bile-duct or of the gall-bladder is simply a "cold" in these parts; while a chronic catarrhal condition of these organs, is the same condition as a chronic catarrh of the nose and throat. Back of each of these conditions are the same causes.

The excessive use of sugar, cakes, pies, bread, cereals, milk, etc., are the chief causes of catarrh. Of course, in all cases enervation must check elimination, else out-go will be made to equal income and health will be maintained.

That person who conserves his nervous energies, who does not indulge in excesses and dissipations, who eats sensibly and moderately, who secures plenty of rest and sleep, who takes daily physical exercise, and who secures an abundance of fresh air and sunshine, will not be troubled with catarrh or any other disease.

A cold does not produce other diseases as is popularly taught and generally believed. The constitutional derangement, enervation, toxemia and intestinal indigestion which brought on the crisis (cold), also builds the other "diseases," even the organic "diseases." Not one cold but many colds and other crises develop over the long period of time during which organic disease is developing.

Nephritis is a disease of infancy and youth. It occurs largely from the ages of one to ten, following usually upon the suppression of scarletina or other febrile disease, and from twenty to thirty when the dissipations of young men reach their maximum. Degeneration of the kidneys belongs to middle age and beyond, when the "habits of life begin to tell."

A man goes along in average health until he reaches the age of forty. There are occasional headaches, colds, perhaps gastritis, and constipation for which he uses laxatives, but he feels well most of the time, is "never sick," has a good appetite, is never forced to be absent from his work because of illness, and he therefore considers himself in good health. Then at forty from one cause or another he has an examination made and discovers that he is suffering with diabetes which is considerably advanced. Nature's repeated warnings had gone unheeded and now he is paying the penalty. These pre-clinical symptoms—discomforts and mild functional disturbances—Orthopathy regards as marking the commencement of the second division of the descending pathological transition: the first manifestation of waning vitality. This is the answer to the question once put to Dr. Jennings: "My wife has a *fever*, what has that to do with *living?*"

A lady became sick enough to call in a doctor. Her trouble was palliated in the usual way. Trouble after trouble developed while others remained. For years she suffered with intestinal catarrh when ulceration developed. During this time she was operated on eight times. Gall-stones and probably the gall-bladder were removed, the appendix and coccix bone were each removed. Three operations were performed on the rectum and two sinus operations were performed. Finally cancer of the intestine developed.

Her physicians regarded each of her affections as distinct diseases, of local origin, and the removal of the affected organ was supposed to cure the disease. That they represented local manifestations of a general or systemic condition, that they all stemmed from the same basic cause, were mere steps or stages in the progressive degeneration of the woman's body, did not enter into their considerations. That there was any connection between intestinal catarrh and the gall-stones, appendicitis or ulcer, or that intestinal catarrh and sinusitis were the same condition in two locations did not enter into their philosophy.

Chronic disease may begin in the liver or pancreas or kidney and develop gradually and insiduously until the affected organ is beyond repair before the owner of the organ becomes aware that there is anything wrong with him. He may consider himself to be in good health. He practices certain destructive habits for years. He is apparently in good health. His friends indulge in the same habits. His doctor and nurse do likewise. Nothing arouses his suspicions that he is not in good condition. He does not even suspect that his habits are not all right. Then, at forty he begins to fail rapidly. Perhaps there is a sudden development of uremia. An examination shows him to be in the advanced stages of chronic Bright's disease with his kidneys beyond repair. He suddenly finds that all the time he was boasting that "nothing hurts me, I do as I like," "I can eat anything," "I always enjoy three square meals a day," "tobacco never hurts me," "alcohol won't harm one if he takes it in moderation," and imagining himself in good health, he was really standing with one foot in the grave, and the other on a banana peel.

Such a condition does not develop suddenly. It is the result of causes that operate in the daily life of the individual. These causes are found almost wholly in the voluntary habits of the person. Back of the first observable symptoms of decline were many small aches and pains, colds and periods of not feeling very well. One crisis after another arose and subsided, but these were considered unimportant and their causes ignored.

Back of these signs of developing chronic disease is another period in which the disease is developing but not making itself felt. During this stage no method of examination now known can detect the developing disease, although a knowledge of cause will enable one, by analyzing the person's mode of life, to declare that some forms of disease is developing.

Back of the clinical signs, back of the pre-clinical signs, when the disease is developing but not manifesting itself in any manner, there are its causes. Disease is a development. It no more comes into existence full-blown than flowers or trees do, the germ theory to the contrary notwithstanding. Its beginnings are small, imperceptible; its development slow, gradual, insidious. The disease begins where cause begins and persists where cause persists. The clinical phenomena of disease, the pre-clinical phenomena of disease and the unobservable phenomena of disease are not separate and distinct stages of disease. They are all of a piece and all shade off imperceptibly into each other. They are all evolutions out of the same causes and are continuous because their causes are continuous.

Men who study disease, that is its symptoms and results, and who look upon these as causes or as entities are led into many rather serious blunders. They regard a given affection as being due to the failure of some organ and treat the organ.

When eating habits are such as to crowd the liver functions—impair its functions of urea formation, detoxification, and preparing sugar for use or for elimination—kidney troubles arise as a consequence. But the failure of the liver's functions is not the cause of the kidney trouble. It is one of the causes, but is secondary to the primary cause, overeating or imprudent eating. Rational treatment would correct the eating instead of treating the liver or kidneys.

The same mistake is made with regard to constipation. There is hardly a disease in the nosology which this common complaint is not accused of causing. By some it is even considered to be the chief cause of cancer.

It is not correct to say constipation causes this or that disease, headache, rheumatism, cancer, etc. It is rather nearer the truth to say that the causes of constipation are also the causes of these "diseases." We must get away from the prevalent manner of viewing constipation as a cause and learn to see it as an effect. It may be objected that when the constipation is cured the headache ceases or that no cancer will develop. It would be equally as correct to say that when the headache is cured the constipation is cured also. They are concomitant effects of the same cause or causes and not one the cause of the other. When the causes of constipation are removed the causes of cancer are also removed.

Those who regard constipation as the cause of their ills attempt to cure their ills by the use of purgatives, laxatives, enemas, wheat bran, etc., while those who regard constipation as part of their ills, a mere symptom, get rid of all their troubles by correcting and removing the common cause of all of them. Thus it will be seen that in practice it makes all the difference in the world which of these views we adopt.

Under the first view the very means employed to cure the constipation invariably make it worse. They irritate, depress, enervate and further inhibit function, and if continued long enough cause a complete cessation of function.

Two "diseases" (tonsilitis and metritis, for instance) existing together or successively are concomitant or successive effects of a common cause, an extension of effects of one cause, and not cause and effect of one another. It is the state of the blood that goes to both the affected organs that causes the disease in each and not the inflammation in one organ that causes the inflammation in the other. The recurrent development of crises in an organ or tissue is due to the continued operation of the original producing causes. The subsequent or concomitant development of a crisis in another organ in a remote part of the body is due to the extension of these same causes.

Obviously, if the causes which result in some bodily disorder or local inflammation, or which lead to the formation of some growth or to the hardening of some tissue, are permitted to continue acting after the inflammation or disorder has subsided, or after the growth has been removed, either a recurrence of the disease or the development of some "other" and, what is most likely, more extensive disease or a worse growth must develop. How often do we see people suffer from repeatedly recurring "attacks" of some disorder! How often does this condition continue to extend and grow worse and "other" diseases develop! The individual who has sore throat or bronchitis or gall-stones or headache may and usually does get another and another "attack" of the same trouble, because, as soon as one crisis is over he begins to build another. A simple ovarian tumor is removed. A few months or a few years later it is followed by another or by the formation of a cancer about the stump of the simple tumor. This indicates that the operation of the same causes that produced the first tumor, when not corrected, produce a second and that the primary causes of simple tumors and of malignant or cancerous tumors are the same.

The blood circulates throughout the whole system, and, if it is abnormal in any respect every part of the body must suffer more or less as a result. It is not accidental which part or parts of the body are affected most. If the blood is normal the parts of the body will be well nourished and properly cleansed, and, in the absence of some more or less accidental local causes, which may momentarily disturb some part, will be able to maintain their structural and functional integrity. Should they be subjected to local irritation, this will soon be remedied, by the circulation of healthy blood in the part, and very soon all traces of the former irritation will be gone. The irritation will be in proportion to the magnitude and duration of the exciting cause, the resistance of the part being great because of its soundness and because of the wholesomeness of its blood supply, so that the suffering caused by the irritant is comapratively slight.

But let the blood be foul—toxic—that is, loaded with waste and refuse and the effects of such an irritant will be much greater and more slowly recovered from. It will occasion greater suffering. Take, for instance, a wound of the leg which heals readily and with little suffering in those of sound health and pure blood, but which, where health is impaired and the blood is foul heals slowly, or not at all, and occasions great suffering. The suffering in such a case would be "proportionate to the magnitude of the injury and inversely as the healthiness of the blood, or proportionately to its unhealthiness." A. Rabagliati, M.A., M.D., F.R.C.S., Edin, a reformed British medical man declares:

"Most local ailments are only local expressions of general states. The specialist is by implication here relegated to his proper place, and is informed, if he has wit enough to read the lesson presented to him, that it is not sufficient to remove an ovarian tumor, e. g., and that if nothing is said at the same time or subsequently as to the causes which induced it, a positive damage may be done to the woman, who may, therefore, while considering herself cured, proceed to manufacture one on the other side, or may find herself in a few years suffering from cancer in the stump of the previous one. Or the child who has tonsils removed, and adenoids cleared away, may and certainly will subsequently suffer from colds, bronchitis, broncho-pneumonia, and the like, and bye and bye probably from rheumatism or rheumatic fever, etc., unless at the same time or subsequently to the operation, his mother is advised to treat him differently from the way in which she treated him before. For, if she does not, a worse thing may happen to him in the future, and so the operation which was intended to benefit may eventuate in damage and not in good. Evidently the same causes which enlarged the tonsils and caused the adenoid growths, on the soft palate and nose will, if they are allowed to go on, tend to make the child ill again either in the same or in some other way. Or the middle-aged woman, who has a chronic discharge from her nose, may get it stopped, indeed, by having her nose cauterised by a platinum wire made white hot by the electric current, only to find herself in a few months suffering from a cancer of the breast, which, being in turn removed, eventuates in cancer of the liver, for which there is no relief. These illustrations are, I may say, by no means imaginary, but are drawn from exeprience of cases in practice."—*Air, Food and Exercises*, pp. 129-130.

Local affections or local inflammations are far more serious as being marks of the general condition of the blood, than they are as being mere local affections. If then, a sick person presents a number of "local diseases" they are not to be considered as independent or idiopathic diseases, nor yet as symptomatic diseases, one derived from the other, but as concomitant or succesive effects of a common cause. Thus when a man

217

presents arthritis in one or more joints, valvular heart disease, or myocarditis, and tonsilitis, the first named local affections are not to be considered as having been caused by the tonsilitis, and as curable by removal of the tonsils, but these affections and the tonsilitis are to be regarded as being due to a common fundamental cause and all, alike, curable by correcting or removing this common cause. Patients often develop endocarditis first, then arthritis and then tonsilitis last. It is a bit hard to make tonsilitis responsible for these other two conditions when they develop in advance of the tonsilitis. It is just as logical in such a case to say that the endocarditis or arthritis caused the tonsilitis as, in other cases, to hold tonsilitis responsible for these other conditions. The only tenable view is that the three conditions have a common origin, even if this does knock the idea of specific diseases due to specific causes into a cocked hat and support our contention for a unitary cause, and the unity of disease. That disease, from first to last is all of a piece was declared by Jennings in the following words:

"There is no propriety in the common mode of computing physical defection—that part of it that obtains the appelation of disease. Whatever name is given to physical degeneracy should be made to include the whole of it, first, second, and third stages. It is all a damaged state, alike needing recruit and replenishment. The gradation in the line of degeneracy, from the elevated point of perfect structural and vital soundness to the commencement of the second stage where functional disturbance begins, must always be a lengthy one; for the distance between the two points is immense, and cannot be traversed by noxious agencies in one or two generations. It would be impossible by any mode or degree of abuse to reduce a sound body to a condition in which fevers, pleurisies, bilious affections, colds, etc., could be manifested. The vital economy might be broken up and destroyed by a great variety of violent methods, and the different parts of the body might be reduced by long-continued and excessive exercise to a tired weary point; but the individual organs could not be made to take on the ordinary forms of impaired health. There are men in this degenerate age—men, too, who fall far short of physical perfection—who go on to a very advanced period of life under a constant strain upon their vital machinery from noxious agencies and practices: who never have colds, coughs, fevers, or any serious illness—'are never sick a day in their lives' They are proof against 'the pestilence that walketh in darkness, and the destruction that wasteth at noon day.' These men have vital force enough within call in every department of their systems to guard against injuries and repair damages without the necessity of making a palpable demonstration of unsoundness.

"These cases, however, instead of constituting the universal rule, as ought to be the case, are but slight exceptions among the great bulk of mankind that are near the lower border of the first grade of degeneracy, verging toward the second grade, constantly liable, from a low state of vital powers, to be hurried into it."—*Tree of Life*, pp. 117-18.

Dr. Page agrees with this statement and expresses it as follows·

"The fact is that there is a process of degeneration going on throughout the entire structure of the man, even to the last tissue, and the symptoms are all indicative of this; and this is more or less strictly true of all disorders. The naming and classifying of 'disease' is calculated to mystify and mislead; sickness is the proper term for describing them all: self-abuse, in the broadest sense of the word, is the cause of them; and obedience to law, the only means of prevention or cure."—*The Natural Cure*, p. 131.

Page, who regarded diphtheria as "only a phase of albuminuria," quotes one Dr. Grasmuck as saying· "Another peculiarity of the scourage is its fondness for children of a certain condition—the fat, sleek, soft, tender, 'well-fed' children so generally admired—such children can offer but slight resistance to this disease; being in fact, chronically diseased, they are predisposed to 'attacks' of all kinds; and, living to adult age, furnish the greater proportion of cases of tuberculous disease. On the other hand, I do not know of a single instance where the disease proved fatal to—rarely attacking—a child of the *genus* 'Street Arab'—children who spend most of their time out of doors, are thinly clad, sleep in cold rooms, have a spare diet, and who have no one to pamper them unwisely."

Inflammation of the respiratory organs—pleurisy, pneumonia, bronchitis and MEMBRANOUS CROUP—often accompany Bright's disease. Whether these conditions and diphtheria are phases of albuminuria and whether or not we accord any place to germs in their production we must recognize those prior causes which prepare the body for the development of these troubles. And we must cease repeating the old error about fat, sleek, ruddy, well-fed children being healthy. Jennings said:

"Let it be remembered that no variety nor degree of 'rosy cheek' is an indication of health, but contrawise, a mark of a very serious constitutional defect "—*Medical Reform.*

Upon this same point Graham declared:

"There is another thing concerning which a general error of opinion prevails. It is a common notion that a florid countenance, when not produced by intoxicating liquors, is a sure sign of good health, and that a pale complexion is an invariable indication of poor health. It is true that there is a kind of sallow, sickly paleness which is a pretty sure sign that the functions of the system are not all healthfully performed; but it is far from being true that a ruddy countenance is always the index of good health; and still farther from being true that it is always the index of that health which is most compatible with long life. 'Too much ruddiness in youth,' says Hufeland, 'is seldom a sign of longevity.' As a general fact, at all periods of life, it indicates that state of the system in which, either from disease or from intensity, the vital expenditure is too rapid for permanent health and for longevity. The clear complexion in which the red and white are so delicately blended, as to produce a soft flesh-color, varying from a deeper to a paler hue according as the individual is more or less accustomed to active exercise in the open air, or to confinement and sedentary and studious habits, is by far the best index of that kind of health and of that temperament which are most favorable to continued health and length of days."—*Science of Human Life,* p. 495.

And lastly, Page says of this common error:

"This symptom (red cheeks) popularly regarded as a sign of health, is simply evidence of plethora when it is habitually observed in robust individuals, young or old, and denotes a predisposition to febrile disease. *Congestion of the cheeks is,* of course, not dangerous, in itself considered, but it is no more a sign of health than is congestion in the bowels, lungs or kidneys: It is a note of warning and should be promptly heeded. The plethoric, or full-blooded, robust subject should be more abstemious in diet—taking less food as a whole, perhaps, or adopting a less stimulating and non-irritating diet. The frail, delicate, or anemic patient's flushed cheeks are not apt to be misinterpreted."—*How to Feed the Baby,* p. 136.

Hale looking men with a moderately full and florid countenance live fast and die prematurely. The florid countenance is due to a moderate and habitual distension and congestion of the capillaries of the face. It is an evidence of plethora or the full habit, of over-stimulation or what Graham called *vital intensity.* How frequently do we meet with fresh, hale looking men who go on to forty or sixty years of age, apparently in good health and then who sink rapidly and die!

A total abandonment of all irritants, other things remaining the same, is always followed by the establishment of a better and more permanent state of health accompanied by a corresponding abolition of the facial congestion.

If the stimulant user possesses a sound, vigorous constitution, and no other overpowering causes intervene, "very good health" will be enjoyed for years, with occasional slight interruptions such as colds, pains, bowel disturbances, etc., but the constant action of irritating matter upon sensitive organs will at length call for reparation.

Where this condition is due to overeating, it will be necessary to eat more moderately and perhaps to revolutionize the diet. For, it should be remembered that considerable quantities of meat, eggs, bread, condiments, spices, etc., will produce such a countenance until the health is so impaired that the blood is impoverished and one takes on the appearance of anemia. A knowledge of the conditions of health will enable us to avoid disease

The study of the pathological changes which occur in an organ in chronic disease, let us say in the kidneys in Bright's disease, is all very well for the technician, although as Dr. Page observes, "If *too much time* is devoted to it, and to the *relation of drugs* thereto, by an individual, he may be, probably will be, the very least fitted to advise an inquirer who desires to know what he can do to be saved from disease and the supposed necessity of taking medicine."

Now "From a practical standpoint" as Page says, "when a man's sickness is attended with a certain set of symptoms, as albumen in the urine, final suppression of the urine and uremic poisoning—occasioned by a peculiar degeneration of the kidneys,*** we care nothing about the kind of change taking place in the kidney, but rather ask what kind of change in our habits will keep this, and all other organs of the body in a healthy condition." To put this more simply, the study of the conditions of health is of far greater importance than is the study of pathology after this has developed from a failure to comply with the conditions of health.

Medical men usually begin at the finish to diagnose a disease. After the patient is dead they hold a post-mortem and their findings are handed out as a diagnosis. They find a cancer, a fibroid tumor, an abscess and these are given as the cause of death. But these things are effects. They are the results of causes that are not discoverable at the necropsy, causes that have ceased. They see the finished product, not its initial beginnings and hence, are not able to learn anything that is of value in preventing such developments.

Tumors and cancers have long been a serious problem in medical circles. Little is yet known in these circles of their causes and development and this we feel is due largely to the fact that they continue to regard them as specific entities requiring specific causes for their production and fail to recognize their oneness with the other pathological states of the body and their origin out of the pathoferic causes which produce these other pathological states.

They are regarded chiefly as a disease of middle life and old age. They are seldom found in children and young people and there must be a good and sound reason for this.

It is probably correct to say that children do not suffer from cancer for the reason that their habits have not had time to produce it. A few cases do develop in children, who must be predisposed to its development, and the number who develop the disease increases as age increases, due no doubt to the fact that the causes which produce the disease continue to accumulate and grow in power as age advances. The causes operating to produce cancer take time to act and it is for this reason that cancer becomes more common as age increases.

In childhood and early life irritation in the body is accompanied by intolerance. The young organism vigorously resists the causes of irritation and throws them off. This gives rise to the fevers, inflammations, sudden and fierce, and frequently of short duration, so characteristic of childhood.

As age advances and the tissues harden they cease to offer such violent resistance to irritation, but tolerate it, so that the diseases of middle life and beyond are not so fierce as in childhood and youth. The ever increasing cause begins to weigh down and depress the powers of the body. The ordinary powers of resistance to toxins and irritants and the usual means of disposing of surplus food are impaired and the body is forced to defend itself and dispose of its surplus food by some more or less unusual means. New growths of all kinds are composed of cells and in order to grow it is necessary that more food material be brought to them than is necessary for the sustenance of the normal tissue of the part. Long continued local over-nutrition due to irritation or circulatory obstruction would seem to be necessary for the immediate production of a neoplasm.

There are many kinds of tumors but these are broadly grouped as (1) connective tissue tumors, (2) epithelial tissue tumors, and (3) mixed tissue tumors, that is, tumors composed of mixtures of various tissues. Wood defines a tumor as "a more or less circumscribed collection of cells arising wholly independently of the rest of the body, in general growing progressively, and serving no useful purpose in the organism." He admits that this definition is entirely descriptive and adds "as we do not know the cause or causes of tumors it is impossible to define these structures more accurately." In dealing with their classification he makes a similar statement, saying: "Inasmuch as we do not know the cause of tumors, it is impossible to make a strictly scientific classification of them. It is, therefore, most convenient to use a purely morphological basis for classification, drawn from the microscopic appearance of the tumors and the tissues from which they originate. Cysts are included with tumors because of their genetic relationship to new growths rather than to any other pathological condition."

We object to two features of this definition—we do not see how it can be maintained that tumors grow independently of the body; and, we are certain that they do serve a useful purpose in the organism. It will not be denied that those portions of a cyst, or at least some cysts, which are genetically related to neoplasms serve a very definite and eminently useful purpose. A cyst which forms around a foreign body, a parasite for example, is definitely useful and protective.

From our standpoint a "strictly scientific classification" of tumors is not necessary, for they represent the same condition, or the same process in different tissues and are the results of the same causes acting on the different tissues. Tumors may develop in any organ or any tissue of any organ in the body and they derive their names from these organs and tissues. Thus, myoma is the name given to a tumor of muscle tissue; endothelioma the name applied to a tumor developing in the endothelium of some of the body's cavities; osteoma a bone tumor, etc., etc. These names relate to tissues, organs and locations—the differences in these tumors are those derived from the differences that exist in the tissues in which they originate. When the variation from the normal type of tissue in which the tumor originates passes beyond a certain more or less indifinite line the tumor becomes malignant. This represents merely another stage or step in the pathological evolution and not the addition of some new element. It is the result of the continued action of the original producing causes.

From these considerations it is evident that tumors are a unit just as inflammation is a unit. Furthermore, they do not represent distinct and specific "diseases," but are merely links in a long chain of causes and effects which extend backward in the life of the individual to infancy, perhaps, beyond.

A female infant suffers with colic, frequent colds, constipation, frequent diarrhea and "hives" or frequent skin rashes of one form or another. As she grows older there are colds, sore throats, enlarged tonsils, "children's diseases," frequent spells of nausea and vomiting, etc. With the arrival of puberty there occurs painful and irregular menstruation. accompanied with headaches, styes on the eyelids, pains in the back, nervousness, loss of appetite and other symptoms. Later indigestion develops and this is palliated, as were all the preceding troubles, with no attention given to cause. The palliative measures afford her immediate relief, but remotely aggravate the indigestion they were used to relieve. She now has frequent recurrences of some one or more ailments like headache, or neuralgia, or colds, or "bilious attacks," or rheumatism, or she is constantly fatigued, and finally becomes chronically ill. Finally at about the age of thirty or thirty-five she is discovered to be carrying a large ovarian tumor. Now it seems hardly correct to single out the tumor from among all the train of symptoms and ills which this woman has suffered, beginning in infancy and lasting throughout her whole life, and decide that its development has no connection with these prior troubles, that it is a distinct and specific disease depending on some specific cause and wholly unrelated to the causes which have been producing her ills from infancy onward.

Multiple tumors, that is two or more tumors in the same individual supply us with an interesting confirmation of our theory of the unity of tumors and the unity of cause. These may develop in any tissue in the body or in several different tissues in which case they resemble the tissues from which they arise.

Irritation—mechanical, chemical, thermal, actinic, etc.—is among the undoubted causes of cancer. But irritation alone is not sufficient to produce tumors or cancer. Tumors of the skin on the face are frequently multiple. So also are tumors arising from x-ray burns or from irritation from coal tar. In such cases a unitary cause is recognized. When there is long continued chronic irritation over a large area the tumors are usually multiple. Unity of cause is here again recognized.

But it is argued that the presence of a carcinoma of the uterus and of a carcinoma of the stomach must be based on different irritants. When tumors are found to exist in some portion of the intestinal tract and also in one or both ovaries, the intestinal tumor is regarded as primary and the ovarian tumor as secondary, being derived from the primary one by *metastasis*. Metastasis is the name applied to the theory that particles of tumors break off or are detached from the parent body and are carried by the blood or lymph to other parts of the body where they attach themselves and begin the development of another tumor.

All of this, I regard as a fanciful hypothesis supported only by the artificial production of tumors—that is the occasional production of a tumor in an animal by inoculation with particles of tumor from another animal. Such experiments can throw no light on the causes of tumors for the very simple reason that no human being ever develops cancer by any such method.

Wood records a case of epithelioma of the lip "which remained fairly localized and was successfully removed by operation with no recurrence at the end of a year." However, by this time there had developed a very large carcinoma of the thyroid, all the lmyph-nodes of the neck being involved along with the surrounding tissue. The patient died. At autopsy no traces of the epithelioma of the lip were found in regional lymphnodes and adjoining parts of the face but numerous small carcinomata were present. Both carcinoma and sarcoma may develop in the same individual concomitantly or successively, and some instances are recorded in which both types of these tumors have existed together in the same organ. These are especially found in the uterus.

Now all of these phenomena we regard as arising out of the same primary cause. The development of a tumor in one organ or tissue is due to the same cause that produces a tumor in another organ or tissue. Instead of multiple tumors, when these exist in different organs, being due to metastasis, we regard them as originating out of the same primary cause. They are not primary and secondary to each other, but concomitant or successive developments from a common basis. Wood records a case of development of carcinoma of the uterus ten years after the removal of a carcinoma of the breast and says that "Metastatic connection between the tumors could be ruled out."

If the irritants that help to produce tumors are to be regarded as always acting from without, and never from within, then it may be right to say that carcinoma of the stomach and carcinoma of the uterus arise from different irritants. But this assumption is by no means necessary and besides, the irritant is a secondary and not the primary cause of the tumor. I do not doubt that sexual self-abuse, eroticism, excessive intercourse and most, if not all contraceptive measures tend to the production of tumors of the female genital organs.

Carcinoma and sarcoma are the two chief forms of cancer and represent special forms of hyperplasia of epithelial and connective tissue. Epithelioma or carcinoma is cancer of the epithelial tissues; sarcoma, as distinguished from carcinoma is cancer of the connective tissues. Sarcoma and carcinoma are doubtless both due to the same causes acting on different tissues. These causes occasion an overgrowth of these structures, two or more cells appearing where before was only one. Once this process has started it continues, under the continued operation of the producing causes, "constantly spreading, ulcerating or fungating by advance and recession. The advance, however, preponderating through necessity until ultimately its break down results in death."

Hypertrophy, hardening and hyperplasia are due to over-nutrition and to irritation. These processes pushed beyond what we may term physiological limits, give rise to ulceration and cancer. They begin as conservative or defensive measures and they continue as such. There is no doubt, in the writer's mind, that except for the development of those conditions known as tumors and cancers, the causes which necessitated them would destroy life much sooner than they do. In other words the development of tumors and cancers prolongs life. I have no doubt that their development is in the highest degree orthopathic; that they develop only when there is an urgent necessity for just such developments. No laws are violated in their development. I am equally confident that if their causes are corrected before they have grown too large, nature will tear down these conservative measures, for they, like all conservative measures, are only intended as temporary measures.

H. W. S. Wright, M.S., F.R.C.S. says: "There can be no doubt that in nearly all cases there is what may be called a precancerous stage. It is moreover a long standing chronic condition which, as a rule, gives rise to very little inconvenience on the part of the patient. After this precancerous stage there appears what may be called early cancer, often indistinguishable to the naked eye from the original precancerous lesion, but giving rise to great suspicion in the eyes of the initiated on account of its hardness, 2nd tendency to be fixed."

In a handbook of *Essential Facts about Cancer*, prepared for the medical profession by a special committee of the *American Society for the Control of Cancer*, I find the following words, "A factor which, during the last ten years, has proved to be of great importance in the causation of cancer, is chronic irritation. As the various theories of the parasitic origin of cancer have been disproved, chronic irritation has been found increasingly to be an important factor in the incidence of cancer in one region or another." This is the opening paragraph of a chapter devoted to "precancerous conditions," and among these conditions are listed and discussed such things as fissures, chronic ulcerations and indurations (hardenings), irritation from gall-stones, erosions and lacerations of the cervix of the womb, chronic cystitis, old burns, scars, the effects of x-rays and radium, etc., while "many tumors which are essentially benign in character" are said to be "capable of malignant transformation, especially in the later years of life."

Cancer at the start is not cancer. It may be a gastric ulcer, or an x-ray or radium burn, or a fistulous rectum, or a torn cervix, or a hardened fundus or a chronically inflamed ovary. What produces this change? Why does last year's ulcer, for instance, become this year's cancer? Obviously, it is an evolution out of the prior condition and due to the same causes perhaps intensified, that produced the prior condition.

Premature ageing, or sclerosis of the tissues and blood-vessels may exist to such an extent that they can offer but little resistance to the causes of ulceration. This is undoubtedly a factor when essentially benign tumors undergo "malignant transformation in the later years of life." Other causes may intervene to cut off oxygen and nourishment so that putrefaction sets in followed by systemic infection. Or, drainage may be cut off forcing absorption and the development of blood-poisoning—cancerous cachexia. Poisoning by cancer is a form of sepsis slowly generated and liberated in the system.

Whatever the cause of the development of a cancer out of a pre-cancerous condition, an ulcer, induration, fistula, benign tumor, etc., it is only another step in the *downward pathological transit*, a condition that would not have developed had the pre-cancerous condition not first developed, and so closely related is it to the preceding condition that it is not possible to tell just where the pre-cancerous condition ends and cancer begins. The folly of attempting to prevent cancer by the surgical removal of the pre-cancerous state should be obvious when it is realized that the causes of the condition lie back of it and cannot be removed by the knife. Indeed the knife frequently occasions the rapid development of a cancer.

The tissues of some people are more susceptible to the development of tumors than are the tissues of other people, and some tissues in the same person are more susceptible to its development than others. Dr. Bulkley thinks there is a *cancer-diathesis* just as there is a *tubercular diathesis, a gouty diathesis*, etc. When a chronic irritant is applied to those tissues of an individual which are "susceptible" to cancer such a condition is much more apt to develop than when applied to other tissues or to the same tissues of another individual. But this state of susceptibility is not, beyond a weakened state of the tissues, due to any inherent predisposition to tumor development. It is undoubtedly due to toxemia of a virulent character.

Irritation causes an extra amount of blood to be sent to the point of irritation causing congestion and inflammation. In all cases of inflammation there is rapid cell proliferation and an overgrowth of tissue. But, where the system is sound and the blood pure the irritation is soon overcome, the inflammation subsides and the excess of tissue is broken down and carted away. Where the blood is foul its accumulation at a point of irritation increases the irritation and, unless the condition of the blood is changed, tends to perpetuate the low-grade inflammation that is thus set up in old people. Those tissues which are most resistant to the toxins and are not killed by these multiply as in all inflammations and as the irritation is continuous, the inflammation is continuous and growth is continuous. Irritation, inflammation, ulceration, induration and cancer is the order of development.

Tilden thus traces the development of a fibroid tumor:—

"A young woman develops intestinal indigestion from imprudent eating. The catching-cold habit, with catarrh of the mucous membranes, follows. Soon there is developed intestinal putrefaction, which being absorbed, causes infection. The pelvic lymphatics become involved. As there is more or less congestion of the mucous membrane lining the uterus and its neck, this condition is made more pronounced each month because of menstruation and the toxins being absorbed in the bowels. The uterine engorgement causes longer and more profuse menstruation; painful menstruation begins, growing more pronounced month by month. Pain forces the calling of a physician, who on examination finds a flexed womb. The flexion is caused by a thickening of one side of the womb, which forces a flexion to the opposite side. The more thickening the more obstruction to the circulation and the more bent is the neck of the womb; and the more bent is the neck, the more the canal is obstructed to the menstrual flow.

"As the womb is flexed more and more, the circulation is more and more interfered with. The flexed side fails to receive the proper amount of nourishment, and the thickened side receives all that the uterine and other vessels can bring; but the return vessels fail to carry back the full amount, and, as a result, hypertrophy takes place—the parts are overstimulated. Nature undertakes to organize the surplus; and she does —and we call it a fibroid tumor. These growths grow rapidly or slowly according to the amount of obstruction.

"A growth may fill the pelvis and abdomen in five years; and again in some other women it may require twenty years to develop a tumor the size of an orange.

"Injuries at childbirth often become the first cause of tumor, next to putrefactive infection from intestinal indigestion.

"Another cause: A catarrhal inflammation locates at an old placental site, as a result of toxemia. Thickening and induration follow, impeding the efferent circulation. The more growth, the more pressure and obstruction, until the new growth—fibroid tumor—is large enough to become a cause of its own growth, by impeding the circulation through its weight and pressure.

"This work of overgrowth is pushed along rapidly by overeating, which means over-nourishing; the surplus being organized into tumor.

"Overeating and improper eating often cause gas distention of the bowels. The pressure from gas crowds and misplaces the womb. From such misplacements enough obstruction to uterine circulation may take place to cause hypertrophic enlargement, which is fibroid enlargement;

"Constipation may cause enough pressure on the womb to start imperfect circulation, and later fibroid growth.

"Wherever there is impeded circulation, new growth must take place; and that means tumor. The kind of tumor will depend on the character of the tissues involved.

"Add to these causes sclerosis, and malignant diseases may follow. That is, the benign tumors may become malignant."—*Impaired Health*, Vol. 1, pp. 255-6-7.

A tumor is not only composed of cells of the same kind as those composing the tissue from which it is derived, but these cells are frequently functioning tissue. Carcinoma of the thyroid often secretes the specific thyroid material, a tumor of the breast is apt to contain structures which remind us of the secreting glands of the mamma; a uterine tumor is likely to contain involuntary muscle fiber, carcinoma of the bowel often contains glandular structures which closely resemble the normal structures of the intestine, and which secrete mucous.

However, the tumor as a whole does not resemble perfectly normal tissue. In a fibroma, for instance, its connective tissue cells are absolutely identical with those of the tissue in which the tumor is situated, but the general structure is usually more or less cellular than the normal connective tissue. Blood vessels have thin walls, or in dense tumors, are almost entirely absent over considerable areas. The lymph channels are defective, while the nervous structures present have no relationship with the tumor. These latter merely pass through the tumor to the normal structures which they innervate. In tumors in cartilaginous structures (chondioma), the cartilage is not so regular in structure as in normal cartilage. In tumor of the bone the bone cells and lamellae are not so systematically arranged as in normal bone.

From this it should be evident that these structures will break down more easily than normal tissue once their nutrition is cut off or their drainage is impaired. They would undergo decomposition and sepsis would develop.

The degenerative changes which occur in the various types of tumors, benign and "malignant," do not differ from the alterations which occur in normal tissues when the blood supply is diminished or ulceration and cachexia have developed. Due to the imperfect character of their capillary circulation, and to the usually insufficient blood supply, and to thrombosis which results usually from pressure or stasis, tumors are more liable to hemorrhage and subsequent degeneration than is normal tissue. Hemorrhage, various types of degeneration, often beginning with fatty degeneration of its cells which may progress to calcifications or even bone formation, and leading ultimately to necrosis or gangrene result from pushing the tumor beyond the boundary of safety. And this is done by the continued operation of the producing causes. If these causes are corrected in time these changes will not occur and the tumor will be reduced somewhat or, perhaps, be completely absorbed.

A lady, age fifty-six, came to the writer in the early part of 1926, suffering with a variety of ailments, digestive disturbances, headaches, high-blood pressure, constipation, pains in the back, excessive weight (she was over forty pounds overweight), and multiple myoma of the uterus. Thirty days on no food but water followed by two months on a diet of fruits and green vegetables, resulted in the loss of all of these affections including forty pounds of weight and the myomata. At this writing, fifteen months from the time the case was dismissed there has been no recurrence of any of her troubles, nor of the myomata. She was saved from a hysterectomy which was urged upon her by four different physicians, and since she is living an entirely different life to what she formerly led, I am confident she will never experience a recurrence of the tumors, unless she returns to the former mode of living.

However, I believe we are correct in general when we say that, when the body has reached such a low state of deterioration and degeneracy that it develops cancer it is next to impossible for regeneration to take place to an extent necessary for the restoration of health. In a large majority of those cases operated on recurrence occurs in from six months to four years, while in the few where recurrence fails to occur there is grave doubt about them ever having been cancer.

I have seen numerous small tumor-like developments quickly disappear under a hygienic regimen and I have seen many enlarged and hardened lymph glands, which had been diagnosed as tumors, soften and become normal in size, often doing this very quickly. I have saved many women from needless operations on their breasts for supposed cancers.

There are five considerations which we would leave with the reader:

1. Those pathological phenomena called tumors or cancers are merely links in a syndrome of causes and effects operating in the life of the individual and are genetically connected with the pathology which precedes them.

2. They constitute a unit, one form of tumor with another form, and also with preceding pathological developments.

3. They are conservative and protective measures and serve to prolong rather than to destroy life.

4. These conditions while undoubtedly easily eradicated in their early stages, in most cases, by remedial hygiene, are not curable by any means after they have advanced beyond a certain stage.

5. They are easily preventable, the prevention depending upon a hygienic mode of living.

FEEDING

Chapter XX

ALL parts and products of the body are elaborated from the blood, and all the functions of the body depend upon the blood for material supplies. The blood is elaborated from air, water, food and sunshine. These are essential and all that are essential, so far as materials are concerned, for the production of good blood and sound tissues and organs, and functional results. We are here chiefly concerned with but two of these items—food and water. No effort, however, will be made to go over the grounds of food composition, digestion, absorption, etc., in this chapter. The reader who is not already familiar with these things is referred to the author's Food and Feeding, or to any other good work on diet.

We are chiefly concerned here with the practical application of the principles of feeding and shall address ourselves to these at once. These principles began to be developed with Graham, Allcot, Trall, Lamb, Densmore, Page and others and have been slowly worked out during the past one hundred years. There yet remains much to be learned about diet and it is to be hoped that with the attention of almost the whole civilized world turned to this subject, there will come a time, in the not distant future, when we can truthfully say that a science of dietetics exists.

My good friend, Dr. Wm. F. Havard, has suggested the following very practical classification of diet: (1) The building diet; (2) The Mature diet; (3) The curative diet It is intended here to discuss each of these in the order given and indicate their application in daily life.

THE BUILDING DIET, or the DIET OF PHYSICAL GROWTH,—which is also the diet of convalescence, reconstruction and recuperation. There are certain periods of life when those foods that enter into the composition of the tissues of the body are needed in greater amount than that required to maintain *status quo.* These are (1) During periods of growth; (2) During pregnancy and lactation; (3) Following a long fast; (4) During convalescence from a wasting illness.

The amino-acids (proteins) have been termed the building stones of the body, since these, next to water, form the largest part of all the tissues of the body. Protein and certain salts, such as calcium salts, and a few others, form the materials out of which the body is constructed. These are naturally required in greater quantities when rapid construction is going on than when the body is merely attempting to maintin equilibrium. However, the old protein standard has been shown to be far too high, even for growing children, while nature had long ago indicated her needs in the normal composition of milk, which, when compared to meat, eggs, etc., is really a low protein food. Eggs are adapted to the needs of the very rapidly growing embryo's of birds.

The diet of growth must meet the following requirements:

1. It must contain a sufficient amount of the proper proteins to both maintain repairs and provide for the needs of growth.

2. It must contain a sufficient amount of those food factors which have been labeled vitamins and completins, to meet the needs of growth.

3. It must contain a sufficient amount of mineral elements, or organic salts to supply the body with enough of these to carry on its daily functions of secretion and excretion, to maintain normal blood alkalinity, and to provide material for tissue growth and repair.

4. It must contain enough carbohydrates and fats to supply heat and energy.

In a general way it may be said that if we live upon natural foods, that is, if we live upon those foods to which man, as a class, is constitutionally adapted, and eat them as nature prepares them without altering or adulterating them, these requirements will be met without difficulty. There are all the organic salts, organic acids, vitamins and completins that the body requires at any time, in fresh fruits and green vegetables. There are all the proteins the body needs in vegetables, fruits and nuts. The so-called heat and energy foods (carbohydrates and fats) are present in abundance in these. It is the perpetual tampering with these in the processes of manufacturing, preserving, canning, pickling, cooking, bleaching, coloring, flavoring, etc., that creates the chief problems of modern dietetics.

The element of foods most discussed and to which most attention is usually directed is the protein element. There are numerous proteins in the various substances, plant and animal, used for human food. Some of these proteins will serve well in supporting life and growth, others are very inadequate for this. However, since no one lives on a diet composed of but one article of food, at least not after being weaned, there is little likelihood of anyone ever lacking sufficient proteins.

The assertion is frequently made by experimenters that animal proteins are superior, as growth promoters, to vegetable proteins. This assertion is based on the results of animal experiments, and in a general sense, is more or less accurate. One thing, however, should be kept in mind—*animal protein does not mean, simply, meat protein.* The term includes the proteins of milk, cheese, eggs, animal blood and various portions of the animal, as well as the muscle proteins.

Lean meat is not adequate to the support of life and growth. Meat eating animals, eat the blood, bones, cartilages, liver, etc., of their prey as well as the muscle and fat. They eat it raw so that none of the mineral elements are lost.

Milk, which is designed by nature to meet the requirements of a rapidly growing animal, and is perfectly adapted to the young of the species producing the milk, changes with the changing needs of the growing animal. Human milk, designed by nature for the human infant, is far superior to cow's milk, or any other milk as a food for infants. Taking two factors only, of many, the milk of the human mother is much more easily digested by the infant than is cow's milk, and, while human milk is much lower in total protein than cow's milk, it contains much more of the two amino-acids, cystin and tryptophan, and is a much superior protein than the protein of cow's milk.

Berg, experimenting on humans, found that when only so much milk is given to these as is required to supply them with the bodily protein requirement, the excess of alkalies in the milk did not suffice either for the growing youth or adult human being. Berg says "natural milk contains acid-rich proteins, and unless these proteins are fully utilized by the body (as they are in the suckling undergoing normal growth) the total surplus of bases is not placed at the disposal of the organism." Lyman and Raymund, experimenting on rabbits, which are very sensitive to acids, found that on a diet of cow's milk, the animals died of *acidosis;* but when sodium citrate was added to the food, the *acidosis* disappeared and the urine contained less ammonia. "Milk," says Berg, "is well known to be adequate in respect to inorganic constituents (minerals) only for the earliest period of life; but for adults is rendered adequate by the addition of a little iron. In my own experience, however, as far as adults are concerned, the richness of milk in protein makes the excess of alkali in this food inadequate."

These facts show that animal proteins, on the whole are but little superior to vegetable proteins, after infancy, and in the case of certain animal foods, are not so desirable as we are often led to believe. Soy beans, potatoes, carrots, bananas and seeds, like maize, wheat, etc., have proven adequate growth promoters, when suplimented with certain mineral elements, at least, so far as animal experiments go. That a diet of fruits, nuts and green vegetables, to the exclusion of all animal foods, will suffice to sustain life, health and growth in human beings after the suckling period is past admits of no doubt. Whole tribes have lived on such for generations and demonstrated this to be so.

FEEDING INFANTS AND CHILDREN: All children, except sick ones, should be fed upon a diet of growth. It is during this period of life when growth and development are proceeding rapidly and nutrition is at its highest (except during pregnancy) that the greatest amount of building material is needed. At only three other periods are such food requirements the same or nearly the same. These are after a fast, after an acute disease and during pregnancy.

And yet, Nature teaches by her own prescription for a diet of growth that orthodox standards are much in error. Nature produces milk for the young mammal that is perfectly adapted to its needs for growth and development and has placed in this fluid all the factors and elements supplied by food that are necessary to maintain normal health, growth and activity. She has not, of course, arranged that the young animal ⸜e fed upon this food during its entire period of growth. In fact, no animal in a state of Nature partakes of milk after it is weaned. So after the young animal is weaned it is forced to supply its food requirements from other sources and this food, except in the case of the carnivero is a low protein food, with the green non-starchy foods preponderating. This should furnish us with a clue to how to feed our own young but probably this does not appear scientific enough to the laboratory gentlemen, who can learn nothing from animals in a state of nature but must have them under artificial conditions.

If Nature has prepared milk for the young animal it is quite obvious that milk is its natural diet during the period in which it is provided. The fact that shows most clearly and convincingly the splendid food value of milk is that during the period of most rapid growth in the lives of mammals, milk is the sole food. So efficient is it as a food that a baby ordinarily will double its weight in 180 days with no other article of food. A calf or colt will double its weight in sixty days and a pig in ten to fifteen days on milk alone. It is equally apparent that the milk of the species to which any young animal belongs is the one best adapted to it. That this is very true in the case of human infants is amply demonstrated by the following facts:

Statistics compiled by the Child Hygiene Association of Philadelphia covering 3,243,958 infants who died during their first year of life showed fifty out of every one hundred bottle fed babies died during their first year of life as compared to but seven deaths during their first year out of every one hundred breast-fed babies.

This fact caused one eminent woman specialist to write the following: "The first and most important duty of motherhood is the breast-feeding of her baby. Next to the right of every child to be well born comes the right to his best food, his own mother's breast milk. Mother's milk is the only perfect infant food; it cannot be imitated; and anyone who advises a mother differently is guilty of a serious crime against a helpless baby.*** When a baby is denied his mother's milk and put upon a bottle he loses half his chance to be kept alive, and nine-tenths of his chances to grow up into a normal healthy man or woman."

Statistics show that only two breast-fed babies contract the so-called contagious diseases where five bottle-fed babies do so, and that where such diseases are contracted the chances for recovery are greatly increased in the brest-fed baby as compared to the chances of the bottle fed ones. Adenoids and enlarged tonsils are also more common among bottle-fed than among breast-fed babies.

From war town Europe came unmistakable evidence of the superiority of breast feeding over bottle feeding, which was equal to that which came from Paris in 1871. During the siege of Paris at that date no cows milk was available, and infants had to be breast fed with the result that the infant death rate took a big drop.

Just before the entrance of the United States into the war in 1917, Lucas reported that the infant death rate in Belgium was unusually low. This he ascribed partly to the fact that the scarcity of cow's milk had forced an increase in breast feeding.

Shortly after the evacuation of Lille, Calumet of the university faculty wrote about infant welfare in that city under German occupation. The German's had confiscated all the cow's so that breast feeding became almost universal. Those mothers who were unable to supply sufficient milk for their infants got other mothers to aid them. So marvelous were the results and so deeply did Calumet feel about the subject that he pleaded against the establishment anywhere in France of any infant welfare depot that would give away or sell or in anyway promote the use of cow's milk.

Following the war Dr. Gini of Germany issued a report on infant welfare in that nation during the war. In normal times only 15 to 20 per cent of the babies in Berlin and Breslau are breast-fed. In August and September of 1914 there was a heavy death rate. After October of that year the percentage of breast-fed babies in these two cities almost doubled. With this increase in breast feeding came a corresponding fall in the infantile death rate. The reports from Dusseldorf, Bremen and Wiesbaden were to the same effect.

No such improvement was noted in the rural districts of Germany due to the fact that the farmers had cows and continued to supply milk to their families and to the further fact that the campaign for breast feeding did not extend to the rural districts.

Dr. Gini thinks that in every warring nation in western Europe except Italy the infant death rate was low during the war.

As superior as the mothers own milk is to any other food for the baby it can be so impaired as to be actually harmful. As an instance of this; experiments by the Pediatricians Society of Chicago showed that many cases of colic in babies stopped when the mother ceased eating eggs, meat and other protein foods.

Proper nutrition is the health and life of the baby. Its own mother's milk is far better for it than cow's milk, however cleverly and "scientifically" modified. The fact that it must be modified to adapt it to the baby evinces the unfitness of cow's milk for infants.

Bottle-fed babies often look normal and well when compared with breast-fed babies. But the future frequently reveals the difference. The bottle fed baby has less chance of survival and is more subject to disease. Do not be deceived by the fact that the baby grows fat on an artificial diet. This does not mean that its vitality is being increased or that its resistance to disease is great. Indeed, a fat infant is a diseased infant, ALWAYS.

Give your child breast milk if possible. If you do not have sufficient milk give it the breast milk anyway and supplement this with cow's or goat's milk. If the child must be fed wholly on cow's milk this should be supplemented with fruit juices.

The only way in which the milk should be modified is by diluting it with plain water. No sugar should be added. Sugar causes fermentation, irritation, a false appetite and an abnormal thirst. No lime water should be added. Lime acts as an irritant and is of no value to the child. *So long as the child is given milk it should be taken from a bottle through a nipple. This will insure thorough insalivation and prevent gulping it down.* Orange juice may be given from the second week on. It may be necessary to dilute this at first. The amount allowed may be rapidly increased until the baby is taking four to six ounces a day. Grape juice, made from fresh grapes and given the child without being cooked, will supply all the sugar needed by the child. This can be made at home by placing the grapes, after they are cleaned, in a vessel and crushing them. The juice is then poured off and strained. This juice will also insure normal bowel action. If grapes are out of season the syrup from stewed figs will answer instead. The unsulphured figs should be used. No sugar should be added.

Do not feed the child more than four or five milk feedings a day. Few will require over four milk feedings. Never feed at night. It teaches the child to eat at night. It soon learns to wake up about the same time every night and demand food. No child should ever be fed at night. Night feeding is bad for the mother as well as for the child. It disturbs her sleep and impairs her health. This impairs her milk. Never feed a child if it is feverish or "out of sorts." Let it fast or, at most, give it diluted orange juice. Little disturbances that would last but a few hours, if this plan were followed, are often converted into formidable diseases because feeding is continued.

Nature fits the milk of each respective species to meet the needs of its young. Cow's milk is designed to meet the needs of the calf; mare's milk to supply the needs of the young colt, sow's milk to supply the nutritional requirements of pigs; dog's milk to meet the needs of puppies and mother's milk to supply the needs of infants.

Mother's milk is more assimilable, more nutritious and of greater efficiency in invigorating and controlling the activities of the infant's organs than any other milk that can be fed to the child. The breast-fed child has greater resistance to disease, grows and develops more naturally and has greater chances of living. It is less prone to colds, tonsilitis, adenoids, measles, scarlet fever, diphtheria, etc., and is less likely to develop rickets than the bottle-fed child.

The chemical composition and physical characteristics of the milk of the various species varies greatly. It also acts differently when acted upon by the digestive juices. Human caseine (the protein of milk) acted upon by the gastric juice of the baby's stomach is reduced to soft tender flecks which are easily digested. Cow's milk forms large curds in the infant's stomach and are very difficult to digest. Gas and constipation are the first evil results. Boiled cow's milk offers still greater resistance to digestion. Boiled milk is worse than raw milk. The intense heat causes it to undergo chemical and physical changes that more or less unfit it for food. Its caseine is coagulated and toughened. Its mineral contents and its vitamins and completins are spoiled for use by the baby. Condensed milk is worse yet. Condensed milk usually has sugar added to it. If cow's milk is to be used, it should be fresh and clean. Pasteurized milk is spoiled by the heat and besides this pasteurization cannot be made to take the place of cleanliness,

A few years ago (in Physical Culture for April, 1914, to be exact) Alfred W. McCann advised:

"Where there is doubt about the cleanliness of the milk it should be pasteurized, but pasteurized milk is justifiable only where there is reason to believe that the milk is contaminated with pathogenic (disease breeding) bacteria and dirt.

"It is better to give the child tubercle bacilli or other pathogenic organisms after they have been killed by pasteurizing than to give them in a living, active state, in dirty, raw milk to the child."

This reveals pasteurization as just another attempt to make unclean living safe. If the milk is dirty, pasteurize it and use it. If it comes from sick cows, pasteurize it and use it. To what foolish stunts the germ theory leads!

Pasteurization does not destroy the filth. It does not kill the germs even if they were dangerous. It does spoil the milk. It does permit the milk dealers to sell you unclean milk. It is an outrage. McCann, in this very article tells of visiting, with the inspectors of the Department of Health of New York City, one of the oldest, largest and most famous pasteurizing plants in the city. He said it was dirty and imperfect and added: "The average brewery compared with such an establishment is a model of sanitation."

If there are vitamins (they are probably enzymes) the animal also can manufacture them. Mother's milk, cow's milk, sheep's milk, all natural milk is rich in them. Cod-livers and other livers are said to be rich in them. Worms, insects, etc., are rich in them. These are undoubtedly manufactured by the animals. Given sunshine and proper food and all animals, man included, will manufacture their own vitamins.

Sugar eating by the mother if carried to excess disturbs the balance between proteins and carbohydrates, delays starch digestion resulting in indigestion followed by fermentation and analkalinity. This reduced alkilinity of the mother's blood causes her milk to build a fat baby with a lowered resistance to disease.

In severe and instrumental deliveries resulting in injuries, infection and the breaking down of much tissue, the blood and tissues, including milk, are so deranged and impaired that the baby is often made sick. The baby may suffer with convulsions, and in such cases, if no other cause is discoverable, every effort should be made to find if the mother's blood is deranged by septic poisoning. If there is septic infection or pyemia (pus in the blood) the child should be taken from the breast at once. If the mother is dysemic (a deficiency of mineral or other elements) her milk will not be of advantage to the child, although, as long as there exists in the mother's body any mineral reserves to be drawn upon these will be sacrificed to the child.

Nearly all diseases affect the quality and quantity of the mother's milk. Mother's should for this reason, if for no other, keep themselves well and strong. The mother's diet should be of a character that insures a normal, wholesome milk supply. Drugs affect the milk.

Before the coming of the white man to America there were no milk animals here. (The deer and buffalo were here, but were not domesticated.) Indian mothers were forced to nurse their children and because they had no milk from other sources to aid in weaning their children nursed them for two to three years. Among the Sioux Indians it is said mothers were sometimes known to suckle two children at the same time. This same thing has been observed among the Guiana Indians of South America who as a rule nurse their children three to four years.

However, American and English mothers are fast loosing the capacity to nurse their babies. Investigations have shown that only 12 per cent. of American babies are entirely breast-fed, while 28 per cent. are absolutely bottle fed and the residue from both breast and bottle, but many of these insufficiently from the breast. These young citizens get a bad start in life and the results show up very plainly when the call for men comes as in the recent war. Less than fifty per cent. of the young men of this nation were found physically fit. In New Zealand where breast feeding is the rule the infant death rate is only half of that in America. This is significant and should lead mothers to a more wholesome mode of living to enable them to suckle their own children.

It is as natural for a mother to supply milk for her baby as for the cow to supply milk for her calf. If the mother is unable to do so it is because she is not normal in some way. Perhaps the most common cause for this deficiency is the denatured, demineralized diet upon which so many mothers live. The mineral salts are absolutely essential to normal secretions. Aside from this they must be supplied to the child and if the mother's diet does not contain them her own tissues will be robbed of their minerals. This deranges the mother's health and impairs her milk. Milk deficient in these salts gives rise to rickets. No calf ever has rickets but human infants often do.

There is good reason for believing that the wide-spread practice of vaccination is partly responsible for the inability of mothers to supply sufficient milk for their babies.

We may say, aside from their frequent failure to suckle their young, that the civilized mothers do better after the baby comes, while the savage mothers do better up to the time of birth. After that ignorance and lack of sanitation work for a high mortality.

If civilized mothers will learn to do as well or better before baby comes as the savage mother does and learn to suckle her child as well as the savage mother, this, coupled with her tremenduous sanitary and hygienic advantages and greater knowledge will enable her to reduce the infant death rate to but a small per cent. of what it now is. It goes without saying that they should learn how to care for the baby in every way.

Cow's milk forms a large, very hard, tough curd which is very hard of digestion, and constipates the baby. It is excellently adapted to the digestion of the calf. It often forms, when fed to infants, such large, hard curds that they have great difficulty in passing them. Painful bowel movements are the result. It is a terrible thing for a mother to fall down on the job of feeding her baby.

Scurvy, rickets, anemia and malnutrition are often caused by the use of artificial foods. Many children seem to thrive on such foods for a while and then disaster overtakes them. Be not deceived by the advertisements of those who have infant foods for sale. These concerns exist for profit and not for baby's welfare.

If the mother is normally healthy and is properly fed her own milk will be all sufficient for the baby. It will be a complete food and there will be no necessity of feeding orange juice or other fruit or vegetable juices to the baby. However, if there is reason to doubt that the quality of the milk is normal, orange juice may be given between milk feedings.

The chief cause of digestive disorders in infants and of all those other complaints that grow out of these is overfeeding. The habit of feeding babies every two hours during the day and every time it wakes up and cries at night is a ruinous one. Such feeding overworks the baby's digestive organs and introduces an excess of food into the alimentary tract to ferment and poison the child. It weakens and sickens the child producing diarrhea, colic, skin eruptions, and more serious disorders.

Feeding the baby at night prevents both mother and child from sleeping and teaches the child irregularity in sleep. When the mother's sleep is disturbed in this way she is weakened and normal secretions are interfered with resulting in an impairment of her milk. The impairment of the milk reacts unfavorably upon the child. Feeding at night is not only unnecessary, it over feeds and sickens the child.

This method of feeding which is also the popular one is what really makes the problem of infant feeding a difficult one. There is no way to adapt even the most wholesome and easily digested food to an infant when it is fed in such quantities. With proper feeding it is but little trouble to find a food that will "agree" with the baby.

Three to four feedings (never over five) in twenty-four hours is enough for almost any baby. Exceptional cases that actually require more are rare indeed. No feeding should be done at night. Regularity in feeding as in other things teaches the child regularity in habits. Babies fed in this way develop faster than those stuffed in the old way. Over nutrition actually inhibits function and retards growth and development. No feeding should ever be done between meals. Every time a child cries it is not hungry.

If the child is sick, if there is fever, diarrhea, etc., it should fast until these are gone. Don't be afraid to let the baby fast. It will not starve to death.

231

No other food except milk or milk and fruit juices should be given the child for the first year of its life. At about one year of age fruits and vegetables may be added to the diet. These should form one or part of one meal a day. If four feedings have been indulged in up to this time one of these should now be stopped.

No starchy foods or cereals should be given under two years. The sweet fruits may be added at about one year. These should be run through a fine sieve and fed to the child once a day. About an ounce at each feeding. Artificial sweets—candies, cakes, pies, sugar, etc., should never be fed to children.

Nuts and salads may be gradually added to the diet. Meat and eggs, if used, should not be given to children under five.

Children should be taught early to thoroughly masticate all food and to avoid over eating. If the child does not relish or desire food it is folly to force or persuade it to eat anyway. If the child is uncomfortable wait until comfort returns before feeding. Children fed in this way will grow up strong and healthy and miss the so-called children's diseases. Over feeding, and wrong food combinations are responsible for most of the diseases peculiar to children. A little intelligent attention to proper feeding will avoid all of these.

It goes without saying that all food fed to infants and children should be fresh and pure. But we do well to remember that the most wholesome food soon becomes poisonous if taken in excess.

After the second year children may be fed one meal of fruit and milk or fruit and nuts (breakfast), one of green vegetables and starch, and another of green vegetables and protein. Plenty of raw food should always be included in the diet of both child and adult, if indeed, it is not all raw.

DIET DURING PREGNANCY: In general it may be said that the diet during pregnancy does not differ essentially from diet at other times. It should be a diet of growth, but by no means should the pregnant woman attempt to "eat for two" as this is commonly understood. If she is eating in the conventional manner she is eating for two before she becomes pregnant, and then, if she attempts to eat more during pregnancy she will injure herself

Morning sickness, sour stomach, gas, constipation, headaches, varicose veins, over-large abdomens, premature births, premature rupture of the "bag of water," and many other of the ills of this period are almost wholly attributable to over eating during this period. Moderation should be the practice.

Any craving for sweets should be satisfied with sweet fruits and not with candies, cakes, etc. Cravings for something sour should be satisfied with acid fruits instead of pickles. The properly fed woman does not develop these cravings, which are undoubtedly demands of the body for lacking nutritive elements, and in no sense abnormal cravings.

The pregnant mother should eat an abundance of fresh fruits and green vegetables. These will supply the child with the needed mineral elements for tissue development and will save the mother's teeth and other tissues.

DIET DURING LACTATION: The diet at this time need not differ materially from that of pregnancy. It is customary to decry fruits and vegetables at this time and advise plenty of meat, eggs, and cereals. This is a serious mistake, one that often causes much harm.

The nursing mother need not eat either meat or eggs. If they are taken at all they should be taken in moderation as should all other high protein foods. An excess of protein in the mother's diet causes colic, convulsions, delayed and faulty development and even death in the child. Eliminating meat and eggs from the mother's diet is often the end of colic in the infant.

It is doubtful if mothers, or any one else, for that matter, should ever eat cereals or cereal foods. Breakfast foods, bread, even whole grain breads, etc., are vicious. More harm is now being done by the excessive consumption of these foods than was ever produced by the excessive consumption of meat and eggs. The bread eating habit is especially vicious and one of the most difficult habits to break which man has cultivated.

DIET IN CONVALESENCE:—Feeding in convalesence is usually a very simple affair. One must feed cautiously at first, in order not to overtax the weakened powers of digestion. A diet of growth is demanded. Due to the fact that the work of the disease process used up a large part of the body's alkali-reserve, plenty of fruits and vegetables, or their juices, are required to restore the alkalinesence of the blood and tissues.

Moderation should be the rule. The patient is not in condition to take a full diet at first. Due to the weakened condition of his digestive organs, it is necessary to feed gradually. Combinations should be of the simpliest. Do not attempt to employ a diet of growth until normal secretion is established.

FEEDING AFTER A FAST: After a prolonged fast a diet of growth is again required to make good the loss of tissue incident to the fast. Sufficient protein to supply the great demand for building material and sufficient fresh fruits and green vegetables to replenish the body's mineral reserves, should be fed, after the fast is properly broken. I do not favor the exclusive milk diet for this purpose.

GAINING WEIGHT: A weight gaining diet should be a diet of growth and not one designed to build fat. However, such a diet should not be given until one is sure the body is able to utilize it. People who are underweight are so, not because of lack of food, but because of impaired nutrition. Correct and remove all causes of impaired health first and see that health is restored before attempting to increase the patient's weight. In most cases a further loss of weight may be necessary before a gain can be registered.

Do not stuff the patient. Over feeding will produce trouble. Digestion cannot be crowded with impunity. Often patients will gain weight merely by eating less than they have been in the habit of doing.

LOSING WEIGHT: This is more easily accomplished than gaining weight. It may be accomplished either by a fast, or an eliminating diet or by a compromise between an eliminating diet and a diet of growth, omitting all fats, starches and sugars.

THE MATURE DIET, or the DIET OF MAINTENANCE— DIET OF ADULTHOOD: After complete physical maturity is reached and growth has ceased, ones food requirements are very different to what they were in youth. It requires much material to construct and complete a building but after it is completed it may. be kept in repair with but small amounts of material. Just so it is with the human body. It requires less building material after maturity is reached in order to maintain it in repair than it required to build it up from a tiny infant to a mature man or woman.

The adult body requires only a sufficient amount of building material (protein) to maintain repairs and this amount is extremely small if the body is rightly cared for. We have already shown that the amount of protein required by the growing boy or girl is not great. The adult requires much less. But we do not often find them consuming much less and this is one of the chief reasons why we so seldom find one enjoying normal (not average) health and why the average person is usually broken down at 45 to 50.

The diet of maturity should then contain but little protein. We can safely say that if the adult person never touched any of the more concentrated protein foods he would never fail to secure all the protein, required by his body, to maintain repairs.

The diet of maturity should contain enough of the heat and energy foods to enable one to perform his daily labors efficiently. No hard and fast rule can be set down as to the amount required. This is largely an individual matter and the amount required varies from time to time and with the seasons even with the same individual.

Above all, the diet should contain an abundance of those food elements so essential to elimination and normal secretions—the organic salts. This is imperative if one is to maintain health, strength and youth. These keep the body sweet and clean and ward off those disagreeable and annoying symptoms and disorders that usually accompany "old age."

As age advances it is usually best to decrease the amount of food consumed daily. The reduction will have to depend on the amount of activity indulged in. If one eats properly and cares for the body intelligently there will not be any necessity for being placed on the shelf at forty and Oslerized at sixty. The weakness and decrepitude that accompanies old age results, not from the turning of the earth on its axis, but from the habitual and daily abuses to which we subject ourselves. It is not so much the length of time that a man lives as the kind of life that he lives that ages him. As the old saw has it, it is the pace, not the distance that tells on us. A fast life is usually a short one and is intersperced with much sickness and suffering.

Eating should always be for health and strength, to supply the needs of the body and should not be indulged in merely for social pleasure, or for the gratification of taste.

At present it is the general rule for summer tables to be loaded down with a lot of heavy, greasy, heating foods, just as in winter. Meat, eggs, beans, cereals, pies, cakes, etc., weigh down the dishes no matter how hot the day.

Nature furnishes an abundance of "cooling" foods in the nature of non-starchy vegetables and juicy fruits but these form a very insignificant portion of the meal of the average person. Many are the times we have seen men come in from work at noon when the sun's rays were beating down upon them with intense heat, and eat a large meal of heavy, "heating" foods and return to work. Many times have we seen these men grow suddenly "sick at their stomachs" shortly after resuming work and have to stop. They are usually relived by vomiting but seem never able to learn the lesson Nature is trying to teach. For they repeat the same eating performance next day. Many a man has been "knocked out" by the heat and forced to stop work whose whole trouble was caused by eating a big dinner of such foods. Farmers, mechanics, laborers, all do this.

This eating a winter meal in the summer time is a thing that should be avoided at all periods of life. Much "summer complaints" diarrhea, nausea, etc., will be avoided in this way. Man requires more heating foods in winter than in summer whatever his age. Every one who handles milk knows that any cow's milk will yield more butter in winter than in summer. This is usually attributed by farmers and dairymen to various things but is most probably a provision for supplying more heat producing material to the calf at this time. Whether or not the sugar content of milk is greater during winter than in summer we are not in a position to say. It seems likely that it would be.

In summer one should make it a rule to practically exclude all the concentarted heat producing foods. Meals should be light and consist principly of juicy fruits and succulent vegetables.

THE CURATIVE DIET or DIET OF ELIMINATION: There are two sides to the story of nutrition. One side deals with the building up of the body and the manufacture of secretions. The other side deals with the elimination of waste matter from the blood and tissues. This latter part is accomplished by the use of food substances that never really become part of the body but are held in solution in the blood. The protein wastes of the cells are carried to the liver where they are combined with the above mentioned elements (positive organic mineral elements) which converts them into soluble salts. These salts are then easily eliminated by the kidneys and skin.

The kidneys, as organs of elimination, are engaged largely in the work of excreting the end-products of protein metabolism. There are various of these end-products, and as they come from the cells, they are highly irritating and poisonous acids. Another source of poisons and irritating acids is gastro-intestinal decomposition. The most destructive of these are also of a nitrogenous character. They are the end-products of bacterial decomposition of proteins.

The kidneys, in their work of elimination, are limited largely to the excretion of substances previously prepared for excretion, in the lymph glands, liver and muscles. Before any of these toxins—whether resulting normally, from the usual activities of the cells of the body or coming from bacterial decomposition in the stomach and intestine—can be eliminated by the kidneys with any degree of efficiency and without great harm to the kidney cells, they must first be changed or neutralized by being combined with some other element or elements. Diseases of the kidneys arise largely from the effects of poisons brought to them by the blood for elimination. If these poisons are first properly neutralized or de-toxified they do not injure the kidney cells and do not produce disease.

This work of de-toxifying organic poisons by chemicalization is accomplished by the lymph glands and liver, but largely by the liver. If the lymph glands and liver

234

do their work efficiently little damage can ever come to the kidneys, except from drug poisons.

This work of detoxification carried on by the lymph glands and liver is accomplished by combining the poisonous acids with certain alkaline mineral elements. The result of this union of an acid with a mineral is a salt and another acid, and in each instance in the body, the resulting salt and acid are virtually, if not actually non-poisonous and but slightly irritating. They affect the kidneys but little and do not destroy the kidney tissue.

These alkaline mineral elements are derived from the food eaten. They cannot be received from any other source. If they are taken into the blood in sufficient quantities to serve the needs of the body the lymph glands and liver will have an adequate supply of these to carry on their work of detoxification. If they are not supplied by the food eaten, then the body extracts them from its own tissues, beginning usually with the hair, nails and teeth and then with more vital tissues. Although the body as a whole suffers greatly as a result of this, the work of the liver and glands will be more or less efficient as long as the internal supply of alkaline minerals holds out. Once this supply becomes inadequate to meet physiological needs, the liver and glands falter in their functions and the blood carries the un-detoxified poisons to the kidneys. Destruction of the kidney cells then begins.

But this is not all. The liver cells, not having sufficient detoxifying elements with which to combine the toxins that come to it from the cells and from the intestine, are also subjected to the injurious and destructive effects of these and are impaired and destroyed themselves. Liver disease and kidney disease, one or both, usually both, although, perhaps not to the same extent in both, thus result from a lack of the alkaline mineral elements of food.

The matter does not end here either. The other organs and tissues are involved, both in the loss of their own mineral elements and in the destructive effects of the toxins. The degeneration is more or less general—every organ in the body partaking of it more or less. Portions of the pancreas may be destroyed producing diabetes, the lungs may be so impaired and destroyed that consumption results, or tuberculosis of the bones or the glands may develop. Almost any other chronic dstructive process is a possibility under such circumstances. Those organs of the body that are weakened most by the previous drain upon their mineral elements and which, therefore, offer least resistance to the toxins will suffer first and suffer most. All tissues or organs do not yield up their fixed alkali with the same ease.

Normally, the blood is slightly alkaline in reaction. The waste from the cells is acid in reaction. If this is not neutralized and eliminated it reduces the alkalinity of the blood, producing *analkalinity*.

There is only one source from which to obtain the minerals or organic salts and this is from the food eaten. If there is a deficiency of these, the body is forced to draw upon its own reserves contained in the blood and tissues, in order to neutralize or detoxify the toxins. If this process is carried too far, the tissues are devitalized and weakened. Orthodox "science" considers foods to be "nutritious" and "non-nutritious" according as they yield much or little nitrogenous, carbohydrate and hydrocarbon substances. In keeping with this idea foods are classed as (1) proteins, (2) carbohydrates and (3) hydrocarbons. Fruits and green vegetables are practically unclassified "The wonderful vitalizing acids (organic acids) and salts" which they contain, are relegated to the "ash" column, and practically ignored.

Dr. Trall declared, that "all good fresh fruits and vegetables are antiscorbutic" which is equivalent to saying that they are "base-forming" or anti-"acidity." Fruits and green vegetables yield to the blood more activating acids and bases than all "nutritious" foods together, and yield them with almost no tax upon digestion, absorption and assimilation. "These particular acids and bases readily travel to the blood and are quickly utilized to build up and repair tissues, to promote immunity to and recovery from disease."

During the prodromal stage of acute disease, say of pneumonia, there occurs an impoverishment of the patient's blood in alkali; then follows an impoverishment of the tissues in alkili. This occurs more or less generally, but localizes itself more specifically in the lungs, or in the organ most affected. These alkali-elements are used in neutralizing and detoxifying the toxins causing the trouble. Some have, indeed, advocated the employment of fruit juices in acute disease to supply the body with alkaline elements and some have recorded cases of acute disease in which there was a definite and distinct call for lemons or oranges or other acid fruits. Whether the general use of fruit juices in acute disease is or is not to be recommended, it is obvious that the diet of convalesence should be rich in alkaline elements to restore those that have been used up in the work of cure. It should be equally obvious that the alkali-depleted diet usually fed to patients is not calculated to help, but must always injure the patient.

The conventional diet is more or less deficient in alkali-elements due to the fact that it is made up largely of the concentrated proteins, carbohydrates and hydrocarbons, and to the further fact that these have usually been deprived of most of their alkaline elements in the processes of manufacture and cooking. Practically all the "staple" articles of food as used in America today show a relative predominance of acid-forming over base-forming elements.

It has been shown that when meats are boiled, from 20 to 67 per cent. of their salts are found in the broth. When these are baked 2.5 to 57.2 per cent. of the mineral matter is found in the drippings of the meat. The meat is already predominantly acid-forming, before subjected to these processes.

When potatoes are peeled and soaked in cold water before boiling 38 per cent. of their mineral matters are lost. Green vegetables, when boiled and the water in which they are boiled is poured off or rejected, lose practically all of their soluable minerals. White flour, denatured corn-meal, polished rice, and all other denatured or de-mineralized foods have lost most of their minerals. Beans and peas, cooked in the usual manner lose much of their mineral content.

Such a diet cannot maintain health. Still less can it restore health. It is predominantly acid-forming and does not contain a sufficient amount of base-forming elements to maintain normal excretion. To bring about increased elimination in a sick body an entirely different diet is required.

A diseased body is one heavily encumbered with toxins and wastes which must be eliminated before health can be restored. The cure must begin with the elimination of these morbid accumulations. Often they are retained due to no fault of the liver, skin, lungs, etc., but to incomplete metabolism. The organs of elimination are confined in their work to such products as have previously been prepared by the liver and other glands for elimination. If these glands fail in their work of preparation the depurating organs must also fail in their work of elimination. If perfect metabolism is to be secured it is essential that the blood maintain a certain alkaline reserve which can be done only if we consume daily a sufficient amount of those foods that are rich in the alkaline mineral elements.

In disease the processes of growth, development and repair are slackened or stopped altogether, indicating that the body is in no condition to properly care for the normal amounts of proteins, starches, etc. And we find by actual experience that when these are eliminated from the diet of the sick they immediately begin to improve in health. On the other hand those patients that consume the protein and carbohydrate foods always improve very slowly, if at all. A true eliminating diet is one that is rich in mineral salts and lacking in the acid-forming proteins and carbohydrates. The base-forming elements must greatly predominate in such a diet.

Most people, due to their eating habits, are carrying around a burden of excess proteins, carbohydrates and fats. They are being poisoned by this excess. We cannot make headway in cutting down this surplus unless we cut down the intake. So long as the intake equals or exceeds the outgo, there can be no clearing out of the accumulated surplus. It may be said, then, that an eliminating diet must meet the following specifications:—

1. It must be a "light" diet, that is, the amount of food taken must be very small so that the combustion and excretion of material from the body will exceed the amount of new material.

2. It must be practically devoid of the acid-forming proteins and carbohydrates.

3. It must be rich in the base-forming or alkaline elements.

Such a diet may consist wholly or partly of the acid fruits, or it may be made up of the green leafy vegetables, or else, it may be a combination fruit-vegetable diet.

The orange diet, or the orange juice diet, the grapefruit diet, the grape diet, and similar fruit diets are of this class. Almost any of the fresh fruits and berries except bananas, may be employed in an eliminating diet. Or, melons may be employed.

Among the vegetables that are especially serviceable in this respect are: celery, lettuce, cabbage, spinach, dandelion, endive, chard, kale, mustard, turnip tops (greens), beet tops (greens), cress, field letture, romaine, radish tops, etc. These may be used either raw or cooked, but if cooked, should be cooked in their own juices and the juices eaten.

In the fruit diet oranges, lemons, grapefruit and acid grapes are the fruits most commonly used. The fruit chosen is taken at regular intervals during the day in varying quantities depending on the individual case.

These fruits are rich in organic salts which are liberated during digestion and supply the body with the elements necesary to the neutralization and chemicalization of the toxins preparatory to their elimination. They are at the same time, extremely limited in the amount of proteins and carbohydrates which they possess and are well adapted to a curative purpose. There is absolutely no foundation to the old medical delusion that acid fruits should not be given in "acid diseases." We often find that to give acid fruits where hyper-acidity of the stomach is present increases the distress in the stomach and for this reason are forced to use a diet of a different kind. However, hyper-acidity of the stomach is not "acid blood," and fruit acids (organic acids) do not enter the blood as acids.

The fruit diet proper consists of the exclusive use of any juicy or acid fruit. The orange, because of its palatableness, is the most popular, at least, in this country. Grapefruit is very popular with some. From three to sixteen oranges (or their equivalent in some other juicy fruit) per day is the usual amounts given. These should be taken at regular intervals, such as: one orange every hour or two oranges every two hours. In cases where but few oranges can be given one every two to six hours are given. The general effects of such a diet are:—

1. The digestive system is permitted to rest.
2. The blood is alkalinized and normalized.
3. They promote elimination resulting in a purified blood and lymph stream.

Vegetable broths are sometimes used instead of fruit and with practically the same results. These are used to distinct advantage in those cases where the digestive tract is so sentitive that the acid fruits cause a burning sensation.

Vegetable broths are of two kinds—cooked and uncooked. The cooked broths are made by chopping—one or a combination of the succulent vegetables—up fine and boiling it. It is usually strained after cooking to remove the cellulose.

The uncooked broths are made by finely chopping one or a combination of the succulent vegetables and pressing their juices out.

The grape diet has won great renown in Europe in the Nature Cure institutions there. It consists in living for several weeks on nothing but grapes swallowing the seeds and skins. Five to eight pounds of grapes are taken daily, beginning with a pound and increasing the amount used each day until the capacity of the patient is reached. Such a diet purifies the system very rapidly. It thoroughly improves digestion, increases the action of the kidneys and reduces blood acidity. General Booth used this diet to cure inebriates. He was not only successful in breaking the drink habit in this way but found that his patients gained in weight.

Grapes are rich in iron and have been found very beneficial in anemia and chlorosis. Such diseases as dyspepsia, constipation, catarrh, rheumatism, gout, stones and gravels, malaria, liver and lung troubles, including consumption, yield very quickly to the grape diet.

Obviously a diet composed exclusively of oranges or grapefruit or lemons could not be continued as long as the exclusive grape diet. However, they can usually be continued long enough to bring about the desired results. Or else they may be employed for a period and followed by a less frugal diet after which they may be resumed again.

In feeding these diets the rules for eating should be strictly observed. No attention can be given to combinations since no combining is done. The diet is strictly a mono diet.

There should be no great hurry about breaking away from a diet of this nature. The one who is actually desirous of regaining health will stick to the diet long enough to secure the desired results. After the body has been thoroughly cleansed and the forces of the organism recuperated; when all symptoms of the disease are gone, then a gradual return to a normal diet should begin.

Perhaps the diet most often used is as follows:—

After the fast is properly broken the patient is placed upon two or three meals a day of fresh fruits and green leafy vegetables. Meals are small in order to secure the maximum of elimination. Much uncooked food is included. No protein and carbohydrate food is allowed unless figs, or raisins are included for their laxative effects. A diet of this kind would be fruit for breakfast, a large uncooked vegetable salad and one cooked non-starchy vegetable at noon and fruit for supper. This diet may be used in hyperacidity of the stomach.

A diet of this kind may be continued indefinitely. The meals may be varied from day to day to avoid monotony. The number of articles of food taken at each meal should be limited to two or three. It should be constantly borne in mind that a diseased person cannot be fed like a harvest hand if he or she is to recover health rapidly.

There are many articles of food that the well man and even the sick man may eat without killing him instantly, and many patients think they should be allowed to indulge in these. They hold to the popular idea that they should eat anything that agrees with them, meaning by this, anything that produces no immediate discomfort. However, the problem of the dietitian is to feed what is best for the patient, and not merely the thing that the patient may eat without immediate evidence of injury. This same rule should be adhered to by the patient after the cure is completed. He should realize that the same course of conduct in eating, and otherwise, that made him sick the first time will do so a second time, if he returns to it. We can maintain health only by healthful living. Therefore, after the cure is completed, observe the rules for eating and combining and no disease as a result of dietetic indiscretions will arise.

Almost everyone thinks diet is the treatment par excellence for all digestive troubles, but few are able to see any connection between diet and lumbago or gout or pneumonia, etc. But diet alone will seldom cure so simple a digestive disorder as indigestion. This is due to the fact that indigestion is not always due to dietetic errors and seldom, if ever, due to these alone. Indigestion may be due to enervation brought on by any cause. It may be due to worry, to lack of sleep, overwork, or other causes as well as to dietetic errors. Or it may be due to any combination of these. Consequently, before the indigestion can be cured the enervating influences must be corrected. Temporary relief may be secured by carefully adjusting the diet to the digestive capacity but such relief is never cure. Coincident with the dietary adjustment must go the correction of all enervating influences.

Here is a rule that should always be followed in feeding a patient or in treating him in any other way: MAKE THE FUNCTIONAL ABILITIES OF THE WEAKEST ORGAN OR PART THE PHYSIOLOGICAL STANDARD. Suppose we have a bridge that in its strongest parts is capable of sustaining a weight of fifty tons, but in its weakest parts will sustain only ten tons. Now suppose we use the strongest parts of the bridge as our standard and start across with a load weighing forty tons. When we come to the weak part, that is only capable of sustaining ten tons, there is a collapse, and we go down with our truck and its cargo into the river.

This would be similar to feeding a patient with strong digestive powers as though all parts of the body were equally as strong. If we make the functional abilities of the strongest organ our physiological standard and feed accordingly we will have a break down of our physiological bridge in its weaker parts. If the skin is inactive a heavier burden is thrown upon the kidneys and these suffer. If the lungs are weak, these are not able to perform the work required to furnish oxygen enough to properly metabolize the meal. If the pancreas or the liver is weak, carbohydrate metabolism suffers. If the heart is weak, it suffers under the burdens, etc.

Never stuff a patient merely because his stomach can stand it. Never stuff a patient because no apparent ill effects follow. The breakdown may not come for a week or a month or more. If distress follows a meal—distress in any part of the body—take the hint and do better next time.

Observe these two rules—eat only to supply the actual needs of the body, and eat only fresh, clean, wholesome, natural foods—and all other rules of diet become of secondary importance. However, if we observe these other rules they will aid us in observing those two primary rules—of moderation and naturalness.

The first rule in any truly natural system of feeding should be: EAT ONLY WHEN HUNGRY. If we do this we eat only to supply the demands of the body. We cannot repeat too often the admonition, do not eat if not hungry.

Hunger is the voice of nature saying to us that food is required. There is no other true guide to when to eat. The time of day, the habitual meal time, etc. these are not true guides.

But there is a vast difference between hunger and what is called appetite. Appetite is a counterfeit hunger, a creature of habit and cultivation, and may be due to any one of a number of things; such as the arrival of the habitual meal time, the sight, taste or smell of food, condiments and seasonings, or even the thought of food. In some diseased states there is an almost constant and insatiable appetite. None of these things can arouse true hunger for this comes only when there is an actual need of food.

One may have an appetite for tobacco, coffee, tea, opium, alcohol, etc., but he can never be hungry for these since they serve no real physiological need.

Appetite is often accompanied by a gnawing or "all gone" sensation in the stomach, or a general sense of weakness, there may even be mental depression. Such symptoms usually belong to the diseased stomach of a glutton and will pass away if their owner will refrain from eating for a few days. They are temporarily relieved by eating and this leads to the idea that it was food that was needed. But such sensations and feelings do not accompany true hunger. In true hunger one is not aware that he has a stomach for this like thirst is a mouth and throat sensation. Real hunger arises spontaneously, that is without the agency of some external factor and is accompanied by a "watering of the mouth" and usually by a conscious desire for some particular food.

The hungry person is able to eat a crust of dry bread and relish it. One who only has an appetite must needs have his food seasoned and spiced before he can enjoy it. Even a gormand is able to enjoy a hearty meal if there is sufficient seasoning to whip up his jaded appetite and arouse his palsied taste. But he would be many times the better for it if he would only await the arrival of true hunger before eating.

If this plan were followed, what would become of our present three meals a day plan? It would be relegated to oblivion where it truly belongs. It should be known that the three meals a day custom is really a modern one. So far as history records none of the nations of antiquity practiced it. At the period of their greatest power the Greeks and Romans ate only one meal a day. Among the many things that have been offered as an explanation for their physical, mental and moral decline has been their sensuous indulgence in food which came with power and riches. Whatever other factors may have contrived to bring about their decline (and certain it is there were more than one factor) there can be no doubt that their excessive indulgence in the pleasures of the palate contributed its fair share.

Dr. Oswald says that "during the zenith period of Grecian and Roman civilization monogamy was not half as firmly established as the rule that a health-loving man should content himself with one meal a day, and never eat till he had leisure to digest, i. e., not till the day's work was wholy done. For more than a thousand years the one meal plan was the established rule among the civilized nations inhabiting the coast-lands of the Mediterranean. The evening repast—call it supper or dinner—was a kind of domestic festival, the reward of the day's toil, an enjoyment which rich and poor refrained from marring by premature gratifications of their appetite."

Herodotus records that the invading hosts (said to have numbered over five millions, but probably slightly over-estimated), of the Persian General, Xerxes, had to be fed by the conquered cities along their line of march. He states as a fortunate circumstance, the fact that the Persians, even including the Monarch and his courtiers, ate but one meal a day.

Those were in days when men and not machinery did the heavy work of the world. There were no trade unions and no eight hour work days. Labor was hard and the days long. Soldiers marched and fought in heavy armor. It has been said that the armor of a Roman soldier would crush the soldier of today.

Gastronomic atheletes, who imagine they would faint and soon perish if they did not have their three and four meals daily, might think on these things, if their over-burdened bodies will permit them to think.

Dr. Page proved that a little child may be taught to guzzle day and night, or to content himself with two to four meals a day. The baby that has been in the habit of guzzling milk a hundred times a day and night, will howl the roof off if you attempt to cut him down to seventy-five guzzles, but after a time he will become satisfied with three to four milk feedings a day.

We teach children glutteny in infancy. We build in them morbid appetencies. We teach them to eat at all hours of the day and night. We encourage them to over eat. Then we wonder why they become sick—why they have colic, colds, diarrhea, constipation, fevers and other troubles. We wonder why they are troubled with enlarged tonsils and finally become anemic.

Children are the most abused elements of our population. Ignorant parents and even more ignorant "child specialists" abuse them more in feeding and drugging than in other ways.

There is no more reason why human babies should be always ailing than there is that puppies, young lions and eagles should be always calling in the doctor—except that the instincts of these animals lead them aright in caring for and feeding their young, while the "science" and superstition of man leads him astray. Man distrusts his instincts. He believes in total depravity.

The Jews from Moses until Christ ate but one meal a day. They sometimes added a lunch of fruit. We recall reading once in the Hebrew scriptures these words (quoting from memory) "Woe unto the nation whose princes eat in the morning." If this has any reference to dietetic practices it would indicate that the Jews were not addicted to what Dr. Dewey called the "vulgar habit" of eating breakfast. In the oriental world today extreme moderation, as compared to the American Standard, is practiced.

Sylvester Graham used to say: "A drunkard may reach old age; a glutton never." The truth of this statement is borne in upon us daily, hourly. Such outstanding examples of "good eating" as the late Wm. J. Bryan and Theodore Roosevelt and other men of public life come readily into mind. Our public men are wined and dined as a part of their social and political life and they soon become veritable gluttens, if indeed, they are not already such before they become public men.

Drunkards are often saved a glutten's grave from the very fact that their "booze" deranges and impairs their stomach and prevents them from eating. The use of tobacco also often prevents glutteny. Many men and women possess digestive organs that are stronger than the rest of the body and which, in the absence of intelligence and self-control, constitute a positive danger to their lives. Their over-indulgence in food works all the other organs of the body to death and wrecks the whole system long before their digestive organs begin to show signs of weakening. Such people may develop diabetes, bright's disease, diseases of the heart and arteries, tumors, etc., as a result of over eating and all the while they may be proclaiming to the world that their food never disagrees with them. They are laboring under the prevailing delusion that unless food causes distress in the stomach it produces no harm.

More people are destroyed by surfeiting than by starving, by feasting than by fasting. Simplicity of habits and moderation in eating are the prime requirements of healthful living. When the lives of old men and old women are studied, it is found that, while they have had their pet vices, they have led simple lives and, particularly, have been moderate eaters. They may have used tobacco, but this, by putting a check upon eating, prevented them from killing themselves with glutteny. While, if they attained to old age in spite tobacco they used tobacco in "moderation."

Heavy eating causes rapid heart action just as heavy muscular effort does. The heart works faster if one is awake than if asleep; if excited than calm. Light eaters who avoid stimulants have a heart beat of about 60 a minute. Heavy eaters and those who consume stimulants have a heart beat ranging from 72 to 95 or more a minute. The average of 72 heart beats a minute that is considered normal is too high and is the average standard for overstimulated, overfed individuals.

But more rapid heart action is not the only evil of overeating. All the functions of the body are conducted more rapidly than they should be until the overwork forces them to stop. This does not mean that the overfed man or woman is in better health or has more energy or endurance or more brain power. Rather the reverse is true.

The light eater has muscles of better quality. His strength and endurance are greater as shown by repeated tests. He thinks quicker, more acurately and clearly. The light eater has more reserve power and due to the fact that his light eating conserves and does not expend his powers in excessive physiological activity, he lives longer. He also escapes the aches and pains that fill the lives of the heavy eaters. Overeating does not merely overwork the body, it also poisons it.

One should always seek to eat at such times and under such conditions that will insure the best results in digestion. Some things enhance digestion while others impede it. If the following two rules are adhered too this condition will be met.

Rule No. 2. NEVER EAT WHEN IN PAIN, MENTAL DISCOMFORT OR WHEN FEVERISH.

Any or all of these hinder the secretion of the digestive juices, divert the nervous energies away from the digestive organs and impair digestion. If pain is severe or fever is high all desire for food is lacking. If these are not so marked a slight desire may be present, especially in those whose instincts are perverted. Animals in pain instinctively avoid food. Any food eaten, while there is fever will only add to the fever. The feverish person needs a fast not a feast.

Certain mental states enhance digestion while others retard and impair the process. The illustration is an old one of the person who sits down to enjoy a hearty meal, after a hard day's work. He has a ravenous desire for food. Just as he is about to begin eating someone brings him the news of the loss of a loved one through death, or of the loss of a fortune. Instantly all desire for food is gone.

Why is this? Because the body needs all its energies to meet this new circumstance, and it requires much energy to digest food. Food eaten under such conditions is not digested. It will ferment and poison the body.

A very interesting experiment once performed upon a cat will be of aid to us here in making this rule clear. The cat was fed a bismuth meal after which his stomach was viewed by means of the X-ray. The stomach was observed to be working nicely.

At this point a dog was brought into the room. Instantly, fear seized hold upon the cat. His muscles became tense and motionless, his hair "stood on end." The stomach was viewed a second time and seen to be as tense and motionless as the voluntary muscles. Digestion was at a standstill. The dog was taken from the room whereupon the cat became calm and settled, with the result that the stomach resumed its work.

These facts, more of which could be given, illustarte nicely the effects of the mental state upon digestion and teach us, very forcefully, the folly of eating when in mental distress. Worry has a similar effect. It practically stops the flow of gastric juices and inhibits the normal peristatic movements of the stomach.

Allow me to repeat: Never eat when in pain, mental or physical discomfort or when feverish. If the eating of a meal is followed by bodily discomfort or by distress in stomach and bowels do not eat until this is past. This is the natural way and is instinctively followed by the lower animals.

Rule 3. NEVER EAT DURING OR IMMEDIATELY BEFORE OR AFTER WORK OR HEAVY MENTAL AND PHYSICAL EFFORT.

Many who read this rule will throw up their hands in holy horror and exclaim: "But I cannot work without food! I must eat to keep up my strength!" All of which reveals how little real knowledge of food and feeding they possess. The ancient Romans displayed more knowledge when they said: "A full stomach does not like to think."

The fact is, if digestion is to proceed normally almost the entire attention of the

241

system must be given to the work. Blood is rushed to the digestive organs in large quantities. There is a dilation of the blood vessels in these organs to accomodate the extra supply of blood. There must be a consequent constriction of the blood vessels in other parts of the body in order to force the blood into the digestive organs and to compensate for their own loss of blood.

But if the brain and muscles are to work they, too, require an increased blood supply. In order to supply them there is a dilatation of the blood vessels in the brain or muscles and a constriction of the blood vessels in the viscera.

Every part of the body cannot be supplied with extra blood at the same time. If one part gets an extra supply some other part must get less.

The same is true of the nervous energies. Those organs that are working must be supplied with nerve force. If one is engaged in mental or physical effort his nervous energies are diverted from the digestive organs and digestion suffers.

The animal in a natural state lays down and takes a rest, perhaps some sleep, after eating a meal. Some years ago an experiment was made by feeding a dog his usual meal of meat and then taking him out for a fox hunt for a few hours. The dog was then killed and the stomach opened. The meat was found to be in the same condition as when eaten. Another dog, fed at the same time and left at home to rest, had completely digested his meal.

The dog in the chase was using all his blood and nervous energies in running. Digestion simply had to wait. In spite of the fact that this principle is well known there are still many who pose as diet experts who advise that the heartiest meal of the day be taken in the morning. The reasons given are (1) The body after a night of sleep is better albe to digest the meal than in the evening after the day's work is done, and (2) The food eaten at this time will supply energy for the day's work.

It is true that we have more energy after the night's rest than after the day's work. It is not true, however, that the digestive organs have rested during the night. It is also true that real hunger is not produced by a night of restful repose and to eat a heavy meal in the absence of hunger would be contrary to the first law of natural dietetics. All of this aside the digestion of a meal eaten in the morning would have to wait upon the other work. We can force our mind and muscles to act and thereby withdraw the blood from the stomach but the stomach cannot force these other organs to cease their activities and permit the blood and nerve force to be sent to it.

If food supplies energy, it can do so only after it is digested and absorbed. Under normal conditions the digestion of a meal in both the stomach and intestines requires from ten to sixteen hours. If one is working, either mentally or physically much longer time is required. Food taken in the morning could not, therefore, supply any energy for the day's work. On the contrary, if the food is to be digested, that part of the energy required to do the work of digesting it is taken from the day's work. Anyone who will test this out may soon satisfy himself of the correctness of this principle. Let him give up the morning meal for a few weeks and note the results.

The morning meal is best omitted altogether. At most it should consist of an orange or unsweetened grape fruit. The noon meal should be very light. The evening meal should be the heaviest meal and should be taken only after one has rested a little from his days toil.

During sleep the blood is withdrawn from the brain and muscles. So, also, the nerve force is withdrawn from the muscles. The viscera receive the blood and much of the nerve force. Digestion may proceed without hindrance. If one is sleeping there is no fear, worries, anxieties, etc., to interfere with the work of digestion.

Of course, if one has had a full meal for breakfast and a full meal for noon he has already had too much food and will be very uncomfortable if another full meal is had in the evening. Three dinners or three banquets in one day are two too many. But this is the popular practice, especially among the laboring classes. As a result, they become old and stiff and worn out early in life.

If one goes into a restaurant in the early morning in any one of the larger cities and observes the clerical and professional world breakfasting he at once discovers one of the reasons why there is so much inefficiency, weakness and disease among this class.

They may be seen in large numbers eating a breakfast of eggs and toast or rolls, with coffee. No time is taken to properly masitcate the food. It is washed down with coffee, while the "eater" nervously fingers the pages of the morning paper. After a breakfast of this kind they rush off to work and get through the morning some way. It is from this class we get most of our patients.

Eating between meals is a common practice. Often we hear people say they do not eat much. Indeed, they don't compared to what is usually consumed by others, if we compare only what they eat at meal time. But these people often eat more food between meals than at any other time. A cow with seven stomachs and eating grass requires the larger part of a day to consume enough food. But a man or woman with only one stomach and consuming concentrated foods may eat in this way in one day enough food to satisfy the actual needs of the body for a whole week. The digestive organs are given no time to rest.

Rule 4. DO NOT DRINK WITH THE MEALS.

This is a very important rule and should be adhered too strictly. It has reference to the use of water, tea, coffee, cocoa or other watered drinks while eating. Milk is a food, not a drink.

Laboratory tests have determined that water leaves the stomach in about ten minutes after its ingestion. It carries the diluted and consequetnly weakened digestive juices along with it, thereby interefering seriously with digestion. It is often argued that water drinking at meals stimulates the flow of gastric juice and thereby enhances digestion. The answer to this is (1) It is not the natural way to stimulate the secretion of digestive juices and results sooner or later in an impairment of the secretory power of the glands; and, (2) It is of no value to digestion to increase the secretion of the digestive fluids only to have them carried out of the stomach into the intestines before they have had time to act upon the food.

Water taken two hours after a meal enters the stomach at a time when the gastric juice is there in abundance and the reactions are proceeding nicely. The water sweeps these on into the intestine and retards digestion. Take your water ten to fifteen minutes before a meal and at least four hours after meals.

Drinking at meals also leads to the bolting habit. Instead of thoroughly masticating and insalivating ones food the one who drinks with his meals soon learns to wash it down half chewed. This practice should be avoided at all costs. Milk is a food and should be slowly sipped and held in the mouth until thoroughly insalivated before swallowing. No other food should be taken in the mouth with the milk. Thoroughly chew, insalivate and taste all food before swallowing. Food that it treated in this way can be swallowed without the aid of a liquid.

Cold drinks, water, lemonade, punch, ice-tea, etc., that are often consumed with meals impair and retard digestion. Cold stops the action of the enzymes which must wait until the temperature in the stomach has been raised to normal before they can resume their action. When the cold drink, is first introduced into the stomach, the stomach is shocked or chilled. After it is sent out of the stomach and the reaction sets in there is a feverish state resulting in great thirst. Ice-cream acts in these same ways. Eating an ice-cream is like putting an ice-bag to the stomach.

Hot drinks weaken and enervate the stomach. These destroy the tone of the tissues of the stomach and weaken its power to act mechanically upon the food. The weakening of its tissues in this way often helps in producing prolapsus of the stomach.

Water in coffee, tea, cocoa, lemonade, etc., is water still. These drinks also stimulate the appetite and lead to over eating. Aside from this the first three named each contain powerful poisons that act as stimulants. Their habitual use impairs digestion, wrecks the nervous system and injures the kidneys. The coffee and tea user, as a rule, perspires excessively in summer.

Drinking with meals is not natural and is not practiced by any of the lower animals. Anyone who would have the most perfect results in digestion will find the pursuance of this rule of not drinking with meals, will do much to give these desired results.

Rule 5. THOROUGHLY MASTICATE AND INSALIVATE ALL FOOD.

This is our last, but by no means least important rule for eating.

Digestion really begins in the mouth and if we neglect this important step in the process we cannot hope to secure ideal results in the remaining steps. We have learned that the flow of the gastric juice of the stomach depends largely upon the taste of the food. Experiments have shown that if food is put into the stomach and this has not been tasted no gastric juice is secreted. If, however, the food is tasted and not allowed to reach the stomach there is an abundant secretion of this juice. This should emphasize the importance of thoroughly tasting the food before it is swallowed. It should be known that food must be chewed and thoroughly insalivated before it can be properly tasted. In fact, the longer one holds the food in the mouth the more taste he discovers.

Certain substances arising as by-products of salivary digestion aid in accelerating gastric digestion. These by-products cannot arise if there is no salivary digestion. It is therefore very necessary that we thoroughly masticate and insalivate our food before swallowing it.

Food that has been completely broken up by chewing is readily accessible to the digestive juices but foods that are swallowed in chunks require much longer time for digestion. Much energy may be saved in the digestive process if we but take a little time and chew the food. Besides, this, swallowing food without chewing it leads to overeating, hurried eating and all the train of digestive evils that arise from these. Allow me to repeat: Thoroughly masticate and insalivate all food before swallowing.

Let us now turn our attention to food combinations. Much that is written upon food combinations is untrue and misleading. Too much effort has been spent in trying to make it appear mysterious and hard to understand. While almost everyone who writes upon food combinations have varying rules, the truth is that the rules for combining food are few and simple. These are based upon the facts which we know about foods, their digestion and use. In the following pages we shall try to make the rules so plain that a child may understand them.

The best rule for combining food that has ever set down is "don't do it." That is the rule advocated by many of eating only one article of food at a meal or as it is termed the mono-diet. There can be no doubt about this practice assuring best results in digestion and if due care is exercised in selecting the food for each meal a sufficient variety can be had to supply all the needs of the body. At the same time this method of eating would tend to prevent over eating.

To follow this rule is not absolutely essential to health and strength; besides by giving a little attention to how we combine our foods and by eating according to the rules laid down above we may get practically the same results.

The greater the variety of food eaten at any one meal the more it complicates the digestive process. The number of articles taken at one meal should be limited. Simple dishes and few of them—not more than four. This is not the general practice. But the general practice leads to disease. The average person has learned that we require a variety of foods and attempts to obtain his variety all at once.

The enzyme ptyalin acts only in an alkaline medium. It is destroyed by a mild acid. Therefore: NEVER EAT CARBOHYDRATE FOODS AND ACID FOODS AT THE SAME MEAL. By this we mean, do not eat bread or cereals or potatoes, etc., with oranges, grapefruit or pineapple or peaches, etc. The acid not only prevents carbohydrate digestion by destroying the ptyalin but it favors carbohydrate fermentation. The fermentation destroys the food and gives rise to carbon dioxide and alcohol.

The flow of gastric juice depends chiefly upon the taste of protein food. If no protein is tasted no gastric juice is secreted. If much gastric juice (which is acid) is poured into the stomach it prevents carbohydrate digestion. For this reason: NEVER EAT A CONCENTRATED PROTEIN AND A CONCENTRATED CARBOHYDRATE AT THE SAME MEAL. That is, do not eat meat or eggs or cheese, etc., with bread or cereals or potatoes or cakes, etc. To do so will not only cause the suspension of carbohydrate digestion in the stomach but the carbohydrate is forced to remain in the stomach until protein digestion is completed. It is then poured into the intestine in a half prepared state, not having undergone salivary digestion. It will likely have already begun to ferment.

An acid process (gastric digestion) and an alkaline process (salivary digestion) cannot be carried on at the same time in an ideal way in the stomach. In fact, they cannot proceed together at all for long as the rising acidity of the stomach contents soon stops carbohydrate digestion completely. Carbohydrate fermentation then ensues.

The eating of two concentrated protein foods at the same meal complicates the digestive process and and leads to over eating of proteins. There are grounds for believing that when two proteins are eaten together the enzyme responsible for their digestion will not attack one protein until the other protein is digested.

Certain it is that if two such foods are taken at the same meal we are sure to consume an over supply of that kind of food. For this reason: NEVER EAT TWO CONCENTRATED PROTEIN FOODS AT THE SAME MEAL. This is to say: do not eat meat and eggs or meat and cheese or eggs and cheese at the same meal. The eating of meat and milk or eggs and milk is also to be condemned.

The practice of eating starches that have been disguised by sweets is also a bad way to eat two carbohydrates. If sugar is taken into the mouth it quickly fills with saliva but no ptyalin is present. Ptyalin is essential to starch digestion. If the starch is disguised with sugar, jellies, jams, syrups, etc., the taste buds are deceived and carbohydrate digestion is impaired.

Soups, which are usually swallowed without mastication and insalivation should not contain starch. Mr. Fletcher advocated masticating soups.

Finally, THE BULK OF EACH MEAL SHOULD CONSIST OF FRESH FRUITS OR FRESH GREEN VEGETABLES. This for the following reasons:—

First: It prevents over eating on the concentrated foods.

Second: It assures an abundant supply of the positive organic mineral elements without which the other elements cannot be utilized.

Third: If such things as vitamins exist, it will supply an abundance of these.

Fourth: These foods supply the bulk to the food so necessary to normal peristalsis.

Fifth: Neither last not least, these foods resist putrefactive changes in the stomach and intestine thus helping to keep it clean and aseptic.

All fresh fruits and green vegetables should be taken uncooked if the above results are desired as the cooking impairs the food. They may be eaten separately or a salads. No dressings or other means of disguising these salads and deceiving the sense of taste should be used on them.

Some uncooked food should be consumed at each meal. A good rule is to eat a large fruit or vegetable salad at the beginning of each meal as this will prevent over eating of the more concentrated foods.

Any vegetables or fruits that are cooked should be cooked in their own juices, and these juices should be retained and eaten. We once read of a lady who ate spinach to supply her system with certain mineral salts which were lacking in her diet. She boiled the spinach and poured the water it had been boiled in down the sink. Most of the soluable salts in the spinach went down the drain pipe with the water. The lady got very little of them.

As a general rule the chief meal of the day should consist of a fruit or vegetable salad (all salads should be uncooked and devoid of all dressings, condiments, seasonings, etc.) one or two cooked non-starchy vegetables and then the protein or starch food that is to accompany the meal. Either fruit or vegetable salad will combine well with all non-starchy foods, including all protein foods. Fruit salads should be combined with the protein meal but never with the starch meal. Acid fruits may be taken with milk contrary opinions notwithstanding. Hunger makes the best sauce to spread over a meal. Use it, but no other.

Do not become a "diet bug." Once your meal is swallowed let it digest. To be continually worrying because you did not get a correct combination, or couldn't get the food you wanted and had to take what you didn't want, or for some other cause, does not help matters one bit, but it does interfere with digestion.

CONDIMENTS: To a normal person, the attractiveness of alimentary substances (food and drink) is proportioned to the degree of their healthfulness and their nutritive value. No normal person is ever misled by an innate craving for unwholesome food, nor by any instinctive aversion to wholesome foods. However, by beginning a carefully graduated plan of "education" the sense of taste can be so demoralized that

245

it will reject wholesome foods and demand the most unwholesome substances. Among those pernicious substances demanded by the perverted taste are condiments and "relishes." These things possess little or no food value and there does not exist a single excuse for their use.

They blunt and deprave the sense of taste, so that the natural flavors of foods are neither detected nor appreciated or relished. They overstimulate and weaken the glands of mouth, stomach and intestine. They irritate the lining membranes of the alimentary canal causing these to thicken, toughen and harden and thus impairs their functional powers. They create a fictitious desire for food and induce overeating. They create a false thirst, one that cannot be satisfied with water. They retard and derange digestion.

They disguise the food eaten. The precise adaptation of the digestive juices to the character of the food eaten is accomplished by nerve impulses set in motion by the taste of the food eaten. Where the food is camouflaged by salt, pepper, mustard, horse radish, vinegar, oil, various dressings and seasonings, nutmeg, spices, sugar and other condiments and "relishes" this adaptation of digestive juices to food is imperfectly accomplished. Digestion suffers as a consequence.

No one need ever develop a craving for these substances and where it is already developed it can be easily overcome if one will give up their use and persist in abstaining from them for a time. When the sense of taste is restored to normal he will then find fine, delicate flavors in foods which he never knew existed.

IDIOSYNCRACIES: It is no doubt true that the normal individual is able to eat anything that anyone else may eat. However, few are normal, and we frequently meet with those who cannot eat certain foods without suffering.

Some people develop skin eruptions after eating strawberries and some other foods. These people should be placed on a diet of strawberries and fed strawberries exclusively until the trouble ends.

Some people are constipated by cheese. This indicates enervation, correct the causes of enervation.

Oranges cause gas with some. Pears and apples do the same for others. Cooked cabbage and cauliflower produce gas in some. Many will have catarrh and a coated tongue as long as they use milk, even if it is but one glass a day. Some fruits cause diarrhea in some patients. Eggs and meat often bring on asthmatic attacks in certain individuals. This is, however, only after such individuals are already poisoned with an excess of protein. Many patients are made uncomfortable (have a heavy feeling in the stomach) when they eat spinach.

All these things have to be considered in planning a diet for a patient. When normal digestion is re-established these things disappear, but while digestion is still impaired, those foods that cause trouble are best omitted from the patient's diet. Often, however, a patient thinks that a certain article of diet causes him trouble, when it is only the wrong combination that produces the trouble. A patient will complain that acid fruits cause gas. Upon inquiry you find that these have been taken with a breakfast of cereal and sugar, and egg on toast. You put the patient upon an acid fruit diet and no trouble results. Wrong combinations are often the causes of trouble.

WATER DRINKING: One of the dogmas of modern so-called science is that man should drink so much water a day. People are advised to drink at least a given amount daily regardless of the quantity of their diet, the nature of their environments (climate, season, occupatoin, etc.) and without consideration for the instinctive demands of their bodies. If they are not thirsty they are advised to drink anyway; to cultivate the habit of drinking a glass of water at regular intervals. The advice usually given is to drink at least six glasses of water between meals each day.

A peculiar feature about this dogma is that it is held by those who advise one never to eat unless truly *hungry* as much as by those who preach the belly's gospel of three squares plus and go by your *appetite*. One should not be surprised to hear medical men advise their patients to drink so much water a day even in the absence of thirst, but one is naturally a bit surprised to find others doing this same thing. Why should one drink without thirst? Is this more appropriate than eating without hunger? Does not the body know when water is needed?

I shall not censure the advocates of this dogma, for I once believed it and practiced it myself. Now, however, I often go for as much as a week with but one glass of water. For several years I have avoided drinking when not thirsty and I am convinced that this is best. More than this, I caution all my patients to cut out their water drinking habit. Benefit always follows the adoption of this advice.

Excesive water drinking water-logs the system. The power of the blood to absorb and carry oxygen is lowered and one becomes meakened. One sweats more when he drinks more, but excessive transpiratoin is weakening. If you will observe, you will readily see that those who suffer most from the summer's heat are the ones who drink the most water. You naturally conclude that they drink more because the heat causes great thirst. If you can induce these individuals to drink less, you will find that their suffering will decrease, thus showing that the excessive drinking was largely responsible for the suffering.

How much should one drink? I don't know. How much should one eat, or breathe, or sleep? You answer—"All that nature calls for." Suppose we say the same in regard to water drinking—how much does nature call for? This will depend on a number of circumstances and conditions, such as: the amount and character of food eaten, amount and character of work performed, climate, age, sex, etc.

The more food one eats the more water will his system demand. The fasting individual has little thirst. The person whose diet is chiefly fresh fruits and green vegetables gets large quantities of water in its purest form from these. He needs to drink less water than the man whose diet is largely dry. If milk is taken with meals this supplies considerable water.

The man who is engaged in active physical labor in the summer's sun requires more water than the office worker who sits in the shade, perhaps near an electric fan, and pushes a pencil or operates an adding machine. We require more water in summer than in winter. More during the day's activities than during the night's slumbers.

No hard and fast rules can be set down in this matter. The intelligent person will not attempt it. It is often stated that our bodies require a certain minimum of water daily. This is doubtless true, but it by no means follows that we should always drink this amount. We may get two-thirds or all of this amount in our diet.

This objection to the excessive use of water is no new one. In 1815, Dr. Wm. Lambe published a work in England entitled "Additional Reports of the Effects of a Peculiar Regimen in Cases of Cancer, Scrofula, Consumption, Asthma and Other Chronic Diseases" in which he ably contended that man is not, by nature, a drinking animal. In 1850 this work was republished in America with notes and additions by Joel Shew. It has now been some fourteen years since I came into possession of a copy of this work and read the annoying evidence against water.

Dr. R. T. Trall declares: "Hydropathic Encyclopedia," in vol. 1, p. 307:—

"IS MAN A DRINKING ANIMAL?—The question whether man is by nature a drinking animal, or whether the water required by his organism is supplied by his natural foods, has been raised within the last half century. Dr. Lamb, of England, has very ably argued the negative of the first proposition; but the majority of dietetic writers hold the opposite opinion. It is, however, perfectly certain—and the fact has been proved by the direct experiments of Dr. Alcott and others—that those who adopt a regimen exclusively vegetable, and make a large proportion of their food to consist of succulent fruits and watery vegetables, can be healthfully sustained and nourished without water-drinking."

Again, in vol. 2, p. 58, he says:—

"Drs. Cully, Johnson, Wilson and Rausse, very severely and justly repudiate the indiscriminate practice of large water-drinking, which is so highly and extravagantly recommended in some works on Water-Cure. I have seen not a little mischief result from it; in home practice water-drinking is particularly liable to be over done. Some persons have boasted of the 'ravenous appetite' produced by drinking twenty or thirty tumblers of water a day; but I cannot understand the advantages of ravenous appetites; they are generally indicative of excessive morbid irritation of the stomach."

Shall we, then, affirm that all the water should be taken that instinct calls for?

If so, how much does instinct call for? What is an instinctive call for water? How much of our present thirst is due to habit? How much to irritation? What part is normal? Is an abnormal thirst any better guide than an abnormal appetite?

Would we say to the glutton: Eat all your appetite calls for; or to the satyr and nymphomaniac: Indulge as much as your desires demand? If not, then, why shall we say to the man of perverted thirst: Drink all your thirst calls for? Such advice could be beneficial only where thirst is normal.

The eating of salt, spices, condiments, greasy dishes, concentrated foods, meats, eggs, cheese, starches, etc., creates an irritation that is usually mistaken for thirst. But water will not allay such a thirst. One may inundate his stomach with water every five minutes and still be "thirsty." If he will refrain from drinking he will find that his supposed thirst will be satisfied much sooner. It is often argued that people turn to strong drink because water will not allay such a thirst. Perhaps it is often true. If the supposed thirst is endured it will be satisfied with the normal secretions and this almost irresistable desire for water will pass away. On the other hand, if water is taken, these secretions are not used to allay the "thirst," while the water, upon leaving the stomach, carries the secretions that are there along with it.

Those who seek to do the body's work for it and are afraid of letting it do its own work in its own way will object to allowing these secretions to be used for this purpose and will maintain that it robs the system of that much water. The objection is unsound from first to last. The secretions can satisfy the "thirst" while water will not. Besides this the secretions will prevent putrefaction and fermentation in the digestive tract while water will favor these very processes. Lastly, the secretions are not lost to the body, but are reabsorbed.

Just here a few remarks about drinking with meals will not be amiss. Many advocate drinking with meals although there is not an animal in nature that does this.

Drinking of water and beverages leads to bolting of food. The food is washed down instead of being properly masticated and insalivated. Many foods are dry and require much insalivation before they can be swallowed. Washing them down with drink prevents the completion of this first and necessary step in digestion. Forego the drink and the glands of the mouth will meet the demand for fluid by a copious supply of digestive fluids.

While one is eating, large quantities of digestive juices are being poured into the stomach. If drink—water and beverages—is taken these are diluted. But more, water passes out of the stomach in ten to fifteen minutes and carries the digestive juices along with it. The food is deprived of these juices and digestion is greatly retarded. Fermentation follows.

The drinking of water with meals and directly after meals leads to dilatation of the stomach. Chronic indigestion, gastritis, ulcers, and even cancer follow in their logical order.

If thirst following a meal is not satisfied with water, it will be satisfied with digestive secretions and these will bring along enough enzymes to prevent fermentation and accomplish digestion in good order. The intake of fluids with meals and immediately after meals interferes with all the digestive secretions and results in indigestion. One may safely drink fifteen to twenty minutes before and four hours after meals.

However, that person who eats fruit, green and succulent vegetables, and avoids condiments and has overcome his drinking habit, will have little cause for drinking at any time and no cause for dringing at meal time or immediately thereafter. Let him not fear that his health will suffer therefrom. I can assure him that it will improve and quickly at that.

DIET NOT ENOUGH: Nutrition is the sum-total of all those processes and functions by which growth and development, maintenance and repair of the body, and reproduction are accomplished. Proper food is not even half of nutrition. To be properly nourished means more than to "eat proper foods in proper combinations;" it means being able to properly digest and assimilate the food and to adequately rid the body of waste and refuse. And into this complex process there enters many other factors than that of food and food combinations. It is often claimed that life is chiefly a matter of nutrition, although the reverse of this is true. For, in the absence of life, nutrition is impossible. However that may be, nutrition is not chiefly a matter of food. A world of wisdom is contained in the Biblical statement that "man shall not live by bread (food) alone." There are many factors which profoundly affect nutrition.

The available supply of energy with which to carry on the nutritive processes is, perhaps, the largest factor. If energy is low, that is, if the person is enervated, nutrition cannot be normal. Enervation is produced by many things. Any habitual practice or indulgence, any influence that uses up nerve force in excess of the daily supply brings on enervation and thus lowers organic function. The result is, every process and function of the body suffers. Secretion and excretion are impaired, nutrition and drainage are lessened and poor health results. When secretion and excretion are impaired nutrition cannot be normal, digestion must always suffer. If elimination is checked the resulting retention of toxins in the body also interferes with nutrition.

Sunshine, oxygen, rest, sleep, work, play, exercise, mental states, sex habits, damaged organs, and many other things influence, one way or another, the nutritive processes, and when any of these are damaging nutrition, it must be corrected before the best of diets can be properly utilized by the body to the fullest.

FASTING—PHYSIOLOGICAL REST

CHAPTER XXI

BY fasting is meant voluntary abstinence from all food except water. Restricted or limited diets are not fasts. The so-called fruit fast is a fruit diet, not a fast.

Fasting had its origin in the dim uncertainties of the long forgotten past when the first wounded animal found that it had no desire for food. From that time to this both animals and man have instinctively resorted to fasting when sick. Ancient physicians well understood the value of abstinence from food in acute disease.

Dr. Oswald says: "A germ disease, as virulent as syphilis, and long considered too persistent for any but palliative methods of treatment (by mercury, etc.) was radically cured by the fasting cures, prescribed in the Arabian hospitals of Egypt, at the time of the French occupation. Avicena already alludes to the efficacy of that specific, which he seems to have employed with similar success against smallpox, and Dr. Robert Bartholow, a stickler for the faith in drugs, admits that 'it is certainly an eminently rational expedient to relieve the organism of a virus by a continuous and gradual process of molecular destruction and a renewal of the anatomical parts. Such is the hunger-cure of syphilis, an Oriental method of treating that disease. Very satisfactory results have been attainde by this means.'"

The conception of fasting as a means of purging the soul is found in all the ancient religions and is practiced in many religions even to this day. This is particularly true in India. Religious fasts ante-date recorded human history and probably had their origin in instinctive fasting in disease among our more normal prehistoric progenitors. who perhaps also noticed its effects on the mind and passions.

At the dawn of human history, the "Ancient Mysteries," a secret worship or so-called "wisdom religion"— a religion that flourished for thousands of years in Egypt, Greece, India, Persia, Babylon, Thrace, Scandinavia and among the Goths and Celts—required a long probationary period of fasting and prayer before the candidates for various degrees could advance. In the mithriac of Persia a prolonged period of fifty days of fasting was required. The Druids among the Celts were also required to undergo a prolonged fast. These "mysteries" in various nations had much in common and were all derived originally from the Egyptians. Fasting was common to all of them.

Among the Hebrews, whose religion was a mixture of Chaldean, Babylonian, Egyptian and other "mysteries," religious fasts were common. The Kabala, a secret "science" and mystic "philosophy" of the Jews endorsed fasting.

Moses, the Hebrew lawgiver, prescribed and employed fasting. He fasted for forty days upon one occasion. Elijah, the Hebrew prophet, fasted forty days. In second Chronicles, twentieth chapter and third verse, we are told that a fast was ordered throughout Judea. David, the Hebrew poet, fasted frequently, one fast of twelve days being recorded.

Jesus, another great Jew, fasted forty days. On one occasion, in explaining to his disciples why they had failed to cast out a devil (overcome hysteria) from a patient, he said: "This kind goeth not out but by prayer and fasting." Luke, one of his faithful disciples and himself a physician declared: "I fast twice in the week."

The cure of disease was not the aim of every fast undertaken by these religious devotees. But we may very properly assume that they were intended to accomplish some great good. Were this not so, the great self-control and denial a fast entails would have prevented them from resorting to this procedure so frequently and giving so much prominence to it.

The doctrine of total depravity taught men to mistrust the promptings of their natural instincts, and while this doctrine is slowly fading from religion, it is as strong as ever in medicine. The proptings of instinct are ignored and the sick are stuffed with "good nourishing food" to "keep up their strength."

"There is a very general concurrence of opinion, says Jennings, "that the aversion to food that characterizes all cases of acute disease, which is fully in proportion to the severity of the symptoms, is one of Nature's blunders that requires the intervention of art, and hence enforced feeding regardless of aversion."

Dr. Shew declared: "Abstinence is by far too much feared in the treatment of acute disease generally. We have good reason for believing that many a life has been destroyed by the indiscriminate feeding which is so often practiced among the sick."

To Jennings, Graham, Trall, Shew, Walter, Densmore, Oswald, Page, Dewey, Tanner, Macfadden, Hazzard, Tilden, Carrington and others in this country and to Keith and Rabagliati in England, we are indebted for the revival of trust in the dependability of our instincts in disease—particularly the instincts that relate us to food or abstinence from food. · These men have sounded the *back to Nature* cry with regard to fasting in disease.

"The fasting-cure instinct," says Oswald, "is not limited to our dumb fellow-creatures. It is a common experience that pain, fevers, gastric congestions, and even mental afflictions 'take away the appetite,' and only unwise nurses will try to thwart the purpose of nature in this repect."

Fasting above all other measures can lay claim to being a strictly natural method. There can be no doubt that it is the oldest of all methods of treating disease. It is much older than the human race itself since it is resorted to instinctively by sick and wounded animals.

It is said that the elephant, if wounded, and still able to travel, will go along with the rest of the herd and can be found supporting himself beside a tree while the remainder of the herd enjoys a hearty meal. The wounded elephant is totally oblivious to the excellent food all around him. He obeys an instinct as unerring as the one that brings the bee to his hive; an instinct which is common to the whole animal world, man included.

A dog or cat if sick or wounded will crawl under the wood shed or retire to some other secluded spot and rest and fast until well. Occasionally he will come out for water. These animals will, when wounded or sick, persistently refuse the most tempting food when offered to them. Physical and physiological rest and water are their remedies.

A sick cow or horse will also refuse food. The author has seen this in many hundreds of cases. In fact, all nature obeys this instinct. Thus does nature herself teach us that the way to feed in acute disease is not to do it.

Domestic cattle may often be found suffering from some chronic disease. Such animals invariably consume less food than the normal animal. Every stockman knows that when a cow, or horse, or hog or sheep, etc., persistently refuses food, or day after day consumes much less than normally, there is something wrong with that animal.

In the human realm the same rule prevails to the extent that we permit. One of the first things Nature does to the person with acute disease is to stop all desire for food. The well meaning friends of the sick man may encourage him to eat, these may bring in tasty and tempting dishes designed to please his taste and excite an appetite but the most they ever succeed in doing is to get the patient to nibble a few bites. The wise physician may insist that he must "eat to keep up strength" but mother Nature who is wiser than any drug peddling biped that ever lived continues to say do not eat.

The man who is sick but who is able to be about his work complains of having lost his appetite. He no longer enjoys his food. This is because his organic instincts know that to eat in the usual way is to increase the disease. The man thinks the loss of appetite a great calamity and seeks ways to restore it. In this he is encouraged by physician and friends who alike erroneously think that the sick man must eat to keep up his strength. The doctor prescribes a tonic and stuffing and, of course, the patient is made worse.

Nature indicates both in animals and man that in acute disease no food but water should be consumed, while, in chronic disease, the amount of food eaten should be much less than that consumed in normal health. If this rule were adhered to by all, an untold amount of suffering would be avoided and many would be saved from an untimely death. But, thanks to the medical delusion that "the sick man must eat to keep up strength," this rule is not likely to be adopted by the great majority for years to come.

251

Many who suffer with chronic disease have a ravenous appetite and feel that it should be satisfied. They overlook or do not know that bad habits will, in the end, dominate and pervert our instincts. Recently a young man visited me who complained of headaches, catarrh of the stomach and nose and throat, hyperacidity of the stomach, constipation and nervousness. He had a reavenous appetite but could digest nothing he ate. A few days before coming to see me he had arrived home from work with an almost irresistable desire for food. He ate a hearty supper and started for the Y. M. C. A. where he was to play in a basket ball game. About six blocks from his home he suddenly became dizzy, everything became black and he fainted. This was followed by vomiting, which brought up not only his supper but food he had consumed at noon the day before. It had not been digested. It seems the height of absurdity to claim that appetites such as he had before he ate supper that evening should be satisfied. To me such claims are on a par with the claim that the cravings for opium, alcohol, tobacco, arsenic, etc., should be satisfied.

I placed this man on a short fast, then taught him how to live with the result that his catarrh, hyperacidity, indigestion, constipation, headache, nervousness and morbid appetite all ended. The demand for instinctive eating, instinctive fasting and instinctive living is fundamentally sound, but we must learn to discriminate between instinctive demands and morbid cravings. Morbid cravings are strengthened, not overcome, by appeasing them.

Dr. Walter says, *Life's Great Law*, p. 209:—

"No process of treatment ever invented fulfils so many indications for restoration of health as does fasting. It is nature's own primal process, her first requirement in nearly all cases. As a means of promoting circulation, improving nutrition, facilitating excretion, recuperating vital power, and restoring vital vigor it has no competitor.**** In chronic diseases fasting is hardly less important than in acute cases. Obstruction of the vital organs, and especially of the process of nutrition, is the rule. Giving rest to these organs is of utmost importance, in order to improve nutrition, and restor vigor. The secondary effect is the exact opposite of the primary.

"Extremes of practice, are, however, to be avoided. Men are always prone to indulge forcing processes. A fast for a few days or at most a week, will often be comforting and valuable; but to compel the organism to live for a month without food is an unnecessary violence. But in acute diseases the fast may continue for weeks because nature cannot appropriate the food; we only object to arbitrary fasts for long periods. Fasting is not a cure-all; it may do evil as well as good; but it *should always be employed in connection with rest of the general system.*"

Jennings says:—

"It is of no advantage to urge food upon the stomach when there is no digestive power to work it up. There is never any danger of starvation so long as there are reserved forces sufficient to hold the citadel of life and start anew its main-springs.

"For when sustenance becomes a prime necessity, the digestive apparatus will be clothed with power enough to work up some raw material, and a call made for it proportioned to the ability to use it. And if there is not power within the domain of life to save the organism, it must perish."—*Tree of Life*, p. 230.

Further explaining the rationale of fasting, he says, while writing of a case that passed under his care:—

"The child has taken no nutriment for a number of days, and may take none for many days to come; if it should live; yet there is nothing to be feared on this account. Take a healthy child from food while its vital machinery is in full operation, and it will use up its own building material and fall to ruin in two or three weeks; but in this case the system has been prepared for a long suspension of the nutritive function. There is now little action of the system generally, and consequently there is but little wear and tear of machinery; and like the dormouse, it might SUBSIST FOR MONTHS ON ITS OWN INTERNAL RESOURCES, if that were necessary, and everything else favored. THE BOWELS TOO HAVE BEEN QUIET FOR A NUMBER OF DAYS, AND THEY MIGHT REMAIN AS THEY ARE FOR WEEKS AND MONTHS TO COME WITHOUT DAMAGE, if this were essential to the prolongation of life. THE MUSCLES OF VOLUNTARY MOTION ARE AT REST

AND COST NOTHING FOR THEIR MAINTAINANCE, save a slight expenditure of safe-keeping forces to hold them in readiness for action at any future time, if their services should be needed. So of all other parts and departments; the most perfect economy is everywhere exercised in the appropriation and use of the vital energies. It is an 'extreme case' and calls for extreme measures; but they are all conducted under a perfect law, which adapts with the most punctilious minuteness the means to the end."—*Philosophy of Human Life*, p. 159-60 (caps. mine, Author).

The body's reserve stores are designed for use in just such emergencies and may be utilized in such circumstances with greater ease and with less tax upon the body than food secured through the laborous process of digestion. As Jennings explained:—

"There is one particular in relation to the lymphatic system of vessels, that deserves special notice and remembrance. In some forms of impaired health, when the nutritive apparatus is disabled, either from defects in its own structure, that require suspension of its action for recuperative purposes, or because the only organic forces that can be used to sustain its action, are, for the time, either exhausted or employed more advantageously in other duties, the lymphatic vessels interpose their kind offices to supply the deficiency by taking up the adipose and fleshy substances wherever they can find them, or any matters that they can work up into nourishment, and throwing it into the general circulation to be distributed among the weary and hungry laborers according to their several necessities,—for they that work must eat. Indeed this expedient is often resorted to in severe cases of illness, particularly in those of protracted general debility; FOR IT IS LESS EXPENSIVE TO THE VITAL ECONOMY TO FURNISH THE REQUISITE SUSTENANCE IN THIS WAY, IN EMERGENCIES, THAN TO DO IT BY THE NUTRITIVE MACHINERY FROM RAW MATERIAL. This wise provision for sustaining life under critical circumstances, should allay all fears and anxieties on the score of eating when there is a lack of appetite; for when there is demand for nourishment, and the nutritive machinery is in working order, and the necessary forces can be consistently spared to operate it, there always will be appetite, and just in proportion to the necessities of the system for nourishment: for real genuine appetite is simply and only nature's appeal for something with which to supply a want, and if she makes no call, it is either because there is no want to be supplied, or she is not in a condition to meet it, and in either case it would be useless and worse than useless to urge food upon the stomach, either in repugnance to obvious indication, or after having provoked an unnatural appetite.

"In an extreme case, when it is expedient to make dependence on the lymphatic system for nutrimental aid for a long period, until all the material suitable for supply through that medium is exhausted, and starvation becomes the alternative to digestion and assimilation, if it is a remedial case, the nutritive system will be clothed with power sufficient to make a call for food, and on its reception, commence operations; it may be in a very slight degree for a while, and at intervals of some hours, just sufficient to sustain the essential organs in working condition, and may need extreme care in feeding, in quality and quantity, lest feeble vitality should be smothered and destroyed. But, if under these circumstances, with proper treatment in other respects, no effort is put forth by the nutritive organs to stay the utter extinction of life, it may be regarded as inevitably a fatal case; for neither the incitement nor power to effort in this direction can be increased by artificial means."—*Philosophy of Human Life*, p. 57-7-9. (caps. mine. Author).

Recording another case he declares:—

"There has been no nourishment taken into the stomach for a number of days, and none will be taken for a number of days to come, for it would be a waste of power to compel the nutritive apparatus to work up raw material under present circumstances, if this could be done."—*Philosophy of Human Life*, p. 166.

It will be interesting to note some of the losses and changes which occur during the fast. In death by starvation the following losses have been observed by some investigators:—

Fat	91%	Spleen	63%
Muscle	30%	Blood	17%
Liver	56%	Nerves	00???

According to Chosat, the losses sustained by the various tissues in starvation is as follow:—

Fat	93%	Blood	75%
Muscles	43%	Nerves	2%
Liver	52%	Pancreas	64%
Spleen	70%		

This table was made from animal experimentation, and agrees very well with the observations of others, except in the loss of blood. Others have given this as less than twenty per cent. The International Encyclopedia, under Fasting," gives a table showing the losses sustained by an animal while fasting for thirteen days. This table gives the loss of blood for this time as 17.6% and the loss to the brain and nerves as, none. Yeo formerly gave the losses as: fat, 97%; muscle, 30%; liver, 56%; spleen, 63%; blood, 17%; nerve-centers, 0%.

It will be observed that during the fast the tissues do not all waste at an equal rate; those that are not essential are utilized most rapidly, those least essential less rapidly and those most essential not at all at first and only slowly at the last. Nature always favors the most vital organs. The fat disppears first, and then the other tissues in the inverse order of their usefulness. The essential tissues obtain their nourishment from the less essential, probably by enzymic action, a process which has been termed *antolysis.*

There are alimentary reserve stores in the body gathered to guard against times of need. These nutritive reserves are ready for use at short notice and with little energy expenditure by the body. They are capable of supplying all essential needs for the time being, and can be replenished at leisure, after the work of reconstruction has been completed. "With no digestive drudgery on hand," says Oswald, "Nature employs the long-desired leisure for general house-cleaning purposes. The accumulations of superfluous tissues are overhauled and analyzed; the available component parts are turned over to the department of nutrition, the refuse to be thoroughly and permanently removed."

Cases of the repair of wounds, broken bones and the healing of open sores during a fast are too numerous for us to doubt for one instant that even during a fast there is still constructive work going on. Aron is reported to have discovered that the brain and the bones actually grow during a fast. Dr. Oswald records a case of a young dog which fell from a high barn loft onto the pavement below and broke two legs and three ribs and apparently injured his lungs. He refused all food except water for twenty days, at the end of which time he took some milk. Not until the twenty-sixth day would he take meat. The bones knit, the lungs healed and the dog was able to run and bark as lustily as before. Cases of knitting of bones in the absence of food are very common in the animal kingdom and numerous cases are on record as occurring in man. This shows unmistakably that the body utilizes the less important tissues to support the most essential ones. "I saw in human bodies," says Dr. Dewey, "a vast rserve of predigested food, with the brain in possession of power so to absorb as to maintain structural integrity in the absence of food or power to digest it. This eliminated the brain entirely as an organ that needs to be fed or that can be fed from light diet kitchens in times of acute sickness. Only in this self-feeding power of the brain is found the explanation of its functional clearness where bodies have become skeletons."

Pashutin records the case of a girl 19 years old who starved to death after ruining her digestive tract by drinking some sulphuric acid. He says her "dead body was like a skeleton, but mammary glands remained unaffected." He also records that in cases of hibernating animals, the growth of granulation tissues in wounds continues during the deepest slumber, even when every other function seems almost to have ceased. The heart may beat as slow as one beat in five to eight minutes, and the blood circulation be so slow that cuts made in the flesh bleed very slightly, yet the cuts heal. Hibernating animals take no food during hibernation.

One important feature about fasting has been entirely overlooked by all the so-called scientific investigators of fasting. I refer to the manner in which it causes the breaking down, absorption and elimination or use of abnormal growths, effusions, exudates, deposits, etc. The "scientists" have conducted all their experiments upon healthy animals or healthy men and are, for this reason, in no position to know its effects in the sick body.

They learned that useless fat and the less essential tissues are consumed first, and the most essential tissues of the body are hardly touched, even where death from starvation results. But, never having watched the process, they cannot know anything of the rapidity with which dropsical fluid, for instance, is absorbed from the cavities or tissues and utilized as food. They cannot know how tumor-like growths are often rapidly absorbed and how, even large tumors are reduced in size. Resolution in pneumonia is hastened, the process taking place so rapidly, often that it would be difficult to believe unless one should see it. Diseased tissues are broken down; exudates, effusions and deposits are absorbed and either used or eliminated. The body utilizes everything it can dispense with during a fast in order to preserve the integrity of the essential tissues. The useless and least essential things are sacrificed first.

THE MUSCLES: During a fast, as has been shown by investigators, the skeletal muscles may lose 40% of their weight, whereas the heart muscle loses only 3%. Glycogen and fat disappear first, and lastly, some of the proteid, but the heart is fed off the less essential tissues. The loss of fat or muscle might occur at any time without impairment to health.

THE HEART: The heart muscle does not diminish appreciably, deriving its sustenance from the less essential tissues. Its rate of pulsation varies greatly, rising and falling as the needs of the system demand. That fasting benefits the heart is certain from the results obtained in functional and even in organic heart disease during a fast. This arises from three chief causes—namely, (1) it removes the constant stimulation of the heart; (2) it takes a heavy load off the heart and allows it to rest; (3) it purifies the blood thus nourishing the heart with better blood.

NERVES: The brain and nervous system are supported and lose little or no weight during a fast, while the less important tissues are sacrificed to feed them. The brain and nervous system are apparently able, if given rest and sleep, to maintain their substances unimpaired and without injury during a most protracted fast. But this is not all, their condition may actually be improved by fasting. In cases of nervous diseases the effects of fasting must be seen to be fully appreciated.

The common practice is to feed these patients all the "good nourishing food" they can be induced to swallow. If they are deprived of food and their accustomed stimulants, there follows a period of depression and an increased nervous irritability Feeding and drugs smother these symptoms just as a dose of morphine relieves the addict who is suffering from forced abstinence from his drug, and this leads physician and patient to believe he is improved thereby. Yet, these very measures, so frequently employed to cure, are often the cause of the nervousness.

If such patients are permitted to fast for a few days a remarkable change occurs in their mental and nervous symptoms. One example must suffice. Recently a young lady consulted me. She was so extremely nervous that if her husband only pointed his finger at her and said "boo!" she would become hysterical, laughing and crying alter-nately for some time before she would finally regain composure. A little noise in the house or outside at night frightened her. She was placed on a fast. It only lasted a week, but her nervousness was completely overcome in this short time. Nothing frightened her any more and nothing would cause her to become hysterical.

Insanity is frequently overcome while fasting. Max Nordau declared: "Pessimism has a physiological basis." It really has what we call a pathological basis and this is removed by fasting.

All the purely mental powers of man are improved while fasting. The ability to reason is increased. Memory is improved. Attention and association are quickened. The so-called spiritual forces of man—intuition, sympathy, love, etc.,—are all increased. All of man's intellectual and emotional qualities are given new life. At no other time can the purely intellectual and aesthetic activities be so successfully pursued as during a fast. To add to the religious power of the fast, sexual desires disappear and thoughts of sex cease to obtrude upon the mind. In India the priests connected with the sacred temples are pledged to the strictest chastity. The Hindu High Priest is forced to undergo a long period of training and purification—and to pass through many severe

255

trials to prove that he has thoroughly conquered his sexual appetites and passions and has them well under control of the higher powers of mind, before he is admitted to the priesthood. In these days when the fallacies of psychology and psycho-analysis are on the lips of everyone and when feminine leaders declare chastity and continnence to be neither desirable nor practicable and insist that they would be harmful if put into effect, methods of attaining self-control in matters of sex are frowned upon. This feature of fasting may not, therefore, appeal to many who read these lines. Fasting does increase one's control over all his appetites and passions, and this will account in some measure for its use by high priests and others in the religions of old.

A few words about the effects of fasting upon the so-called spiritual powers may be appropriately introduced here. In detailing his experiences during his forty day fast taken some years since, Dr. Tanner said:—

"My mental powers were daily augmented, to the very great surprise of my medical attendants, who were constantly on watch for mental collapse, which was freely predicted, if I persisted in the experiment until the tenth day. About the middle of my first experiment I, too, had visions; like Paul of old, I seemed to be intromitted to the third heaven and there saw things which not even the pen of a Milton or Shakespear could portray in all their vivid reality. As a result of my experiment, I came to comprehend why the old prophets and seers so often resorted to fasting as a means of spiritual illumination."

That the mental powers of the faster are elevated instead of being decreased by the fast, I have shown, but I pause here to express my opinion about these visions that fasters see. They are, I beileve, due to hysteria, or autohypnosis. They are seen by people who are called psychic which means they are easily swayed by suggestion, particularly by auto-suggestion. Fasting tends to increase temporarily this suggestibility and for this reason was and is employed by all mystic religions for purposes of "illumination." Auto-suggestion, during these religious fasts, takes the form of frequent and repeated prayers.

The old Roman proverb, "a full stomach does not like to think," well expresses a fact that is known to all mental workers. A full meal leaves them dull, unable to think clearly and continuously and often makes them stupid and sleepy. Mental workers have learned to eat a light breakfast and lunch and have their heavy meal in the evening after the day's work is done. When I was a high school boy I used to miss a meal entirely when I knew I had an examination ahead. At that time I knew nothing of fasting, but I had learned that I could think better on an empty stomach. These facts are due to physiological causes. Large amounts of blood and nervous energies have to be sent to the digestive organs to digest a meal. If these energies are not required there they can be drawn upon by the brain in thinking.

However, in our experience with fasting we seldom see any increase in mental powers at the beginning of a fast. This is because we deal with the sick and these people are all inebriates and addicts—food inebriates, coffee and tea inebriates, tobacco and alcohol addicts. As soon as these things are taken from them they suffer a period of depression with headaches and various slight pains. After a few days, that is, when the body has had sufficient time to readjust itself and overcome the depression, then, the mind brightens up. The special senses also become more acute. I shall speak of these first.

There can be no doubt that all of man's special senses are more or less dulled and weakened by civilized life and by his disease and degeneracy. In fasting without the recorded exception of a single case the senses are remarkably improved. Indeed, so distinctive a sign is this that we look upon it as evidence that our patient is fasting. I have seen hearing restored on a fast. Catarrhal deafness of long standing, where there are no adhesions in the Eustachin tube, is always improved or overcome. Hearing in those who considered their hearing normal becomes so acute that sounds that ordinarily are never heard are noticed often to the extent that the faster is annoyed by them. People who have been deaf for years are enabled to hear the ticking of a watch and low sounds that before was impossible. I have seen the senses of taste and smell, which had been long paralized, restored to their normal condition while fasting. The sense of smell becomes so acute that the faster is often annoyed by odors in his daily environment that he never knew existed before. People who have worn glasses for years and who could not read without them are frequently enabled by a fast to discard their glasses and find their sight to be as good as ever. The eyes also become clear and bright. The sense of touch becomes very acute.

The weakening and deadening of man's sense perceptions is due chiefly to depleted vitality and the accumulation in the tissues of excess food and retained waste matter. The fast by cleaning out the excesses and wastes and eliminating them from the system and also by permitting nervous recuperation, removes the causes of dulled senses.

THE BLOOD: Dr. Rabagliati pointed out that the first effect of the fast is to increase the number of red blood corpuscles, but if persisted in sufficiently long, decreases them. This increase of erethrocytes, during the early part of the fast, he regarded as due to improved nutrition resulting from a cessation of overeating. This increase in red blood cells has been noted even in anemia.

Prof. Francis Gano Benedict, whose *The influence of Inanition on Metabolism* and a Study of *Prolonged Fasting*, are accepted as authoritative by orthodox scientists says:—

"Senator and Mueller, in reporting the results of their examinations of the blood of Cetli and Briethaupt, note an increase in the red blood corpuscles with both subjects. In a later examination of Succi's blood, by Tauszk, the conclusions reached were: (1) that after a short period of dimunition in the number of red blood corpuscles there is a slight increase; (2) that the number of white blood corpuscles decreases as the fast progresses, (3) the number of mononuclear corpuscles decreases; (4) the number of eosinophiles and polynuclear cells increases, and finally (5) that the alkalinescence of the blood diminishes."

Later experiments agree almost entirely with these results. The Carnegie Institute Bulletin, 203, page 156-7, says: "The results of the above studies (of fasting) are conspicuous rather from the absence than the presence of striking alterations in the blood picture," and adds, "The final conclusions as to the effects of uncomplicated starvation on the blood to be drawn from the results of examinations of Levanizin, are: In an otherwise normal individual, whose mental and physical activies are restricted, the blood as a whole is able to withstand the effects of complete abstinence from food for a period of at least 31 days (the lenght of Levanzin's fast), without displaying any essentially pathological change."

Pashutin records the case of a man who died after four months and twelve days (132 days) without food and says that two days before death the blood contained 4, 849, 400 red and 7, 852 white corpuscles in one cu. mm.

The decreased alkilinity of the blood due to prolonged fasting is often urged against it. It is contended that fasting produces *acidosis*. Fasting does not produce *acidosis* and the decreased alkilinity is never great enough, even in the most protracted fasts, to result in any deficiency disease, unless the frequent cases of impotency are to be regarded as due to a loss of vitamins or mineral salts.

LIVER, KIDNEYS AND SPLEEN: The losses to the liver and spleen during a fast are chiefly water. The benefits they receive are mainfold. The losses to the kidneys are insignificant. The increased efficiency of the liver and kidneys as organs of elimination is quickly seen. They receive an added supply of nervous energies due to the fact that fasting conserves energy. Since no food is being consumed, they are allowed an opportunity to catch up with the work of elimination. They are also enabled to repair any damages they may have sustained; that is, heal and cure themselves.

THE BOWELS: After the digestion of the last meal prior to the fast, the bowels practically cease to function. They take a rest. Dr. Oswald says: "The colon contracts, and the smaller intestines retain all but the most irritating ingesta." Sometimes they will continue to move regularly for the first three to four days of the fast. In rare cases a diarrhea will develop even after fifteen days of fasting. Mark Twain describes cases of starving shipwrecked men whose bowels had not moved for twenty and thirty days. For this reason, most advocates of fasting insist upon the daily or almost daily use of the enema. I feel that this is a distinct evil and should not be employed.

The stomach, intestine, and colon are given a complete rest by the fast and are enabled to repair their damaged structures. Piles, proctitis, colitis, appendicitis, enteritis, enteric fever (typhoid) gastritis, etc., speedily recover under the fast

THE STOMACH: The stomach is given a rest. It is afforded an opportunity to repair itself. A distended and prolapsed stomach shrinks and resumes its normal size and tone. Its morbid sensibilities are overcome. Appetite becomes more normal. Digestion is improved.

THE LUNGS: That these are greatly benefitted is shown by the cure of lung diseases, even tuberculosis, during a fast. Shorter fasts are usually required in lung disease than in diseases of other organs and Mr. Carrington thinks this is due to what may be a fact that lung tissue "possesses the inherent power of healing itself in a far shorter time, and more effectually, than any other organ which may be diseased."

THE SEXUAL ORGANS: The sexual energies seem to be almost invaribly absent during a prolonged fast. This was not the case, however, with Mr. Johnston whose fasts I shall mention later, nor did he become impotent. It seems to be the rule, however, for impotency to develop, during a prolonged fast, but sexual powers usually return with full vigor upon the return of hunger, although, sometimes they are delayed.

Both male and female organs are enabled to cure and repair themselves during a fast. Menstruation is often brought on a week or even two weeks ahead of the regular time.

SECRETIONS AND EXCRETIONS: After the first day or two of fasting the secretion of gastric juice is entirely suspended during all cases of fasting. In cases of gastric hyperacidity, two to three days of fasting are usually sufficient to bring relief from this. The intestinal juices cease to be secreted to any great extent.

In some very foul conditions of the body, the secretion of bile is greatly increased either during the first few days of the fast or at some period of its progress. This often finds its way into the stomach where it causes nausea and vomiting. In such cases the bile is invaribly evil-smelling and tainted. After a crisis of this kind the patient's condition is seen to be much improved. The amount of bile secreted is then greatly decreased in amount.

The secretion of saliva is greatly lessened, and changes from a mildy alkaline fluid to a neutral or slightly acid fluid. In some cases it is very foul and possesses a very unpleasant taste, even causing vomiting. The saliva becomes alkaline with the return of normal hunger if the fast is carried that far.

During a fast some patients wil throw off an almost incredible amount of thick, tough, transparent, white, gelatinous and slimy expectoration. Later this may become gray, yellowish or greenish and pus-like in quality. In cases of diseased and long abused stomachs such matter may be thrown out by the gastric mucosa and vomited. Thus we see how nature adopts every possible avenue of elimination as a means of cleansing the system. In cases of mucous colitis, the amount of long, tenacious, worm-like ropes of mucous that will be passed is astounding. After a time this ceases and the disease is ended. Acid secretions of vagina, leucorrheal discharges, etc., soon cease and the secretions become normal through fasting. The urine becomes "thick" dark, or highly colored, smells foul and strong, with a high specific gravity, and then clears up, as the work of elimination is completed. The sweat is foul and usually profuse. The breath is exceedingly foul, so much so at times that one can hardly remain in the same room with the patient.

THE TONGUE AND BREATH: These are interesting studies during a fast. The tongue becomes heavily coated in almost every instance (I have seen one exception) and remains so throughout most of the fast, gradually clearing up, beginning at the edges and point, until, when hunger returns, it is clean.

The breath becomes very foul and remains so during most of the fast gradually becoming less so as the work of purification proceeds until, with the return of hunger, it is sweet and clean.

The more foul a man's body is, the more foul will be his breath and the more heavily coated his tongue.

GAIN AND LOSS OF STRENGTH: As paradoxical as it may seem to those who have had no experience with fasting, there is a frequent, and perhaps always a gain in strength while fasting. Let me begin with a quotation from a thoroughly orthodox and "scientific" source. Prof. Benedict in his report details a number of experiments upon the strength of Dr. Levanzin during his experimental fast. Then referring to similar tests made by others he says:

"In the tests made by Luciani on Succi in which a dynamometer was used, the strength of the right and left hands showed results seemingly at variance with the popular impression. Thus on the twenty-first day of the fast, Succi was able to register on the dynamometer a stronger grip than when he first began. From the twentieth to the thirtieth day of the fast, however, his strength decreased, being less at the end than at the beginning of the fast. In discussing these results, Luciani points out the fact that Succi believed that he gained strength as the fast progressed. Considering the question of the influence of inanition on the onset of fatigue, Luciana states that the fatigue curve obtained by Succi on the twenty-ninth day was similar to those obtained with an individual under normal conditions."

Macfadden, Carrington and others record numerous examples of increase of both mental and physical strength during the fast. Every one who has had experience with fasting has seen similar results.

In the chapter on exercise we pointed out that strength is a combination of muscle (machinery) and nerve force (motive energy). We should add that the purity or impurity of the blood greatly influences both the muscles and the nerves. Fasting brings about the purification of the blood and also conserves nervous energy, so that there is more energy on hand to be used and the condition of nerve and muscle is improved so that they respond more readily to the will. This increase of strength is, therefore, most marked in those who are most toxic and over loaded with excess food. Such an increase cannot continue indefinitely due to the gradual wasting of the muscles. After these have wasted below a certain minimum, while there is no diminuition of nervous energy, there will be a decrease in strength.

It is necessary to distinguish between one's actual strength and one's feeling of strength. The man who is accustomed to eating three square meals a day of rich, highly seasoned foods and taking tea and coffee along with these, and using tobacco between meals, will feel miserable, weak, languid and shaky when deprived of these. He will feel too weak to sit up, perhaps. This feeling of weakness is due to the withdrawal of his accustomed stimulants. As the fast progresses he will feel stronger and more cheerful. Fainting during the fast usually comes, if at all, during these first three or four days.

The faster who feels weak will find that he feels much stronger after a few minutes of exercise. The feeling of weakness is due to the withdrawal of energy from the muscles. Exercise causes a greater determination of nervous energy to these.

THE PULSE: The pulse varies greatly during a fast. It may run up to 120 or even higher, or it may drop as low as 40, per minute. Indeed Mr. Macfadden records a case in his practice in which the pulse went down as low as 20 and was so feeble it could scarcely be felt. It is the usual thing to have the pulse rate increase at the beginning of the fast and then, after a day or two, to drop. In chronic cases that are confined to bed during the fast, the pulse usually, after its temporary rise, drops to 48, or 40 where it may remain for a day or two days and then mount up again to 60. After a few days it will settle at 60 and remain there until eating and activity are resumed. It is, of course, understood that the pulse is subject to all the variations, while fasting, as at other times of life, and that where there is disease of the heart, or nervous troubles it will often vary greatly from the above standard. Where stimulants are employed during a fast these effect the heart more powerfully than when one is eating.

Discussing what, to the unitiated, are alarming heart symptoms which may arise during a fast, Mr. Carrington says, Vitality, Fasting and Nutrition, p. 464:

"I may here remark, however, that such extreme variations invariably denote some profound physiological change, taking place at the time—a crisis, in fact. The fact that hitherto weak hearts are actualy strengthened and cured by fasting proves conclusively that any such unusual symptoms, observed during this period, denote a beneficial reparative process, and not any harmful or dangerous decrease or acceleration, due to lack of perfect control by the cardiac nerve."

Abnormally high or low pulse rates during a fast are exceptions and not the rule and do not denote any danger from the fast itself. They should cause no alarm so far as fasting *per se* is concerned.

TEMPERATURE: In the matter of body temperature fasting presents us with a very paradoxical series of phenomena. In fever patients, the temperature invariably falls to normal as the fast progresses whereas, in those chronic cases where the temperature is habitually below normal, it will slowly but surely rise until it reaches normal, by the time the fast should be broken. "Thus," says Carrington, "supposing the patient's temperature to be 93.8° at the commencement of the fast, it will gradually rise until about 98.4° F., be reached—though the fast may have extended over forty or more days.*** Time after time, in case after case, I have watched this gradual rise in the bodily temperature of the patient; and in every case the temperature has not failed to rise as the fast progressed. At first, it is true, the temperature sometimes tends to fall, but let the fast be persisted in, and a return or rise to normal will occur in every case."

Dr. Rabagliati made this same discovery, and says of it, *Air, Food and Exercise,* p. 261:

"In point of fact, I raised the temperature of a man who was, besides, thin, emaciated, and attenuated by constant vomiting, lasting for seven years, from 96° F. to 98.4° F. by advising him to fast for thirty-five days. On the 28th day his temperature had risen to normal, and remained so."

Low temperature is often the result of too much food, or lowered vitality due to habitual over eating. The case just quoted from Dr. Rabagliati was, as he remarks "dying on the plan of frequent feeding." He lost 13 pounds during the fast and gained health although he had been sick and taking a "highly nourishing diet" for seven years. Carrington noted a few instances of long fasts where the temperature dropped a degree or two immediately upon resuming eating.

Despite the fact that one maintains normal body temperature on a fast, or even has a rise in temperature, there is a feeling of chilliness in a moderate temperature in which one ordinarily feels comfortable. This is due to a decreased cutaneous circulation.

In many cases, particularly of overfed individuals we have what is called "*famine fever*" when a fast is entered upon. It is a slight elevation of temperature which may last from one to several days. I agree with Carrington that "it is, as in the case of all other diseases, a curative crisis, and should be regarded as a favorable sign, in consequence." Dr. Rabagaliati also regarded it as curative and added: "If we cannot fast without fever, it is because we have been previously improperly fed."

LOSS OF WEIGHT DURING THE FAST: We usually say that a faster loses about a pound a day. However, the loss of weight varies greatly depending on a number of circumstances. Fat subjects lose more rapidly than lean ones. The more active, physically, one is the more rapidly he loses weight. The longer the fast progresses the less rapid is the loss in weight. Losses of five or six pounds a day for the first two or three days are often recorded. But such losses are not losses of flesh. Most of this apparent loss is due to the emptying of the alimentary canal of several pounds of food and feces which is not replaced by more food. In one fast of thirty days conducted by the author the loss during the last five days was one-fourth of a pound a day. The patient was moderately active from 9 A. M. to 7 P. M. each day. During Mr. Johnston's thirty day fast he lost from one-half a pound to two pounds a day. On the thirtieth day of the fast his loss was one-half pound. On the twenty-second and twenty-third days he weighed the same, apparently losing nothing. This, however, was due to profuse water drinking. I have seen cases gain weight for two and three days at a time from drinking so much water. At the beginning of his 30 day fast Mr. Johnston weighed 154½ lbs. At its completion, his weight was 131½ lbs. his total loss being 23 lbs. During the twenty days of walking from Chicago, without food he lost 37½ lbs. or 14½ lbs. more than in the previous fast of thirty days.

It is said that a man may lose forty per cent of his normal weight before his life is endangered. However, we know that many fasting patients lose much more than this without danger or harm. Indeed, Dr. Dewey insists that "when death occurs before the skeleton condition is reached it is always due to old age or some other form of disease or injury and not to strvation." Dr. Hazzard and Mr. Carrington hold to the same view, and, as will be shown later, there are facts which support this view.

GAINING WEIGHT AFTER THE FAST: The gain in weight after a fast is usually very rapid. Often it is almost as rapid as the loss during the fast. People that were formerly always underweight and emaciated, due to impaired digestion and assimilation, will become normal in weight. There is no reason why the emaciated person shall not fast. Indeed there is often every reason why he should.

Special weight gaining diets are not required. The milk diet is frequently employed after a fast to force a rapid gain in weight. This I consider not only not necessary but as tending to actually undo some or all of the benefits derived from the fast.

APPETITE: The first day of fasting is seldom accompanied with any noticeable change in the usual demand for food. On the second day there is usually a big demand for food. By the third days this has greatly abated or entirely disappeared. From the disappearance of appetite onward, for many days, the body ceases to call for food until a time arrives when food must be had. During this period it is not uncommon for a repugnance to food to be present. Nausea and efforts at vomiting may develop at the very thought, smell or sight of food. But a time comes when natural hunger returns, when it is very necessary to avoid over eating.

FASTING VERSUS STARVING: The return of natural hunger marks the dividing point between fasting and starvation. So long as there is no desire for food, the individual who abstains from food is fasting. After the return of hunger, the individual who abstains from food is starving.

THE FAST TO COMPLETION: Mr. Carrington, Dr. Hazzard and others insist on carrying the fast to "completion," that is, until the return of natural hunger. Mr. Carrington declares, "I must contend, and strenuously, that the breaking of the fast prematurely is one of the most foolish and dangerous experiments that can possibly be made. Nature will always indicate when the fast should be broken and there can never be any mistake made by those who are accustomed to watching fasting cases as to when to terminate the fast."

While it is often true that some stomachs will reject food until natural hunger returns it is seldom necessary, in chronic disease, to continue the fast until this time. Hunger will soon return after a little food is eaten and if proper feeding is employed no damage will be done. Indeed not one fast in a thousand now undertaken is ever carried to completion.

The following brief summary will give the main developments which indicate that the body is ready to break the fast—(1) The tongue becomes clean; (2) The breath becomes sweet; (3) body temperature becomes normal; (4) salivary secretion is resumed, (6) the bad taste in the mouth ends, (7) the eyesight becomes clear and sharp; (8) the excreta becomes odorless; (9) there is a return of hunger—felt in the throat and mouth just as thirst is.

DEATH DURING THE FAST: In a letter to Mr. R. B. Pearson, dated Nov. 18, 1919, Dr. Hazzard writes, "in sixteen years active practice" she had "fasted nearly 2500 cases with eighteen deaths, in every case of *death a post mortem never failed to reveal organic defects* which made death the inevitable outcome, fasting or feeding." Then she adds: "I have never turned a patient away."

Dr. Dewey says, *The No Breakfast Plan and Fasting Cure*, p. 31:

"As the months and years went on, it so happened that all my fatalities were of a character as not to involve in the least suggestions of starvation, while the recoveries were a series of demonstrations as clear as anything in mathematics, of evolving strength of all the muscles, of all the senses and faculties as the disease declined*** For years I saw my patients grow in the strength of health without the slightest clue to the mystery, until I chanced to open a new edition of Yeo's *Physiology* at the page where I found this table of estimated losses that occur in death after starvation*** And light came as if the sun had suddenly appeared in the zenith at midnight. Instantly I saw in human bodies a vast reserve of predigested food*** I now knew that there could be no death from starvation until the body was reduced to the skeleton condition*** I could now know that to die of starvation is a matter not of days, but of weeks and months; certainly a period far beyond the average time of recovery from acute disease."

The American Encyclopedia quotes Chosset and Brown-Sequerd as saying: "In man as in animals, the immediate cause of death from starvation is a decline in the animal temperature. Death is accelerated by cold, and delayed by the presence of moisture in the atmosphere." Pashutin mentions the case of a man whose temperature remained normal throughout a 50 days' fast and says: "however, we know from the experiments upon animals that only when the total of the body reserves is consumed the body temperature decreases markedly."

The American Encyclopedia quotes M. Chosset as having:

"deprived a number of animals (birds and small mammals) of all sustenance and carefully observed the phenomena that followed, and his experiments throw much light upon the subject of starvation. The temperature in all the animals was maintained at nearly the normal standard until the last day of life, when it began rapidly to fall. The animals, previously restless now became quiet, as if stupefied; they fell over on their side unable to stand, the breathing became slower and slower, the pupils dilated, the insensibility grew more profound, and death took place either quietly or attended with convulsions. If when these phenomena were fully developed, external warmth was applied, the animals revived; their muscular force returned, they moved or flew about the room, and took greedily to the food that was presented to them. If now they were again left to themselves they speedily perished; but if the external temperature was maintained until the food taken was digested (and from the feeble condition of their digestive organs this often took many hours) they recovered. The immediate cause of death seemed to be cold rather than starvation."

Fasts of long duration are on record. Mr. Macfadden records one of ninety days, the Cork hunger strikers fasted for ninety-six days, thousands have fasted to up to forty days and longer. Many fasts have gone on to fifty, sixty and seventy days and longer. McSweeney died on the seventy-eighth day of his fast. While this hunger-strike was on I heard Dr. Lindlahr tell of a fast of seventy days which he conducted. Dr. Dewey records one of three months.

In none of these cases have there ever developed deficiency diseases nor has death ever been due to so-called acidosis. It would seem that a deficiency disease can only develop where the body is being filled with denatured foods. Its vast store of reserves seems to be well balanced. It is known that the blood has almost unlimited power of resisting analkalinity (acidosis), for it will die before turning acid.

Starvation can come only after the body is reduced to the skeleton condition and comes then more as a result of cold than of anything else. This means that no one will ever starve to death as a result of fasting in disease. If death came at all during the fast it would come as a result of other causes. For, even reduced body temperature would not occur in this time.

Pashutin records the case of a girl who drank sulphuric acid and ruined her digestive tract. He says, "some liquid food was given for 4 months but not believed absorbed as it was eliminated too rapidly and no chlorides in urine at all. Last 16 days no food at all." In this case the body temperature did not begin to decline until the last 8 days of life.

WORKING DURING THE FAST: On general principles working during a long fast is to be severely condemned. It has been done. It can often be done. But it should not be done. Perhaps the first fast of any length in which the faster worked was the twenty-eight day fast underwent by Mr. Milton Rathbun, a wealthy grain dealer, in 1899. Mr. Rathburn took this fast upon the advice of Dr. Dewey and continued his daily work throughout the entire length thereof. According to the New York Press, of June 6, 1899, "he worked and worked hard. He came down earlier to his office and went away later than usual. He made no effort to save himself. On the contrary, he seemed determined to make his task as hard as possible."

Others have done this same thing and some of them were even more remarkable. In 1925 a weaver in Jersey City, N. J., fasted forty days and worked as a weaver throughout the time. On January 18, 1926, Mr. George Hasler Johnston, of New York City, a friend and co-worker of the author, began a fast which lasted 30 days, during which time he was unusually active. Mr. Johnston underwent this fast, under my supervision, purely as a publicity stunt and not because he was in need of a fast. He is an athelete of no mean ability and was in excellent physical condition at the beginning and the end of the fast.

During the entire period of this fast, Mr. Johnston arose each morning at 5 o'clock and went down to a radio broadcasting station where he broadcasted three classes in exercises, each class lasting fifteen minutes. From here he usually walked a distance of twenty-five blocks to the offices of the Macfadden Publications where he entered upon his editorial duties. At 11:30 A. M. each day he visited one or the other of the Physical Culture Restaurants in New York City, where he remained until 2 P. M. meeting the people and answering their questions and giving advice upon fasting, diet and exercise. From the restaurant he would return to the office where, at 3 P. M. he conducted two classes, composed of Macfadden employees, in calisthenics. After this he resumed his editorial duties, remaining at his desk until 5 P. M. During most of the fast he would walk home in the evening, a distance of 72 blocks, and spent his evenings at Madison Square Garden, watching the boxing and wrestling bouts. It was not until the end of the first week of the fast that he gave up his training at a downtown gymnasium and his track work—running.

This fast ended on the evening of Tuesday, Feb. 16, just 30 days after it had begun. On June 2, just three and one-half months thereafter, Mr. Johnston started from Chicago, in an effort to walk from there to New York without food. This stunt, I warned him against, but he made a brave effort and ended it June 20th at Bedford, Pa., having covered a distance of 577.8 miles in the 20 days.

This walk carried him over hills and valleys, through wind, rain and the summer's heat and through crowds that flocked the way. Hand shaking, interviews, posing for pictures and making short health talks consumed almost as much of his energy as the walking. These often delayed him so that his walking on several days began late in the forenoon, although it often extended far into the night. I warned Mr. Johnston before he left to conserve his energies and predicted that he would go 20 days and no longer. He would have covered more miles in the time he walked had he done more walking and less of other things, but he would still have ended on the 20th day.

This thing can be done, but it is damaging, even dangerous, and should never be undertaken. Gandhi, the Hindu Nationalist leader, who has probably fasted more than any other man in modern times, has learned the necessity of conserving his energies while fasting. A painful mistake, which almost left him an invalid for life, taught him this lesson. It was while in South Africa that he took his second long fast, lasting fourteen days that he foolishly imagined he could do as much work as while eating. On the second day after breaking the fast he began strenuous walking. This caused excruciating pains in the lower limbs but he did the same the next day and for several days thereafter. The pains increased. His health was greatly injured by this and he was years in fully recovering from it. Of this he says:

"From this very costly experiment I learned that perfect physical rest during the fast and for a time proportionate to the length of the fast, after the breaking of it, is a necessity, and if this simple rule can be observed no evil effects of fasting need be feared. Indeed, it is my conviction that the body gains by a well-regulated fast. For during fasting the body gets rid of many of its impurities."

This warning against working throughout a long fast does not apply to a short fast. I have on several occasions worked both at hard physical labor and at prolonged and exacting mental labor for three and four days without food and I have had hundreds of patients to do the same up to as high as nine days. But I do not think this should be prolonged beyond the tenth day and, where it is possible to absent oneself from work, it is best that all the time be spent in rest.

Unless contraindicated by other conditions, or unless in acute disease, some light exercises should be taken each day during the fast. The practice pursued by many of spending the whole day in activity retards recovery from disease. Conservation of energy should be the guiding principle.

WATER DRINKING DURING THE FAST: Most fasting advocates advise drinking lots of water during the fast. There is neither need for so much water nor benefit from it. One may rely upon the instinct of thirst. Drink when thirsty. Do not drink when not thirsty.

A frequent development while fasting is a dislike for water. This is particularly true if the water is "hard". "Hard water," that while one is eating tastes pleasant enough, is rejected by the sharpened sense of taste. In such cases we find the use of distilled water or the addition of a few drops of lemon juice to each glass of water to be satisfactory.

THE ENEMA DURING THE FAST: Dr. Hazzard, Mr. Carrington and others regard the enema as almost indispensible during the fast. This arises out of a distrust of the body's powers of self-adjustment. There is no more need for nor benefit to be derived from the enema during a fast than at other times. What is more, if no enema is used, normal bowel action will be established much sooner after the fast than if the enema is employed.

FASTING DURING PREGNANCY: In the previous chapter we have called attention to the fact that chronic disease, even that form called tuberculosis, frequently abates during pregnancy. Great changes, developmental changes akin to those of puberty and adolescence, take place in a woman's body during pregnancy. Weak hearts, weak lungs, weak kidneys, weak nervous systems are strengthened. Glands long dormant awaken to activity. Her whole body undergoes a strengthening, renovating process.

This is the meaning of the nausea, vomiting ("morning sickness") lack of appetite and other symptoms that so many women experience during the early weeks of pregnancy. No woman in good health, who is living sensibly ever has the slightest trace of these symptoms. No woman who has undergone a thorough renovation just prior to becoming pregnant and who lives sensibly during this time ever experiences these "symptoms of pregnancy."

They are not symptoms of pregnancy. They are symptoms of renovation. They indicate that nature is undertaking a house cleaning, that the body is to be put into its best shape preparatory to pregnancy and parturition. If they are heeded all will be well. If they are not heeded, nature will usually succeed in her work in spite of opposition and interference. Sometimes she fails. Always her success is more complete and more satisfactory if we cooperate with her.

The development of these symptoms is a sure sign that a house-cleaning is necessary. When anorexia, nausea and vomiting develop, absolutely no food but water should be taken until these have disappeared and there is a distinct call for food. There should be no fears about fasting. You can be sure that these symptoms will end and nature will call for food as soon as her renovating work is completed and long before there has been any damage to mother or foetus. A fast is just what she is calling for in the plainest possible manner, and a fast she usually gets even if she has to keep throwing the food back into your face as often as you eat it, for days. Rest is called for as loudly as the fast and should be had.

If this renovating work is allowed full sway and the woman will eat and live sensibly, there will be no necessity for another fast during pregnancy. She will continue in good heath. But if she "eats for two" (six), and lives the conventional unhygienic life, she will suffer from a sour stomach, gas, dizziness, headaches, constipation and frequently more serious difficulties. She may develop an acute disease.

In such a case the hygiene of the disease should not vary from the hygiene of the disease were it to develop in any other period of life. The pregnant woman should not hesitate to fast for as long as nature indicates if she is suffering with an acute eliminating crisis. Let her be assured that to do so will shorten her period of illness, and that it will harm neither her nor her child. On the other hand, to eat will not help either her or the child.

Chronic disease should not be handled differently during pregnancy to the manner in which it is handled at other times. The author would object to a long fast in chronic disease during this period, however. There can be no objection to a short fast, or a series of short fasts, but a long fast involves elements that one should seek to avoid. Dr. Hazzard says:

"When a pregnant woman fasts, her tissues, even including such essential ones as the heart and brain, will be utilized as may be necessary to properly nourish the child."

264

This is true, but it is not something one should seek. Of course, true to the principle that the tissues are sacrificed in inverse order to their importance, the essential organs are not damaged until it becomes necessary to sacrifice them for the child. But a woman does not even want to lose her hair, or nails, or teeth, nor should she be asked to, where this can be avoided. Under the modern plan of feeding most women lose a tooth and develop a few cavities during pregnancy anyway.

A short fast, where one is necessary, or will be of benefit, should be entered upon without hesitancy by the pregnant woman suffering with a chronic disease, but a long one should be avoided unless acute disease makes it necessary. Feeding in acute disease does not feed anyway.

FASTING DURING LACTATION: If this is necessary it should be done, but if not necessary it should be avoided for the reason that it stops the secretion of milk and even the diminution of this secretion resulting from a fast of three or four days is seldom overcome by a return to eating.

FASTING IN INFANCY: When nature cuts off the appetite of an infant it should be permitted to fast until there is again a demand for food. If there is pain, fever, inflammation, no food should be given. Infants may fast for days without harm. They lose weight rapidly and regain it equally so. They seldom have to fast as long as an adult. I have never hesitated to allow a sick infant to fast and I have yet to see one harmed by it.

Where their troubles are light and there is still some demand for food they will not fast without considerable fuss. In such cases, fruit juices or vegetable juices (raw or broths) may be allowed them. At one period I attempted to use diluted milk (50-50) instead of these juices but it was never satisfactory. A short fast, when baby is irritable, "out-of-sorts," or feverish, instead of the usual feeding and drugging will save them much future suffering and discomfort, besides preventing the little discomforts from developing into more formidable bonfires.

"In childhood," says Dr. Oswald, "chronic dyspepsia is in nearly all cases the effect of chronic medication. Indigestion is not an hereditary complaint. A dietetic sin per excessum, a quantitative surfeit with sweet-meats and pastry, may derange the digestive processes for a few hours or so but the trouble passes by with the holiday. Lock up the short-cakes, administer a glass of cold water, and, my life for yours, that on Monday morning the little glutten will be ready to climb the steepest hill in the country. But stuff him with liver-pills, drench him with cough-sirup, and paregoric, and in a month or two he will not be able to satisfy the cravings of the inner boy without 'assisting Nature,' with a patent stimulant."—*Nature's Household Remedies,* p. 60.

HOW LONG MUST THE FAST BE: The controversy between the advocates of the short fast and the advocates of the fast to completion is interminable. After all their controversies, which give rise to more heat than light, each case will have to be considered by itself. Individual considerations in each case will determine the length of the fast.

FASTING IN ACUTE DISEASE: Nature indicates in the strongest possible manner her desire to fast in acute disease. Anorexia, nausea, vomiting and the absence of all relish for food should convince anyone who is not a convert to the doctrine of "total depravity" that no food should be given.

Let us see what happens if we feed in acute disease. The first thing the patient and physician notes is an increase in symptoms. The fever goes up, the pulse increases, pain and other symptoms become more intense. The patient is caused much unnecessary suffering and the patient's relatives are caused much needless anxiety.

Food taken under such conditions is not digested. Nature has temporarily suspended the digestive functions. This is necessary in order that her undivided attention can be given to the task of cure. Energy that is ordinarily consumed in the work of digesting, absorbing and assimilating food is now being used to carry on the curative processes. The muscles of the stomach and intestine are in about the same condition as the muscles of the arm.

There is an almost total absence of the digestive juices. What little of these that are present, are of such poor quality that they could not properly digest even small

265

amounts of food. Along with the absence of the power to digest and the absence of the digestive juices, there is lacking the keen relish for food which is so essential to normal digestion. Pain inhibits digestion and secretion. Fever inhibits these. So does inflammation.

If the food eaten is not digested of what value can it be to the sick man or woman? A two hundred pound man may become sick with typhoid fever. He will loose weight no matter how much he is fed until when he is well he is but a shadow of his former self. In fact, the more he is fed the sicker he becomes, the more prolonged is his illness and the more he will loose in weight. What more conclusive evidence is needed to prove that the food eaten does harm and not good? What is true of typhoid is also true of other diseases.

Food that is not digested undergoes fermentation forming a mass of toxins more or less of which are absorbed to further poison and sicken the patient. A vertible cesspool is formed under ones diaphram that is much more dangerous to the individual than any cess-pool that may be in the neighborhood.

To get rid of this rotting fermenting mass of food and the toxins it has formed requires a needless expenditure of energy. Nature is trying to conserve energy. This is precisely the reason she has temporarily suspended the digestive functions. It is little less than criminal to force the organism to divide its energies and attention between the work of curing and the added task of eliminating a rotting septic mass from the digestive tract.

The only sensible thing to do is to keep the digestive tract free of all such matter. Nature herself indicates this in the strongest possible manner, for not only is all desire for food cut off, but the most tempting dishes are not relished by the sick person. There is a positive disinclination to take food.

The amount of work done by the heart, liver, lungs, kidneys, glands, etc., is largely determined by the amount of food eaten. Why should these organs and the stomach and intestines be given more work to do by eating? Haven't they enough work to perform under the circumstances? Nature demands physiological rest not physiological over work. Her call for rest comes in unmistakable terms. Why, then, shall the organs be forced to do extra work by the use of stimulants or by feeding? To stop the use of food for a time affords the most complete rest to the whole vital economy.

In disease the body is encumbered by a mass of toxins that must be eliminated before a return to health is possible. One of our rules for treating the patient is to stop the absorption of all toxins from the outside. Feeding during disease does just the opposite. It keeps the digestive tract full of decaying animal and vegetable matter which is constantly being added to the poisons that are producing the disease. Fasting eliminates all this.

Elimination of toxins is absolutely essential to recovery. There is no known method by which elimination can be so effectively hastened as by a physiological rest or fast. During a fast the processes of elimination reach their maximum point of efficiency. The bowels, skin, kidneys and lungs are each and all enabled to work with more efficiency. Even the digestive tract which before was busy with the work of digestion and absorption becomes actively engaged in the work of elimination. The process has been likened to a sponge. During health the sponge (intestines) are busy absorbing, during a fast the sponge is being squeezed. Pains that seem unbearable without the use of narcotic drugs rapidly lessen while one fasts so that within a few days the patient is comfortable. Acute diseases are cut short and made very comfortable. I have seen the almost unbearable pains of acute articular rheumatism subside and the patient become comfortable after three to four days of fasting. The fever rapidly abates and the inflammation quickly subsides. After a few days of fasting, if the patient will live properly and eat sensibly, he will never again suffer from rheumatism in any of its many forms.

Typhoid fever patients become comfortable in three to four days if the fast is instituted at the "onset" of the disease, and in from seven to ten days are convalescing. The patient will have such a comfortable sickness and recover so speedily that friends and relatives will declare he was not very sick. And, indeed, he wil not be very sick.

266

It requires feeding and drugging to convert those simple natural processes we call acute diseases into serious and complicated troubles. It is not possible to have a typical case of typhoid fever, as described in Allopathic text-books, without typical text-book treatment. Unthwarted nature never builds such complications and such serious diseases as are described in Allopathic works. All this mass of pathology is built by drugging, serum squirting and feeding.

FASTING IN CHRONIC DISEASE: In chronic disease digestion is not suspended. Appetite may and may not be present. There is not the same necessity for fasting in chronic disease as in acute disease. Yet, if a fast is begun, nature usually signifies her willingness to undergo a long deferred fast which she has probably asked for, but did not receive, times without number, by cutting off the appetite on the second or third day and perhaps by developing nausea, vomiting and a repugnance to food.

The length of time the fast will last will have to be determined by each individual case. In most cases there can be no sound objection to a fast to completion although this will seldom be necessary.

DOES FASTING CURE DISEASE: We do not claim that fasting cures disease but simply that it enables the organism to cure itself. What then does fasting do?

(1) It gives the vital organs a complete rest.

(2) It stops the intake of foods to decompose in the intestines and further poison the body.

(3) It gives the organs of elimination an opportunity to catch up with their work, and promotes elimination.

(4) It promotes the breaking down and absorption of exudates, effusions, deposits, diseased tissues and abnormal growths.

(5) It permits the conservation of energy.

(6) It increases the powers of digestion and assimilation.

(7) Clears and strengthens the mind.

CONTRA-INDICATIONS FOR FASTING: These are:

(1) Fear of the fast on the part of the patient. Fear may kill where the fast would be of distinct benefit.

(2) Extreme emaciation. In such cases a long fast is impossible. A short fast of one to three days may often be found beneficial, or a series of such short fasts with longer periods of proper feeding intervening may be found advisable.

(3) In cases of extreme weakness or degenerative cases. Even in many such cases a series of short fasts as mentioned above may often be beneficial. In the latter stages of consumption and cancer the fast can be of no value except to relieve the patients suffering. It may prolong life a few days. However, fasting is of distinct benefit in the earlier stages of both these diseases.

(4) In cases of inactive kidneys accompanied by obesity. In such cases the tissues may be broken down faster than the kidneys are able to eliminate them.

COMPLICATIONS: These may take the form of uncontrolable vomiting, extreme weakness, persistent hiccoughs, a very eratic pulse that remains eratic, fear of starvation or an *unreasonable* and persistent determination to the break the fast. Any of these should cause us to terminate the fast. However, one should be certain, before breaking the fast, that such symptoms are really lasting and are not mere temporary annoyances. An eratic pulse may arise and last but a few minutes, or hiccoughs may develop and continue for a few minutes and then cease. These should not cause any alarm or apprehension. Be sure the symptom is to be lasting, then break the fast.

Complications are extremely rare. Indeed in my years of experience with fasting I have met but two cases.

In certain quarters much is said about the development of abnormal psychism during the fast. This is something I have yet to see and I note that it is not mentioned among the *complications* or *crises* by those who have had most experience with fasting. I am of the opinion that such developments, if they do occur are due to other causes. They do develop in people who are not fasting. Many fasting patients have lost their abnormal mental conditions while fasting.

The nearest approach to such a condition that I have found recorded in fasting literature is one recorded by Carrington. He says:

"The patient became practically *insane* from the second to the fifth day of the fast—normal conditions being restored on the fifth day! When once the crisis was passed, no indication of such a condition ever recurred; the mentality became, on the other hand, far clearer than in years—indicating that the condition was transitory and merely a curative crisis; one aspect of the vital upheaval, affecting, by chance, the mentality. In this case, the condition was undoubtedly brought about by the excessive, morbid action of the liver, which was greatly deranged, causing an excessive flow of bile; and to a disordered circulation. This was undoubtedly the cause, since the patient, also, turned almost *green* during these few days—her complexion becoming normal as the fast progressed."—*Vitality, Fasting and Nutrition*, p. 535.

I have often thought these cases of so-called abnormal psychism might be crises and once asked Dr. Lindlahr if he had ever considered them in this light. He evaded my question and gave a long talk on his many years of experience.

CRISES: Crises developing during a fast are not different to those developing at other times and are not to be cared for any differently. Fasting frequently revives the symptoms of old troubles which have been suppressed. There is also, in chronic disease, sometimes an immediate, though temporary aggravation of symptoms. Sometimes eruptions are made "worse," temporarily.

Fever, dizziness, fainting, headaches, vomiting, nausea, are frequent developments especially during the first few days of a fast. Cramps in the bowels develop rarely. Very rarely there may be diarrhea. A cold may sometimes develop near the beginning of a fast.

Insomnia is really due to the lack of a need for sleep. The fasting patient requires but little sleep and should not worry over the fact that he does not sleep as much as when eating. He will get all the sleep his body requires.

"Pain in the heart" and palpitation are due to gas in the stomach and intestines.

HYGIENE OF THE FAST: This does not differ from the *hygiene* of *acute disease*, or the *hygiene* of *chronic disease*. Rest, warmth and a proper mental attitude are the chief requisites. Fear of the fast, or broodiness and other phases of mental depression are especially to be combatted. Observations made during the fasts of Succi and others show that the body wastes less rapidly when the patient is kept warm and at rest.

OBJECTIONS TO THE FAST: The two chief objections to the fast are, (1) it produces "acidosis" or decreases the alkalinesence of the blood; and (2) it weakens the patient, and lessens his chances of recovery while rendering him more liable to other diseases.

The first of these objections has been noticed already and can only have any force when applied to a long fast in chronic disease. It could not apply to a short fast, nor to a fast in acute disease. It remains only for us to notice the second objection.

It is claimed that the sick must eat to "keep up their strength," that food cures disease, and that it increases resistance to disease. If food cures the sick, how did they become sick? If feeding increases resistance to disease how do the well-fed fall ill? If food is essential to recovery, how do fasting patients ever recover? Why do not all fasting patients die? Why do they have more comfortable and less protracted illnesses and shorter convalescences? Why do they recover without complications and sequelae? If people who are taxed to death by excess food become sick how will more feeding help them? Why does feeding make them worse? Why does temperature run up and discomfort grow more pronounced after eating?

A patient in a sanitarium with which I was connected a few years ago was too weak to walk up the steps at the time he entered the institution. He was placed upon a fast and did not taste food of any kind for eighteen days. Before this time was up he was able to run up the steps. If food gives strength why was he so weak while eating and why did he gain strength when he ceased to eat?

Food is not nutrition. Overeating with continued wasting of the body is an every day experience of life. Reduced eating with gain in weight and health is becoming a more common experience as people learn that gluttenous indulgence is not conducive to health and clearness of mind. The most important element in nutrition is the living, active body that utilizes the food and not the dead, passive food that is utilized. When the body is not in a condition to carry on the processes of nutrition, it is worse than idle waste to feed such a body. Such an organism should fast.

Fasting not only does not reduce resistance to "disease" but, on the contrary, it increases resistance. Resistance is the product of pure blood and an abundant nerve force. Fasting, because it increases elimination and conserves nervous energy adds to these qualities. I have known fasters to be subjected to all kinds of unfavorable influences, but I have yet to see any disease develop as a result. I know that disease recovers much more rapidly in fasters than in those who eat. The following words of Geo. S. Weger, M.D., a reformed medical man, agree perfectly with my own experience with fasting:

"In all of my personal experience with fasting, I have yet to see a case of tuberculosis develop as a result of it. On the other hand, I have seen many patients recover from tuberculosis who made their first improvements after a fast followed by moderate feeding.

"Real vital resistance is very rarely lowered by fasting. Temporary muscular weakness should not be classed as lowered vitality. Indeed, I have seen many cases of infection of different kinds recover completely on a fast. Take for example an advanced case of sinusitis after five or six painful operations—frontal, ethmoidal and antrum—with surgical drainage and irrigations two or three times a week, continued over a period of two to five years, with no relief or amelioration of symptoms. After almost unendurable suffering, such patients are, as a rule, thin and physically and mentally depressed. When they make complete recoveries after a prolonged fast, as the great majority of them do, is this not sufficient proof that fasting somehow or other raises the power of the organism to overcome infection, rather than that fasting renders them more susceptible? What is true of sinusitis is equally true of other infections, even those so situated anatomically that they cannot be surgically drained and must therefore be absorbed."—In Defense of Rational Fasting.

Dr. Weger says concerning the effects of the fast in improving the blood condition:

"We quite agree that considerable iron and proportionately other necessary elements may be consumed during a prolonged fast. However, the needful materials in the body are not lost to the same extent that the unusable waste is lost. It should not be forgotten, as previously stated, that the human body has within itself the power to use and refine the materials it has on hand during a reasonable fasting period.

"The writer has witnessed in a case of anemia, actual rejuvination of the blood during a twelve-day absolute fast, during which time the red blood cells increased from 1,500,000 to 3,200,000, Hemoglobin increased from fifty per cent to eighty-five per cent, and the white cells reduced from 37,000 to 14,000.

"This is but one instance of many that have impressed the value of fasting in cases where to some practitioners it might have been contradicted. If the body, because of its crowded nutrition, cannot assimilate vitamin bearing food, it can be brought into condition to do this by a purifying fast."—In Defense of Rational Fasting.

There are times when fasting is not only beneficial, but when it is demanded by nature, and only those who distrust the instincts of the body would object to fasting at such times. There are cases in which a suppression of this instinctive demand for a fast has been accomplished so often and a morbid appetite created, that food is "demanded" when a fast is needed.

Whatever may be the source of vital energy, it is certain that no food can supply any of this energy until after it has been digested, absorbed and assimilated. It requires much vital power to digest, absorb and assimilate food, or to maintain it in a state against decomposition, hence it is worse than folly to urge food upon the patient in cases of debility of the stomach or of the whole body, or when there is no natural demand for food. For, beyond a natural call for food there is no power to make profitable use of it.

Mr. Carrington wrote:

"It has been said that an acid condition of the body fluids and tissues (acidosis) is sometimes brought about by fasting. I cannot concede that this is ever the case, in true fasting. As a matter of fact, all the evidence seems to prove that, as Dr. Haig expressed it, 'fasting acts like a dose of alkali'. If there is acidity in the system, fasting will remove it and restore the chemical balance of the system. Therapeutic fasting never created acidity, but on the contrary removes that state when existing. Of course, protracted starvation may do so, but then, who ever advised starvation.

"The medical as well as the general idea is that starvation begins practically immediately when meals are discontinued. The impression is that at once the blood and solid structures of the body begin to break down, and that organic destruction has begun. Such is far from the case, as results have proved in scores (thousands) of cases. The vital cells of the organs and glands—those doing the active physical and chemical work of these parts—do not begin to disintegrate until *actual* starvation begins."

During a fast the body lives on its reserves. Starvation does not begin until these reserves are exhausted. What is more, these reserves contain sufficient alkaline reserve to prevent the development of so-called acidosis.

BREAKING THE FAST: The care that must be exercised in breaking a fast is in proportion to the length of the fast and to the general condition of the fasting individual. The approved plan is to break the fast on liquid food, using for this purpose fruit juice, or tomato juice, or water melon or vegetable broths. Fruit juice—usually orange juice—is used most often. Orange juice and water may be used for the first meal and then followed by more such food two hours later.

After the first day, fruit may be employed and then other foods. After three to four days a normal diet may be returned to.

After a short fast in chronic disease, it is usually desirable to keep the patient on an eliminating diet for a few days or weeks before a normal diet is resumed.

For gaining weight after a fast, the same foods that are used for this purpose at other times are all that are required. Glutteny, however, for the purpose of gaining weight, should be avoided. The milk-diet, which is an exceedingly gluttenous procedure, does not meet with the approval of experienced Orthopaths nor with that of the more advanced Naturopaths.

LIVING AFTER THE FAST: The results of the fast will be more or less temporary unless one lives properly thereafter. Fasting will not make one disease-proof. Orthobionoic living is essential thereafter if one desires to remain in good health.

REST, SLEEP, RELAXATION
Chapter XXII

"THE Rest-cure is the only scientific form of cure known to our day." These are the words of Dr. Walter in contrasting the "rest-cure" with the tonic practice which was then and is yet the vogue. The most important and most essential factor in the preservation and restoration of good health is an abundance of vital or healing power. A knowledge of the means or conditions of the conservation, accumulation and recuperation of this power is, therefore, of more importance than any other thing discussed in this book. There is a broad sense in which the whole subject of health and disease is involved in this knowledge, and in which the conservation and recuperation of vitality is the "all-inclusive condition of good health and the very first step in the direction of hygiene." Rightly did Dr. Walter say:

"Even causes or occasions of disease fail to produce disease as long as the power of health is abundant. For which reason we easily persuade ourselves that bad habits are not so bad after all. If tobacco may be used for sixty years and we still survive, it must be a very slow poison. If one may keep himself soaked with alcohol for the greater part of a century and still live, it cannot be as bad as it is painted. The true answer is that we had such an inheritance of vitality, or what is called constitution, that we could continue for long years to waste our substance and still have enough for moderate use."—Life's Great Law, p. 191.

The processes of cure are the processes of health. This fact has been abundantly proven in previous chapters. Repair is a necessity of living existence. It is always in process in every living thing. The power of repair is the same power whether in health or disease. The object of repair is also the same in these two states of the body. The essential difference between health and disease is the extent of the repairs requiring to be made. Health, if one possesses it, is easily maintained by healthful living. If it has been impaired it is to be restored, repaired, in the same way and by the same agencies that maintain health. Special conditions require special applications as dictated by normal, undepraved instinct, but the condition called disease never calls for processes of treatment that will produce disease in a well man. The employment of means that make well men sick in an effort to make sick men well is not only unreasonable and based upon delusions, but is damaging and deadly.

Whether it is a wound or a broken bone that is to be healed or a body tired from a day of toil that is to be repaired and restored to normal vigor, rest is the prime requisite. Rest is the condition of repair and recuperation. Whether the body is but slightly enervated from a day of toil or profoundly enervated from weeks, months or years of living in such a manner that vitality is greatly depleted, rest is the first and most necessary condition of recuperation of energy and repair of tissue. Whether one is exhausted by prolonged excitement or prostrated by shock, rest is the prime essential for recovery. Stimulants invariably retard recovery and prolong the condition of vital impairment.

That we better understand this subject I shall attempt to formulate:

THE LAW OF REPOSE: Whenever action in the animal body has expended the substance and available energy of the body, rest is demanded and received in order to replenish the substance and for recuperation of power.

The intervals and periods of healthy repose are proportioned to the kind and amount of work performed by the particular organs. If you would do efficient work you must have abundant power to do work with. If the power is lacking it must be recuperated through rest. If you are exhausted you must first be reinvigorated through rest. If you would be active you must first be willing to sleep. If you would be strong you must first be willing to be weak.

A tired man may feel strong in the presence of danger. He may forget his fatigue under excitement. A cold plunge or a hot shower may exhilirate him for the moment. A cup of coffee or a dose of some drug may increase his strength. A few snappy exercises may "pep him up." But these things do not recuperate power nor repair tissue. On the contrary, they exhause power and destroy tissue. "An evil indulgence," says Dr. Walter, Life's Great Law, p. 192, "instead of obviously depleting our powers,

271

produces, on the contrary, an increased consciousness of power, often a pleasing exhiliration, due to the vital resistance which it arouses, thus giving an appearance of vigor at the very time and by the means that it is exhausting the power and providing for a reduction of vigor."

The more injurious a habit, agent or indulgence is, the more dangerous and the more delusive it is. "Opium and alcohol, in comparison with tea and coffee, are the illustrations." The first named two are much more delusive than the latter, because they are correspondingly more deadly. Energy which is manifest only through work, through expenditures, makes its manifestations correspond to its expenditures. Tonics, stimulants, food, work, excitement, etc., call out and make manifest, the powers of the body and thus appear to give us the very power which they cause to be expended. Recovery of health must, therefore, come through opposite practices, that is, practices that conserve and do not deplete the powers of life. Dr. Walter says, *Life's Great Law*, pp. 192 to 198.

"The Rest-Cure is not simply the proper cure for disease in its varied forms, but for all the ills that afflict humanity. Only power in abundant measure can produce vigorous health or enable one to do successful work; incompetence, disease, and especially chronic disease, are due to depleted vital resources, which depletion is very apt to be increased, rather than diminished, by the methods in vogue of sustaining one's powers. 'He that would save his life shall lose it.' It is always a dire misfortune for any one to feel his want of power, and to commence to supplement or sustain it under present-day methods. The overworked, 'run-down,' well-nigh exhausted portion of the community is a large one, each individual being analogous to a locomotive, whose steam-pressure is greatly reduced. It is not steam that drives the steam-engine, but the intensity of the force in the steam. Exhausted vitality, like exhaust-steam, can do little work. And yet too many are trying to carry forward life's work upon partially exhausted vital resources, always trying to make up for deficiency of power by the use of stimulants and other forcing processes.

"The folly of all this is well illustrated by the folly of the engineer who would do his work with steam at fifty pounds pressure when he should have one hundred pounds. An engine with fifty pounds pressure can do some work, at sixty pounds it may do the work of forty horses, at eighty the work of fifty horses, while at one hundred pounds it is a sixty-horse-power engine. Just so the ability which any one possesses for work is determined chiefly by the intensity of his powers. Half-dead men are altogether too common, waiting unconsciously for some disease-germ to gather them in. For the principles we are advocating show that contagious and epidemic diseases result from the depleted powers of the patient more than from any other consideration. It is a remarkable fact that epidemics rarely increase the total death-rate of a community, if we extend out statistics over a sufficient length of time. A contagious disease is only a form of taking off. Highly vitalized men don't die, even if they should contract the disease, which they rarely do, it is the enfeebled, depleted, poisoned ones that succumb to infection. If they had not died of LaGrippe, smallpox, or other such ailment, they would surely have fallen a victim of pneumonia, typhoid, or the like.

"The question before us, therefore, is not simply how to regain or maintain health, and not alone how to preserve life, but how to live well, feel well, enjoy life, do efficient work, and be entirely free from the habits and indulgences which so frequently enslave men. To this end we recall that it is nature that cures, as she does everything else in the natural world; in this matter of cure we are called upon to deal with an important department of natural existence, known as the vital. This department, like each of the others, is presided over by its own inherent force, controlled in its operations by its own great law, which force under conrtol of its law performs all the functions of its department and produces all its phenomena. *Vitality, called also vital force, produces, repairs, heals; the rapidity and certainty of its work correspond chiefly to the amount of power; all processes should be employed to recuperate the patient's powers, and nothing done to deplete them.* Though temporary relief may be secured by depletion, as by purging and blood-letting, because the power of the disease is the patient's vital power, so that reducing the one always reduces the other, all physicians of all schools now agree that such practice is destructive to the patient's best interests. No one now believes it to be wise practice to cure diseases by destroying health, no matter how persistently he may ignorantly continue the method.

"The opposite theory of cure is the one now everywhere advocated. Sustain the patient's strength is the cry everywhere heard. Support the vitality and the patient will surely rally. *The theory we hold to be true beyond all peradventure; it is the application of the theory that is erroneous.* If the real is the opposite of the apparent; if we are deluded by appearances which are generally the opposites of the realities; if substances administered to give strength to the patient appear to do so only by taking away his strength, who cannot see how utterly destructive and fallacious a practice based upon observation must be. If disease, instead of being an enemy, is really nature's effort at cure, who fails to perceive ample justification for the alarming increase of nervous diseases in our time, as the result of the use of the tonics and nervines so generally employed. Something does not come out of nothing; no effect exists except from an adequate cause; the facts of today prove either a failure of the theory that nature cures, or a failure of its methods of application. The latter error is the true one. Because of a theory of vital force and its source, which is equally opposed to the facts, men proceed to produce the diseases they imagine they are curing, and to exhaust the power they are trying to sustain. The consequence is the more one is cured the more he needs to be cured; and the more he is sustained the greater his need to be sustained; or, to put it in concrete form, the more whiskey or other stimulant or tonic we administer to the patient, the more he needs it; the more we sustain him by the methods of the schools, the weaker and worse he gets. We turn our attention to the accumulation of vital power as the true means by which obstructions shall be overcome, disease rendered unnecessary, and good health be restored. The methods of recuperation that we shall advocate are all based upon the theory that life is an inheritance and not a product. If life could be manufactured there would at least be some excuse for exciting into action the organs which are supposed to manufacture it, but having absolutely disproved the transformation theories, and shown that life comes only from life, we are shut up to the alternative of securing recuperation of power through cessation of its use. We cannot recuperate by increasing its use. Recuperation must come through rest and sleep, and the necessity for these in every living thing is the best proof that it cannot be obtained in any other way. If we could manufacture vitality for horse or man, what need of sleep and rest half the time; if hay and oats could take the place of sleep, the horseless age would still be far away.

"The word recuperate, which means to recover, is a term chiefly employed in connection with living things, or at least with such things as spontaneously recover their powers. We may recuperate our health or our strength; an orchard or a farm may recuperate, and of late years the term has been applied to electricity, as in the recuperation of a battery. But no matter in what connection it is employed the leading idea is rest. Under the Mosaic law the necessity for rest in order to recuperate was everywhere recognized. Even the land had its sabbath. Man and horse and ox are expected to recuperate every night, in addition to the rest of every seventh day. The battery also recuperates when we cease its use; but no matter in what department we use the term, the leading, if not sole idea, is recovery through rest. We do not recuperate a steam-engine, a wagon, or a plow; we repair these; we recuperate only those things which have within them the power of recovery when we cease to use and expend the power. The battery recovers its powers by cessation of work; the orchard and farm recuperate so as to produce a harvest after a season of rest; man and horse are always reproducing, and therefore, recovering their powers. It is properly said also that the spendthrift recuperates his fortune when he ceases to spend it. But this is a true use of the term only when his fortune is an inheritance. If he is a self-made man, his fortune being the product of his own labor, we would not think of his recuperating his fortune by rest; we would speak of him as making his fortune by greater activity and vigor. Just so with the vital organism; we may recuperate its powers because they are an inheritance which we receive as an income, that may be squandered by ceaseless activity, riotous living, or accumulated to great abundance by rest and waiting. But if it be true that man manufactures his vital powers, then recuperation is an entirely improper word to use in connection with this increase. If tonics and stimulants and food and drink and air make for us vitality, then accumulation of power must come through increased work, as during the day, while sleep and rest would prove to be not

273

only useless but destructive. If power could be manufactured out of food or drink or medicine, what excuse would there be for holidays and sabbath days as well as for nightly rest. Where is the necessity for rotation of crops on the farm if fertilizer will answer all purposes. Why not heavy fruit crops every year if feeding the soil can take the place of rest. Once let it be shown that vital power can be manufactured, and rest is at once proved an unnecessary indulgence. If increased work can produce vitality for any one, sleep becomes a reckless waste; if we can give strength to an invalid by the use of a drug, we ought to be consistent and repudiate sleep as a contribution to senseless fashion.

"But men are seldom consistent. They seek to give strength from without at the very time they admit the importance for the invalid of rest and sleep. Recuperation means the hoarding of power through its non-use; a statement which, if true, shows the absurdity of the attempt to give power by its increased use through increased activity. Both these plans cannot be true. We recuperate through rest or we manufacture power through active work; but we never have done, and never can do, both at the same time. There is a dilemma here, and we may take either horn we please; no one can ride two horses at the same time when these are going in opposite directions.

"The primal thought of the system we advocate, therefore, is rest—rest of body and of mind, of muscle and of nerve, of heart and lungs, liver and kidneys, stomach and bowels. This system might thus be called Scientific Rest-cure. It is Rest-cure because it inculcates and promotes rest as the *sine qua non* to recovered health, and it is scientific because it is a logical development, not from supposed facts, but from established first principles, to the elaboration of which development future chapters are devoted."

Work is not only desirable, it is necessary. Power is useless unless we may expend it or employ it. But it is extremely important that we distinguish between processes of expenditure and processes of recuperation. If we know these processes and the conditions of these we may secure either at will. In this connection it makes all the difference in the world whether vitality is manufactured by food, oxygen, exercise and tonics, or expended by these, and recuperated through rest. Do tonics, and stimulants, really strengthen us or do they take away the strength they appear to give? Is the athlete strengthened while he exercises or while he rests and sleeps? Does he recuperate while active or when passive? If vitality is the product of the action of the vital organs and not the power back of their action, then, indeed, should the athlete live forever and never become exhausted. Indeed, the more active he becomes the more vitality should he acquire.

The law of dual effect knows no exceptions. It applies to all departments of life. Labor or exercise arouse vital activity and give the appearance of increased vigor. This is the first effect. The secondary effect is fatigue and exhaustion. Very often the invalid is told that he must keep up, because, if he goes to bed, he will lose strength. This is the first effect. The secondary effect is a gain in strength. Travel or excitement makes the invalid feel stronger and better as a first effect. But the secondary effect is languor, weakness, exhaustion. Rest and sleep, on the contrary, produce as their first effects, weakness and languor; but no one doubts their recuperative value. Rest and sleep are the only means whereby recuperation and invigoration can be secured. But these are secondary effects. *The invalid must become weak that he may grow strong.*

By many sleep is regarded as a waste of time. They seek means of doing away with its necessity. However, we know that no action can occur without a corresponding reaction; effort must be followed by rest. Human energy is not an inexhaustible quantity. The pendulum of human energy cannot swing always in one direction. Man must cease his activities and recharge his vital or nervous batteries. Body, mind and special senses must rest.

Every vital action is necessarily attended with an expenditure of vital power and waste of organized substance. The functions of sensibility, voluntary motion, expression and of the conscious mind cannot be indulged in indefinitely. After a period of activity a condition arises, due to this expenditure and waste and the consequent need for recuperation and repair, known as fatigue. After a time—the length of which is determined somewhat by habit and the general condition of the organism—the contractile powers of the muscles begin to diminish, and if action is continued long enough, they cease to contract at all. What is true of the muscles is equally true of the brain and special senses. A temporary cessation of activity is enforced. If only voluntary action ceases, this is rest; if mind and special senses also suspend functions, the result is sleep. Sleep may be said to be rest of body, mind and special senses, or complete rest of all voluntary activities and the functions of external relation. The involuntary functions also secure a certain amount of rest during this period. The nutritive functions of the body—digestion, respiration, circulation, secretion and excretion—continue throughout life with but little abatement or modification. Where they are temporarily suspended we have *suspended animation*. And, this, I believe, serves a definite end just as rest and sleep do, is merely rest and sleep pushed to the greatest possible limit. Ordinarily, however, for the vegetative functions of life, there is no cessation, and scarcely any dimunition of activity, except in disease, from the beginning of life until death.

The state of sleep has been compared to the foetus in utero, which, by some, has been described as being in a perpetual sleep until aroused at birth. The foetal existence of an animal is the period of its most rapid growth and development and also its period of least activity. Rest is essential to growth and development and equally as essential to repair, renewal and renovation. During the whole of rest and sleep, a process of renovation and repair goes on throughout the whole of the organs of animal life. It has been long known and recently shown by experiments that the first two to four hours of sleep are the *deepest* and *soundest;* that more effort is required to awaken a sleeper during this period than subsequently, and that durir.g this time one derives most benefit from sleep. The *sounder* or *deeper* the sleep the more efficient is the renovating process.

Healthy sleep differs from the state of coma and apparent death induced by disease, drugs, asphyxiation and drowning, in that, when the animal arouses from sleep, he feels refreshed and renovated and is ready for action, whereas, the animal aroused from coma, from whatever cause, is languid and exhausted and not fitted for action. This, however, is not the fault of the coma, but of the causes that induced it. They are greater than the causes that induce sleep and their effects are not so speedily and effectively overcome. There can be no doubt that coma is a defensive measure as will be seen from the description of the primary and secondary effects of anesthetics given in another chapter of this work.

By expending and exhausting our powers, but rendering us conscious of them in the process of expenditure, stimulants, tonics, and other measures delude us by making us believe they communicate to us the powers they are taking from us. The more of a drug one uses the more he feels the need of it. It produces the very ailment it is intended to cure. Nervines produce nervousness, cathartics produce chronic constipation. The more epsom salts one employs the larger the dose he must use. The same is true of all drugs for all purposes.

A cold bath is a wasteful process. It stimulates powerfully and robs one of the strength it appears to give. It is a developing process in that it forces the body to develop its resistance to cold. Some exposure to cold is not only necessary but unavoidable. But the cold morning bath brings no adequate returns for the expenditure. Sea bathing is a summer indulgence along the sea coast. It is an utterly wasteful process. It invariably results in enervation necessitating long weeks of lassitude in which to recuperate. Athletics are processes of development. As indulged in today in school. college and professionally, they waste life. Processes of development are processes of expenditure, and when carried to excess necessarily result in exhaustion. Such things call forth power. They never produce or communicate power. If great development communicates power, the powerful and fully developed gymnast or strong man should live forever. If lungs, and stomach, and heart manufacture vitality, if food and air and exercise are the sources of life, then hearty feeders and powerful atheletes should never die.

"We urge," writes Dr. Walter, "the largest development in all right ways, but to secure it we are sure that recuperation is the important prerequisite. The secondary effect is the opposite of the primary. Recuperation provides for development; we can never get out of a man what is not in him. Let us fill the reservoir with power, and the work of getting it out in scholarship, athletics, or business, will prove a delight, not a hardship. Social, political, or financial triumphs will be real enjoyments whenever the vital reservoir becomes bubbling over with the animation which belongs to abundant vitality."—*Life's Great Law*, p. 227.

Activity expends power. There can be no doubt of this. Activity exhausts and tears down. Whether it be of body or brain, of stomach, or liver, heart or lungs or any other organ of the body, work exhausts that organ. Activity is the process of expend-ing power.

Inactivity (rest, relaxation and sleep) is the process of recuperation. A return to the passive state is the only legitimate process of recuperation. If invalids are to be restored to good health, if strength and vigor are to take the place of debility and weakness, we must save life by saving power. The conditions of recovery are conditions of conservation and recuperation. This principle applies to every organ and function of the body. Rest for each organ is as imperative as rest for the whole body. The heart requires rest as much as do the muscles of the arms. The stomach must have rest the same as the eyes. The glands of the body have the same need for rest as does the brain. Rest, by reducing activity, is the first requisite of recovery.

But it is the height of folly to urge the importance of rest upon a patient and, perhaps send him to bed, and then administer tonics and stimulants which promote activity and prevent rest. It is the practice in medical rest-resorts to give the patients drug stimulants or hot and cold baths, massage, electrical stimulation and the like. Such patients do not rest—they are exhausted. "Whether it be calomel for the liver, digitalis for the heart, or whiskey for the general system—whether it be cold baths or hot baths, electricity or anything else, whatever arouses vital activity, and especially vital resistance, is exhausting to the patient's power, and is preventive of recovery not promotive of it," wrote Dr. Walter—*Life's Great Law*, p. 201.

All processes and measures that promote activity in the present invariably neces-sitate reduced action in the future. Rest must follow work. Recuperation must be commensurate with expenditure else the vital forces are permanently lowered. The pendulum of human energy cannot swing always in one direction. The law of *dual effect* is absolute. Those measures which, while occasioning increased action in the present, do so by doing violence to the body or to the vital instincts, call for the greatest reduction of activity in the future. For this reason, drugs are the worst of all stimu-lants (irritants).

There is only one way to secure rest for overworked organs or for an overworked body—this is to stop working them. How can an organ be rested by lashing it with tonics and stimulants (irritants) as is the prevailing practice today? In acute disease there is increased action in the system Frequently patients feel better than usual just before the "onset" of acute symptoms. This is due to irritation. Irritation occasions increased action, so that the patient feels stronger and more vigorous while he is getting sick. But when he is getting well, that is after the "onset" of symptoms and during convalescence, he is weak. Disease begins with irritation which occasions an exhaltation of function so that the individual is deluded into the belief that he is growing stronger and getting well, and this, at the very time and by the very means that his health is be-ing impaired. This condition of irritation is called *stimulation*. "All stimulants and tonics," says Dr. Walter, *Vital Science*, p. 290, "cause increased function because they are irritating or exciting in their nature, and tend to destroy health instead of re-cuperate it. Recovery, on the contrary, is being effected by rest and consequent reduced function of the organ or of the organism as a whole."

Rest, like sleep, reduces function and restores health. Rest in bed is of tre-mendous importance. But of even greater importance is as complete rest of all the organs of the body as it is possible to secure. This may be obtained by cutting off all sources of stimulation, resting in bed and ceasing to eat for a few days. The work of the liver, lungs, kidneys, heart, stomach, glands, etc., is determined largely by the amount and kind of food one eats. To cease eating for a time affords the most com-plete rest to the vital organs and permits them to carry forward their work of replenish-ment and repair very perfectly so that they are soon restored to normal condition. Rest and sleep are the great representative restorative processes. The excitement of irritation (stimulation) wastes power and substance.

"After an organ has been lashed by overstimulation," says Dr. Tilden, "until its nutrition is perverted and organic change has taken place, it may come back to normal if all stimulating influences are removed and sufficient rest—physical, mental, and physiological— is given. If nutrition is very greatly impaired, and the organ broken down to the extent of adding infection to toxemia, even a million-dollar remedy may not cure."—*Philosophy of Health,* p. 399, Nov. 1922.

The necessity for rest after shock is theoretically recognized by all. But its practical dismissal is everywhere the vogue. Instead of rest, tonics and stimulants and madcap endeavors to restore function are employed in a frenzied round of *doing something.* Dr. Tilden aptly describes the modern method and contrasts it with the right method in the following words:—

"There is a difference between disease and injury. A body that is not diseased—toxemic—takes little offense at injuries, unless the injury destroys the function of an organ, or shocks the system so greatly as to enervate profoundly. After profound enervation from shock, rest—physiological, physical, and mental—allows the return of the functions of secretion, excretion, or elimination; but if stimulants—drugs and food—are given, reaction is prevented, and death ensues.

"To illustrate my meaning: An accident occurs. Someone is shocked into insensibility. A doctor and an ambulance are called. The proper treatment is to stop the hemorrhage first. Place the patient in the shade with a folded coat or something soft under his head--not too high. Leave someone in charge, and send the idle and curious away. The patient should not be disturbed until reactions take place; then he may be removed to his home or hospital as gently and quickly as possible, there to be kept quiet, without drugs and food, until normal.

"The way such cases are usually treated is to rush to the doctor pell-mell, who administers a dose of stimulant hypodermically. The patient is bundled into an ambulance, and rushed, with the speed and noise of the fire deparment, to a hospital —it may be a mile or it may be two or three miles. Then he is rushed to a receiving ward, where he is pawed over—and what else, God only knows.

"Rest! Modern medicine has no such word in its dictionary. It is supplanted by stimulation and narcotization. Time is another word that has been eliminated. Care given to the injured is much like the Chinaman's description of the first electric car he ever saw: 'No pushee, no pullee, but run like hellee.' Such treatment has prevented the reaction in thousands and thousands of cases. But the public is satisfied; for something is done, and done speedily, and neither last not least, the patient is done to a finish.****

"If shock is not profound, lack of proper rest may prevent a full return of secretion and excretion, or elimination. Then toxemia will be increased, and a long-drawnout convalescence may be experienced, in which organic change may take place; which means that the most vulnerable organ of the body will give down, and, unless a skillfull letting-alone policy is followed, death may end the victim's misfortune."—*Philosophy of Health,* August 1924.

It does not matter whether enervation and impaired or suspended secretion and excretion are due to shock or to long continued abuses of the body, it does not matter whether enervation develops quickly or slowly, rest—mental, physical and physiological —is the means of recuperation and of restoration of normal function. REST AND REPLENISHMENT OF POWER IS THE FIRST STEP IN THE CURATIVE WORK, as Dr. Jennings declares in the following quotation:—

"In the lowest depths of adynamic disease, when the last glimpse of life seems fading quite away, there still lingers, lives and reigns the 'law of cure' which will secure a restoration to health, if, under existing circumstances, such an event is possible. Rest and replenishment of power is the first step in the ascending pathological transit; removal of useless matter by the decomposing function, with its activity and force increased by resting, constitutes the second step, and the third consists in a repair of breaches by the accretion of new well wrought material. These three steps form the first grand division in the ascending pathological transition, the removal of *structural* derangement, or *cure* of *organic* disease. The next grand step in the ascending pathological work consists in the re-establishment of regular or natural *functional* action."—*Philosophy of Human Life*, p. 102.

After emphasizing that the tendency of the movements of life in disease, "all and singular, is to save life, as far as that may be in danger," he says:—

"The first object aimed at in this treatment (Orthopathic), is to shut down all unnecessary waste-gates; to place the system as far as possible, under circumstances in which there shall be no unnecessary expenditure of power, in order that the departments of labor that are now deficient in force, may receive an accession to their strength."—*Philosophy of Human Life*, p. 169.

The resting invalid is the recuperating invalid. Invalids do not recover so long as they are being stimulated and worked. They only recover after they have given up hope of recovery and abandoned all efforts at cure. Seizing the opportunity nature begins silently and gradually to recuperate the expended power and repair the damaged structure. Silently and unconsciously the power accumulates. It may be then, that some miracle monger comes along with a catchy little metaphysical ditty or a persuasive personality and, having persuaded the patient of his marvelous and unusual powers, begins his experiments with her. She responds. She feels her strength "returning." Hope and expectancy are renewed. Greater efforts are made and health is soon hers. Why? Because the power of health once in her, it is an easy thing to call it out. The power of response is her own power—power gradually, silently and unconsciously stored up through rest and resignation. *She began to get well as soon as she ceased to try to get well.* All the essentials of recovery must be completed before the miracle monger comes along, else he fails.

Before offering any examples from my own experience I desire to present the following from Dr. Walter's *Life's Great Law*, pp. 222-3-4-5:—

"Two important cases, further illustrative of these truths, which occurred in our own practice, must be here recorded. These cases were so like each other that it was hard to distinguish them. They were of the same age, victims of the same occasions, afflicted with the same ailments, the results alone differing. H. C. was an orphan boy, commended to our care by two former patients, who impressed upon his friends that our treatment was his last chance. Depression, melancholy, weakness, were the prominent symptoms; dyspepsia, neurasthenia, even melancholia, were the diagnosed diseases. The patient arrived in good time, was put in care of a nurse, all stimulants, tonics, and anodynes were withdrawn, and he continued to lose flesh and strength until he was confined to bed. A mild massage, for exercise, a bath to keep him clean, only healthful food at proper times, and good nursing, were the things done for him. For weeks he was lifted from bed to rolling-chair and wheeled into sunshine and fresh air. As he never used his strength he continued unconscious of its possession, until after six months he became restless and moaned out, "Doctor, I am sick and tired of this bed. I can't stay here longer.' 'Well, why do you stay here? Get up and go out.' 'May I?' he inquired. 'Certainly you may.' That day he crept out to the scales and got weighed, and never afterward went back to bed to stay there. He gained flesh and added fifty-five pounds to his weight during the following six months, and was restored to excellent health. He returned to his home vigorous and hearty, and greatly alarmed his friends by his apparent recklessness. They thought surely he would break down again, but our answer to all inquiries was, 'Never mind, Harry, he is alright for anything that he undertakes.' After a happy and active summer he returned to school, graduated with honors, and was made valedictorian of his class. Soon after he engaged in business, got married, and for nearly ten years has enjoyed uninterrupted good health. The gentlemen who advised him to us, one seventy and the other eighty, are still apparently in their prime, actively at work illustrating the value of a system of healing that operates upon the plan of keeping the power *in* and allowing business and social requirements to get it *out* as needed.

"We turn now to the counterpart of this case, as alike the other as two peas are alike each other, except in the results. This patient, like the other, had broken down at school, and while the severe mental depression was absent, he was nevertheless a very sick boy. The first attempt to restore him, we were informed, was by development

278

through gymnastics. Though under the care of a skilful teacher he grew steadily worse under this plan. Then sea-bathing, boating, and swimming were tried with the same result. The patient grew worse rather than better; it was vainly imagined that development could be secured without reference to whether the power of development was present or not. At length a noted specialist was called in, who changed the methods of the development, but still continued to squeeze the dry orange. Tonics, general and special, especially strychnine, were the means employed, and the patient seemed to gain a little strength. Finally, his friends were advised that he was substantially well, and required nothing further than out-door life in the country, and he would soon return to his studies.

"It was under these circumstances that the boy was brought to The Walter Sanitarium. One peculiar fact of this coming was that a journey of one hundred and fifty miles completely exhausted him, and he continued for a long time greatly prostrated. We demurred to continuing his tonics, and for nearly three months he had no medicine but a little homeopathy, while he lay substantially confined to his bed and his cot under the trees. No attempts at development were made, there was little to develop. A daily massage, oil-rub, or bath were administered, but the patient made no apparent progress. Like the other case, he continued almost helpless, but comparatively comfortable. Soon an additional complication arose; the patient became afflicted with a diarrhea which often belongs to the 'dog-days.' This prostrated him much, and his parents, becoming alarmed, determined to remove him to his home, and put him once more under the care of the specialist. This doctor came to assist in his removal, and of course began at once to develop and sustain his powers. The results were surprising to everybody; the patient responded with an ease and certainty that was very encouraging. Father and then mother wrote that the patient gained strength every step of the way, and returned home in better shape than he left it.

"The reader who comprehends these principles will agree with us that there was no reason for surprise. The results were to be expected. Three months of recuperation could not go for nothing, even if it was broken off in the middle. The patient continued to gain, and the father wrote nine months afterward, 'Our son has about recovered. At times he is nervous but this is disappearing,' etc.

"Another year has passed away, and the early promise has not been fulfilled. The father now writes, a year later: 'Our son has had a very slow recovery, getting up and going down again from time to time. He is now, I think, getting firmly on his feet, but is not yet able to return to school!

"We are sorry to note that this new hope sounds very much like the one of the year before, and we are not sure that a year from now the same hope will be cherished, but the same disappointment be recorded. Building a house upon the sand is wiser than to build human health on strychnine; we can only imagine how desperate the physician must become who has been hoping and promising for these years, only to be disappointed. Desperate prescriptions are possible in such a case, and a desperate prescription is a dangerous thing.

"The conclusion to be drawn from these varied examples which might be duplicated a thousand times, is that it is an easy matter to develop human beings in any direction one chooses provided only that the power of the development is in him. It cannot be supplied from without. Capacity cannot be bought, no matter how much one is prepared to pay for it. And it all leads us back to the orginal proposition that recuperation of power is the first and most important element in its development. For a hundred years at least men have directed all their efforts toward development until the facilities, social, intellectual, physical, and moral have become one of the wonders of the world, while not even the slightest effort toward recuperation is exhibited. Sleep is a waste of time in the thought of many, and thousands cheat themselves out of it all they can, not knowing that they are preventing, not promoting, development."

Time is an important element in recuperating power. Rest is the means of recuperation, but time is required in which to recuperate. Invalids must learn to live by faith and not by sight. Patients, their relatives, friends, physicians and nurses, like to feel and see the improvement of the patient or the increase in his power. But the very act of making the increased power obvious, also decreases his power. The patient can only become conscious of his power by expending it and he loses it by expending it. Stimulants and tonics, which call out the patient's powers, while they make him feel and appear better for the time, leave him weaker in the end. They thus impede or prevent recovery. The manifestation of power can never exceed its source. No more power can be gotten out of a man than there is in him. When his power is all out, he goes out with it.

A case that came under my care in a sanitarium with which I was once connected, will well illustrate this point. A lady, about forty-five, of good constitution and, although profoundly enervated, not seriously deranged organically, was given daily stimulating treatments consisting of massage, chiropractic, hydrotherapy, electrical stimulation, and traction with radiant heat to the spine. After a few days of this she became too weak to be out of bed and was unable to eat. A few days in bed secured enough recuperation to enable her to be up and around and to eat as well as before. Then the stimulating treatment was resumed and she was forced to go back to bed again in a few days and to again discontinue eating. This process was continued for some time—periods of feeding and stimulation necessitating periods of rest in bed without food or stimulants—until she died. The little power she recuperated through rest was soon dissipated through stimulation. All the stimulation she received was of a drugless character. She was given no drugs.

A lady suffered with a variety of complaints. Rest in bed with moderate feeding brought about gradual improvement. After three months of this, unavoidable excitement, altercations and much opposition to her course, on the part of friends and family, caused her to suffer the first "attack" during the time. The "attack" was not severe and on the following day she motored to a town four hours distant. This fatigued her. She motored home again next day. This fatigued her more. That night she remained up late. Another "attack" was the result. The lady said of her experience: "Until last Tuesday I had been piling up energy, it seems—for I felt strong enough to go on that trip and out to dinner, etc. One is so apt to forget quickly when one feels momentarily strong, and I outdid my slowly acquired energy very rapidly."

I once had under my care in San Antonio, Texas, an aged man who had suffered for over forty years from the abuses that both he and his physicians heaped upon his long suffering body. A druggist by trade, he had tried about all the drugs in the pharmacopea. Physician after physician had prescribed for him. In despair he finally turned to Osteopathy, then to Chiropractic, then to electroterapy. Each of these appeared to help but he soon found himself worse than before. He turned to new thought and other mental methods and then to Naturopathy. Four Naturopaths had treated him. But he had not improved. The apparent improvement which came with each system was short lived. He then placed himself under my care. All stimulation was stopped. REST, REST, REST was enjoined. One by one his symptoms disappeared, and for three months he went steadily forward toward health. At this time I left San Antonio and came East. Despite my warnings and despite his past experiences he again placed himself in the hands of a Naturopath. There followed massages, manipulations, sweat baths, etc. His next report to me was a glowing account of how rapidly he was improving under these forms of stimulation. Three months of recuperation could not have gone for nothing. He now had power in reserve with which to respond. But the response was its expenditure. The improvement was not of long duration. He next sought out an electrotherapist. Again he seemed to improve and wrote me that he had now found a man who really understood electrotherapy and was rapidly recovering. Some people never learn by their experience. A few weeks later he was again lamenting his failure and complaining that he was then worse than before going to the electrotherapist. He again turned to Chiropractic but after a short period of apparent improvement grew still worse. He was back now to about where he was when I started him to recuperating but he had not learned his lesson and was still seeking for a cure that would restore him to health.

A young sweat-shop worker in New York City came to me. She had symptoms of tuberculosis, and was afflicted with what are called female disorders. A brief rest enabled her to return to work but the work was hard and the hours long. She soon grew worse again. She went away to the country where she improved rapidly, but due to the necessity of earning her way, did not secure as much rest as she should have had. After three months she returned to the city and resumed her old work. In a month's time symptoms of T.B. again appeared. I then sent her to a Health School where she secured the needed rest and in three months returned, a new woman. She was able to work hard for fourteen hours a day without fatigue.

A gentleman journeyed from New York to Chicago to enter a well known sanitarium of "Natural" therapeutics located there. When he arrived there he was able to walk and his bowels were moving daily. They began the work of stimulating his vitality away. Cold sitz baths, the cold "blitz-guss" electrical stimulation, massage and manipulation—some one or the other of these twice daily. In two weeks ne was too weak to walk and his bowels refused to act. He remained in the institution five more weeks confined to his bed, but being stimulated as above, stuffed with food and given a daily enema. He was sent home at the end of this time too weak to sit in the train, suffering with severe attacks of pain in the abdomen, very badly constipated and very nervous. Agar and mineral oil were handed him, as he left, for his bowels, bell-ans for the gas and cod-liver oil in pellet form to be taken regularly.

When he arrived home I was called. I stopped all feeding, all drugging and all enemas and said, REST. In a week he was able to walk. In four to five days his bowels began to act normally. He developed a ravenous appetite and suffered with no more attacks. His nerves grew steadily better. Such are the comparative results of the stimulating practice and the recuperative practice. If the "Natural therapists" would only accord to Nature the opportunity as well as the power of cure and cease their damaging fads and fancies, their successes would be greater.

The mode of living in this age produces such a waste of power and such a sense of weariness that only the limited few ever know the supreme delights and the enviable luxury of power in reserve. They keep their semblance of vigor up by means of stimulation and seldom take sufficient time to re-change their vital or nervous batteries. Nights are turned into day, while mental and nervous poise is exceedingly rare. All poison habits, all excesses, the indulgence of any or all of the passions constitute distinct drains upon the vital resources and are fruitful sources of diminished vitality, crippled usefulness and shortened life. Modern life presents us with an almost unlimited variety of means of stimulation, excitement, thrills, and dissipations chiefly orginating in the clever but perverted ingenuity of those who reap rich financial rewards from these things.

Enervation, nervous prostration, melancholia, and other forms of insanity are always close at hand. "For years," says Dr. Felix Oswald, "the infinite patience of Nature labors every night to undo the mischief of every day," but when people spend half their nights in feverish activity, nature cannot fully succeed in her recuperative work. The functions of the body begin to lag. It is, of course, a natural sequence that the decadence of an entire organism must follow the waning functions of the individual organs.

Throughout all nature repose alternates with activity. Back of every action is a great repose. Nature has her resting times. Civilization attempts to do away with these and supplant them with stimulation. When disease results, instead of returning to the quiet, perfect way of Nature, man resorts to every conceivable artificial means as a rapid transit back to health and strength, and, as a logical consequence, only succeeds in getting farther away from health. Man quiets his protesting nerves that he may continue to abuse them. He palliates a diseased stomach that he may continue misusing it. He seeks strength in stimulants that he may use this in greater dissipations. He does not obey the laws of life from which alone he can obtain the strength he craves. All of his efforts to stimulate health injure his health. Every artilcial means of increasing functional activities depletes his powers.

A "rest-cure" is not the ultimate cure. What is the advantage of a rest to restore you to normal vigor if you are only going to return to the former dissipating mode of living and again exhaust your vital fund? Unless you learn how to live properly, and then live what you have learned, you will be forced to go back occasionally for another "rest-cure." Rest is only a means of recuperation. It cannot be expected to make you disease-proof.

We divide rest into three classes—*mental*, *physical* and *physiological*. This classification is more or less arbitrary and only serves as a convenience.

MENTAL REST is secured by poising the mind, and removing all sources of disturbance and annoyance—noises, talk, fears, anxieties, worries, etc. People in civilized life have lost that poise and mental and emotional relaxation and repose that characterizes the animal and so-called savage world. They must be taught to re-cultivate poise and self-control.

PHYSICAL REST is secured by ceasing physical activities and going to bed. In bed one must lie quiet. Relaxation and repose are essential. A tensed, contracted condition of the body is incompatible with rest. Rolling and tossing on the bed prevents rest. A hard, comfortable bed, a comfortable temperature, with not too much cover, are essential to rest.

PHYSIOLOGICAL REST is secured partly as a result of the above two forms of rest, partly as a result of stopping the food intake. Food works the stomach, intestine, liver, lungs, kidneys, glands, heart, etc. and when the amount of food consumed is reduced, the amount of work these organs must do is decreased. If all food is abstained from their work is reduced still more. All stimulants overwork the organs of the body When these are abandoned these organs are allowed to rest.

No greater or better condition or combination of conditions can be brought to—gether to promote recuperation and, through this, invigorate and increase the efficiency of all the organs and functions of the body, than that of mental, physical and physiological rest. Nothing will promote elimination as these do. Nothing else so effectively hastens repair of tissue and restoration of health.

Certain superficial and not well founded objections to the "rest-cure" have been offered by Physical Culturists, who regard exercise as the panacea for all ills and as the creator of human energy. These objections demand a brief notice at this point.

First, there are the psychological objections. People are said often not to realize that they are seriously sick until they are ordered to go to bed and their ailments are materially aggravated by being ordered to bed. Going to bed is also said to be "giving up" and acknowledging that your ailment has gotten the best of you. It is declared that one should not "give up" but that he must mentally "struggle against" his ailment.

Both of these objections are puerile and very wide of the mark. No patient is frightened or made worse or caused to worry over his troubles by going to bed if the reasons for going to bed are explained to him. If the patient is told "you are a very sick man, you go to bed at once," he may be made worse by such advice but only a fool would give advice in this manner.

An "aggravation" of symptoms does not always mean that the patient is getting worse. It more often means that he is getting better. He who lacks an understanding of the nature of disease will naturally think that the "aggravation" of symptoms means that the patient is growing worse.

An ailment is not something to struggle against. It is not something to fight. This objection to the "rest-cure" is based on the primitive idea that disease is an unseen dragon tearing at the vitals of the patient. Disease is something to cooperate with. "Giving up" to it simply means allowing it to carry forward its work more freely.

Two objections brought forward have not the slightest relation to going-to-bed *per se*. One of these is that three square meals a day in bed would result seriously. It is true that the patient in bed has no need for such food, but it is equally true that many patients who cannot eat one square meal a day while active, without suffering, may consume three square meals a day in bed without discomfort. However, so far as we are aware only medical men and milk diet enthusiasts ever advocate gorging a bed patient. The next of these objections is that people are afraid of a draft and menacing symptoms are sometimes induced by poor ventilation. This is an objection to poor ventilation. I know of no Orthopath who ever advocated keeping patients in poorly ventilated rooms. Dr. Walter had his patients lay on cots out doors. Aside from this, the fear of drafts is much more easily overcome in bed than in a chair. Any man who has had experience with patients knows this. Indeed, people who keep their windows closed through the day, in Winter, sleep with their windows open at night.

It is objected that one should be guided by his instincts and should not go to bed until he desires to. It is claimed that when we ignore our instincts we must pay the associated penalties. This objection is offered by those who advocate exercising even when one is disinclined to; and who advocate drinking so many glasses of water a day and ignoring one's instinct of thirst. It is advocated by those who advocate mixing a little intelligence with one's eating, by those who would put the same patient on a fast without waiting for instinct to demand a fast and who insist that the demands of appetite that persist during the first two to four days of a fast be ignored; who give cold baths when there is a dread of these; who seek means of forcing sleep when nature does not give sleep voluntarily. The inconsistency of such advice and such practices must be readily apparent.

To demand instinctive living on the one hand and reject it on the other is simply ridiculous. The argument that one should be guided by his instincts would be good if those instincts were normal. But if they are not normal knowledge and intelligence may rightly be called upon to help them out. People who keep their bodies lashed with stimulation do not know when they feel like going to bed. Withdraw their stimulants and notice the "let-down," the languor and lassitude that reveal the true condition of their system and their need for recuperation.

It is next objected that the ordinary daily activities "materially stimulate the functions of the body." When one goes to bed he is deprived of this mechanical stimulation. Metabolism is less active. Elimination is retarded. The circulation is slowed down. It is insisted that poisons are driven out of the body more rapidly if one is active.

If these objections possess any validity the proper way to treat a sick man is to make him run at top speed until he is well. If this mechanical stimulation is not an exhausting thing, then the longer he runs the stronger he should become. If the activity purifies the blood, by stimulating elimination, then the more active one is and the longer he is active the purer his blood should become. Instead of a marathon runner dropping within sight of his goal because of the fatigue poisons that accumulate in his body, he should be fresher at the end of the race than at its beginning. We can recognize the basis of fact that exists in the above superficial objections to rest without endorsing the extremes to which the objections themselves would logically lead.

The success of the work of the vital force is *inversely to the degree of its activity.* Men go to bed at night tired and worn out from a day of active toil. A night of rest recuperates and restores them. The "rest-cure" is only a prolongation of this same normal period in bed in order that the patient may recuperate from a more profound enervation and be restored from a more injured state of his or her tissues.

It is objected also that if a healthy man, a strong man, is confined to bed for a few days he will lose part of his strength and if he remains there for several weeks he will be unable to walk. All of this objection arises out of the fallacy that "strength comes as the result of exercising the muscles." It mistakes the muscular machine that is built up when exercise is indulged in for the power back of the machine. Large, well-trained muscles are better able to manifest power, providing there is power to be manifest, but in doing so they expend the power. Exercise does not give us power— it expends power. It consumes energy, tears down tissue and, if continued long enough, produces exhaustion. If exercise were the source of our strength, then the more we exercise the stronger should we become. It should recuperate us and not exhaust us. But the reverse is true; exercise exhausts and we must go to bed for recuperation.

The farmer who turns his well-fed horses out on the pasture after the crops are laid-by knows well that the rest and grass diet will weaken, (soften) his horses and that when he again puts them to work they will not be able to do as much work as before going to the pasture. Their formerly hard muscles will have become soft and flabby. Their tough shoulders will have become tender. But the farmer knows, also, that after a few days of work, his horses are stronger and can do more work than before he sent them out to rest. They are all the better for the rest. He also knows that he cannot work them indefinitely. He would soon kill his horses.

283

I know a strong man, a weight lifter, who is a careful liver. He spent the summer of 1921 in a summer cottage on a lake in Ohio. The summer was spent in the water. He stuffed himself with milk. He was over two years getting to the point where he could lift as much weight as before he went to the lake. He took plenty of exercise and little rest. The results speak for themselves. He maintained the condition of his muscles, but depleted his nervous energies.

One writer, who calls the conclusion that going to bed conserves one's energy for the work of disease "the silliest conclusion that has ever been promulgated," fully recognizes the value of that form of rest that is secured by fasting and insists that a prolonged rest of this kind improves and does not weaken digestion. The contradiction is apparent.

The strong man confined to bed does grow muscularly weaker. His muscles become soft and flabby. He is unable to lift as much weight or run as fast and as far. But muscular strength is not the thing we use in overcoming the causes of disease. The kidneys need nervous energy, not muscular strength if they are to increase their functions. Nothing increases elimination like rest—not even exercise. Exercise does increase elimination temporarily, but at the same time it creates more to be eliminated, while, in the reaction, elimination is decreased.

It is admitted that if one is "so weak and depleted that he desires to remain in bed" he should do so. This admission if fatal to the above objections. If strength comes from exercise, the weak and depleted should exercise vigorously and often. If going to bed really weakens one, I mean, if it really subtracts from one's fund of vital power, then the weak and depleted would commit suicide by going to bed.

All these objections are further offset by the fact that we do not, except in cases where exercise would aggravate the condition, permit the chronic sufferer to lie in bed without taking some exercise. The human body does not require to be physically active, at work, play or exercise, twelve hours a day in order to maintain structural and functional integrity. Those who attempt to discredit the "rest-cure" should first take the trouble to acquaint themselves with it for patients get well through rest, and recoveries are more satisfactory, than through the methods advocated by physical culturists.

In previous chapters it has been clearly shown that the living organism, in disease, reduces activity in some of its organs in order that the power ordinarily expended through these channels may be utilized where its need is more urgent. This is not merely true of acute or primary disease, but of chronic or secondary disease, as well. The chronic sufferer is tired, dull, listless, feeble, lacks energy and "pep," his appetite is frequently lacking. He does not awake refreshed after a night of sleep. Very little physical or mental effort is required to exhaust him. He gives every evidence of the need of rest and when he secures this he begins to improve.

By resting he recuperates. By resting he enables the body to utilize the energy, usually expended in mental and physical work, but which is conserved through rest, in the work of elimination and repair. Functions which have been lashed to impotency by overstimulation are slowly restored to normal. Structures that have been damaged by overstimulation or by toxins are slowly repaired. Energies that are at low ebb are recuperated. Muscles that grow weaker, while at rest, become stronger than before the rest, after they are judicisuoly exercised, because there is more power back of them. Development is the outgrowth of power within. If the power of development is lacking no development will occur. Recuperation of power is the prime requisite of development. The invalid cannot develop health if he lacks power to do so. He must recuperate his powers.

SUNSHINE AND SUN-BATHING

CHAPTER XXIII

"LIFE is a sun-child," says Dr. Oswald; "nearly all species of plants and animals attain the highest forms of their development in the neighborhood of the equator. Palm trees are tropical grasses. The python-boa is a fully developed black snake; the tiger an undiminished wild cat. With every degree of a higher latitude, Nature issues the representatives of her arch-types in reduced editions—reduced in beauty and longevity, as well as in size and strength."—*Nature's Household Remedies*, p. 79.

That was back in 1885. It was still *heresy* of the rankest kind to say such things at that time. "Science" had not put the seal of her approval upon the "quackery" of sun-bathing and the learned ones of the dominant school of therapeutics only mocked and derided and denounced such statements. A great change has come in medical circles since then, with regard to the value of sun shine and, as is their usual custom, they now pose as the discoverers of the value of and claim exclusive rights to the use of the sun-bath. They first denounce everything, then claim everything. It is quackery until forced upon them, after which it becomes "science." "Quackery" has triumphed many times in her battles with "science."

In her *Materia Medica and Therapeutics* (1916) a Text-book for nurses, Linette A. Parker, B.S. of Columbia University says (p. 295-6) :—

"The first series of observations as to the effect of sunlight on disease was made by Dr. Loncet of Lyons, France, about 1890-1900, in cases of tubercular affections of the joints. He obtained excellent results, some of which were almost miraculous, and became convinced that the benefit extended also to the internal organs. In 1911 Dr. Rollier, a Swiss physician, followed Dr. Loncet's method under very different climatic conditions with equally good results."

Another name frequently mentioned as a pioneer in what is called heliotherapy, is Dr. Niels R. Finsen, of Denmark, who experimented with sun-rays and the rays of "artificial" light at the same time Dr. Loncet was making his observations. The work of Finsen is largely responsible for the inundation of the market with a vast array of elaborate and costly apparatus for treating disease by means of artificial light, which light, although it is controlled by the doctor and can be charged for at high rates, is by no means as effective as sunlight.

It would be a fairly safe guess if one were to say that probably both these men borrowed their first ideas on the employment of sunlight in disease from Arnold Rickli whose sun and air cure institution in Switzerland attracted patients from all over the world. Rickli, who died in 1907 at the age of 97, wrote seven books about his methods, the principal ones, of which were translated into Spanish, French, and Italian. Rikli's work grew out of his childhood experiences in sun-bathing. The story is told of him that when a boy, he would run away from his father's field, where he aided his father and brother in rasing potatoes and when they would find him he would have all his clothes off basking in the sun. When asked why he did such things he would only reply "I like it." His institution at Weldes Krai on the Adriatic Sea is still conducted by his grandson. Dr. A. Montenus of France tells us in his work on *Air, Light, and Sun Baths*, (Rothwell's translation, 1907); "Arnold Rikli is regarded as the inventor of these baths; for over half a century he has been prescribing atmospheric treatment." This grand old Nature Curist of Germany who lived to be nearly a hundred used to go up the mountain each morning and take a sun and air bath himself. He believed in his own "medicine." He took it.

Rikli declared: "Man is made to live in the open air; therefore when exposed to the action of light, air and sun, he is in his real element. As a natural agent, water takes only an inferior place, above it comes air, whilst light takes precedence of every other natural agent, and is the greatest esesntial wherever organic life exists. The nervous system, which is an inherent principle of our organism is acted upon by light, especially through the skin. The purpose of the air treatment is the strengthening of the skin by restoring its natural functions and vitality and elasticity it has absorbed from its primitive state when directly in contact with the skin."

285

Saleeby quotes the French students as saying:—

"Baths of water are good, baths of air are better, baths of light are best." This is but a shortening of Rikli's statements above.

Waldvogel, of Bohemia, in 1715, had advocated sun-bathing. Dr. Lahman, of Germany employed the "sun and air cure" in his institution. Bilz, of Germany employed the sun cure in his world-famous institution as early as 1872-73.

Rikli gave his sun-baths on the tops of two hills, the "Hill of women" and the "Hill of men," in the early morning hours before the sun became too hot. The wisdom of this program is now, at least partly understood. It is now known that in the more rarified atmosphere of the mountains, less of the beneficial rays of the sun are deflected. It is also known that more benefit is derived from the sun when it is not too hot. The heat is greatly enervating.

Finsen and Loncet could not have been ignorant of the above facts. Indeed, Lawrason Brown, M.D., of Saranac Lake, N. Y., in an article entitled "Natural and Artificial Light in Tuberculosis," published in the *Journal of the Outdoor Life,*—April 1926, says:—

"During this period the clinicians had not been idle. A physiotherapist, who was not a physician, Arnold Rikli, (1855) of Veldes, Austria, subjected patients to sun baths in the course of his treatments."

Rikli was not a physiotherapist, but then, no "regular" would dare give him credit without, at the same time concealing the fact that he belonged to the nature cure "quacks" of Europe.

It is known that the Ancient Romans and others used the sun bath while the ancient Greeks practiced nudity, but the value of the sun and air in maintaining health was lost sight of in that awful period in human history known as the Dark Ages when it actually came to be believed that the filthier a person was the more saintly he was. The body was looked upon as a vile, sinful thing to be tortured and execrated in every possible way.

Before coming to the American side of the matter, a few words regarding the sun-bath in ancient times may, therefore, be in order. Man was a nude animal before he learned to make clothes. His first clothes only covered portions of his body and, at first was worn chiefly during the more inclement months of the year. Man learned the genial powers of the sun when, after a spell of cold, or cloudy inclement weather, it came forth again to cheer and warm. He even learned to look upon it as a god and sun-worship was prevalent throughout the world. Indeed in the Third Century A. D., Mithraism, or sun-worship came very near becoming the universal religion. It was so like Christianity in every essential respect that it became its chief opponent. The final triumph of Christianity and its extreme reaction against everything "pagan" practically ended the sun-bath, so widely employed by well and sick alike in ancient times, just as it destroyed the Roman thermae.

Akhenaton of Egypt, Zoroaster of Persia, Hippocrates of Greece—these men had elevated the sun to the dignity of a god and a force. The great sanitarium of Hippocrates' on the Island of Cos was equipped with a large solarium for the use of the sun. The Roman thermae were all equipped with solaria for those taking sun-baths. Pliny says that in these hot-houses the sun is very helpful.

The Incas of Peru treated "syphilis" with sun-baths. In Haiti, similar procedures are still employed. Certain Germanic tribes placed children with fever in the sunlight on the tops of their houses. On the shores of the Bay of Gascony sunlight is still employed in rheumatism. Among the Greeks places called helioses, were usually constructed along the seashore, where the people walked nude in the sun. Herodotus, according to Oribasissus, wrote of the necessity of exposure to the sun and especially emphasized its value for those who were run-down and who needed to gain weight. He thought Fall, Winter, and Spring the best time for such exposure, cautioning against the great heat of summer.

In Rome, Pliny the younger tells us of Vestricius Spurina, that, "as soon as the hour of the bath had come, he went to walk completely naked in the sun if the air was calm, then played with a ball a long time. Celsus, Galen and other Roman physicians are said to have recommended the sun-bath. During that millinium of anti-natural madness, we call the Middle Ages more appropriately the Dark Ages; the only physicians who employed the sun-bath were among the Jews and Arabians.

In his *Lectures on The Science of Human Life*, pp. 638, Graham, while discussing the evils of clothing, shocked the Prudish American Conscience by declaring:—

"My object is not to advocate bodily nudity in society; though I cannot doubt that morality would be greatly improved by it, in the course of two of three generations, if in all other respects mankind conformed to the true laws of their nature;****.

"If man were always to go entirely naked, the external skin, the anatomical structure and functional character and relations of which we have fully contemplated, would be preserved in a more healthy and vigorous state, and perform its functions more perfectly, and thereby the whole human system in all its properties, powers and interests, would be benefitted; the circulation, and particularly the venous circulation which is near the surface, would be more free and unobstructed; respiration or breathing would also be more free, full and perfect; voluntary action would be more unrestrained and easy; the bones would be less liable to disease and distortion; all the muscles of voluntary motion would be better developed and more powerful; in short, the anatomical development and symmetrical proportion, and the physiological power, and functions of every part in the whole system, would be more perfect; and, as a natural consequence, the sensual appetites would be more purely instinctive, and exert a less energetic and despotic influence on the mental and moral faculties, and imagination would be deprived of its greatest power to do evil."

Dr. Trall laid great stress upon the powers of sunlight, both in health and in disease, as will be seen from the following, taken from his *Hydropathic Encyclopedia*, pp. 304-5-6-7, (vol. 1):—

"RELATION OF LIGHT TO ORGANIZATION: The hygienic importance of light is not sufficiently understood by the people nor its remedial influence sufficiently regarded by physicians. Whether it be a distinct imponderable entity, a property of electricity, or something else, it would be idle here to speculate; but it is certain that the light which this earth derives from the sun and the fixed stars, has a powerfully modifying influence on all the functions of its animal and vegetable kingdoms.

"Some plants thrive best when exposed to strong sunlight, others in a moderate light, and others when considerably shaded, yet all of them, without exception, require a good degree of the influence of light to become hardy, firm, and vigorous. Those which grow in deeply-shaded situations or dark cellars are comparatively colorless, slender, and friable. Light is the cause of color in all bodies; it is entirely reflected by white surfaces, and completely absorbed by black.

"Many insects and fishes while living are constantly luminous, in consequence of the rays of light being constantly emitted from various points of their bodies; the fire-fly emits its sparks from two oval spots at the side of the thorax; in the glow-worm a phosphorescent brilliancy issues from its abdominal rings; luminous insects are supposed to absorb light during the day, like the Bouonian stone, and impart it in the evening.

"PHYSIOLOGICAL INFLUENCES OF LIGHT: Plants absorb carbon, and give out oxygen or vital air in the light; but during the night this process is reversed, so that they absorb oxygen, and give out carbon; hence it is injurious and even dangerous to sleep at night in a situation which is closely surrounded with dense foliage, and not well ventilated. The nutritive process is materially checked in all vegetables and animals when deprived of light for a considerable time; in this case vegetables are said to become *etiolated*, a condition analogous to that called *anaemia*, or *hyperaemia*, in man—a state of debility, bloodlessness, and inanition. In some of the lower animals the process of metamorphosis is arrested by deprivation of the solar influence. The tadpole, for example, instead of developing into the frog, either continues to grow as a tadpole, or degenerates into some kind of monstrosity; and the specimens of human monstrosities, developed abnormally, in consequence of the absence of a due degree of 'Heaven's first-born,' are neither few nor far between in the underground tenements of large cities.

"The operation of light on the animal organism has always been recognized as urging to exercise, and increasing the activity of both the bodily and mental powers; while its absence or privation disposes to indolence and obesity. Animals are more readily fattened when kept in obscurity, because the diminished activity of the depurating functions favors the accumulation of adipose matter. Poultry are often confined in dark places to augment their store of oil; and the heads of geese and turkeys are sometimes covered by a hood, or their eyes put out, in order to procure from them fat and greasy livers, as choice morsels for depraved epicures.

"Almost the entire population of our large cities, who occupy backrooms and rear buildings where the sun never shines, and cellars and vaults below the level of the ground on the shaded side of narrow streets, is more or less diseased. Of those who do not die of acute diseases, a majority exhibit unmistakable marks of imperfect development and deficient vitality; and, in fact, as with animals and vegetables in like circumstances, often run into deformities and monstrosities, not more reproachful, however, to those parents who propagate under such disadvantages, than disgraceful to that city, state, or national government which either *compels* or *permits* any class of its citizens to live in such abodes.

"These facts show us that light, and an abundant supply of it, is indispensable to a due development of all organized bodies.

"THERAPEUTIC CONSIDERATIONS: Medical men have always noticed that diseases of all kinds, from the most trifling toothache, quinsy, or rheumatism, to the severest attack of fever, scrofula, or consumption, are much less manageable in low, dark apartments. And it is notorious that, during the prevalence of epidemics, as the cholera, the shaded side of a narrow street invariably exhibits the greatest ratio of fatal cases.

"The observations of Dr. Edwards, on the influence of light in promoting the perfect development of animals, led him to conclude that in climates where nudity is not incompatible with health, exposure of the whole surface of the body to light is favorable to the regular conformation of the body; and he, therefore, has suggested insulation in the open air as a means calculated to restore healthy conformation to children affected with scrofula, whose deviations of form do not appear to be incurable.

"Pereira says: 'As in bright solar light we feel more active, cheerful, and happy, while obscurity and darkness give rise to a gloomy and depressed condition of mind, so we employ insulation in the open air as a mental stimulus in melancholy, low-ness of spirits, and despondency."

"SANATORY INFERENCES: The inferences deducible from the foregoing considerations are sufficiently obvious. All persons, in order to acquire and maintain the best condition of health and strength, should be frequently exposed to the light of the sun, except when oppressively hot. Children are generally maltreated, more especially in cities, in being kept almost entirely excluded from sunshine. Many good mothers are more fond of the delicate faces and pale complexions of their little ones, than intelligent in relation to their physiological welfare. A little sun-browning occasionally of their faces, necks, hands, and feet, and, finally, of their whole bodies, would not only render their development more perfect and enduring, but tend to the production of the greatest symmetry and beauty in manhood and womanhood. Parents should not be too careful in putting umbrella-hats and bonnet-sun-shades on the heads of their children every time they run out of doors.

"Almost all persons, young or old, who live in cities can invigorate the skin and improve the general health, by frequent exposures of the whole body to the air of a well-lighted room, applying moderate friction to the surface at the same time. Light as well as air is generally excluded from the surface by too much or too tight clothing, which evil such exposures in some degree would counteract.

"Dwelling-houses ought to be constructed with especial reference to light. Those rooms which are most occupied should be the best lighted, as the kitchen and sitting room. The sun should be allowed free access to the yard and out-grounds. Shade-trees and shrubbery, useful to some extent around the dwelling, should never be so thick as to shut the direct rays of the sun out entirely. The influence of light in dissipating and decomposing noxious vapors and deleterious gases, which collect in and around low grounds and dark places, is very great.

"The sudden exhilaration and invigoration experienced by the pent-up denizens of our large towns, when they go from their dim counting-rooms, gloomy offices, and basement workshops, to rusticate a few days in mountainous regions, is due nearly as much to the greater strength of the natural light as to the greater purity of the air."

Trall again wrote in his *Water-Cure for the Million* (1860) :—

"The importance of light as a remedial agent, is not sufficiently appreciated. Nearly all forms of disease are more severe and unmanageable in low, dark apartments. Many persons who live in elegant and expensively furnished houses so darken many of the rooms, in order to save the furniture, as to render the air in them very unwholesome. The scrofulous humors which prevail among those inhabitants of our cities who live in rear buildings and underground apartments, sufficiently attest the relation between sunshine and vitality. Invalids should seek the sunlight as do the flowers—care being taken to protect the head when the heat is excessive. Exposing the whole skin in a state of nudity, frequently, to the air, and even to the rays of the sun, is a very invigorating practice. For scrofulous persons this is particularly serviceable."

Among the conditions in which Trall declared that "abundant sunshine" should "be allowed especial prominence in the remedial plan," he lists, in this same work (p. 38); "CACHEXIES—Scrofula, including its various forms of humors and tumors, glandular enlargements, white swelling, cutaneous eruptions, fever sores, RICKETS, LUMBAR ABSCESS, HIP-DISEASE, otitis, opthalmia, etc., as well as plethora, SCURVEY, elephantiasis, CANCER, etc." He added: "The air bath is admirable in these cases." Plenty of pure air, out-door exercise and a "rigidly physiological" diet with cleanliness were given equal prominence with the sun in remedying such conditions.

Dr. George H. Taylor, Trall's co-worker, lays great stress upon the value of sunlight both in health and disease, in his *Health by Exercise* (1883), first published in 1856 under the title *The Swedish Movement Cure.* He regarded light starvation as a chief cause of rickets, scrofula, tuberculosis, and other troubles, and employed the sun as a means of overcoming these. The following quotations from this work will suffice to show the reader what emphasis he placed upon sunlight:—

"The scrofulous diathesis manifests itself in a great variety of symptoms, differing according to constitution and age. In children, it is denoted by a peculiar pallor of countenance, dullness of complexion, hypertrophied or inflamed mesenteric glands, and tumid abdomen, bowels alternately loose and costive, capricious appetite—frequently too urgent—shrunken limbs, fetid breath, indisposition for play. Eruptions of various kinds may occur upon the skin of the face or other parts of the body, and swellings upon or about the neck of an indolent character often appear. The scrofulous child often presents a haggard, almost wild appearance, and its blue veins are painfully prominent. Sometimes the head becomes abnormally developed, accompanied occasionally by a precocity of intellect,**** while the extremities are at the same time illy nourished.****

"In youth, the most striking symptoms of the affection are enlarged glands of the neck, fragility of form, narrowness of the chest, and a strong tendency to cough, and lung disease, which not unfrequently terminate in pulmonary consumption.

"In adults, the morbid action is apt to center in the lungs, in disease which, as commonly treated, is generally incurable."

He then declares that the intelligent reader should perceive that there was a period anterior to the appearance of these symptoms during which the "latent disease" was being developed by its producing causes, and during which time "sufficient knowledge and a correct practice would furnish an effectual bar to its further progress. But as such knowledge is only acquired under the spur of feelings resulting from the presence of the disease in its developed state, we must be content to bring into requisition a *curative,* means that ought to have proved *preventive.*" (p. 278)

This doctrine that the means that prevent the development of abnormalities are the means with which to correct or cure them, is still foreign to the Heteropathic schools. He explained that the condition, above described, results from a failure of the vital processes to complete their work,—"imperfect nutrition," failure of the skin and lungs in excretion. "Disease being essentially incomplete or ineffectual action (pathology being simply modified physiology), it can occur only through defect of

289

the conditions essential to perfect development of the system in all it parts and functions. The nature of the mischievous agents that concur in the production of these conditions is learned only by a study of the disease during its development and subsequent progress." (p. 279). This proposal to study the disease during its development and progress and the conditions under which it develops and progresses is the opposite of the present age-long method of studying end-results, largely after the patient is dead.

"In this way," he continues, "we discover among the prominent causes of this disease, *insufficiency of pure air, light, and exercise, and want of cleanliness.*

"We have only to look into the abodes of poverty and squalor for confirmation of this statement. Every city physician has abundant opportunities for studying all forms of this disease in connection with these causes.

"But the wealthy, and those who have it in their power to command the conditions of health, are quite as apt to be afflicted with scrofula in one or other of its forms, and in their case it is evidently the result of the same causes that produce it among the poor. For the real hygienic condition of those whose circumstances and social position are so different, are often very much alike. For while the one class is deprived of fresh air and sunlight by being confined in low crowded localities, the other suffers an equal deprivation through the agency of shutters, heavy window-drapery, and interior rooms, aggravated by the choking dust and corrupt air, which are the inevitable concomitants of fashionable upholstery and carpeting. In both cases, respiration is rendered ineffectual through lack of healthful motion and purity of the air, and these effects are aggravated by want of exercise and good habits on the part of the persons thus exposed." (p. 279).

Coming to a more detailed discussion of sunlight he declares (p. 438-9-40) :—

"The fact that light has powerful hygienic, and even remedial properties, is one too much overlooked. Light is well known to be a most potent chemical agent, both in nature and in the arts. It arouses the vegetable world into life and perfects its products, and without it all animate nature would soon perish for lack of sustenance. In the arts, modern science has wonderfully economized its powers, and makes it serve the most important uses. It is a most potent agent for determining the chemical state of bodies, readily decomposing numerous chemical compounds, and re-combining their elements in new forms.

"That peculiar property of light whereby it is rendered a most important hygienic agent, is manifested in its power to destroy noxious vaporous bodies existing in the atmosphere. The surface of the earth, covered with vegetable and animal matter in a state of decay, sends forth under the influence of heat and moisture an abundance of gaseous matter, which, mingling with the air, enters the lungs to poison the blood, and produces various forms of disease. Though existing in quantities too minute to affect the sense, or any known chemical test, yet, through the lungs, these particles are constantly being conveyed into the system, where they accumulate and exert their chemical power in full force, in opposition to the conditions of health. It is well known that in those localities characterized by a degree of heat and moisture favorable to the most rapid vegetable decomposition, fevers of various kinds abound. These effects can occur only when the noxious products in question are produced more rapidly than they can be destroyed by the agency of sunlight.

"We receive the most injury from insidious and disregarded causes. We seldom give a thought to what may be the consequences of denying to the rooms in which we dwell, the wholesome and vivifying influence of sunlight, but on the contrary take the most unwearied pains to exclude it. In the absence of light, the invisible causes of disease, entering by the windows and doors, or generated from the gaseous matters eliminated from our bodies, operate with all their force. It is useless to try to counteract the effects flowing from these causes with drugs, or to combat them in any other way, while the causes themselves are operating in full force. Commonly the air and light are shut out together, which is much worse than if the air, newly acted on by the strong light, were freely admitted.

"The influence on the constitution of this custom of living in darkness is most favorable to the production of that condition of the blood and of the vital habit from which springs scrofula. The pale and dusky complexions, eruptive skins, flabby and

290

weak muscles, and generally sickly aspect, which are so frequently witnessed in young children, are, in many instances, mostly attributable to this cause. Of course, light is a most important agent to be employed in the cure of affections of this class. It is wonderful and delightful to see how soon a pale, attenuated, miserable child, after being freely exposed to the sunlight for several hours every day, will begin to improve, and the symptoms here described to disappear. Even scrofulous swelling of the glands of the neck, or other parts of the body, will quickly succumb under the magical influence of sunlight and pure air.

"Nursing mothers, especially, need these hygienic influences to maintain the purity and vigor of their system, that they may not lay the foundation for lasting disease in their offspring, for the child is sure to suffer, even sooner than the mother, the grievous consequences of her physiological errors.

"Is it necessary that the parlors and sitting-rooms of our dwellings should be kept so dark and unwholesome? The first reason always assigned by the housekeeper is, that only in this way can she preserve the colors of her carpeting and upholstery, as if the color of a carpet or a curtain was more precious than that of the cheek and lip. In a hygienic point of view, one is led to feel that these household comforts and elegancies do more harm than good, that their advantages are rather more than balanced by their ill effects. However beautiful and costly, they are necessarily uncleanly. However well kept, they are the inevitable receptacles of impalpable dust, which yield invisible clouds at every touch, besides, being the reservoirs of air contaminated in the way we have noticed. Carpets, so common a luxury here, are but little used in Europe, except in England, and it would undoubtedly greatly promote the health of our own people were they to be abolished by statute from every habitation in the land."

Dr. Lust says that "the first sun-baths given in America were at Butler, N. J., at the Yungborn, in 1897." This statement must be incorrect in view of the use of the sun-bath by Trall and Taylor at a much earlier date. Nevertheless, it reveals that the sun-bath has been employed here continuously since a time before Loncet had advanced very far with his investigations, for they are still given at the Youngborn as well as at many other drugless resorts and sanitariums. Dr. Lust's place is modeled after the German "Nature" cure institutions and is not Orthopathic.

All three of these men, Graham, Trall, and Taylor, recognized the great part played by sunlight in nutrition both in health and disease. Sunlight was, to them, a hygienic necessity in all states of the body. Its influence on the skin, blood, muscles, bones, instincts, mind and health are all noted. It was studied as food is studied—not as an essential in certain states of disease— but as an indispensible elemental condition of continued active life and normal development and function. Its anti-septic powers were also stressed, although in this they differed from the present day conception of this in that they regarded sunlight as an agent in destroying poisonous gases arising from decomposition while today it is claimed, probably erroneously, to kill germs.

But, even in allopathic circles, where the germ theory is strongest, the idea is growing that light is less valuable in killing the germ than in raising the body's resistance to it. When the germ theory has completed its passing the fact will then be clearly recognized that sunshine is an essential factor element in normal nutrition.

The mere enumeration of a few of the effects of sunlight upon nutrition will be enough to emphasize its nutrtive importance. It enables the body to assimilate calcium. It is through this that it is of value in the prevention and cure of rickets and tuberculosis, in both of which there is a lack of calcium. A few minutes exposure daily to the sunlight will double the quantity of phosphorus in a baby's blood in a fortnight. It rapidly increases the number of red-blood corpuscles in the blood and is indispensible in overcoming anemia. The haemoglobin in the blood is increased. This increases its oxygen carrying power. The circulation of the blood itself is improved. The blood's power to build and repair tissue is increased. The growth of hair is stimulated. Ulcers, sores, skin diseases, etc., heal more rapidly under its influences. The muscles grow larger and firmer and acquire greater contractile power, even without exercise.

Sunlight dominates the chemistry of the blood. On a simple, natural diet, with sufficient sunlight, the blood will contain all the elements it requires for life and growth. Pills, capsules, and liquid drugs of lime, iron, sulphur, phosphorus, etc., are of no earthly value to the body, well or sick, whether given in the sun or out of it. Nature Curists have for years advocated eating sun-cooked foods. "Eat the sun's rays" was a favorite expression with them. Recent experiments have shown that their instincts and reason had not led them astray. Plants or animals raised in the sun have better health and more food value. Milk from "sun-fed animals contains more vitamins."

Theory has it that a new arrangement of the molecules that constitute cholesterol, a "fatty" substance which is pretty well distributed through the animal and vegetable kingdoms, is brought about by the exposure of foods to ultra-violet radiations which gives rise to vitamin D. Nobody knows what vitamin D is, but the trend at present is to have a vitamin for each letter in the alphabet. However, the fact that sun-ripened and sun-cured foods are superior to indoor-ripened or kiln-dried foods, long known to hygienists, has now become known to the "scientists." Experiment has shown that sunshine cured hay has more growth-promoting potency than that dried in cloudy weather, while clover, growing in the sun, lacks its supply of vitamin; it must also be dried in the sun.

A vitamin is probably not something different from the rest of the food. It is probably not a distinct chemical substance, but merely a peculiar element-grouping, brought about by the action of the sun's rays, which renders the food, or some part of it, more easily assimilated and used by the body.

Not vitamins alone, but minerals, are concerned in this problem. Milk in pasture-fed cows is not only richer in vitamins, but contains much higher percentages of phosphorus and calcium and fifty per cent. more citric acid. Cows and mothers can produce perfect milk only when given green foods and exposed to the sun. Young animals fed exclusively on milk from cows fed in the shade on dry fodder lose weight and die. Similar animals fed on similar quantities of milk from cows that run in the pasture, getting both sunlight and green foods, grow and thrive.

Dr. J. Bell Ferguson, a medical health officer, of England, had a school-room glazed with a form of quartz glass that permits 50 to 65 per cent. of the ultra-violet rays of the sun to pass through. Another room of the same size and same exposure was glazed with ordinary lead glass. At the end of nine months, the children who had studied under the quartz glass had gained an average of an inch more in height and three and a quarter pounds more in weight than the children under ordinary glass. The result was that this glass is now used to glaze London's zoo, while a few hospitals are putting it in. At least the animals will be cared for.

A few years since, some experiments were performed on rats at the Johns Hopkins University. Eighteen rats were fed a diet which was known, from previous experience, to produce in rats, rickets which resembles in every way the same disease in man. Twelve of these rats were sent to New Haven, Conn., where they were exposed to the sun shine for about four hours daily for about two months. The other six rats were kept in Baltimore and reared in well ventilated, but poorly lighted rooms.

At the end of the period the rats were all killed and examined. The report states that in the rats exposed to sun no evidence of rickets were found. Their condition was normal with the exception of the bones, which were more delicate than in rats of a corresponding age which had been reared on a more satisfactory diet. An abundance of fat was present. The rats reared in Baltimore, out of the sun, presented but scant fat, as well as the evidences of rickets.

Are we to conclude from this experiment that sunlight can be made to take the place of a proper diet? Shall we conclude that the sun's rays supply the lacking food elements? Not at all. We can only claim that rickets are due to a combination of "causes" among which is lack of sunlight. It is evident that the required food elements were present in the diet but that the rat out of the sunshine was not able to extract and assimilate them. The other rats under the beneficient effects of the sun's rays were enabled to extract the food elements and assimilate them.

The favorable effects of sunlight upon nutrition, its action as a vital or *compensated stimulant* upon growth and repair are plainly apparent in this experiment and the facts enumerated above. It is for this reason that we declare that the highest degree of health and strength can be attained and maintained only by adequate contact with the sun. Housing and clothing have deprived us of our normal supply of sunlight, so that we are suffering from light starvation and etiolation.

The phosphorus and calcium content of an infant's blood is known to rise and fall with the season, there being less in Winter and more in Spring and Fall. Hens kept out of the sun lay eggs with thinner, softer shells than those kept in the sun. They also lay fewer eggs.

With an insufficiency of light, specifically, the non-illuminating ultra-violet rays, the fibrine and the red blood corpuscles become diminished in quantity, The serum or watery portion of the blood is increased, inducing leukemia, a disease characterized by a great increase in the number of white blood corpuscles. A total exclusion of sunlight induces the severer forms or anemia, originating from an impoverished and disordered state of the blood.

Tenement house districts in large cities to which sunlight has no access have the greatest infant mortality and are the chief breeding places of rickets and tuberculosis.

Inhabitants of southern mountain slopes are stronger and healthier than those living on the northern sides.

C. W. Saleeby, M.D., Ch.B., F.Z.S., F.R.S.E., of England, declares, *Sunlight and Health*, p. 166:—

"Phosphorus is a good thing in a child's blood, so is calcium. No child nor man can live without these things; nor bones nor teeth can be formed without them. We supply them copiously in medicinal form, therefore, and the idea, is excellent. Very often we fail however to get the results we desire. But the Americans have shown, and our own workers are conrfiming them, that, without any amelioration of a thoroughly vicious and defective diet, the amount of phosphorus in the blood will be doubled after a week or two of daily exposure, lasting a few minutes only, to sunlight. Some chemical process is thus begun, some ferment, or internal secretion, or 'harmone,' constructed which enables the body to take and keep and use, from the diet, what it would otherwise have to go without. And the children at the school in the sun, most inexpensively and simply fed, without medicine or cod-liver oil, flourish and grow strong and straight, and remain so, doubtless because these mysterious and as yet unexamined vital processes are set going in their bodies by the prime source of all life and health."

It is asserted by some that sunshine enables the body to manufacture vitamin A. The theory has been advanced by Saleeby that the skin is an organ of internal secretion and that as suggested by Sheridan Delepine, under the influence of sunshine it contributes to the making of haemoglobin. He insists that in the pigmented skin, under the influence of sunlight, very active chemical processes are occurring. If this view proves correct, it will justify Graham's attachment of so great importance to its effects upon the skin. Others think they have found that by the aid of sunshine the body manufactures a substance called cholestrian which is essential to calcium metabolism. Whichever way we turn the emphasis is on nutrition.

Hess showed that milk from cows fed on pastures in the sunlight maintains the health and growth of young animals, whereas milk from cows maintained out of the sun and fed on fodder will not maintain life and growth. The *American Review of Tuberculosis*, vol. XIII, No. 2, Feb. 1926, says: "something also may be accomplished in this direction (the prevention of rickets) by improving the hygienic condition of Milch cows. At present many of these furnishing the best grade of milk are kept throughout the year in sunless barns, are allowed a very limited amount of exercise, and receive little or no fresh green fodder."

It seems not to have occurred to them, as it did to Taylor, that the nursing mother would also be benefitted by sunshine and that it would enable her to supply more and better milk for her child, so that she would not be forced to depend on the cow to mother her offspring. Indeed the subjection of the pregnant woman to daily sun-baths will benefit both her and the developing foetus, and, I am convinced, will also do much toward lessening the pains that now make childbirth a harrowing ordeal in so many cases. Girls brought up in the sunshine properly fed, and normally active should develop so well and normally that normally painless childbirth should be the rule instead of the now rare exception.

It is notorious that the clad races, and especially those who live in the cities, and are in the sun but little, are unable to supply their children with milk that will sustain them. Babies that are themselves light-starved, and which are fed on milk from light-starved mothers or light-starved cows are at a double disadvantage.

It is also worthy of note that those mothers who are in the sun-light least are the ones who have the most difficult deliveries in childbirth. When mankind deprived itself of the sun it took a long step in its progressively downward course—its course of degeneration.

Dr. Carl Sonne, experimented with the light bath on guinea pigs to determine its action or diphtheria toxin in the body. He, of course, employed experimental "diphtheria," that is cultures of the supposed diphtheria germ, and not diphtheria. However, his findings are of value for the introduction of this material into the body is the introduction of toxins. He found the bath tends to the rapid destruction of the toxin. Saleeby declares:—

"The destruction in the course of a single light bath lasting two hours, without the production of any fever (rise in the general body temperature) is as great as that caused by a general fever of 40° C. lasting several days and nights. The possible significance of this remarkable result for the treatment of such disease as diphtheria will be evident to the reader."

Take away the sunlight and all life upon the earth would soon perish. However, this does not mean that the sun is the source of life as the materialist claims. For the same thing would happen if we took away all water or all air or all carbon, etc. Sunlight is as we hope to show, only a powerful and necessary factor in plant and animal nutrition just as water and air are necessary factors in nutrition. It does some of the things that vitamins are said to do. Its absence produces some of the results that vitamin insufficiency is claimed to produce.

If a plant is deprived of sunlight it either dies outright or puts forth a sickly, colorless growth. If any rays of light chance to filter through the covering of the plant it will bend towards it in the effort to get the light. If it fails it soon withers and dies. Its tissues are deprived of the mysterious but none the less actual influence of the sun-light. What the cave, the box or other covering does for plants, clothes and houses do for man. Our pale (dead) white skins are signs of disease not of health and are tolerated only because a long persistence in the error that caused it has degenerated into a custom. Custom holds us in its powerful grip.

No one would attempt to raise ferns or roses in the darkness nor to raise plants under a box, yet they attempt to bring up their children and maintain their own health with their bodies always in darkness. Would that we could learn the truth of Michelet's statement: "Of all flowers the human flower is the one that needs sunshine most." Man clothed and housed becomes pale and anemic and a prey to every disease influence. In the tropics where sunlight is most abundant life exists in the greatest profusion. On the other hand, in those portions of earth where nights are longest and days are shortest and where long winters prevail life is either absent altogether or it consists of poorly developed forms.

The chemical rays of the sun are the most powerful of all vital stimulants. If a piece of black cloth be tacked over a grass plot for a few days and its effects noted one may easily see the effect of the deprivation of these rays upon plant life. To fully appreciate the evils of wearing dark clothing tack a piece of white cloth of the same texture over another grass plot and let it remain an equal length of time. Other colors may be experimented with. It will be both interesting and instructive. In general, we may say that the darker the color the less of the sun's rays will be allowed to pass through.

Plants may be grown under artificial light. But they lack the rugged constitution of plants grown in the sunlight. They do not possess the same organic quality, are not as sturdy and strong. They may be made to grow more rapidly than plants in the sunlight, by subjecting them to light for longer hours than our revolving world does, their rate of growth increasing or decreasing with the increase or decrease in light, but forced growth of this kind proves to be defective in more ways than one. The plants do not have the same color, nor equal structural soundness, nor are their flowers and fruit equal to those of plants grown in the sun. The sun has no rival, neither with plant or animal. Artificial light cannot supplant or substitute for the sun's rays. Higher prices may be charged for it—that is all.

The ultra-violet rays destroy bacteria and animals with bare, unpigmented skins. Snails die in twenty four hours after exposure to these rays. Tadpoles and flies become torpid after an exposure lasting three hours and are killed in five hours. Young grass-hoppers die in two to three days. These facts reveal the dangers that lie in the use of the powerful ultra-violet rays from the doctor's lamps, when compared to the more beneficial rays from the sun which do not so easily or quickly destroy bacteria and young animals.

Plants grown in the dark lack color, and are unable to flower and fructify. Some of them, like the potato, are unable to put forth leaves. They are of very poor quality, breaking easily, and short lived. Every cell and fiber in the plant and animal body is strengthened by the sun's rays.

I quote the following from *Rational Diet*, (p. 25-6) by Otto Carque:—

"Of the many experiments which have been made so far to demonstrate the beneficial effects of sunlight, that of John Blayton is the most remarkable and significant. In order to determine whether the indirect or diffused daylight, perhaps during a longer period of time, has the same effect as the direct sunlight, he selected twelve bean plants of the same variety and in the same stage of development. Then he planted them in such a way near one another, that six always had full direct sunlight, while the others received only the diffused daylight. In October the pods were harvested, and the weight of those exposed to the sun rays was found to be in the proportion of 29:99, that of the dried beans 1:3.

"This result was to be expected, but in the following year, when all the plants grown from the same seed received the full amount of sunlight, the surprising fact was ascertained that those which had been raised in the shade only yielded half the amount of the previous year's harvest, while in the fourth year, they blossomed but did not mature. The deprivation of sunlight during *one* summer weakened the stock to such a degree that the species became extinct after four years."

Etiolated plants are structurally weaker, possess less resistance to weather changes and to disease influences. They are unable to fructify and often unable to put forth leaves. Etiolated animals are the same. Their bones are more delicate, tissues less firm and resistant. They are short lived, subject to disease and possess less resistance to weather changes. But the above series of experiments reveal that the absence of sunlight has a harmful effect upon the germ-plasm and is thus an actual cause of racial degeneracy. We are dealing with a more important element of natural hygiene than we have ever before realized.

Dr. Alfred F. Hess, of Columbia University, and Professor Steenbock, of the University of Wisconsin, almost simultaneously announced the discovery that exposure of foods to the ultra-violet rays creates chemical changes in these that makes them better food for children with rickets and also better food with which to prevent rickets. Dr. Hess thinks he has found that this is due to the formation of the "anti-rachitic" vitamin D, when fatty substances of plants are exposed to the ultra-violet radiations. Ergosterol, a fat like substance in plants, has been isolated and is considered the vehicle for this "anti-rachitic" quality. "It was found to bring about a health process of the bones when even as little as .0003 milligrams per capita was given daily," a homeopathic dose.

It seems quite certain that many of the discoveries in vitamins have been made under the influence of alcohol or other strong drug, and it is quite probable that much of the present enthusiasm for ultra-violet radiations is of this same character. However hygienists have long contended that sun-ripened fruits and vegetables grown in the fields possessed greater food value than fruits pulled green and ripened out of the sun, or than vegetables grown in green-houses. We have long claimed that the failure of many who attempted the exclusive fruit and nut diet was due to the fact that they ate fruit not ripened on the trees in the sun. This has been the significance of the advice: "*Eat the sunshine.*".. The above mentioned discoveries may serve to vindicate and explain our contention that tubers and other foods grown under ground are inferior to foods grown on the surface where they receive the sun's rays.

It is only by the aid of the ultra-violet rays that plants are able to make sugar and starch out of carbon-dioxide. When Berthelot discovered that by the use of these rays he was able to produce sugar without the aid of plant life there followed from many quarters, and they are still pouring forth, predictions of a time when synthetic food would take the place of farm and orchid; chemists would supplant the farmer, the secrets of vegetation would be discovered so that trees would shoot up to maturity in ten years instead of a century, vegetables would mature in days instead of weeks, etc. It has been proposed to fit restaurants with ultra-violet lights so that eaters may have these while eating. All manners of costly commercial projects are forecast. With characteristic pigheadedness, the orthodox crowd forget the sun and think only of the inferior machines, which they are exploiting for profit. After the effects of ultra-violet irradiations on food were discovered, "sunshine" pills were put on the market in England. Dr. Colwell of London advocated radiation of cows by ultra-violet lamps, through the winter. It has been proposed to introduce ultra-violet rays directly into the stomach, in cases of indigestion, by means of quartz tubes, to cure indigestion. Quartz tubes for use in the ears, nose, throat, rectum, etc., are already in use. The whole lesson is learned from the wrong end. Sunshine is being ignored and therapeutics is being made to obscure hygiene. About the only practical suggestion thus far offered is that of substituting quartz panes for the glass panes that are now used in our houses and this will not be practical until a cheap method of production is found.

Let us get a glimpse of what the absence of sunlight does for us. Take the example of children who have been imprisoned for some time in dark cellars by cruel, remorseless parents, as has sometimes happened. They become pale, almost corpse like, anemic and emaciated. Their bodies waste away until they are literally "skin and bones." Of course, in such cases, the lack of sunlight is not the only factor in the production of such results but it is one of the largest factors.

We observe the same thing, though to a less extent in those who are constantly indoors and who seldom get into the sunlight. No matter how wholesome their food nor how regular their habits, the effects of a lack of sunlight are apparent.

Then there is the "jail bird" who has been locked in his cell for sometime, as a shining example of what a lack of sunlight will do. We remember one such who had been in jail for three years where very little sunlight ever reached him. He appeared to have been bleached. He was etiolated. His muscles were flabby and had wasted away, he lacked strength, endurance, pep. He was in line for disease.

Now all of these results were not due to lack of sunlight. He was inactive during the time of his imprisonment. His mental attitude was not conducive to health. The bill of fare presented by these county boarding houses is usually not fit to feed a dog upon. These factors and others all contributed their fair share in producing his condition. However, the lack of sunlight was a very potent factor in producing his condition. They demonstrate that the sunlight exerts a profound effect upon human nutrition.

It is an axiomatic first truth that there can be no perversion or impairment of a natural function without resulting in corresponding injury and disease. Man has become so accustomed to looking upon his present unhealthy, degenerate state as natural, and his degenerating practices as harmless, that he is not easily led to see the influence of clothing in impairing his physiological functions, and especially those of his skin.

Complete organs may be removed from the body, not only the arms and legs, but some of the internal organs, and life will continue as before, but if the function of the skin is suspended for only a few minutes, death is the result. The skin serves several very important functions, not the least of which is that of serving as a protective covering for the rest of the body and excluding infectious matters from it. It serves as an organ of elimination and performs a very important part in the regulation of the body temperature. The resistant powers of the normal skin counteracts in a marvelous way those changes of temperature to which the body is so frequently subjected. The skin weakened by clothing is unable to do this very effectively.

Again, the skin that has become weakened by clothing serves as a less effective barrier to infectious matter from the outside. Medical books list about twenty different forms of skin inflammations, about forty different varieties of hypertrophies, thirty-five of atrophies, several forms of neuroses, several varieties of skin hemorrhages, about sixty to seventy kinds of new growths, and many parasitical affections. These skin diseases appear almost wholely among the much clad denizens of the hot house condition we proudly term civilization, and are seldom, some of them never, met with among the unclad races.

Geo. Wharton James, author of *What the White Man May Learn From the Indian,* says:—

"While there is no doubt that the uncivilized and unclothed Indian occasionally suffers from a few forms of skin disease, I can abundantly testify from my thirty years intimate association with the tribes of the southwest, that amongst those who have been least in contact with civilization there is so little skin disease as to make it inappreciable. For many years I scarcely saw a skin disease amongst them, and when the skin would be torn or injured in any way, as I have often seen it, by their falling form a horse, by riding through the forrest after deer and catching the projecting limbs of trees etc., the rapidity with which the wounds healed were both surprising and enlightening. It was enlightening in that it revealed to me the advantage, from this standpoint at least, of their life over mine. When my skin was torn there was a good deal of pain and it took a long time to heal, and yet I was far healthier than many white men. Yet what to me was a severe skin wound they regarded as a trivial affair, paying little or no attention to it, and the rapidity with which it healed justified their scornful laugh at my warnings that they take care of it lest greater evil ensue."

Mr. James also says: "I have never seen an Indian with a poor head of hair or with dandruff or any other disease of the scalp."

Saleeby says:—

"Properly aired and lighted, the skin becomes a velvety, supple, copper coloroured tissue, absolutely immune from anything of the nature of pimples or acne, IN-CAPABLE OF BEING VACCINATED, (meaning its resistance to infection is greatly increased, author), and its little hairs usually show considerable development. When the visitor touches such a skin in the cool air, he is surprised to find it quite warm. The sun was not shining when I did so first, and the patient was, of course, perfectly nude except for a loincloth. Evidently plenty of heat was somehow being produced in that little body, with so large a surface to cool, relatively to its mass. This would seem to be a puzzle, for these patients have, in many instances, never moved a muscle—practically speaking—for months; they have not even had their muscles innervated (sic) by the faradic current; they have not been massaged. But always the muscles are firm and well-developed under the warm skin. 'The sun is the best masseur,' said Dr. Rollier to me; and one realized that the stimulant light, playing upon the nude skin in the cool air, induces and maintains that condition of tone in the muscles which, indeed, moves no points but is yet a form of muscular activity essential for the production of bodily heat and for the proper posture of the bodily parts. Hence we understand how plaster of Paris apparatus is here as utterly unknown as the knife. The tone of the muscles, thanks to the nude skin and the reflex response to the light, is enough to keep the recovering young spine, for instance, in proper position, and to form what Rollier calls the 'corset musculaire.' One sees very little fat on any of the patients. Their condition is more like that of the trained athlete. (He is describing T. B. patients who receive no exercise. Author's note.), and one's ideas as to the importance of fat in tuberculosis go by the board."

It may not be out of place at this point to observe that Rollier "discards meat, except very rarely, absolutely excludes alcohol in all stages of all cases," gives no cod-liver oil, and "detests and scrupulously avoids" "overfeednig, hitherto a cardinal principle in the therapeutics of tuberculosis." Cereals, milk, milk products and vegetables and fruit constitute the diet. Saleeby says:—

"The clinical evidence is clear that, when the sunlight fails, as it not infrequently does at Leysin, the patients are injured, and that they prosper when it returns. The natural process of excretion of rubish—such as a morsel of dead bone—may be observed to cease in obscure weather, and be resumed when the process of insulation is again permitted by the atmospheric conditions."

Such facts make it clear that the sunlight acts in some more subtle and more fundamental manner than that of killing bacteria. This is proven by the fact that it beneficially affects deep-seated local affections, when applied to the skin, and by its beneficial effects upon affections, wounds included, that no one supposes to be due to germs, as well as by all the facts that have been given in this chapter.

The beneficial effect of sunlight upon the bones, glands, etc., is noted in the treatment of tuberculosis of the bones by the sun-bath. The following bit of information from a thoroughly orthodox source confirms many of the claims which hygienists have been making for many years, and for which they have been denounced as quacks and ignoramuses by the regular physicians. In Octorber, 1922, a tuberculosis conference was held in Augusta, Maine. The newspapers for October 3rd printed the following interesting account of the conference:—

"Success of the sun-cure, not only for bone and glandular tuberculosis in children, but for the pulmonary forms as well, was announced at the opening session of the New England tuberculosis conference today by Doctors Cole B. Gibson and John F. O'Brien of Connecticut, who are superintendents of the only two state sanatoria for children in America.

"Dr. Gibson, superintendent at Meriden, where 200 children are treated, asserted that lung tuberculosis yields, like the bone and glandular varieties, to heliotherapy. Dr. O'Brien, superintendent at the seaside of Niantic, asserted in his paper on bone and glandular tuberculosis:

"1. All forms of the disease yield to the sun-cure.
"2. Surgical operations are unwise for the treatment of diseased glands.
"3. Pure sunlight, instead of sunlight filtered through windows is demanded.
"4. The intense suffering which children ill with bone tuberculosis experience, stops speedily under the sun-cure treatment." (This fact is one of the reasons I consider that daily exposure to the sun prevents, in animals and "Primitive" peoples, the pains of parturition, suffered by "civilized" women. Author's note).
"5. The removal of tonsils and adenoids has not led to benefit but to a decided aggravation of symptoms.

"Dr. O'Brien described the Sanatoria on the eastern shore of Long Island Sound where, he said, 'Even when the ground is covered with snow and the ponds with ice, naked children who are winning their uphill fight for health, may be seen romping on the beach or swimming in the ocean.'

"According to our experience, exposure of the entire body to the weather, during both summer and winter, not only does not cause colds, but actually is a most effective means of prevention. (If the reader will take the trouble to read the works of Trall, Rausse, Macfadden, Page, Just, Kuhne, etc., he will find that Nature Curists have been proclaiming this fact for many years. They have been denounced by the regulars for so doing. Author's note).

"Heliotherapy, we have found at the seaside, increases weight, cures tuberculosis, and in a most remarkable manner stops the suffering from pain.

"Even more striking than the gain in weight is the astonishing change in the general condition of the patient. During the fine weather, our bed patients even are carried to the beach where they attend classes, play in the sand, and crawl in the water. One of our patients, who was admitted with both lower limbs completely paralyzed from spinal tuberculosis, actually learned to swim while the power was coming back into his limbs even before he was strong enough to walk. Although he still wears a large calot jacket, during the baseball season he demonstrated his skill as pitcher. The only boy he has been unable to strike out is a little fellow who has one limb encased in plaster of paris, and who, when he goes to the bat, is able to support himself with one crutch and still use both arms for a full swing at the ball."

It is gratifying to see these men arrive at the conclusion that the removal of tonsils and adenoids aggravates rather than helps the condition. Such operations have been condemned by Nature Curists from the beginning on these very grounds, as well as upon the grounds that operations do not remove causes.

Rollier condemns the cutting out of tuberculous glands. In fact Rollier has adopted so much of the Nature Cure program—sunbaths, non-meat diet, no alcohol, no drugs, no cod-liver oil, etc., that one quite naturally suspects that he has been browsing among the books of the "quacks."

In removing these glands the medical profession has always been removing parts of Nature's first line defenses against the spread of infection.

The sun's light is not a salve or an ointment. However, great are its local effects, when applied locally, it cannot be made to suppress a local effect of a general or systemic condition. In London in Aug. 1922, patients who had been given local light treatments applied to the diseased areas, but who had failed to improve, were given general sun baths, without exposure of the diseased areas at all, and they all recovered rapidly. These results serve to further confirm the orthopathic premise that these local effects are secondary to the general effect and that all "treatment" must be constitutional. Those little quartz rods and tubes in the offices of the physio-therapists and physicians, for insertion into and treatment of the nose, throat, ear, and other orifices of the body, are wrong in principle and failures in application.

We wish especially to call the reader's attention to the effects of the sunshine on the development of the bones. Rickety bones are defective, misshapen, brittle, easily broken. The bones of the rats which were given a daily sun-bath (refer to Johns Hopkins experiment previously noted), presented none of these conditions of the bones. This reminds us of the statement of Graham:—

"If man were always to go entirely naked the bones would be less liable to disease and distortion."

Dr. W. T. Bovie, Professor of Biophysics, Harvard University, reared two flocks of chickens in a green house. Both flocks were fed the same food, given the same space in which to run about, both wallowed in the same dust and scratched the same gravel. Their conditions of life were identical except for the fact that one flock was exposed for fifteen minutes a day to the ultra-violet rays of the quartz lamp.

Seventy-five per cent. of those not receiving the light died of "weak legs" (rickets), while the survivors were not normal by any means. All those treated to the ultra-violet rays, except a few killed by rats, lived. These latter were larger and more vigorous than those reared under the glass of the green house but which received no ultra-violet light. Ordinary glass does not permit the ultra-violet rays of the sun to pass through. Basking in the warmth and light of the sun that passes through the window pane is of no value in the prevention or cure of disease. The unfiltered rays of the sun are alone capable of assisting the work of metabolism.

Milo, Hastings, who conducted PHYSICAL CULTURE'S food research laboratory, writes in *Physical Culture*, June 1927: —

"Speaking of bowlegged babies—of course everybody knows that this deformity is caused by allowing the little dears to walk while their bones are still too soft! Yet little chicks can walk the day they are born. If they spend the next six weeks of their lives out-of-doors their legs grow straight. But if they spend that period indoors their legs become bowed out and bowed in and knotty-kneed and twisted and weak. This trouble is called 'leg weakness.' But it cannot be caused by walking too soon or too much, since the outdoor chicks walk much more than do the indoor chicks. Until five years ago poultrymen believed just the contrary about their bowlegged chicks of what they believed about their bowlegged children. Their contention was that lack of use of legs caused the bowlegged chicks, while too much use of legs caused the bowlegged children.

"Five years ago this spring I bought one thousand baby chicks and put them in an airy building at Little Silver, New Jersey. I had previously planted a garden of lettuce and rape and chard. I had a theory that leg weakness in chickens had nothing to do with out-door exercise, or even fresh air or sunshine, but that it was a nutritional disease, and that the reason indoor chickens were more likely to suffer from it than out-door chickens was because the out-door chickens ate more grass and green feed.

"I nursed and nourished those thousand chicks most carefully and never once let them out of doors. But I fed them green leaves galore and far more abundantly than any out-door chicks would have been able to provide for themselves. My chicks thrived for a few weeks and then began to spraddle and sprawl, and developed bow-legs aplenty. One hunderd of them died from their malformations and inability to get around to their food. Then I turned the rest of them out of doors, and they recovered promptly, and the weak legs grew strong, though the worst of them remained twisted and bent at ridiculous angles."

The unnecessary and excruciating sufferings to which animals have been subjected by heartless vivisectionists in dietetic experiments almost equal those caused by animal experiments in the serum and bacteriological laboratories. This cruel torture of animals is being carried on on a world-wide scale. Mr. Hastings once stated in my presence that a scientist should be cold, logical, and devoid of sentimentality. He was denouncing the anti-vivisectionists.

The evidence is clear from animal experimentation and human experience that if you give your child an abundance of sunlight it will thrive on almost any kind of a diet, whereas, if you deprive it of the sunlight it will not thrive well on the best of diets. Sunlight is one of the most important elements of the natural diet. Nor can its place be taken by cod-liver oil. A lot of bunk is being written about this nauseous stuff by those who are interested in building up a huge commercial enterprise, but children are not helped by it and are often made very sick by its use.

Give the child sunlight and no "just-as-good" substitutes. Give it sunlight before birth and it will be a more normal, more healthful child at birth. Every pregnant mother should have a sun-bath every day the sun shines. Not for her sake only, but for the sake of the child as well.

Cartilage is transformed into bone when the calcium and phosphorus salts are properly utilized by it. Without the aid of the ultra-violet rays this assimilation of calcium and phosphorus does not take place in a normal manner. Dr. Bovie gathered statistics which show that about ninety-seven per cent. of all the babies born in our Northern cities are afflicted to a greater or less extent with rickets. These babies, are, many of them, born in the Fall and Winter, instead of in the spring as they should be, and are kept in-doors all winter. In the tropics rickets is rare and maturity is reached earlier.

H. B. Cushman, who was born among the Indians, of missionary parents, while they were still east of the Mississippi, and who went with them when they were ruthlessly driven from their homelands, spending nearly seventy years among them, says in his *History of the Choctaw, Chickasau and Natchez Indians*, (1899), p. 246, that among the Choctaws "deformity was almost unknown, proving that nature in the wild forest of the wilderness is true to her type." Again, "It is said of the Natchez, 'that the sight was never shocked by the appearance of deformity,' such as are so frequently observed among the white race; and with equal truth, the same may be said of all the North American Indians," p. 533.

George Catlin tells us that "amongst two millions of these people" (Indians), he met with very few cases of deformity.

In view of the known effects of sunlight upon health and development it cannot be doubted that their habit of going practically nude was largely responsible for this almost total lack of deformity among this once proud and noble race. It must not be overlooked either, that this condition prevailed as well among the northern Indians. Rickets was unknown among them as was tuberculosis, anemia, leukemia, and, for the most part, skin diseases.

Andrew Combe, M.D., an early English hygienist, quotes an "intelligent old author" in the *Historie Naturelle et Morale des Isles Antilles, Rotterdam, 1658* as saying of the Caribs, 170 years previous, *The Principles of Physiology applied to the preservation of Health*, (1833), p. 130:—

"They do not swaddle their infants, but leave them to tumble about at liberty in their little hammocks, or on beds of leaves spread on the earth in a corner of their huts; and nevertheless their limbs do not become crooked, and their whole body is perfectly well made!" Again, "Although the little creatures are left to roll about on the ground in a state of nudity, they nevertheless grow marvelously well, and most of them become so robust as to be able to walk without support at six months old."

The naivete of this expression of surprise that the Carib infants could grow so marvelously well with only the assistance of nature, and without the aid of stays, swaddling bands, bandages, etc., then so much in use in Europe, shows how artificial was his way of thinking and well illustrates the same condition of mind today. So accustomed are we to depend on art that although we have the strongest evidence of its hurtfulness before our eyes, custom and prejudice prevail over intelligence. Look, for instance, at out present clothing customs, how they prevail in spite of our growing knowledge of their actual hurtfulness.

In Stevenson's narrative of Twenty years' residence in South America, he says of the Araucanian Indians: "the children are never swaddled, nor their bodies confined by any tight clothing." "They are allowed to crawl about nearly naked until they can walk." "To the loose clothing, which the children wear from their infancy, may doubtless be attributed the total absence of deformity, among the Indians."—Vol. 1, p. 9, 10.

It is important, in this connection, that we take account of the fact that there was no tuberculosis, rickets, no hunch-backs, bow-legs, no idiots or lunatics, no defective teeth, no deaf and dumb and almost no deaths either of mother or child in child birth, among the Indians before the white man civilized them—that is clothed them, gave them "fire-water" to drink, cooped them up on reservations and taught them to eat white bread, salt-bacon, black coffee and sorgham molasses. Rickets and tuberculosis, like scurvey, should be regarded as "deficiency" diseases, largely due to lack of sunlight.

Saleeby bursts out into the following bit of poetry about the skin:—
"This admirable organ, the natural clothing of the body, which grows continuously throughout life, which has at least four absolutely distinct sets of sensory nerves, distributed to it, which is essential in the regulation of temperature, which is waterproof from without inwards, but allows the excretory sweat to escape freely which, when unbroken, is microbe-proof, and which can readily absorb sunlight—this most beautiful, versatile and wonderful organ is, for the most part, smothered, blanched and blinded in clothes, and can only gradully be restored to the air and light which are its natural surroundings. Then, and only then, we learn what it is capable of."

Man also breathes through his skin and it is vitally necessary that a constant supply of fresh pure air reach the skin if it is to carry on its respiratory function normally. A healthy skin is essential to normal health and can be had only by giving it the advantage of those agencies which are intended by nature to come in contact with and affect the skin.

No skin can be maintained in anything like a clean condition if it does not come in contact with the sun and air. Anyone who ever had his feet to sweat knows how disagreeable is the odor that exudes from them when his or her shoes are removed. Every one is acquainted with the fact that the feet of the "bare foot boy with cheeks of tan" may sweat the whole day through without producing such a condition. Why the difference? It is because the sun and air disintegrate and carry away the excretions from the skin of the feet. If they are tightly sealed up in those leather sweat boxes called shoes they are not only denied the benefits of light and air but are forced to remain in their own filthy exudations. Someday man will substitute the sun and air bath for the present water bath.

The manual laborer goes to work on a hot summer day and sweats profusely throughout the day. His clothes become saturated with sweat. It gives off a very disagreeable odor. The hands and face which have been exposed to the sun and air do not give off such an odor. If one examines he finds the space between the man's body and his clothes occupied by foul hot air and gases which are very repugnant to the olfactory sense. The man is literally wallowing in his own excretions, he has them bound to him by his clothing so that they escape slowly. This is filthy. This same thing is true of every one who wears clothes whether they are "high collared" financiers or just plain folks. It is not true of those who work without clothing. This condition caused by the clothing weakens the skin. In many cases it is almost dead.

Man's resistance to atmospheric changes is also lowered to such an extent that every time he meets a sudden change in temperature he suffers. The Indian could travel all day in a blinding snow storm or swin frozen streams but if his "pale face" brother attempted this he died a few days later of pneumonia. A skin debilitated by the hot house conditions produced by clothing is not an adequate protection for its owner. The sooner he begins to harden and revive it the better it will be for his health.

But exposure of the body to light and air does not stop with benefitting the skin. It goes deeper at least, the sun's rays go deeper. But we do not wish our readers to understand that there is a sun cure or heliotherapy. We would have you keep in mind the fact that it is the inherent powers and functions of the organism that actually does the curing while the sunlight is simply one of the necessary conditions for cure. But it is more than this. It is a necessary condition for health, and should be used by those who have health.

As might be expected, any influence which produces such marked effects upon nutrition and occasions such profound changes in the deeper, as well as of the superficial tissues of the body, exerts a wholesome influence upon the mind. It is a matter of common observation that on dark cloudy days people are more subject to worry, ill-temper, moroseness, the "blues," etc. and that as soon as the skies clear away and the sunshine returns happiness and good naturedness return. But the influence of the sun on the mind strikes deeper than this. The following account is extracted from an article on *Sunshine for Brains*, by Dr. Edwin E. Flosson, in *Science Monthly*, Nov. 1925.

"It has been known for some years that the ultra-violet rays, whether they come from the sunlight or the mercury-quartz lamp, will greatly benefit and cure children crippled by rickets or tuberculous joints. It is now found that light treatment not only betters their bones and improves their general health, but also brightens their brains and sweetens their dispositions.

"A class of boys from the London slums who were taken to the garden of a private house on Clapham common, where they studied and played all day long, attired in 'very short shorts and no shirts,' showed at the end of six weeks that even such feeble sunlight as London affords had increased their mental capacity and alertness as well as their appetites.

"A comparison of the results of mental tests made in the special schools for physically defective children in London with those made on the children who had taken the light treatment at the Lord Mayor Treloar Cripple's Hospital at Alton showed a marked superiority for those who had the advantage of the sunshine. Both groups of children were naturally retarded on account of their disease, but the mental retardation of the London children was, on the average, 1.95 years, while that of the Alton children was 1.14 years. Both groups were about the same age, 11 years, and the London children had had more schooling."

"A more exact test was made at Alton on a ward containing 200 small children all afflicted with tuberculous disease of the spine, and therefore bound immobile to their beds. The diet and treatment of all were the same, but ten of the children were given systematic treatment with artificial light. Sir Henry Gauvin reports:

"'While the physique of those receiving light treatment showed improvement as compared with the others, the effect on the mentality was even more definite. Those exposed to light were markedly happier, more vivacious, more alert, and I may add, more mischevious.'"

While it is true that in the higher altitudes one receives more of the beneficial rays of the sun, it is also a fact that both plants and animals may receive sufficient of these at sea level or below sea level, to enable them to maintain health, growth and development, and to reproduce themselves. Indeed, there is no known part of the earth where there is not sufficient sunshine to maintain life and in most of the earth, there is sufficient sunshine to supply the needs of man. Even the denizens of the jungle receive sufficient sunlight. Man in the jungle does likewise. It is the over-clad, over-housed, inhabitant of the smoky cities who is deprived of his fair share of the sun. Those who live in the modern caves that line the canon walls of our modern cities and who dress in heavy dark clothing, suffer most.

We must distinguish between the "light" of the sun and the heat of the sun. It is not the sun's heat from which all these benefits flow. Cities like Chicago and Pittsburgh receive plenty of the Sun's heat, but less of it's light, or less of its non-luminious rays, with the result that the blood of their inhabitants is on an average, about twenty per cent. deficient in hemoglobin.

Animals seek the sunlight but avoid its heat. This is to say, they prefer to be in the sun during the cool portions of the day and seek the shade when it grows hot. The extreme heat is depressing and enervating. The guiding hand of animal instinct in avoiding the heat of the sun may be seen in the city's zoological Gardens, the country's pastures or in the untamed places of the earth. The Indian in Mexico, Peru, South America, the negro in Africa all obey this instinct. The fox, the chamois in Switzerland, the cows in the pasture, the hens in the barn lot, the birds in the tree tops all love to bask in the sunlight of morning but retreat to the shade as the heat of midday approaches.

Weariness, fever, headache, inflamed skin, loss of appetite, sleeplessness, and such results from too much exposure or exposure to the hot mid-day sun are not desirable. This is the chief reason why the early morning hours of summer are better for the sun-bath than is mid-day, a thing observed instinctively by animals, birds, plants and so-called savage man.

Begin your sun-bathing exposing your body only three to five minutes a day and gradually increase the length of time of exposure until a half hour to an hour or more, even to three and four hours, are consumed. Make haste slowly.

Efforts are made in medical quarters to convince everyone that the "sun-cure" is a complicated and extremely hazardous procedure that can only be applied by a technically trained man from the laboratory, a physician. This is mere pretense with a commercial basis. Anyone with sense enough to eat or sleep or exercise or breathe pure air may take a sun-bath. It is as natural as either of these things and equally as simple.

In the tropics, the leaves of the plants, trees, etc., are either thick and heavy or have their edges turned to the sun. This is another of Nature's methods of preventing the excessive absorption of sunlight. At mid-day, when the sun is hottest, the leaves of plants curl up . The lesson is obvious. We should exercise extreme caution in beginning the use of so powerful a force as sunshine. Keep in mind that the "sun-cure" is a "light-cure" and not a "heat-cure."

. All stimulants produce enervation if used too long or too frequently. The chemical rays of the sun are no exception to this rule. To prevent absorption of too much sunlight nature has supplied the child of nature with a color-screen called pigment which shields it from this possibility. Those races of men that live in regions where sunshine is most abundant are dark skinned races. Those living in regions where sunshine is less abundant are fairer and are known as the blond races. The Eskimo forms an apparent exception to this rule, living as they do in the far north where the sun shines so little. However, the ice and snow in those regions acts as a reflector and serves to intensify the amount of sunshine that strikes them.

Originally the blond races were perfectly adapted to the climate in those regions of the earth which they inhabit. But the habit of wearing clothes and remaining much of our time in-doors has served to break down and weaken our natural protection. For this reason extreme care must be exercised in giving sun-baths to those unaccustomed to them, if we are to avoid injury. For there is the danger, not only of "burning" the body but of over stimulating the vital functions. The so-called brunettes are able to withstand more sunlight than the so-called blondes. Tanning is a vital reaction, and the better this reaction the more benefit derived. This pigmentation of the skin is very important. Those who pigment quickly and deeply receive most benefit from the sun. Those who only freckle must be more cautious in exposing themselves. Red-haired people require greater caution.

Protection of the head and eyes is usually strongly urged. This is ridiculous. Nature made the head and eyes as she desired them and adapted them to the sunshine. Sunlight is actually beneficial to the eyes and hair. Gazing directly into the sun actually improves sight and aids in overcoming diseases of the eyes. Sun-stroke does not result from an uncovered head and eye-strain is not the effect of lack of eye shades, else would nature have equipped man, and animal with bonnets and goggles.

The chemical rays do not pass through ordinary glass. For this reason a sun-bath taken in a room where the sun is forced to enter through glass is of but little value. The top sash should be lowered. The bottom sash may be covered with a shade or screen to prevent offending passers by.

Although medical men do not employ the sunlight in all conditions, as Hygienists do, they are coming more and more to see its value in many conditions which formerly they did not consider it useful in. When once they have grasped the fact that it is a hygienic and not a therapeutic method and when they understand the unity of disease, they will be better able to appreciate its universal use by Hygienists. Rollier's records, covering over twenty years, include recoveries of extreme cases of spinal tuberculosis, with paralyzed lower limbs, etc., tuberculosis of every part of the body, tuberculosis of the lungs included, rickets, many skin diseases, varicose ulcers, many of these of long standing, war-wounds, non-healing operative wounds, osteomyelitis, bed sores, etc. We are informed that bronchitis, colds in the head and rheumatism do not develop at his place in Lysen, although germs must be plentiful.

It has been found that the sick make more rapid recovery on light days or if placed where they may sit or lie in the sunshine. The discovery by medical men of the value of the sun-bath in the treatment of rickets came about by the accidental finding, in a hospital for treating rickety children, that the child that was fortunate enough to be assigned to a certain cot where he would be exposed to the sun's rays recovered with amazing rapidity. This led to a series of experiments first on white rats, then on children with the result that this Nature Cure method is now recognized by medical men everywhere as a proper procedure in rickets.

If sunlight is so necessary to the perpetuation of life it is equally as necessary to the maintenance of health and the prevention of disease. It is essential to the restoration of health and has been shown to hasten recovery in all cases. I agree with Saleeby when he declares: "Every sanatorium which is not essentially a solarium must today be called a tragic farce."

We again remind you that cure is accomplished by the organisms own forces, processes and functions and not by any external agencies. The sun-cure does not cure. It only supplies the body with one of those important elements that are essential to life and health and thereby renders it possible for the organism to cure itself. We would not say the sun can cure a wound but we know that wounds that are exposed to the sun are healed more rapidly than those that are not.

Sunshine is necessary to life in health or disease, just as air and food are necessary. It is a hygienic not a therapeutic agent. Without it the body must inevitably weaken and become diseased. The highest degree of health that is possible to man is not attainable unless sunshine is supplied his body. Sunlight fills an important need in the organism and when that is done that is as much as we can get it to do without harm. It cannot take the place of exercise or moderation in eating. It is no substitute for sleep or chastity, for self-control or clean living. It has many of the properties attributed to the vitamins but it isn't the kind of a vitamin that will enable one to break all the laws of health with impunity. Combine your sun-bath with other hygienic regulations and measures, using care not to over do it.

The true lesson of all that has gone before is one of hygiene not one of therapeutics. We will have learned our lesson well when we have eliminated smoke from our cities, blinds, shutters, shades, etc., from our windows, remedied the crowded, sunless sections of our cities, provided parks and play grounds for our city children, equipped the roofs of all apartment houses with sun-baths, provided free public sun-parks for the sexes in the cities, and learned to wear clothing that permits the sunlight to reach the body, or else, as suggested by Graham, go nude except in the most inclement weather. In Columbia University experiments with inexpensive mercerized cotton—some white, some black—showed that enough sunlight penetrates the white to "cure" rickets, but through the black it does not.

We believe that the highest degree of health and strength can be attained and maintained only by adding sunshine to our health building measures. Housing and clothing have deprived us of our normal supply, so that we are suffering from light starvation. Man should expose his body to light and air daily.

The present objections to nudity must be overcome. The prudish idea that the human body is vile, vulgar, indecent, obscene, and must be kept hid from public view is the source of much injury. The outcry against present styles in women's clothes, is of course, confined to a few fossil brains that belong to a time that was, but we are face to face with the fact that despite the present styles we are still afraid of a nude body. This is because of our machine-made morality. The prevailing customs, the laws of the land, the thoughts of our neighbors, these determine our standard of conduct.

We are guilty of great offense against the principles of ethics in our blind worship of custom and convention. Whatever is customary in conduct is right. Whatever is not customary is wrong. And yet customs change continually and differ in different parts of the world. It cannot be consistently claimed that the true principles of morality change with time or with the crosing of boundary lines between Nations.

Only a few years ago a woman was arrested and fined for appearing in public in a split skirt that showed a few inches of the stocking on one of her lower limbs. Today the women have cut off their skirts to where they are only abbreviations of grandmother's skirts and show more stockings on each leg than the lady above referred to exposed. And they have reduced the stocking to a mere net.

Some of the ladies one-piece bathing suits cover less territory than mother Eve's fig leaf apron. Thus do customs change. And only a few old fossils kick.

In China the lady dare not expose her wrist. In Turkey she must keep her face veiled in public. Thus custom decrees one thing in one part of the world and another in another part. But the principles of morality and ethics do not change in that way.

The truth is that there is nothing indecent, immoral, vulgar or vile about the nude human body. It is simply natural and the natural is right. Many bodies are ugly and misshapen, lack development, etc., but this does not make them vulgar or immoral. Indeed, the habit of keeping them smothered in clothes has aided in mishaping and uglifying them.

The author saw a little baby sitting nude in a bowl. Everyone was delighted with the picture it presented. No one thought the child immoral or indecent. No one was shocked or horrified. Even the mother forgot to ask herself that hypocritical question: "what will my neighbor think?"

Then, in my mind's eye I pictured the baby as it grew up through childhood, puberty, youth or maidenhood to maturity and wondered at just what stage of its development the body changed into the vulgar and obscene. The little girl and boy goes barefooted. But mother and daddy dare not. It's indecent. What a farce!

This whole attitude towards the body comes, not from any actual wrong in exposing the body, but from a filthy mind. It is the habit of mind to project in imagination its own obscenity, vulgarity, and impurity or its own cleanliness and purity into the things around it. The unclean mind can find an evil suggestion in everything that it hears or sees. Saint Paul struck the keynote when he declared: "Unto the pure all things are pure but unto them that are defiled and unbelieving is nothing pure, but even their mind and conscience is defiled."

This attitude towards clothes will have to pass away if man is again to enjoy the health and vigor that is his by right. In this we have said nothing about the evils of corsets and high heeled shoes worn by women and the worse styles in men's clothing, as we were dealing with clothes as they exclude the light and air from the body. The effects of these two things are indeed bad.

So prone are we to regard those conditions under which we are born and reared as natural and to look upon those things which the majority of mankind do as an average as the best for us to do as a whole that almost everyone regards clothing as both natural and best for man. The fact is, clothing is both artificial and harmful.

In truth man was designed by the Creator to enjoy the direct rays of the sun and the soothing and strengthening influence of the winds over the whole surface of his body. He is by nature a nude animal.

PHYSICAL EXERCISE

Chapter XXIV

ALTERNATE action and repose is the order of life. As sure as rest must follow exertion, activity must follow repose. It is only in this way that the functions of the body may be restored to or maintained in a normal condition.

Cell life in the animal body, is dependent upon nutrition, drainage, warmth and freedom from violence. In order to secure these for all the cells, the fluids of the body, which form the greater part of its weight are, or should be, in perpetual motion. To keep up this grand vital circulation and to give tone to all vital functions and perfection to all vital changes, to secure a proper supply of blood to every part, keep the lymph moving normally and maintain the general health of the entire system, exercise or voluntary activity is very essential. Exercise through its various effects, serves to impart vigor and activity to all the organs and to secure and maintain the healthful integrity of all their functions, and the symmetrical development and constitutional power of the whole system. Exercise may be truly considered the most important vital tonic of the body. If it is wholly neglected, the body will become weak, and all its physiological powers will be diminished; but regularly and properly indulged in, the whole system will be strengthened and invigorated. It seems a law of the vital economy that a certain relation should always be observed between the quantity of food received and the amount of exercise taken.

Exercise is more than muscle-building. It is body-building in the complete sense of the term. Every cell and fiber in the body is involved in the consequences of exercise, both in the efforts and in the effects. The lungs, heart, arteries, liver, kidneys, skin, stomach, bowels, glands, etc., as well as the brain and nervous system are each and all accelerated in their functions and strengthened in their structures.

Exercise does not merely improve the tone and quality of the voluntary muscles. The tone and quality of every tissue of the body is improved. The size, strength and quality of the bones depends very much upon the amount and kind of exercise the body receives. The development of the chest, the powers of digestion and assimilation, the strength of the heart and efficiency of elimination, all depend largely upon physical exercise. The blood vessels are strengthened, the circulation of blood and lymph improved, respiration is deepened and the lung capacity increased through exercise.

If one receives no physical exercise for some time, his muscles become soft, flabby and weak. They lose tone and their fibers deteriorate. In time they waste away. A similar condition develops throughout the body. This weakness is not merely functional, for there is an actual weakening of the structures of the various organs, similar to that which takes place in the muscles. By an irrevocable law of life, growth, development and strength of mind and body are acquired through exercise. Exercise is as essential to physical vigor, strength and development, as air is to life.

If any part of the body is called into action, more blood is sent to that part and there is an increased determination of nerve force to it. The quickened and increased circulation results in the improvement of nutrition and drainage. Metabolism is increased with a consequent improvement in the tone and quality of the tissues involved. No other method is known which will increase the circulation to a part more effectually and quickly than exercise. Proper physical exercise of the whole body brings about this result throughout the entire system. A muscle that is regularly exercised and given periodical rest, will, if subnormal, grow in size; if normal in size, it will develop a finer grain or texture. The fibers of the muscles improve in quality.

Strength and endurance are builded, coordination and agility are developed, there is an increased flexibility of the joints. Proper posture which assures a correct relationship between bones, muscles, organs and other tissues, is established and maintained. Grace and poise are acquired, beauty and symmetry of the body developed, and neither last not least, there is a feeling of fitness and a joy of living that cannot be had without exercise.

Shortened muscles and ligaments may be stretched, adhesions broken up, contracted muscles relaxed and nervous efficiency increased by exercise. By this, is not meant that nervous energy is increased, but that nervous transmission is improved. Exercise hastens the absorption of exudates and deposits and effects the body temperature. It also aids in developing the mind.

For the man in health, exercise is a very simple matter. Let him decide what he desires to develop, that is whether great strength, endurance, agility, flexibility, speed, etc., or all of these, and then he can easily choose those exercises that develop these. If a deformity is to be corrected, special exercises that are designed to correct it are required. Instances of such deformities which may be corrected by exercise properly and persistantly used are; round or stoop shoulders, spinal curvature, innominate abnormalities, bow legs, knock knees, club foot, flat foot, rupture, visceroptosis, such as "fallen" stomach, "floating" kidney, "fallen" or prolapsed womb, etc. Exercises for these purposes are best performed under the care of an expert. We have proven in our years of experience with spinal exercise (spondylokienetics) that a sure and permanent correction of most spinal curvatures may be accomplished by exercise alone.

Exercise is a most valuable and effective means of restoring health and no patient suffering from chronic disease or convalescing after some acute disease should omit this health builder.

Man was once forced by stern necessity to secure plenty of physical exercise but with the increasing development of civilization a large class of sedentary workers has grown up whose duties do not call for physical exertion. Like the well-fed dog, these become fat and lazy and develop a dignified look. Labor has been rather unequally divided so that many men are forced to overwork their bodies thus injuring them. On the other hand, specialism in work results in the over use of some parts of the body and neglect of other parts.

So long as the present unequal rewards for service remains in vogue, this must continue. So long as a cartoonist can get more for one drawing than a farmer may get for a whole year's work in raisng food, so long as the members of the marry-and-divorce-for-fun colony out at Hollywood get more for a year of making fools of themselves than a coal miner earns in a life time, just so long are these unequal conditions going to exist. So long as the pugilist can obtain more money for one fight than the men who build our homes receive in a life time, just so long will there exist a parasite class that "toil not neither do they spin" who will continue to live off the products of the overwork of others.

This parasite class is the "better class" the "intelligencia" and despise the members of the common herd who do the really productive work of the world. The better class, it should be known, is composed of those who fight the "struggle for existence" through a substitute. That is, they get the common people to do it for them—they mine the miners, farm the farmers, and work the workers.

In our present hyper-civilization some substitute for the work of securing food and defending oneself and family against foes has to be used. For Nature demands exercise. If an arm is placed in a sling, or should we cease walking, Nature will gradually remove the muscles, rendering the inactive limb entirely useless. But if we make strong enough efforts to use it again she will graudally restore what she took away. Intelligent exercise is therefore not only necessary to the sedentary worker, but to the manual laborer as well for these latter must counteract the one-sided tendencies of their work.

Before offering a few general rules for the application of exercise, I desire to combat two prevalent fallacies. First, that exercise is the power of development, and second, that the cultivation of the body is wasteful and unnecessary.

Exercise never, under any circumstances, imparts the Principal of strength, the power back of the action, but on the contrary, always consumes more or less of it. We do not know what vital power is, nor what its source is, but we can be as certain as we are of anything in the universe, that its use is not its accumulation or generation.

"If we were to look," said Jennings, "at a set of large, well-formed muscles, full of vital energy, we should say that they were strong muscles, that the man who possessed them in that condition was a man of strength. Deprive those muscles of the

307

vital power, and the man is deprived of his muscular strength. Here then, we have the Principle of strength, and also learn that it is a Union of this Principle with muscles that constitutes muscular strength. Without good muscles, no man could be strong, however much of the vital power he might have, and without vital power, no man could be strong, however much of well-formed muscles he might possess."— *Medical Reform*, p. 335.

Suppose we say the body is a power machine and compare it with the electric motor. The strength of the motor depends on its size and the amount of force it receives. A small motor with a large current is not a strong motor, while a large motor with a weak current is not a strong motor. But a large motor with a large current gives us a strong motor. But no one would think of confusing the current and the motor as one, or of confusing the activities of the motor wtih the production and distribution of the motive force—the electric current. These activities expend and exhaust that force.

Large, well developed muscles plus sufficiency of vital or nervous force, gives great physical strength. But exercise neither produces the vital force nor the muscles. Growth and development are from within. The power that built the muscles in the embryo, is the power that develops them after birth. How much development will take place will depend upon conditions. "No man ever became a Hercules without Herculean exercise," declared Jennings.

If the conditions of the Growth or Development of a character or part, are taken away, the character or part becomes reduced or suppressed. Exercise is a condition of development. The greater activity does not Cause the functional or structural increase. That is but a condition. Causes are inherent—within.

Theory has it that the use of an organ or part develops it. This is very narrow in conception and far from correct. This theory was manufactured by the evolutionists to account for their theoretical evolution. Theory must always be invented to sustain a theory. Facts are often stubborn things, but theories can be made to suit any situation. So development of parts by use came into existence to uphold a theory.

We often hear that "evolution has supplied us with an explanation," etc. But have we ever stopped to consider whether or not the explanation is a correct one? Can a better explanation be given—one that accords with known facts rather than with manufactured theories? "Nothing is ever settled until it is setted right," and it cannot be too strongly emphasized that conclusions based upon assumptions are themselves assumptions.

The evolutionist accounted for the development of parts by use. This necessitated that the part be past the rudimentary stage before use could begin to develop it. It must needs exist before it could be used. The inquiry is a pertinent one; what originated the part and what developed it from the rudimentary stage up to a useful stage? Not use. Use cannot develop organs or parts that do not exist for the simple reason that they are non-existant. Use cannot develop rudimentary parts because these are not useful. We must insist, therefore, that development is from within outward and since something cannot come from nothing, that which is not in a thing cannot be brought out.

The capacity for development must be inherent else no development is possible. Development and growth are practically the same and are subject to the same laws. If we assume a certain capacity, for development, to start with, how can that be exceeded until the capacity to exceed it be provided? It simply cant' be done for the very good reason that something cannot come out of nothing.

"Nature puts forth efforts to meet demands." Yes, but Nature cannot meet demands or requirements that are beyond her capacity. Nature's powers of accomodation are not limitless, not absolute. The law of vital accommodation is the law of development. Vital force, or life, is the power back of that development. Use and other factors in our environment only serve to suppress or call forth that which is in us; they cannot get out what is not there. Kick a bull dog, a feist and a stone and you get an entirely different result in each. It all depends on what was in the objects kicked. The kick was only an occasion for the action. So exercise or use is only an occasion for development.

There is a story told in the south of an old negro slave who was sent, by his master, for a load of rails. Taking a wagon and team he drove to the woods for these. After having loaded on what he considered a load, he began to reason "if they can pull those they can pull one more," so he put another on. He then decided if they could pull that one they could pull another, so he put it on. He continued this until he had rails stacked as high as he was able to stack them. Mounting the rails, he started to drive home, but the team was unable to move the wagon with its load.

Seeing this inability to pull the load the old negro began to unload the rails and reasoned in the other direction—"If they cannot pull that one they cannot pull this one"—until the wagon was empty. He then drove home and told his master that the team could not pull a single rail.

This represents the evolutionists attitude towards development. He sees that use does a few things and decides it can do all. He proceeds to load his wagon with rails until his team can't pull it. If use develops an organ the limit of the possibility of development in that organ is the limit of its possibility for use. The more it is used the more developed it would be. By this principle the weight lifter who keeps adding weight to his barbells would ultimately reach the point where he could juggle a string of the Rocky Mountains.

The fact is that use is a destructive and exhaustive process; consuming energy and tearing down tissue. All repair of tissue and recuperation of energy takes place during rest and sleep. If the amount of destruction of tissue and dissipation of energy occasioned by activity is greater than the organism's ability to recuperate from, then we have, not development, but exhaustion and atrophy. If the demand made on the organism is greater than it is able to meet, it will seek to accomodate itself to the demand. If the capacity to accomodate itself to the demand is present, development ensues; if the capacity to accommodate itself to the condition or demand is lacking, exhaustion and atrophy are the consequences. The development is from within, the occasion for development is from without.

Use does not develop the brain, nerves, muscles, bones, skin, hair, nails, stomach, eyes, ears, lungs, liver, kidneys, gentilia and other organs of a baby to the stage we see them at birth. They have developed while wholly inactive. They have been formed when there was no need for them. They are fitted for duty, and capacity to perform that duty is implanted independent of use. Design is there with eyes on the future. After birth, the baby that sleeps most and sleeps soundest, develops fastest. The sleepless baby is the sick baby and it develops slowly—maybe abnormally.

It is not use that develops the procreative powers at puberty, or that sprouts the young man's beard. Use does not prepare the young woman's breasts to fulfil their functions at, say twenty-five, when her first child is born. The power and the development are from within.

Development follows definite directions from invisible beginnings to the latest results and complexities of structure, the completed product having previously existed, potentially in the germ. "It is the great peculiarity of organic development, or growth," says the Duke of Argyle, "that it always follows a determinate course to an equally determinate end. Each seperate organ begins to appear before it can be actually used. It is always built up gradually for the discharge of functions which are yet lying in the future. In all organic growth, the future dominates the present. All that goes on at any given time in such growths has exclusive reference to something else that has yet to be done, in some other time which is yet to come.**** The growth of a living organ is always premonitory of, and preparative for, the future discharge of some functional activity. As Mr. Spencer expresses it 'Changes in inorganic things have no apparent relations to future external events which are sure, or likely, to take place. In vital changes, however, such relations are manifest.' This is an excellent generalization. It only needs that the word 'relations' be translated from the abstract into the concrete. The kind of relation which is 'manifest' is the relation of a previous preparation for an intended use. Unfortunately, Mr. Spencer is perepetually escaping or departing from the consequences of his own 'manifest relations,' in a subsequent passage of the same work he says, 'Everywhere structures in a great measure determine

309

functions.' This is exactly the reverse of the manifest truth—'that the future functions determine the antecedent growth of structure.' "—*Organic Evolution Cross-Examined.*

The germ of life—fertilized ovum—is so constituted that it contains within itself certain innate properties of development along definite lines of growth, the issues of which have been forearranged and predetermined from the first. Development is an unfoldment of a purpose and the great rapidity with which these germs can sometimes evolve their inherent or involuted complexities and "develop their predestined and pre-arranged adaptitudes," in the absence of use or of any present need for the exercise of its evolving powers should convince the most ardent disciple of use as the power of development, of the error of his view. Among some of the lower orders, the full development of germs takes place in a very short time. Some birds require but three weeks in which to develop, from an egg, a complete fowl with legs, wings, eyes and instincts, all ready made to lead an adult and independent life. In frogs and toads, the time of hatching ranges from three days to three weeks. In some insects, a few hours are all that are required in which to produce a very highly organized creature with many special and often remarkable adaptations. In numberless other cases, a living creature, already leading a separate life, goes to "sleep within an exterior case or shell of its own making, and, while in that state of 'sleep' is radically transformed in all its organs, and emerges, after a few days, an entirely new animal form, with new powers, fitted for new spheres of activity and enjoyment."

"In the metamophoses of Insects, certain organs of the perfect Insect, or 'Imago,' are sometimes visible as rudiments in the imperfect or larval form, although in that form these rudiments have no use or function," says the Duke of Argyle. "In these cases, all such rudiments have their interpretation not in the past, but in the future." "They are fashioned and prepared not by use, but for it."—*Unity of Nature.*

Life as we know it, is the antecedent or the cause of organization and not its product. The germs of life have now, and have always had, their own predetermined line of development. Existence came before use, and not after it. There never has been any experience before the faculties by which it is acquired have first come into existence and begun to function. There never could be any use before the organs have been formed to be used: They are formed and developed, "NOT BY USE, BUT FOR IT."

Only nine months are required for a human ovum to develop into the very complex structure of the human infant.

The power of development in all cases is obviously within and it is obvious enough that external conditions can never act upon the organic mechanism, to "Produce" (call out) development except through, and by means of, a responsive power in that organism, and that organism will always follow out the direction given from within in response to the external element.

This inherent urge to development carries the individual to a certain point. If he is to develop beyond this there must be some external factor to call forth further development. But the possibilities of development are not infinite. External factors can call forth development until the extent of one's capacity for development is reached and there development must cease. Capacity varies with individuals and is determined at birth. External factors may call it forth to the fullest extent or may hinder development.

Activity and exercise are destructive. Rest and sleep are constructive. Both are required by the living organism if health and strength are to be maintained. Some organisms require less activity than others; some require more of rest and sleep. Plants require less activity than men. Some men require more rest and sleep than others. At all times a sufficient amount of rest and sleep should be taken to maintain the balance on the constructive side. Exercise like eating, should not be carried to excess.

There exists today a class of self-styled intellectuals who affect to despise physical strength and the heavier forms of physical exercise. These pretended worshipers of the highbrow are constantly telling us about "great ugly muscles" that are a menace to health and life and of how much greater importance is the cultivation of the intellect.

However, when we compare the soft, flabby, unshapely bodies possessed by these men and women with the firm, symmetrical bodies of the well-developed man or woman we realize at once that the ugliness is all on the other side. There is no beauty in the body that is so skinny that all the art of the tailor or dress maker cannot hide it, nor in those barrel shaped perambulating lard cans one meets everywhere. There is nothing of beauty in the ungraceful awkard way in which such beings move themselves along nor does beauty reside in the disease their indolence has produced.

Brains! intellect! We beileve in these. We believe in cultivating them to their fullest extent. But we are not convinced by the mental output of these physical nonentities that their intellectual development is a thing to justify our envy. Besides we know that no brain can be clear and capable of putting forth its best unless supplied with pure blood. Man may well be defined as primarily an intellectual mechanism equipped with a secondary nutritional mechanism over which it rules. (We use the term "Intellectual mechanism" for the want of a better term. We, by no means, subscribe to the modern doctrine of materialism; that man is a mere machine and mind the output of the Atom). No intellect can give its best to the world if its body is not functioning properly. The human body is an apparatus or organism for carrying on the work of nutrition— digestion, assimilation, disassimilation and excretion of food and waste. If anyone of the nutritive functions are disordered or impaired the brain, which is the organ of the mind, also suffers an impairment.

There exists the greatest necessity for keeping the body itself in the highest degree of perfection and closely following all the laws and rules, all the requirements of nature, for health and physical strength. We want a powerful intellect backed by a powerful physical oragnism—a body the organs and tissues of which are strong and vigorous enough to sustain that intellect in its most strenuous efforts.

There is a normal and inseparable relationship and co-ordination between mind and body and when the normal balance between these is broken they both suffer. What Nature has joined together, no man can rend asunder without doing violence to the severed parts. The mind is dependent upon the body not alone for the blood that nourishes the brain but for the mental food it receives through the eyes, ears, nose, skin and tongue. It is no more certain that alcohol and opium will confuse the mind than that pure blood will clear it.

The order of Nature cannot be disturbed and broken with impunity. Every attempt to work the intellect independently of the forces and functions allied to it, must end in a miserable and disastrous defeat. Nature has inseparably harnessed body and mind together, to pull together in perfect concord, and so long as they are allowed to do this, only good can come. Mind and muscle perform co-ordinate, not antagonistic functions.

In every age sculptors and artists have chiseled and painted the nude forms of men and women to represent their gods and goddesses, their ideas and ideals. So skillfully did some of the ancient masters do their work that many of their creations seem to us almost sublime in their perfection of outline. But what man or woman in ancient Greece or Rome would have worshipped a pot-bellied god or a scrawney necked goddess.

In our day many men whose fine brains and ripe judgment have commanded the respect and admiration of the world have possessed bodies so disproportioned as to be grotesque. Our artists, who make the statues we erect today represent our heroes in full dress. Dress, like charity, covers a multitude of sins.

Mishapen despisers of the body are seen everywhere and may be heard declaring that all they want is health, as though any degree of health worth having is possible without strength. If these men really possessed health and strength they could accomplish far more than they do and will not be bumped over the great divide just at a time when their judgment, ripened by years of observation, study and experience render them most useful. In this respect note the untimely death of Robt. Ingersol, Henry Ward Beecher, Dr. Talmadge, the late Pastor C. T. Russell, Theodore Roosevelt, the recent death of Pres. Harding, Caruso and others. President Wilson broke down right at a time when the duties of his office required his services most. Neglect of proper body culture was responsible in every case.

Civilized man who boastingly refers to himself as the noblest of all animals is the most unsymmetrical. Still he pretends to admire symmetry of form. The ancient

Greeks and Romans fairly worshipped at the shrine of bodily symmetry and beauty. Wild beasts are seldom badly proportioned, yet many wild beasts would not exercise enough to keep in health if they were not driven by the pangs of hunger to seek food, or by necessity to defend themselves or young against foes. Domestic animals that have their food given to them and are not forced to exercise become fat and lazy. The young puppy may run about and play but the older dog will sit around and look at you in a dignified way when he isn't asleep. He has learned to despise "great ugly muscles" and is trying to cultivate intellect.

Some of our "intelectuals" admit that a certain amount of physical exercise is needed but talk learnedly about the dangers of over development. As a matter of fact, over development is impossible. When exercise is carried beyond the points of usefullness—that is, when it is carried to excess the destruction of tissue and expenditure of energy thus occasioned, is greater than can be renewed and recuperated, with the result that exhaustion and atrophy ensue. If exercise is not carried to excess, it surely cannot produce over-development. If it is not carried to excess it surely cannot harm one.

There is an individual limit to development beyond which the individual cannot go. No two individuals are equal in this respect, although the range of variation is not great. But we fail to find a single fact in Nature that can legitimately be claimed to show that man is injured by reaching his maximum degree of physical fitness and development. Nor have any of the high brows ever given us a reason; although, their own lives of weakness, disease and misery have furnished us with a most excellent proof that the neglect of the body is injurious.

But if exercise served no other purpose than that of building muscles, we would not insist upon it so strongly. Bulk of muscle is by no means a reliable criterion of strength, and still less of health. Quality of muscle is as essential as quantity, and muscles are dependent very much upon proper exercise for quality.

The body that is loaded with toxins is weak no matter how bulky the muscles. The strong man who is prostrated with typhoid is a weak man. Pure blood cannot be maintained without exercise.

Men with large amounts of nervous energy can often perform feats of strength that are far beyond the powers of larger and stronger men. The muscles of men are stronger in proportion to their size than the muscles of animals; chiefly because man has greater nerve force, and is able to concentrate his nervous energies to the highest possible degree. Less nervous energy is required to perform a given movement or feat after muscular co-ordination is established than before. The young inexperienced mechanic works himself into exhaustion in eight hours and accomplishes much less than the more experienced mechanic who has exerted himself much less. Exercise develops muscular co-ordination. This adds to efficiency and efficiency adds to Life.

Exercise is absolutely essential to healthy life and every one should put forth efforts to secure regular daily exercise. Unlike the modern athlete, one should keep in training at all times. The boxer goes in training for a bout and as soon as the bout is over, lapses into indolence and laziness. The fight of life is continuous and one should be always in the pink of condition in order to meet the demands made upon him by modern existence. A resume of the medical and anthropological statistics of the provost Marshall General's bureau at the time of the civil war, will furnish a very impartial insight into the relation of physical activity to physical fitness and disease

Out of over one million men examined, fifty per cent. were rejected for physical inefficiency. Kid ourselves as we may, these figures of the Civil War, when compared with those obtained in the recent war, show that in spite of our boasted advance in knowledge of how to care for the body and prevent and cure disease, we are, if anything, in a worse state physically now than then. Diseases of the digestive system were responsible for more rejections than any other cause, and the professional class— lawyers, teachers, editors, etc.,—furnished the highest percentage of rejects. Seven hundred and thirty per thousand. Next came diseases of the circulatory system including the heart and blood vesesls; and again the professional class furnished the highest percentage of rejections while the unskilled laborer, the iron worker, furnished the lowest percentage: One hundred and eighty per thousand. The iron worker does very heavy work.

Physiological law has not undergone any change since 1865. The examinations in the late war showed that what was true then is true now: The professional classes, the self-styled intellectuals were then the most unfit and are still in this same class. In cultivating their superior(?) intellect they have permitted the foundation to rot from under them. During the Middle Ages, "religious" fanatics denied attention to the body because it detracted from spiritual development. "Intellectual" fanatics of the present, make the same mistake. Whether the body is neglected in the "interest" of the spirit or the mind, physical decadence is the result. However great may be their intellectual attainments, they have not achieved to heights they may have attained had they kept their bodies in the pink of condition. Their flat sunken chests, shallow breathing, sluggish circulation, lazy bowels, inactive skin and kidneys cannot keep the brain in its best condition.

Some of these have tried to offset this by standing before their windows and taking a few deep breaths immediately after rising in the morning. The practice is of little value. First, because a few deep breaths in the morning will not offset twenty four hours a day of shallow breathing and second because in passive deep breathing the blood is not sent to the lungs in sufficient quantities to take up the oxygen contained in the air breathed. A quickened circulation produced by active exercise will demand more oxygen and will receive it. Gymnastics for the chest are very important in any health building regime but passive deep breathing is practically useless.

I realize that those who have machines for "developing" the chest will dispute this, but they do so only that they may sell more of those cheaply construcetd apparatuses at a high price. The sole value of such machines lies in the fact that their use keeps up one's enthusiasm.

Breathing is natural and every one will breathe correctly if he has not cultivated an incorrect breathing habit. Such incorrect habits may be due to habitually sitting in a cramped position, to belts, corsets, and other bands that intefere with breathing or to disease—either of the chest or of the nose and throat. Mouth breathing for instance, may be due to adenoids. Mouth breathing except when undergoing great physical effort, as in sprinting, is unnatural.

Anyone having acquired the shallow breathing habit should cultivate deep breathing. However, this is better done by exercises that lift the chest and create a need for more oxygen than by mere passive breathing. A large powerful chest is the best life insurance one can have.

Through proper physical training, we strive to fit the body to respond promptly, at all times and under varying circumstances to the will; to counter-balance mental with physical work, contrasting throughout the results obtained with the aim in view— healthy development.

Nothing in this world of real value can be had without effort. If we desire health, strength, symmetry and beauty of body, we must put forth the necessary effort. Any exercise that is not of sufficient force to arouse a conscious effort defeats its own end by ceasing to have any appreciable effect upon the physiological and chemical processes of the body. Great strength can be had only by the use of exercise that calls for strength. The bigger and stronger the muscle the greater the resistance which is needed to fully develop it. Flexibility, elasticity and speed can be had only by exercises that call for these. The ideal system of exercise is one that includes all these.

Exercise may be roughly divided into (1) Hygienic exercise, (2) educational exercise, and (3) corrective exercise.

All exercises may properly be termed hygienic exercise unless it is performed in such a manner that it injures the body.

Educational exercise is such as trains the mind and muscles to act in the greatest degree of co-ordination. The voluntary muscles ordinarily obey only the mandates of the *will* and the *feelings*. The highest aim of gymnastics is to so train the muscles that they are the ready and obedient servants of the higher powers. The muscles should be trained to serve the mind.

Unless a movement requires mental concentration in its execution, it is not educational, although it is hygienic. When a movement has been mastered, so that it becomes automatic, it retains little educational value. More complex movements should then be employed. After co-ordination is established and the movement becomes more or less automatic, less energy is expended in its execution. Correct gymnastics lengthens life by conserving energy in work.

Corrective gymnastics means exercise performed for the correction of anatomical defects and deformities.

Movements are divided into two general classes—active and passive. The active movements are performed by the subject either with or without resistance while the passive ones are performed by the operator with the subject passive. This is to say, in passive exercises the operator moves the part while the subject remains passive. These exercises have special value in certain conditions of weakness and deformity, but are of little value otherwise. They should be applied only by one thoroughly trained in their use and only when actually required.

Active exercise may be either "free," "resistive," or "assistive."

By "free" exercise is meant those exercises performed by the subject in which nothing is resisted.

"Resistive" exercises are those performed by the patient in which resistance is offered to the movement of the parts. The resistance may be supplied by the subject's own muscles, by the operator, or by apparatus of some kind.

"Assistive" movements are those in which the subject is assisted by the operator in his movements. These are of use in cases of extreme weakness where full movement of a part is desired but where the subject is too weak to accomplish this alone.

Resistive movements are of two kinds—"aggressive" and "submissive." An "aggressive" movement is one in which the subject makes the movement against the resistance of opposing muscles, the operator or weights of some kind. The patient assumes the aggressive and initiates the movements. A "submissive" movement is one in which the movement of opposing muscles, operator, or apparatus, is resisted by the subject. In this instance, the other forces are on the aggressive and initiate the movement. The submissive forms of exercise have a depressing effect, especially marked upon the timid and should not be employed except upon an aggressive individual.

In beginning, exercise should be light, even assistive in some cases, and the amount of resistance gradually increased as one grows stronger.

Muscles should be contracted to their fullest extent and then thoroughly relaxed. The joint should be carried through its full range of movement. If there is limitation of movement, the part should be carried as far as possible in the direction of limitation and then an effort should be made to carry it further. Movements should be followed by one in opposite direction.

Caution, must be used not to carry the exercise to the point of fatigue, nervous depletion or circulatory embarrassment. If exercise is followed by trembling, fainting, difficult breathing, blueness of lips, or extremities, or prolonged fatigue, it has been carried too far. Except in cases where great endurance is desired exercise should not be prolonged beyond a slight feeling of fatigue.

If resistive movements are given by the operator, these should be slow and resistance even. The amount of resistance should gradually increase toward the middle of the movement and then gradually decrease.

Patients should be given one day's rest from exercise each week. If he is very weak two days of rest each week will be found beneficial. A sufficient amount of rest between treatments is fully as important as the exercise.

In the invalid, the power of recuperation is more or less impaired or limited. Hence exercises that are too vigorous or that are too long continued, are harmful, because they are sure to exhaust the patient, while, due to impaired recuperative powers, and defective organic processes, he is not so quickly restored. The invalid may actually be made worse by our efforts to help him, unless caution is exercised.

Muscular growth is accelerated by work alternated with rest. It is asserted in some quarters that massage can be made to do the work of rest,—that massage will restore the exhausted muscles more quickly and completely, even, than sleep. Repeated experiments have always shown that five minutes of thorough kneading of an exhausted muscle will enable it to repeat, and in some instances exceed the performance that exhausted it. Five minutes of rest has never enabled the exhausted muscle to repeat the performance that exhausted it. If the conclusions that are usually drawn from this are correct, rest and sleep are largely a waste of time. After a day of toil, the tired laborer should get a vigorous massage and go on with another eight hours of work after which he should repeat the performance. The test of the conlcusion that is usually drawn from the above experiment is its ability to keep up the process indefinitely. If it cannot do this, rest and sleep are superior to massage.

If a patient shows loss of weight or energy, the exercises have either been too severe or too frequent. If there is increase of strength but the symptoms are growing worse, this indicates a crisis. After co-ordination is established, less nervous energy is required than at the beginning.

In taking up physical exercise, one should have in view the cultivation of general strength as well as the correction of any defects that he may have. There are many atheletes who possess special strength—that is, they may have tremendous strength of the arms and shoulders, but may have weak undeveloped legs or weak backs. Others may possess strong legs and back but weak arms and abdomen. They have specialized in some particular kind of athletic work and neglected the rest of their body. It is no uncommon thing for atheletes to do this. Trapeze performers for instance, may have powerful arms and shoulders without much leg development. One should avoid such one sided development.

Full health of the body, or efficient functional activity of the whole organism, subsists not in the full development and vigorous activity of some of its parts, but in the full development and vigorous activity of all of them.

Avoid over doing. Do not strain. You cannot develop great strength in any other way than by the use of exercises that offer great ressitance to the contraction of the muscles. As these grow stronger, the resistance must be increased. But you must be content to progress slowly. Don't stuff yourself. Don't try to hurry the matter too much.

Exercise is an excellent aid in reducing weight. But unless it is combined with a rigid control in diet one is more likely to gain than lose weight. Exercise increases the appetite, improves digestion and assimilation, so that if one does not control the food intake, the scales will register an increase in weight.

For this very reason, exercise may be used to put on weight when one is below weight. However, it should be known that underweight is usually due to some disease which must first be corrected before healthy flesh can be put on in satisfying quantities.

Be regular and persistent in your exercise. Results will not come if they are performed haphazzardly. Keep at it, and do not permit yourself to get out of training. Keep in the pink of condition all the time, not just part of the time.

MIND IN HEALTH AND DISEASE

Chapter XXV

OF the medicine man some witty person has penned the following lines:—
"For physic and farces,
His equal there scarce is,
His farces are physic
His physic a farce is."

The steadily growing recognition of the truth contained in these lines has led many to lean more strongly upon the powers of the mind as a means of preventing and curing disease. Mental cults of various shades have arisen, all of which have spread by the "cures" they have accomplished. Thus they have proven the truth of the statement of Paracelsus that: "Whether the object of your faith is real or false, you will nevertheless obtain the same effects."

However, we would not have it thought for one minute that all the so-called cures accomplished by mental healing were really accomplished in this way. All real cures of real diseases are accomplished by the physiological processes as explained in a previous chapter. If the trouble is due to the mental state and the so-called mind-cure succeeds in correcting the mental state, thus removing the cause, cure would naturally follow. However, if cause lies in some other realm palliation only can come through the "mind cure." No real and lasting cure can come by any means so long as the cause is uncorrected.

It is, however, easy to allow oneself to be deceived by mere co-incidences and to exault these to the ranks of cause. As an illustration of this the following story told by Chauncey Depew upon his arrival in America after one of his frequent visits to Europe, will serve. He said:—

"I became lame from rheumatism over there and was recommended to a physician. He treated me by means of what he called an electric battery. I took a handle in each hand and he turned a crank. I didn't feel anything, but I began to improve with the first treatment. After two weeks of this I was cured. Then I was informed that I had had no electricity, and that the handles I held were not connected with anything."

Those not acquainted with the true nature and cause of rheumatism and with the way in which cure is really accomplished will either conclude that the senator either had no rheumatism or that it was cured by imagination. As a matter of fact, the senator had what is called rheumatism and his cure was as real as any cure for rheumatism. In other words, as explained in a previous chapter, the so-called rheumatism was a curative crisis and lasted until the toxins in the body were reduced to the toleration point after which it subsided. This would have occured under any form of treatment or without treatment. But the fake electrical apparatus was used coincident with the recovery therefore the coincidence is referred to as cause. Too many mind cures are on this order.

We hear much of the "power of suggestion," but no one explains this power to us. The fact is that suggestion has no power. The supposed power of suggestion is the power of the patient, and its "effects" depend entirely upon how the patient receives it. We make the same suggestion to three different individuals and get three different effects. One may become angry, one may enjoy a hearty laugh, and the third may be wholly indifferent. All action occsaioned by suggestion is vital action—the out-working of the patient's own power.

No amount of suggestion can overcome the effects of gluttony or inebriety or sensuality or voluptiousness. No amount of suggestion can take the place of exercise or fresh air, or sunshine or sleep. Any effort to cure disease by suggestion is an evil.

In recounting his now famous experiment, Dr. Majendi, the French physiologist said:—

"Let me tell you, Gentlemen, what I did when I was a physician at the hotel Dieu. Some three or four thousand patients passed through my hands every year. I divided the patients into classes: with one I followed the dispensary and gave the usual medicines, without having the least idea why or wherefor; to the other I gave bread pills and colored water, without of course, letting them know anything about it; and occasionally I would create a third division, to whom I gave nothing whatever. The division, to whom I gave nothing would fret a great deal; they felt that they were neglected. Sick people always feel neglected unless they are well drugged, 'les imbeciles,' and they would irritate themselves until they got really sick, but nature always came to the rescue and *all* the *third* class got *well*. There was but little mortality among those who received the bread pills and colored water, but the *mortality* was greatest among those *drugged* according to the *dispensary.*"

No deaths among those who received no treatment! not even the suggestion of treatment, a few deaths among those who, though receiving no treatment, received the *suggestion of treatment* at frequent intervals each day and often at night, would seem to indicate that nature works better without even suggestion to "aid" her. Those who received no treatment, and were not deceived into believing that they were being treated, worried and fretted, but all recovered. This would seem to indicate that *suggestion* is more desrtuctive than worry and fretting. But even worry and fretting would be abolished if people were given the truth about disease. Then, those who are not treated and who are not given *placebos* will not feel that they are being neglected. The truth will set them free.

In his work on "cures" James J. Walsh, M.D., Ph.D., Sc.D., claims that anything will cure the patient when nothing is the matter with him. This is equivalent to the clergyman's assertion that "Christian Science is a real cure for imaginary diseases and an imaginary cure for real diseases." This leaves too much room for real disease to be classed as imaginary. Just as in Senator Depew's case, so other real afflictions that may be cured by nature coincident with the exercise of the imagination, may also be referred to as imaginary.

There doubtless exist imaginary disease. The following story realted by Dr. Abrams in his *Man and His Poisons* is to the point:—

"A butcher slipped in attempting to hang up a heavy picee of meat and was caught by the arm upon the hook. He was at once removed to the office of the surgeon. He said he could not remove his coat, the sleeve must be cut off on account of the excruciating pain from which he suffered. When this was done it was discovered that the hook had passed through the clothing close to the skin, and that the latter was not even scratched."

"A surgeon in a French hospital," according to Dr. Abrams, "gave one hundred patients water for the object of experiment. Then in a state of alarm he told them he had given them an emetic in *lieu* of the proper medicine. The result was that four-fifths of the number became unmistakably sick." We doubt this story, but give it for what it is worth.

Dr. Goddard claimed that: "The idea of disease produces disease in direct proportion to its definiteness and in inverse proportion to the strength of the idea opposing it." If the above cases and many more like them mean anything Dr. Goddard's law is about correct. The imagination can easily produce symptoms of disease. Likewise, the imagination, if changed, would cure, the imaginary disease.

These are unusual cases and are seldom met with in real life. But we are constantly meeting with a very similar occurrence. I refer to the power of the mind to magnify and intensify symptoms that are real. Pains that are slight and "insignificant" in themselves are, by the imagination, very often magnified into formidable pains. The mole hill becomes a mountain. No case of nervous trouble ever came under our care that there were not one or more "insignificant" symptoms that were ruining the life of the patient through an overheated imagination. There was real trouble with the patient, but it was not half so bad as he imagined it to be.

Here is a case from our own practice that well represents this fact. An old lady suffering from what is called rheumatism in her leg and arms called us in for treatment. Her pains were slight but her imagination and desire for sympathy were great. She would howl with pain and ask for morphine for relief. While manipulating the affected parts (This was in the days when we were in the curing business), she would make even more fuss. One day we succeeded in getting her to tell a story in which she was very much interested. She forgot her troubles and laughed very often during the course of the story. We manipulated the effected parts even more vigorously than at any previous time but she did not appear to know that we were treating her. However, immediately, upon completion of the story, she began again to cry with pain.

Well did Emerson write:—

"Some of your hurts you have cured
And the sharpest you still have survived,
But what torments of grief you endured
From evils which never arrived."

Dr. Tuke claimed that: "There is no sensation, whether general or special, excited by agents acting upon the body from without, which cannot be excited also from within by emotional states affecting the sensory centers, such sensations being referred by the mind to the point at which the nerve terminates in the body." Just as the mind, through the emotions, can produce sensations, so the mind, through the emotions, is capable of affecting the functions of the body. This too by way of the nerves.

A few familiar examples that are of daily occurrence will suffice here. The effect of mind upon the circulation is easily recognized in the blushing of the embarrassed maiden or youth. Professor Gates, was able by thinking intently of one of his hands, which was immersed in a basin full of water, to cause enough blood to flow into the hand, to make the water overflow. The effects of fear upon the heart, which appears to come "up into the throat," and upon breathing is well known to everyone. The effects of fear and worry upon digestion has been discussed in another chapter. Fear or anxiety increases the flow of urine while attention directed to the bladder necessitates frequent urination. Thought of food causes the saliva to flow—the mouth "waters." Other emotions such as sorrow, sympathy, and even joy causes the eyes to over-flow with tears. Deep mental attention temporarily suspends respiration giving rise to "breathless attention."

Mind exercises two influences upon the functions and organs of the body— stimulation and inhibition. It may either increase or decrease function and if such influences are intense or prolonged they may result in functional derangement or disease. If this derangement is maintained sufficiently long structural changes may result. That mental influences may be intense enough to cause a great and immediate interferrence with the normal operation of life is instanced by those cases of death due to fear; by the many well known cases of fear causing the hair to become gray in a very short time, and numerous other such changes.

These well known effects of mind are deserving of our most careful attention and should serve to show us that, while the influence of mind over matter is not as great as our Christian Science and New Thought friends would have us believe, nevertheless its influence is of sufficient importance to justify us in carefully avoiding any destructive or harmful effects mind is capable of producing. Fear, anger, jealousy, anxiety despondency, self-pity, worry, envy, etc., should be avoided like the plague. We should cultivate hope, faith, courage, cheerfulness, contentment, love and self-respect. Pride is not self-respect. It has well been called the dry-rot of the soul.

The legitimate office of the mind cure is that of supplanting the destructive emotions with constructive one's and disabusing the mind of the ideopath of his false idea. It should not be thought that mind, because it can influence function so power- fully can cure disease. It may by interfering with normal function cause disease and by ceasing to interfere with such function permit the disease it has caused to be cured. But, it should be understood, that no amount of stimulation or inhibition by whatever method—mental, physical, mechanical, electrical, thermal, or chemical—can ever produce any health worthy the name.

Cause must be removed first, then, the cells of the body will gradually evolve back into the normal state. If one's trouble is due to the practice of sensuality no amount of mental stimulation and inhibition can overcome the effects of the sensuality. First the sensuous practices must be given up and then gradually the organism will return to health. If disease is due to overfeeding, the overfeeding must be stopped. If disease is due to loss of sleep, more sleep is necessary. Whatever the cause or causes, these must be corrected. If the cause is mental, the mental state must be corrected but the cure will not be instantaneous. We may often change the mental state quickly but the effects of the previous mental states require time to be removed.

The idea that one can break all the laws of his being and then by constantly repeating to himself some metaphysical formula—such as, "everyday in every way, I am getting better and better,"—and escape the consequences of broken law is an idea one does not even expect from a child. That one can hurl himself down the sides of a steep cliff and escape injury when he strikes the jagged rocks below by denying the reality of matter and affirming all is mind is an idea belonging only to that ever increasing crowd of unreasoning "reasoners" who call themselves the apostles of "New Thought," "Higher Thought," "Advanced Thought," etc.

If you are over-weight and expect to reduce weight by repeating some metaphysical formula without cutting out your gluttenous eating you are destined to be disappointed. If you are living in such a manner that you have become diseased, and if you expect to recover health by repeating your daily affirmations and denials and without correcting your mode of life you are attempting the impossible. You are asking your mind to set aside the laws of Nature and wipe out the legitimate effects of cause. If you are a reasoning being you will cease this vain effort at once and learn to live for health. If you want health, real health, you can have it by healthful living, but you cannot, by any process, cheat Nature out of the penalty for broken law.

Allow your mind its legitimate sphere, avoid the evil its improper use may cause, then correct any other harmful habits or indulgences you may practice. Put your organism under the conditions essential to its most rapid return to health.

Granting to mind a power over the organism, does not negative the converse of this—that is, the power of the organism over mind. The blood stream that is saturated with alcohol effects the brain and gives rise to all manners of mental disturbances. The brain that is affected by the toxins of disease and high temperature of fevers is subject to hallucinations and temporary insanities. The reaction of the body upon the mind is as certain and as profound as the reaction of the mind upon the body. Even so slight a body ailment as a mere cold effects the mind.

We are proving right along in our work that most cases of chronic worry, fear anxiety, etc., are the result of disease and form secondary causes super-added to the primary causes. So strongly has this fact borne in upon us that we seriously doubt that a truly healthy man would be capable of such an intense or prolonged worry that disease would result. By this we do not deny the harm of worry to the healthy man. We simply say that the healthy man will not worry enough to produce disease. It is extremely doubtful, also, if the really healthy man will be possessed of so deep and intense or so prolonged a fear as to produce disease. The disturbances fear would produce would be only temporary.

A patient comes to us filled with fear—fear of tomorrow, of death, of some impending catastrophe. His fear is wholly unfounded. Nothing has transpired to justify it. It has come into his mind and he has been able to rid himself of it. Rather, it has grown stronger day by day. Invariably we find that the disease with which he is suffering preceeded the fears and that such unfounded fears are but mental symptoms of nervous derangements. The patient is placed on a proper regimen, that is his system is thoroughly cleansed, and built up by natural means and the fears pass away as naturally as darkness retreats before the rising sun. Health is the sun that shines away the darkness of fear in such cases.

The effort to convince these people that their fears are foolish and that their worries are needless and for nothing, or that their jealouses are unfounded is usually a vain effort. The use of suggestion in all its varied forms is of no avail. Something that impresses and sways these people very deeply will sometimes, temporarily overcome their fear or worry, but since the disease state that is responsible for such mental states remains untouched the mental state is very likely to return, unless, of course, the patient is cured before the impression wears off. We may add that things of a religious nature usually have a stronger influence over such minds than most other things. For this reason, the religious "healer" is usually more successful in treating cases of this kind than the scientist.

The influence of the mob effects one profoundly. Mob-psychology is yet a mystery to the scientist. The individual under the influence of the mob spirit will resort to actions and means that he could hardly be driven to under any other circumstances. This explains the "cures" *en masse* of large numbers of the sick by the "healers" at public meetings. After days of sensational advertising which has builded hope and expectancy in the sufferers, comes the psychological moment and the influence of the crowd and "cures" are made—"cures" that are described as "astounding," "miracles." Seldom are such cures lasting or real.

The safer plan is the adoption of a rational or healthful mode of life. Learn to eat right, exercise for health and strength, learn what to do and what to avoid, learn how to control the mind and real health will ultimately be yours. Don't say it can't be done. We are proving daily that it can be done.

When men have health there will be no place for the "healers." Health is superior to any and all forms of "healing." Whether we call it "human healing" or "divine healing" it cannot equal or supplant health. Health is above and beyond any system or method of healing that can be discovered or invented.

Man may have health as soon as he learns to live properly. He does not truly live until he lives as he should. A knowledge of how to live exists now, but it will take a few million years for the average man to get around to this. Just now he is too busily engaged in killing himself in the pursuit of false pleasures.

Other than his love of "pleasure," the belief in cure stands between man and health. This belief is the greatest obstacle to health. So long as man believes that the results of wrong living can be remedied with a pill he will live as he pleases and take the pill. So long as he thinks surgical mutilations can atone for his transgressions of the laws of life he will attempt to substitute surgery for good behavior. Why should man obey the laws of life if they can be so easily set aside? Why should he deny himself the fleeting pleasures and momentary thrills that certain follies provide if he can outwit the evil results of broken law with a pill, powder, plaster or potion?

At the outset, we admit that mind does exercise a profound and far reaching effect upon the processes and functions of life. While we do not believe it can cause health, we are very certain that the evil effects of certain mental states, if profound enough or prolonged enough; can and do result in enervation and toxemia and deranged secretion and excretion although we consider the mental state in most cases of disease, only a contributory factor—one of a multiplicity of causes. To make our meaning a bit clearer, we will say that health is the normal state and always obtains where the normal conditions of healthy life exist. Health is potential in life and always manifests under those conditions. Disease ensues when these conditions are disturbed or interfered with, by whatever cause. Disease, also is potential in life; it is simply a reaction of life against abnormal conditions. Disease is a more or less violent effort of the living organism to re-establish that condition of internal purity and physiological equilibrum which we call health. This effort is made necessary by factors that interfere with the normal processes and functions of life. Disease as a thing *per se* does not exist.

To be exact then we would say that mind causes neither health nor disease; but, that, certain mental states are conducive to normal function while others are impediments to it. Whether the function is normal or abnormal, the function, *per se,* is not produced by mind. Mind may stimulate or inhibit function and either of these influences if profound enough or sufficiently prolonged will induce a condition necessitating disease to overcome. Just as food does not cause health, but does form one of the essential conditions of normal life and just as water and air and sunshine do not cause health but are only essential elements with which life builds its normal state, so mind does not cause health but does influence it. These same things are true of disease, for disease like health is the reaction of the living organism to its environment.

With these principles in mind let us examine a few facts connected with a certain historical "cure" that was of a mental variety although clothed in religion or rather superstition. I choose this particular cure because it is the only one in which I can find an authentic record of a more or less thorough investigation of its patients and results. I have reference here to the cures that were performed at the tomb of Abbe Paris.

320

The Abbe was a wealthy and zealous follower of Jansanius, who gave away his goods to the poor; and, lived, himself, in the most miserable manner, in rags and hunger, sleeping on the bare ground and inflicting painful penance on his poor long suffering body. After his death he was canonized by his followers. Soon it was noised around that miracles were wrought at his tomb and multitudes flocked to the Sacred spot to be healed of their diseases by intercession of the saint. After a time the excitement became so great and the crowds so immense that the government was forced to build a high wall around the tomb. This put an end to the miracles.

Now it happens that the Jesuits were powerful rivals of the Jansanists and they investigated and exposed many of these cures. The archbishop of Paris exposed one instance, and the archbishop of Sens more than twenty. It is authoritatively stated that out of the thousands who crowded the tomb only a few were healed. Montgeron, himself, a strong believer who wrote an account of the matter, succeeded in finding vouchers for only nine.

Of these nine, everyone was gradual in the process of healing; some requiring days, some weeks, and even months. None were instantaneous. It was also shown that some of the cures were only partial and temporary, the trouble soon returning.

The "cures" all taking place under great emontional excitement which often brought on convulsions could mean only that the mental excitement or stimulation had so accelerated or "electrified" the functions of the body that for the time being these people thought they were well. They were in a state of hysteria. There was all stages of hysteria ranging from a near-normal state to temporary insanity. Hysteria is now recognized to be suggestibility. The powerful suggestions of the reported miracles, the great crowds, and prayers, coupled with faith and religious emotions easily brought on such a state. The sick were mentally intoxicated and forgot their diseases. But such mental states do not last. If they did they would soon exhasut their possessor. Therefore we read that many of the cures were "only partial and temporary, returning again afterward."

One young man visited the tomb, with one eye inflamed and the other wholly blind. The inflamed eye was relieved, (not immediately), but the blind eye was not affected at all. But note this, the inflamed eye was improving at the time the young man visited the tomb. Another young man had had his sight destroyed by the puncture of an awl. This eye was being gradually restored before he visited the tomb. The aqueous humor was said to have been replaced by fresh secretions. At the tomb he was gradually restored. These two and many other of the "cures" were permanent.

What is worthy of note in the cures performed at this tomb is:—

1. Not all who visited the tomb were "cured."

2. Of those who were "cured" or improved the cure or improvement in most cases was only temporary.

3. All, or nearly all, the cures were gradual; few if any were instantaneous.

4. A small percentage of the cures were permanent.

5. In all cases where improvement or cure was found, the patients had been improving before visiting the tomb.

These five facts are very significant when viewed in the light of orthopathic principles, but I have found no explanation that adequately meets the needs of the case here. So far as I know, no thorough check up on the cures reported to have been made by E. Coue, during his recent visit here was, or has been, made. No inquiry was made into the actual condition of the patient at the time of his visit to Coue, or to his previous condition and improvement. And with but few exceptions no checking up was done to determine the percentage of "cures" made by him and the length of time the "cures" lasted. A few cures were reported in the daily press that lasted but a few days. Many have passed under the writer's care and observation since, who, though, they did not visit Coue, did try his formula for longer or shorter periods without success.

I recall a case that occurred some years ago in my own home town. I was but a lad and do not know the nature of the trouble with which this particular patient was afflicted, but I do know that, whatever its nature, the patient was forced to walk on crutches. It was bruited about that an old negro man, an ex-slave, who lived seven or eight miles from town in a lonely little cabin in the woods, was possessed of remarkable curative powers. He laid his hand on the sick and mumbled a few sounds that no one understood and they were healed. The patient I am telling of was carried to him, and in some ten or twelve minute was able to walk without his crutches. Possibly he could have done so without going to the negro if he had tried but he did not try. Be that as it may, he was forced to resort to his crutches again next day. Such cures as this one are often reported and since no check-up is made many so-called miracles are claimed to be performed by various "healers" or "relics" or "saints" and allowed to pass unchallenged and therefore form the basis of a great deception. Such "cures" serve to indicate the powerful influence the mind is capable of exerting over the body. On the other hand, those cases where total failure results serve to indicate that the power of the mind over the body is limited.

I have observed many cases of "cures" of precisely this same nature—that is, the patient was apparently cured, but his cure only lasted a few days or a few weeks—to occur under other forms of stimulating and even inhibiting treatment. I have seen many cases "cured" by electrical stimulation, by spinal stimulation, by thermal stimulation but the "cures" were not lasting, although they were often rapid. It is generally known that many of those who write the genuine testimonials published by patent medicine manufacturers, and who, at the time of writing, think they are well, later die of the very trouble the medicine was supposed to have cured. There are many cases on record where the drug manufacturers were still circulating the testimonial long after the disease their medicine cured, had killed the patient who wrote the testimonial.

Such cures, whether from mental, mechanical, chemical or thermal stimulation, indicate that in many cases the sick organism, the impaired functions and palsied nerves, can be whipped into a temporary semblance of health. But the fact that such "cures" are not permanent and that often the condition of the patient after the "cure" wears off is worse than before he was "cured" should indicate to the discerning that such methods form no true part of nature's requirements for a real cure. And these facts should enable us to explain the nature of those apparent cures that are permanent.

These cures that occurred at the tomb of the Abbe were in patients who had been improving before visiting the tomb. Since the cures were not instantaneous but were gradual, requiring time, it is only fair to assume that the improvement that was already under way before the visit to the tomb, continued and brought about recovery. "Cures" that are apparently instantaneous, if investigated, are usually found to be either not cures at all, or were in cases of paralysis or some similar trouble where there was a chance for the patient to be well without being aware of it. In such cases, anything that will cause the afflicted to put forth earnest effort, releasing the mental inhibition born of the belief in the continued inability to do, will produce a "Cure." In such cases the "cure" will be permanent.

A few years ago Prof. Wm. E. Flynn of the Pacific Coast who was called "The youngest old man in America," "The Health Evangelist," "Daddy Flynn," "The Billy Sunday of the Health Movement," etc., stated that "Chronic invalids are people who have been sick, got well, and haven't found it out yet."

Prof. Flynn met the Long Beach wheel chair invalid so well known to all the coast tourists. He was a paralytic who had been wheeled up and down Long Beach for twenty years. Flynn met him and "healed" him. He made the man walk at the first treatment. Flynn was a psychologist along with his other qualifications. He performed "miracles" as well as the rest. His opinions are worth something. Suppose we explain the "miracles" of the psychologists on the basis of his definition: A chronic invalid is one who has been sick, got well, and don't know it.

Let's apply it to case. In Charleston, at the time of the earthquake, there was a woman who had lain in bed for eight or nine years with paralysis. When she felt the earth trembling and the buildings shaking under her she jumped out of bed and ran out of the house. The accounts published of the incident at this time stated that from that moment the lady was cured. Will anyone contend for an instant that the earthquake or the fright cured her? Isn't it more reasonable to believe that she was well already but didn't know it?

In 1921 Mr. Marion L. Erin, of Jersey City, N. J., was reported cured of paralysis by lightening which struck his house. Mr. Erin was a farmer, but a month before the incident was striken with paralysis. It was claimed he would never walk again. However, when the lightening struck the house he jumped from bed and ran out of the house. Up to a late hour that night there had been no return of the paralysis. His physician expressed the opinion that the "cure" would not be permanent.

Dr. Walter records the following in his "*Life's Great Law.*" Speaking of mind power in disease he says:—

"An excellent illustration of this subject occurred in the practice of a brother physician. The patient had been carried from bed to chair for many years, without apparent benefit, until the house caught fire and burnt to the ground. When the cry of fire was heard the patient jumped from her bed, caught up her trunk and threw it out of the window, and ran downstairs and saved herself, and never went back to bed as an invalid. Does anyone believe that the power could have come out of her if it had not been in her? Did the cry of fire put it in her? No, it was months and even years of resting that had accumulated what she needed to restore her to health, while threatened danger appealing to the instinct of self-preservation enabled her to use it."

The truth is, the lady was well but didn't know it. Let us suppose that she was not well; does anyone suppose fright would have cured her? Maybe she would have been able to do what she did but it would not have been recorded that she "never went back to bed as an invalid." On the contrary, she would have collapsed as soon as the excitement wore off and would have been worse than before.

Dr. Walter has the following to say:—

"Let us suppose a case that has proven an utter failure, and we will find him to be one who is tired and worn, or whose constitution has been so depleted by drugs that no response remains, and we can predict with assurance that mind-cure or any other kind of cure will prove a failure if immediate results are expected But let us now suppose a case which has in it the elements of success. That old maid, it may be, has kept her bed substantially for twenty years, and all physicians having failed to confer any benefit, have at length taken their departure, and the patient is left to her own resources. Having tried all remedies she has finally abandoned them in despair, and for years, it may be, she has done nothing. Nature, in the meantime, has been recuperating, silently and unconsciously, but the power has been accumulating. Under these circumstances a new doctor appears, either mind-cure, faith-cure, or Christian Scientist, perhaps even some shrewd medical charlatan, who, having obtained the patient's confidence, begins his experiments. An immediate response follows, because the power of response is in the patient, it matters very little what the agency is, as long as it arouses vital activity. The patient feels her strength returning, new hope and new ambitions are awakened, and she goes along to a complete recovery."

The explanation of the different results obtained in these cases is easy: The first patient failed to respond because of lack of power, the second responded because the power of response was present. Does anyone suppose for an instant that the effects of a lifetime of wrong living can be overcome in an instant by fire, lightning, earthquakes, the mind of a "healer," etc.? Isn't it much more reasonable to think that the work of repair and recuperation had been slowly and silently going on for years so that the patient was well but didn't know it.

In various parts of the world are to be found Catholic institutions where are enshrined some relic of the saints, a "shin bone of St. Anne," a piece of the "cross upon which Christ was crucified," or something of similar nature. These are vested with miraculous healing powers and yearly thousands journey to these places to be healed. At these shrines are to be found large piles of walking canes, braces, crutches, stretchers, etc., that those "healed" left behind as they went out. Those that journey to these places may be divided into three classes, according to the results obtained:—

First: Those who are "healed" and stay well.

Second: Those who are "healed" and remain so for from a few hours to a few months.

Third: Those who come out as they went in—not healed.

Class one was well already but didn't know it. They went to the shrine believing they would be cured and were. What has belief to do with the matter. Let us see A man has some infirmity which forces him to resort to crutches. The trouble lingers on for years. Both he and his physicians give up hope of curing him, so treatment is abandoned. Slowly but surely the silent forces of the organism are at work healing and repairing the affected parts. The man is healed, but not realizing it he continues to use his crutches; he makes no attempt to walk without them. His will does not act in any direction which he does not believe is possible for him to work. He must believe he can walk before he will make the effort.

Take the familiar example of a baby reaching for the moon. The baby believes it can reach it, so makes the attempt. The adult never makes such an attempt because he does not believe he can reach the moon. The disbelief acts as a break to his will and paralyses effort. The child's belief that he could reach the moon did not enable him to do so, but it did enable him to make the attempt. If Columbus had not believed the world to be round, he never would have sailed away to find a water-route to India. Our patient of class one, having faith in the healing powers of the shin bones of Saint Anne or some other such "relic," makes the effort and suddenly discovers that he can walk without his crutches.

Class two is not well, but under the stimulus of the occasion, they are enabled to work up a semblance of health which lasts for a shorter or longer time, after which their old symptoms return. These people visit the shrine after days of expectancy and nights of keenest anticipation of the joys of health which the visit is to bring to them. They read the glowing accounts of the many others who have been healed there and their whole being becomes electrified with faith and expectancy. Then comes the psychological moment, the pent-up emotions are released in an almost uncontrollable outburst, every cell and fibre of the whole organism is stimulated to renewed activity. The patient is "cured." The glands of the body, its nerves and muscles, which have been slumbering for years, are excited and stimulated to their highest pitch. The power, however, is power from within.

A friend of the author's awoke one night and found his home afire. In his excitement he picked up a very heavily loaded trunk, put it on his shoulders and walked out of the house with it. The next morning, his excitement over, he was unable to lift the trunk from the ground. The power to do something unusual under excitement is well known. Similar things are possible without excitement if the individual has acquired the ability to concentrate his whole attention and energies upon the effort. Enthusiasm enables one to put forth extra effort. Sudden and unexpected responsibility helps us to do greater work. But these things do not give us added power. They only enable us to expend the power we possess. These "miracles" are from within.

Patients cured in this way, if not already well, stay cured from a few hours to a few weeks, then have a return of symptoms. They are forced again to resort to their cane, crutches, chair or bed.

This same principle will explain a lot of other cures that are widely advertised. A lady has been ill for years. Her physicians have given up the job. An almanac put out by some patent medicine concern falls into her hands. She reads the glowing testimonials of other women who were afflicted as she is and how they were cured by this wonderful medicine. She sends for a bottle. It comes. She is filled with expectancy and hope. Now, at last, she is to be cured. She feels better, even before she takes the first dose. Then comes the first dose of the magic potion. It contains some powerful stimulant. This, with her mental stimulation, "cures" her in a few days. She, too, writes a glowing testimonial. Alas! Poor woman! In a few days her old trouble returns. The testimonial never says anything about this part. She tries the wonderful remedy again, but this time the results are not so good. She has less power of response.

A man has been sick for years. He has been from physician to physician, and from climate to climate. Finally, when he is about to give up in despair, a booklet falls into his hands in which he finds the wonderful stories of how thousands of others as bad, or worse, than he is recovered health in some drugless institute. He writes for terms and their opinion of his case. The reply offers him great hope. He decides to go. He begins to get better the minute he gets his ticket. He can hardly wait for the train to get him to this wonderful health plant. Finally he arrives. Those in charge inspire him with hope and confidence. The patients all tell him how they have improved and how others were cured and left. He is lifted up into a higher sphere.

Then comes the treatment. It is one long merry-go-round of stimulation. Cold sprays, sitz baths, salt rubs, cabinet baths, steam baths, mechanical, thermal or electrical stimulation of the spine. He feels fine. This stimulation added to the mental stimulation and he is soon "cured." At the request of the physician in charge he too, writes an "unsolicited" testimonial, and returns home.

In a few days or a few weeks his old troubles return. How deceptive are immediate results—appearances. He returns to the Sanitarium or resort for another cure. Year after year he makes the round of such places to be cured all over again.

Another case hears of Chiropractic and its wonderful results. He reads the Chiropractor's own glowing account of how his little punch in the back is snatching people back from the grave, even after they have one foot in it. He, too, reads testimonials whose writers may have wished later that they had not been in such a hurry about writing them. He visits a Chiropractor who explains to him the wonders of this new "science." He is shown pretty pictures of the spinal column and the nerves that emerge from it. It's all new to him and fills him with awe. What's more, it sounds reasonable. He is told of how others who had the same trouble he has were cured by Chiropractic. He decides to try it.

Here is renewed hope. He is filled to the brim with expectancy. He feels better. He gets on the table and is treated. As the Chiropractor gives his thrust he hears a snap in his spine and knows the vertebra has been moved. The punch on the spine is also stimulating. He gets up feeling better. In a short time he is "cured" and writes a testimonial. In a few days or a few weeks his old trouble returns. He resorts to Chiropractic again, but this time the "wonderful science" fails him and he seeks elsewhere.

Thus are we forced once more to insist that immediate results are not always lasting and that the condition of the patient a few months later must be our true guide.

Now we come to class three. These go into the shrine on stretchers or crutches, or are wheeled in on invalid chairs, and are brought out on these things. What was the matter? Was the "relic" unable or unwilling to heal these? No. These were simply not well and did not have the power to respond to the mental stimulus of the occasion. Perhaps if they return home and rest for a few weeks or months and return they will be able to respond.

There are two other ways patients are cured by these methods. We will consider first a case that has been put to bed by the physician. Perhaps he was able to be up and even able to work a little before he was ordered to bed. He rests and recuperates for a few weeks. Silently and gradually the work of repair and recuperation has been going on. But the patient no more realizes that he has grown stronger than the sleeping athlete is aware of his strength. We become conscious of power only by expressing it.

At this stage a "faith healer," a "mental healer," a "metaphysician," or some similar "healer" comes and persuades him that there is no disease, that God is all and God is good. She persuades him to get up. Now for the first time he becomes conscious of his added power. But he gives the credit to the "healer." He announces to his physician that he is well and will not require his services any more. His "cure" may be permanent and it may not. The permanency will depend on how long he rested.

The other method of cure which the "mental scientist" or "divine scientist" uses is well illustrated by the following case:

A little boy, son of Christian (?) Science (?) parents, had typhoid fever. A physician was called. The boy grew worse. The physician gave up, saying the boy could not live. The mother sent for a Christian Science practitioner. The practitioner came, poured out the drugs, and, as my sister who lived in the same house at the time said to me, "from that very day the boy began to get better. The boy recovered and today no one would think he had ever had typhoid."

The reader should note the fact that the improvement began the very day the drugs were thrown out, and that previous to that he had continually grown worse. We explained these results by saying that the poisonous drugs which were being poured into his body every half hour were slowly killing him. As soon as the poisoning ceased he is calculated to begin growing better, and this is just what he did do.

There is one form of "mind" that our "all is mind" friends won't tolerate, one form of "good" that those who proclaim "all is good" have no use for—drugs. There is one transgression of natural law that their denials, affirmations, silent prayers, absent treatments and metaphysical formulas will not atone for, and that is the taking of drugs. These they prohibit all their patients. And it must be remembered that many patients with acute disease are killed by these deadly agents; that many invalids perpetuate their condition by the habitual use of drugs.

A certain well known drugless physician who makes more or less of a speciality of treating blindness with reported great success, succeeds in this same way. Recently, while engaged in conversation with a friend and former co-worker of his, this man, who had been associated, in practice, with the first mentioned physician told me that he had seen him get four of five cures out of hundreds and that these were all in cases where the blindness was only partial and of short duration; that not one of his cures was secured in cases of long standing. He added: "his cases either get well in a few weeks, six to eight, or they do not get well at all." This would indicate that the few "cures" he makes are in functional cases that would get well of themselves and that when he encounters a case that will not get well of itself, no "cure" is performed. Now if we consider the nature of his treatment, which is almost wholly one of stimulation, and the kind of conditions nature requires to accomplish her best work, we would be justified in saying that perhaps some of those cases where he fails to secure results could get well. At least it is just possible that they could recover if properly cared for before injured by his treatments. We would also be justified in saying that the cases wherein he succeeds could have recovered quicker under different conditions.

I recount these facts here simply to show that the cures under other forms of treatment do not differ from those performed by mind cures and that it is the same class of patients that recover under the one as under the other. Note also the permanent or temporary cures are in the same classes of patients whatever the form of treatment.

In previous chapters the reparative powers exercised by plants and animals, whereby they restored lost parts—limbs, tails, hands, eyes, etc.—and whereby a small section of the worm becomes a complete worm, or a small fragment of the leaf of some plants becomes a complete plant, were noted and emphasized. The identity of these powers of repair and those that are constantly exercised during the life of the animal in growth development and maintenance in health, was pointed out. This power exists in the adult man as much as in the morula and operates in the adult without mental influence as in the morula. It operates constantly, even while we sleep or while we are in a coma, or a faint, or while unconscious from a blow on the head. If it could not and did not accomplish its work of purification and repair as well under such conditions when mental influences are suspended as at other times such states would usually end in death.

Mind cure will have to give way to Nature Cure and the little truth the mind cure systems possess will be found to fit nicely into its proper place in Nature Cure—for mind is Natural, not super-natural or extra-natural. Nature Cure cannot say with the mentalist "all is mind, nothing matters" nor with the materialist: "all is matter, don't mind it." The idea that anything will cure that affects the mind of the patient strongly enough and favorably enough is only another of those many mistakes that make up the labyrinth of fallacy the human mind has built up on appearances. It is only an appearance, like the appearance that the earth is flat, and the sun goes around it every twenty-four hours.

Several of the huge religious combines— institutionalized and commercialized religion and superstition—which for years sneered at Mrs. Eddy's grotesque carricature of Christianity and Science have recently realized the large amount of money that can be made from what is called spiritual healing and are cashing in on popular ignorance and credulity while the cashing is good. Those engaged in the regular paid religion trade realize that if the religion business is to be kept afloat they have to do more than bark at the moon.

He who examines the descriptions of the methods employed by the "modern healer" is struck by their resemblance to the work of the medicine man of the un-tutored tribes of Asia, Africa, South America, Australia and the South Sea Islands.

"Healing" has been practiced by the Church from the days of Constantine and all manners of deceptive methods have been resorted to to accomplish cures. "Relics" of the Saints (?) have been popular means of cure. These have consisted of bones of the saints, pieces of their apparel, scrappings from their tomb stones, etc. It has been estimated that in Europe there are enough pieces of the Cross Christ was crucified on to make hundreds of such crosses. These all possess "curative" powers.

The Russian Communists, in their war on religion, opened some of the shrines or tombs of the saints which had "healed" their thousands for the Holy Greek Catholic Church, and found these saints to be made of wood, hay, straw and cotton. If all the thousands, who had traveled long distances and paid their hard earned coin into the coffers of the Church to be cured by these saints, could rise from their tombs and see this straw and cotton and realize how they had been hood-winked in the name of Christ and religion, by the hypocritical religious combine, there is no guessing just what they would do to such scoundrels. We need more "reds" in other countries to expose the saints of wood, hay and cotton that are credited with miraculous powers in these.

Most of the healing business seems to be carried on by Saint Anne, or her shin bones. Saint Anne is said to be the mother of Mary the Mother of Jesus. The Bible no where tells the name of Mary's Mother and no one knows whether it was Ruth or Raechal. Anne, probably was not her name. Nor is it known whether she was a saint or a normal wholesome woman. But all this does not prevent her most holy shin bones from accomplishing wonderful miracles of healing. Shrines of St. Anne exist at Montreal, Canada; St. Anne, Ill., Holywell, England and at various places on the European continent.

On a July day in 1921 according to the New York World, it took four priests all day to apply a relic of St. Anne to the afflicted bodies of the thousands who came to the church of St. Jean Baptiste, in New York City. Of course, no one possesses a single bone or other relic of the grandmother of Jesus and it has been suggested that the Priests used "a chicken leg or an old soup bone" and that they "had an uproarious laugh behind the scenes over the whole farce." It is a damnable practice for those who profess to be followers of the Nazarene to be engaged in.

Bernadette Soubirous claimed to have seen an apparition, claiming to be the immaculate conception, on Feb. 11, 1868, which told her to drink of the spring which is now inclosed within the Basilica of Our Lady of Lourdes, in Southern France. Since that date this shrine has done a thriving business in cures. Its business especially boomed immediately after the war when every sentimentalist went wild over everything French. In May 1923, some 858 Britishers journeyed to Lourdes hoping to receive help but returned un-cured. According to the London Herald over half this number again took the trip in Sept. 1923, but returned without one being cured.

One poor soldier, on the way there, was hobbling along on his crutches and while crossing a railroad track beheld a locomotive coming down upon him at a rapid speed. Fear, not faith, siezed him and he dropped his crutches and ran. His cure was permanent, it has since been reported. Thus a modern locomotive accomplished in this instance what Our Lady of Lourdes failed to do in about 1300 other such cases. Perhaps we should erect a Shrine to Saint Engine.

But the Shrines are losing caste and new "Saintes" are bobbing up. The Anglican Church until recently thought it had "lost" the power of healing; but now has its hat in the ring and is competing with the Christian (?) Scientists (?) Spiritualists, (?) "savage" medicine men and "heathen" "devil" worshipers for first honors in the field of cure. They have the audacity to quote to us the 15th to 18th verses, inclusive of the 16th chapter of the book of Mark in defense of their claims, notwithstanding that every educated man in the Christian world knows that the whole of the chapter from the 9th verse onward is spurious.

Among the modern saints, one over whom the Episcopal Church has grown enthusiastic, is one James Moore Hickson. This man, who has been circumnavigatnig the globe during the past few years, was in New York City in 1919. He claimed to be an instrument of Christ and received the endorsement of Bishop Manning and the Board of Bishops.

Three months after his visit to New Yrok, the Baltimore News said:—

"A sincere effort was made to find some absolute cures resulting from the healing service, but nothing could be discovered that could not be laid at the doors of hypnotism or sudden emotional exaltation and belief."

Later, when he left Melbourne, Australia, a Melbourne Journal had the following to say:—

"Hickson, the healer, passes. About fifty cases of benefit are claimed in Melbourne. The church authorities pay no heed to the unuttered reflcetions of the 3,000 sufferers whose pilgrimage of pain to St. Paul's Cathedral has led them into a pit of despair blacker than the night from which they emerged towards this newly-lit lamp of healing."

THE PEOPLES PULPIT, an Australian religious newspaper, had the following to say: —

"To our certain knowledge, Mr. Hickson laid hands upon thirteen sufferers in the vicinity of Melbourne, none of whom were cured, and six of whom died before the healer left the city."

Hickson claimed that he "found children the easiest to work upon because their minds are absolutely open." On February 14, 1920 he tried to heal a little boy in Pasadena, Calif. The boy, his body undersized and undeveloped and his legs pitifully twisted, was carried out of the church and asked to be taken out on the grass where he "would walk and surprise everybody." He made the effort to walk and fell in a heap.

According to the Denver Times, the Denver District of the Methodist Episcopal Church has formally approved of "faith healing" and urges all ministers to "make this subject an integral part of their ministry." A Rabbi in San Francisco has gone in for the same thing, only he isn't using Christ. The Rev. Evangelist F. F. Bosworth is advocating the same thing. Lewiston, Maine boasted in 1924 of a healer who was only three years of age. Porto Rico had one, a lady, who went into trances and was aroused with great difficulty. New York had a healer who declared that he got his powers by revelation that came to him from heaven in flaming letters. At the same time The Detroit News reported that one prominent faith healer had been ordered back to the asylum.

Mrs. Annie Semple McPherson who became involved in some suspicious circumstances and thus obtained the needed publicity, and who is in the healing business in California, claims no miraculous power but maker her cures dependent upon submission to the will of the healer. This sounds rather like hypnotism and, indeed, as we shall later see, this "great psychological crime" is the ruling factor in all these healing performances.

A three weeks investigation of supposed cures performed by Mrs. McPherson in Fresno resulted in the discovery of twelve cases of insanity and domestic strife following her mission, but no cures. This is a rather poor showing for one who claims so much. She seeks every mesmeric advantage over her subjects and the results speak for themselves.

A certain Mr. Smith Wiggleworth, who worked the religion business for all there was in it, in New Zealand a few years since claimed that some angels appeared before him and commissioned him to heal. His commission was for a limited time only. These spirits or angels demanded, however, that his patients have implicit faith in the trinity before they could be healed. This trinity is that strange doctrine opposed to the One God of the Scriptures, that "the Father is the Son of himself, and the Son is the Father of himself, and (that) each of these is another person, who is the same and yet different from the other two"—The Holy Ghost. No real cures have been traced to this man.

Dr. Chas. S. Price of Vancouver, B. C., attracted considerable attention as a "healer." Of him the Golden Age says:—

"A committee that investigated the basis of the excitement that his meetings have aroused there found that not one miracle of healing had been performed and that no organic lesion or defect had been helped. The only successes were in cases of functional or hysterical disturbances."

John Cudney, who called himself "Brother Isaiah" was at New Orleans in the spring of 1920, where he lived in an old house boat on the Father of Waters. This unassuming me-and-God fledging declared that the very ground upon which he trod became sacred rgound and possesssed wonderful curative powers. Some of this earth sprinkled over a worthless oyster bed caused the bed to become the finest in the South. "Brother Isaiah" worked all the tricks of the conjurers and magicians and hypnotists. He claimed to be able to tell at once the name of his visitors and what they had concealed about their persons. He pretended to be able also to tell what their ailments were.

Cudney was able to mesmerize whole crowds at once. Had he only been French he would have been as popular as Coue. A favorite stunt of his, as reported by the Jacksonville Times-Union, was to change the color of the sun to suit the whims of the herd that came out to see him. A few years ago, when correspondence courses in hypnotism, mesmerism and electrical psychology were cluttering up the mails, the present writer learned quite a bit about how such mental states are induced by the skillful operator. Some greater things than merely changing the color of the sun were then claimed for electrical psychology. These changes are, of course, subjective and are produced by suggestion upon hysterical subjects.

The crowds with scores of ailing and crippled men and women came out in such uncontrolable numbers that five policemen, who had been detailed to keep them in line, were pushed off their feet into the Mississippi river. Indeed the crowds became so great that the newspapers had to print notices requesting other sufferers to stay away as they could not be handled. One editor remarked: "Clergymen almost without exception, agree that 'Brother Isaiah's' work had done good."

What good? Who received the benefit? A careful census was taken after he departed from New Orleans and not a single real cure was found. Discussing this healing business carried on by the professional collection-box passers and referring directly to "Brother Isaiah," himself, the Columbus Evening Dispatch said:—

"All over the world are shrines to which people used to make pilgrimages to be cured of disease; in every age have appeared these healers; always there is a rumored place or person that has mysterious powers of healing. But time reveals the fact that there was really nothing in it. The healers pass away after a brief reign, and it is seen that they did not really heal at all."

I believe that if the people were given a knowledge of the history of such shrines and healers from remote antiquity to now and also a dependable history of the many other systems and methods of cure that have been tried throughout the ages, they would not be so easily led to part with their hard earned dollars by those who pretend to cure and heal.

Emil Coue, a French druggist, visited America in 1922 and 1923. We had not gotten over our sentimental way of slobbering at the feet of everything French at that time, so we went into hysteria over an obscure man who was not known outside of the block he lived in in France. The American press and American hysterics made him famous. There was nothing essentially new or original in his method and he admits that he got his start by spending thirty francs for an American work on hypnotism.

He learned his lesson well for he was able to mesmerize whole crowds at once. Personal magnetism, or power of personal influence, we called this when the country was being flooded with the correspondence courses on hypnotism and electrical-psychology. Suggestion, Coue calls it. Its all the same. So is Auto-suggestion. There is no essential difference between hypnosis induced by the operator and auto-hypnosis and both are induced by suggestion. Modern psychologists and psychiatrists are agreed that hypnotism is hysteria and hysteria is suggestibility. There are all degrees of hysteria ranging from mild "enthusiasm" to apparent or temporary insanity.

Hysteria is an induced state, induced by suggestion, and often causes the sick and crippled to throw away their crutches, or get off their beds, or out of their wheel chairs, and walk or run or do many things they previously thought were impossible. The mental exhilaration often observed in such states causes every organ and gland in the body to increase its efforts. Functions that have long been all but dormant are accelerated, the whole being seems electrified. No doubt the endocrine system is stimulated along with the nerve centres. Marvelous cures, miracles of healing, "instantaneous" recoveries, are common in such states.

These patients are usually prepared for days beforehand, by glowing accounts in the papers, of cures performed. Their days and night are spent in joyous expectancy. Then comes the psychological moment and the wonderful "cure" is accomplished. But alas! and alack! The investigations reveal that few, very few, such cures are real or lasting.

Visits to fifteen of Coue's patients, upon whom he had laid his hands, revealed that his treatments grew less and less efficacious, with his absence, thus showing that the power of his suggestion grew progressively less.

The New York Times reported that Coue had given up reciting his day-by-day formula, and he admitted that as long as the proper mental state is maintained the Litany of the Saints or any other Litany would work just as well. "The proper mental state" is one of suggestibility, a negative mental attitude, then any formula that carries the suggestion will induce auto-hypnosis or hysteria, be this formula the Litany of the Saints or the mummery of a devil worshiper. He may be a medicine man on the Congo or the Amazon or he may minister to the spiritual needs of the head hunters; his little jingles will have the same effect on suggestible minds.

Doctor Reisner, Pastor of the Chelsea Methodist Episcopal church of New York City, said of the Frenchman and his method:—

"Mr. Coue has put before us a wonderful system. Without religion his system is like a motor with no electric power in it. But the church may make his system into a great channel of power for helping humanity. It is a great mistake for ministers and churches to attack Mr. Coue. He has exalted God by enforcing the marvelous gifts with which the Creator has endowed men. It is well that he has not tied his system to any special religious cult or sect, but leaves it open for wise religious leaders to appropriate the truths he has uncovered by showing how religion can be related to these truths."

It is true that these "healing" suggestions are more effective when tied to some religion—whether this is Paganism, Heathenism, Judaism, Mohammedianism, Confiuscianism, Buddaism, Brahamanism, Christianity or Devil worship. And no effort was ever made to separate it from religion until recent modern times. But I can see no reason for calling those things which the church has decried as "works of the devil" until recently, "the truths he has uncovered." The "truths" were in use long before Methusela was born. They cannot be tied to any special religious cult or sect, for they belong to all of them, the "false," and the "true."

Mr. Coue did not completely divorce his practices from religion. He says: "My plan is quite simple. It is just the same as Christ's." This gives him a right to send around the collection plate and declare: "The Lord loveth a cheerful GIVER."

Coue, Hickson, Price and all the rest of these "spiritual" healers employ hypnotism in their work and then declare this is the same as that used by Christ. It can be shown that he condemned this very thing. Witness the mass-hypnotism in the following account of one of Hickson's missions as published in the Cleveland News-Leader:—

"I attended one if the sessions of Hicksin's missions of Healing. I was not in the church five minutes when I felt myself in a most inflamed, abnormal, exalted state. I did not seem to be myself. The sight of the misshapen, the miserable, about me strained my emotions to the bursting-point. I found that I could use my rational faculty only with considerable exertion. I was in a mood to believe almost anything. If a crutch had risen before my eyes and danced, I would not have thought it strange.

I was immersed in the supernatural. I felt I could do something extraordinary if I were called upon to do it. I felt an overwhelming yearning for God to come down in healing upon this tragic and stricken multitude. I cared not how He healed, whether by hands or feet, by straw or star, so long as He stilled the cry of those demented souls! I stood it for an hour, and could stand it no longer. I must leave or bust. I left."

The Melbourne Journal, previously quoted from, said of Hickson:—

"A young priest approaches a group and, in a voice of authority, asks them to desist from doing something—one does not hear what—as it may disturb this 'atmosphere.' It is apparent that the atmosphere plays a very important part in the proceedings. His (Hicksons') appearance indicates phenomenal strength and animal magnetism, but no trace of spirituality."

Still more graphic is the following description of one of the Healing Missions of Dr. Price as reported in the Daily-Star, Toronto:—

"The stage of Massey Hall last evening again witnessed poignant and pathetic scenes of faith healing. Over a score of women together with one man were swept from their feet by the inrush of some force apparently psychic.

"There were no means of estimating whether there were or were not cures. It was obvious, however, that the evangelist's fervent challenge to disease to depart caused severe nervous shocks and sharp physical reactions. The tremors and twitchings, the almost epileptic moans and groans of those subjected to the process of healing, their livid or waxlike features, their facial contortions, were painfully and physically real. Each patient seemingly received what a surgeon would call a trauma, a wounding or rending of physical or mental tissue. There was a suggestion of the abnormal as much as the supernatural. Had the lame thrown away their crutches and walked, had the blind opened their eyes and claimed vision, the evening would have been as joyful as a resurrection. With its results in tearful balance it seems as morbid as a morgue.

"After his platform clinic the evangelist descended the main floor of the hall, and annointed and laid hands on the sufferers in the opera chairs. Again there was an immediate and obvious physical seizure. Their heads fell with a jerk against the back of their chairs. Features became crisped, fists clenched, and muscles cramped. For the most part they closed their eyes tightly. They drew their breath in sharp gasps. Their lips quivered as if in prayer. Their whole being seemed to be drawn inward in some intense affirmation of faith.

"One blind man pressed both hands tightly over his eyes and seemed violently agitated by some superhuman effort of will. Beside him sat a man who was said to be paralytic. When the healer touched him, he crumpled up in his chair. When the healer had passed, he flung back his head, and, sitting on the edge of his seat, thrust his legs straight before him without flexing the knees. One of them kept up a galvanic quivering, which a man beside him tried to quite by placing his hand on his knee.

"At the conclusion of his service Dr. Price gave some description of the healing force. 'Evidently,' said he, 'some kind of spiritual force flowed through the body. Children had spoken of it as a prickly feeling. 'I often feel its presence at once,' said he, 'when I take hold of a sufferer. A paralytic limb is cold. When the spiritual power flows in it at once becomes warm. I have known a withered limb in which the skin had been clinging to become immediately plump with flesh.' "

Evidently the reporter was also a bit hypnotized or else he was "half-shot" for he has probably recorded things he saw that were only subjective impressions and not objective realities, at all. Under the magic "spell" of the hypnotist, whether he uses "scientific suggestion" or religious flumdummery, the sick can be made to feel that they have been cured while in reality they have only been deluded.

What must be the attitude of the natural hygienist toward this so-called spiritual healing? We deal here with a problem that involves religious prejudices, psychological theories, therapeutic hypotheses and the testimony of experience. It is inevitable, then, that there shall be almost as many attitudes as observers. But this much is certain, if the basic principles which underlie orthopathic philosophy and practice are correct, this healing business that is carried on by the "Priests who pray for hire" is a gigantic delusion and swindle.

In the preceeding chapters, I pointed out that curative actions are constantly going on in the body and that they work slowly, silently, unobservedly; often bringing about a cure of the physical trouble without the mind becoming aware of it. In such cases, what are apparently instantaneous cures are made. The real truth, as already pointed out, is that the really essential part of the cure was accomplished before the healer or relic, etc., came along.

This is simply saying as Dr. Jennings did over seventy years ago: "In the recuperative process a certain series of changes must necessarily take place in the part before it can be restored to soundness, and that these changes must necessarily occupy a certain time," or, as Dr. Dewey so admirably put it: cure, "is an evolution in reverse." If we let perfect health be represented by the summit of a hill, average health by a line at its base and the physical condition of a patient be represented by the foot of a long stairway leading down into a pit or quarry, we will know that in getting back to average health, the patient will have to reverse his steps and climb the stairs, step by step, over the same road he descended, until he reaches the base of the hill. There are no elevators to health—nothing that will enable us to jump up the stairway and land at the top in one bound, any more than it will enable us to jump to the summit of the hill to perfect health.

By the above, I do not mean to say that the Deity cannot supply an elevator to health. I would be equally as much of a bigot were I to attempt to place a limit on God's power as is the fellow who tells you all that He can do. What God can do and what the "healers" can do are not the same things and should be kept apart. The me-and-God crowd of professional collection-box passers may not all agree with this; nevertheless, it remains a fact that to question their infallibility and wisdom is in no sense a reflection upon the God of the universe.

Certain religious sects regard the whole thing as manifestations of spiritism or demonism. This method of disposing of one's unnecessary adversaries was common in the Middle ages. Anything one didn't like was of the devil. Even the movements of the stars as revealed by the telescope was attributed to the devil, by those who knew the earth to be flat and the stars to be chandeliers stuck in the "firmament." Many refused to look into a telescope because it was the work of the devil. This method of solving problems was a very convenient substitute for thought and still serves this purpose.

Demons and devils may exist. The spirit mediums, and institutions for "psychic" research have been trying for years to convince us of the reality of these super-human, invisible beings. Sir Olive Lodge, Conan Doyle, Cammille Flammarian and other notables have endeavored to convince us of their reality. But, so far, the evidence is far from convincing. Until we are sure of their existence we are not justified in explaining natural phenomena by an appeal to these assumed beings.

Hypnosis is an induced state and is mentally destructive; but I can see no logical reason why this cannot be induced by the operator or the subject himself without the intervention of spirits or demons. Even if we grant that these demons exist, that they are capable of influencing the human mind, or even of taking possession of it, as in what is claimed to be demoniacal possession, or spirit obsession or delusional insanity (hysteria), I can still see no reason why one human being cannot influence the mind of another or why auto-suggestion cannot do the same.

THE STIMULANT DELUSION

Chapter XXVI

THROUGHOUT all systems and methods of therapeutics there runs the basic error that what they call the therapeutic actions of their various procedures represent the beneficial actions of these things upon the body, or that they call out actions on the part of the body that are beneficial or useful in overcoming "disease." The truth, as the student is now ready to understand, is that these so-called "therapeutic actions" of "remedies" are REACTIONS OF THE BODY AGAINST THE "REMEDIES." The living organism reacts to everything in its environment—to useful and salubrious agents and influences to assimilate and make use of these; against non-usable and destructive things to throw them off and defend itself against these. The reaction against harmful substances and influences is proportionate to their harmfulness and commensurate with the power of reaction possessed by the affected organism. These two factors—the amount and destructiveness of the agent or influence, and the powers of the organism—are the determining factors in every reaction except where toleration has been established.

Mistaking the defensive reactions of the sick body as evidences of the beneficial actions of drugs and other supposed remedies has led physicians of all schools into the most serious and egregious errors. Perhaps in no other field of "medicine" archaic or modern have greater blunders of this nature been made than in the delusion that "stimulation" is a beneficial or strengthening thing. We know of no portion of the human race in any age or in any part of the world that has not been mislead by the *Stimulant Delusion*. No greater delusion ever possessed the human mind than the stimulant delusion. Like the ancient idea that the earth is flat and the heavens a great chandilier-studded canopy stretched over it, the *stimulant delusion* is based on appearances. Man lives in the appearance of things until ratiocination dawns, after which he attempts to get back of the scenes and find out what it is that makes the wheels go around. It is then that he makes the, at first, shocking discovery that the real is the opposite from the apparent. Most people in civilized countries now know that the world is round and not flat, but how many of them know that stimulants take away the power they appear to give?

Before defining stimulants and explaining their "action" it will be well to draw a sharp distinciton between what I shall call the *compensated*, or necessary vital stimuli; and the *uncompensated*, or unnecessary and accidental stimuli—*natural* and *artificial* stimulants, these are usually called.

What the vital or organic force is we may never know, but we do know that it is not independent of certain conditions. The necessary elementary combination of the vital principle may be present, and yet not manifest as life. This quiescent state of life as observed in the impregnated germ of the egg before incubation and in the seed before germination and in cases of hibernation and suspended animation is not to be mistaken for death. The manifestations of the organic force or life begin under the influence of certain necessary conditions such as warmth, air, moist nutriment, etc., and these conditions never cease to be necessary for the continued manifestation of life. Whether life or vital force is passive or active, depends upon the conditions under which it exists and its essential manifestations are modified by differences in these conditions.

The ova of animals and plants remain in the state of "germ" only so long as they are maintained perfectly quiescent and beyond the influence of the external factors essential to their development. They remain capable of development, and retain the creative force of the germ, but this force is latent or dormant. It passes from passivity to activity only under certain essential conditions. The ova of some animals will, if withdrawn from the influence of the atmosphere and warmth, retain their capability of development for a long period. Thus the productive power of the ova of many insects are preserved through the Winter. The same is true of the germinating power of seeds. Under favorable conditions this power is preserved in the seeds of many plants for many years. As, soon, however, as these are subjected to the external influences necessary to call this power into activity, the germ, if still capable of development, becomes developed; if not still capable of development, they putrefy.

It should here be observed that however favorable to life the conditions are, if the vital principle is lacking in either seed or ovum, no life will be manifest. The infertile egg, for instance, when supplied with warmth, instead of developing into a chicken or a duck or some other bird or reptile, depending on the kind of egg it is, putrefies and succeeds in producing nothing more than gases with a foul odor. The vital principle is the essentially causative factor, the external conditions being only necessary conditions to its activity. These latter call forth but do not produce the action. The cause which produces growth is always inherent in the living organism, true growth being a process found only in the organic domain. External factors—environment—may hasten or retard or even divert the process. Warmth, light, air, food and moisture are conditions that render growth possible and are undoubtedly necessary factors in the process, but, these are not the causes which produce it. However favorable to and well adapted for growth an environment may be, an organism will not grow or develop unless it contains within itself the power to do so. The organism which contains the power of growth within itself will readily grow, within certain limits, even in an unfavorable environment, so long as it retains its inherent vital force, although it may become abnormal. The vital principle is the true cause, environment but the condition. It is essential that causes and occasions be kept apart, for, by the loose manner in which occasions are converted into causes today many false teachings are made to appear true.

The already developed organism, when the conditions for its further growth and maintenance fail, either falls into a state of apparent death, as in hibernation or suspended animation, or else it actually dies. In the passive states of hibernation and suspended animation, when all the life processes appear not to exist, it is not possible always to apply successfully the criteria of life. This quiescent state found in both plants and animals, both in the seed or ova and in fully developed plants and animals, requires no external stimuli for its maintenance and may be considered as a state in which the living organism becomes capable of withstanding conditions unfavorable to activity. Some animals have been observed to lie in this dormant state for periods up to fourteen years, during which time there was nothing to distinguish the living organism from one recently killed. However, when these were introduced into favorable conditions, they became active. Certain conditions such as cold, dryness, darkness, absence of food, etc., tend to induce this passive state, while warmth, light, moisture, food, etc., form the necessary stimuli in restoring and maintaining active life.

Stimuli may be regarded as the external factors which call into activity the life principle and the living organism and, without which, the life principle which has produced the organization necessary to life, is incapable of manifestation. All forces are dormant or active as the case may be depending on the conditions under which they exist. The general essentials of life, the vital or renovating stimuli, are common to plants and animals, and, unless in excess, are salutary in their influence.

There is, however, an evident difference in the degree to which living beings are dependent upon different vital stimuli. For instance, new warm-blooded animals have most need of external warmth and cannot live without it, while cold-blooded animals are capable of existence in much less heat. Many animals, such as mollusca, and insects, serpents, tortorses, scorpions, etc., have been kept for months without food. Fungus requires little or no light. Many animals require but little water. The duration of excitability without external stimuli is generally in inverse proportion to the complexity of the organization. The simplest animals can live longest without these stimuli. The greater the complexity of the organization the greater the dependence of the organs on each other and of the whole organization upon the individual organ. The more simply organized animals, therefore, live longer after injuries than the higher animals do. Revival from a state of apparent death, as in drowning or asphyxiation, is much easier in the lower orders.

To every species of plant and animal life there is a congenial and favorable temperature, although great variations exist in this respect, as well as in the power of adaptation to extreme conditions. As an example, many plants perish with a slight frost while many more endure year after year the extremely cold Winters of the far North, and the little fungus which we call the yeast plant, does not lose its vitality at 76° below zero, although it requires a higher temperature for its active growth. Many experiments have shown that a moderate increase in temperature quickens the movements of living matter while a corresponding depression retards them. However, the action of these stimuli vary. The activities of the ameba are arrested in iced water and recommence only after the temperature has been raised. The segmentation of trout eggs proceeds nicely in iced water, but they soon die in a warm room. Animals have been frozen and revived, and there are instances on record of men enduring for some time with little inconvenience, the heat of ovens raised to 500° F. If the change of intensity of the stimuli be made graudally, and not suddenly, the living organism can sometimes adapt itself to it without serious disturbance. To a certain extent, indeed, the cell may exist unaffected by the influence of its environment, by virtue of its own inherent properties, but the range of independence is very limited. If the external conditions deviate from the normal by more than a certain small amount disturbances of cell-functions at once manifest.

Electrical, mechanical and chemical stimulation have similar effects to heat but are not necessary to life and are injurious and destructive in their nature. A great error has been committed in classifying the necessary and vivifying stimuli with other unnecessary or accidental stimuli. These latter do not really contribute to the normal composition of organic bodies, nor to the necessary conditions of normal function, and do not renovate their powers. A mechanical stimulus—for example, pressure—which modifies the condition of a membrane endowed with sensibility, excites, it is true, vital phenomena—sensation and, perhaps, motion—but does not vivify or invigorate the organic forces; while on the contrary, the essential vital stimuli really contribute to the formation of organic matter and form essential factor elements of its normal functions. Nutriment, for instance, is not merely a stimulus of living matter, but is capable of being transformed into living matter and thereby vivifying it. Nutriment is the material with which growth, repair, reproduction and the manufacture of functional products are accomplished and, in the absence of all nutriment, these processes and functions cannot be carried on. Man in a healthy state is absolutely dependent upon food and cannot continue to exist for long without it. Water and air both serve similar purposes to food and are indispensible to life. Life, in the higher animals, cannot continue many days in the absence of water. The complete absence of the oxygen of the air produces death in but a few minutes. Heat, which is not a substance, is especially important to life. Among the warm-blooded animals, if the animal is unable to generate its own heat in sufficient quantity as is often the case with the young, or in disease, external heat is essential. Both plant and animal require heat to varying extent if their life processes are to continue. Even among cold-blooded animals, if the temperature falls below certain points the organic processes are suspended until there is a rise in temperature. Under the influence and by the use of the vital stimuli—heat, light, air, water, food—the organic being is developed from the germ and by these same forces and agencies it carries on its processes and functions, repairs and maintains its parts, thus, the phenomena of life are equally as dependent upon the vital stimuli as upon the vital principle itself.

It should not be inferred from the above that the vital stimuli are always salutary in their effects and are never harmful under any circumstances or in any amounts. Such an inference would be far from true. Heat in excess of the organism's power of adaptation is decidedly injurious. Light in excess of the body's needs or in excess of its powers of adaptation is also injurious. These things act as stimulants and in excess they over-stimulate. Over-stimulation wastes the body's substances and powers beyond its powers of recuperation. The same can be said of food, water and oxygen. The amount of any of these stimuli required by the body at any time depends upon various conditions. Its requirements vary from day to day, from hour to hour or even from minute to minute. There are conditions, as will be shown in another chapter, in which it is dangerous and injurious to feed the body. Forcing vital activity, beyond the recuperative abilities of the organism is a ruinous process, even when done with normal stimuli.

Making an effort to define the vital and non-vital stimuli we would say: Vital (compensated) stimuli are those substances, agents and influences which are essential to the normal existence, development, maintenance and active life of organisms and which contribute either directly or indirectly to the formation of the organic structure and to the processes and end-results of what we call organic functions. These stimuli consist of such things as air, food, water, warmth, light, exercise, rest and sleep.

Non-vital (uncompensated) stimuli are such substances, agents and influences that will arouse or excite action in the living organism but which are not essential to the normal existence, development, maintenance and active life of such an organism and do not contribute either directly or indirectly to the formation of organic structure nor to the processes and end-results of organic function. These consist of pressure, electricity, vibration, concussion, all drugs or poisons, etc.

In an effort to define stimulation, by which is meant *uncompensated stimulation,* Herward Carrington says: *Vitality, Fasting and Nutrition,* (1908), p. 38:—

"We know that it is an induced condition in which the organism can, temporarily, perform a greater amount of muscular, vital or mental work than would normally be performed in the same period of time and the increase in its ability to work is undoubtedly traceable to the 'stimulus' it has received."

This definition is only partially correct. There can be no doubt that the stimulus occasions the rapid expenditure of power but it does not necessarily increase the functional output, or if it does, the output is deteriorated—that is, of poor quality A skilled mechanic may turn out a given amount of work a day of the highest order, but if he is forced to turn out more work the quality of his work will suffer and, if he is hurried too much, he becomes excited and confused so that he turns out less work than normally and of an even poorer quality. If we attempt to hurry a book-keeper he makes mistakes and his work is valueless. That this analogy is applicable to the practice of stimulating the organs of the body will be made apparent as we proceed. One example will suffice at this point. Alcohol is claimed to stimulate the flow of digestive juices. Dr. Trall accurately described what it does do when he wrote, *Alcoholic Controversy,* p. 68:—

"When alcohol or other poison is taken into the system, we have instead of the digestive juices, an outpouring of a watery viscid fluid (serum and mucous) from the whole mucous membrane, contemplating the expulsion of the enemy from the system."

Carrington writes, *Vitality, Fasting and Nutrition,* p. 38-39:—

"There is a greater capacity for work (implying a greater nervous force being expended in such action), and it is generally known that there is invariably a 'reaction' or prostration, more or less profound and noticeable, following upon such stimulation. But beyond this, how much is known of the *rationale* of stimulation? Is it known how this extra force is imparted or given to the system? What is the real nature of such action? And why does the reaction invariably follow? In what manner is the (apparently) added force related to its source—its stimulus? In short, why do stimulants stimulate at all?"

A completely satisfactory explanation of this increased action cannot be given until we understand the true relations of living and dead matter. It is essential that we know that the action of stimulation is vital action and the power of this action is vital power. A stimulant is an agent or influence that occasions the expenditure of power, and not an agent that supplies the power. But in this very act the power expended is lost so that the condition of the individual after the stimulant ceases to occasion this loss of power is one of weakness.

Alcohol is a stimulant. I am well aware that it is now regarded as a depressant and so it is. But, so are all stimulants. Alcohol is a protoplasmic poison. It cooks (coagulates) the protoplasm of the cells just as it will coagulate the white of an egg. In small quantities it acts as an *irritant. Irritation* and *stimulation* (by means of non-vital stimuli) are the same. Being extremely volatile, alcohol readily reaches all the tissues so that the irritation it causes is general throughout the system.

At this place it may be well to attempt to formulate the *Law of Stimulation,* before proceeding to a few remarks about irritation:—

THE LAW OF STIMULATION: *Whenever any toxic or irritating agent* or influence is brought to bear upon the living organism this occasions vital resistance and excitation manifest by increased and impaired action, which, always necessarily diminishes the power of action and does so in precisely the degree to which it accelerates action; the increased action is caused by the extra expenditure of vital power called out, not supplied, by the compulsory process, and therefore the available supply of power is diminished by this amount.

In those cases where stimulants *appear* to do the most good they *actually* do the most harm. The harm they actually do is proportioned to the amount of energy they expend and the good they *appear* to do is also proportioned to the amount of energy they expend.

All excitants operate on this principle. They *seem* to do much good. They *actually* do much harm. Their *real* and *lasting* effects are the equal but opposite of their *apparent* and *temporary* effects. The *exhiliration* which they occasion is followed by a depression due to the waste of power that causes the *exhiliration*. Excitants, stimulants, tonics, all act on the principle of *irritation* or *excitement*. The part or parts acted upon rally to their own defense. Reserve forces are thrown into the field to resist the excitant. Habitual stimulant users are always in danger of terminating their lives by pushing this process too far, and drawing, unwarned, the vital current below the point of recovery.

Stimulating or "toning up" the body, by the drugs of the physician is, from first to last, of a piece with those means that are responsible for the break down of the system and that produces the disturbance. Drugs or "medicines" act on the system on the same general principle and produce the same general and particular effects as do tea, coffee, cocoa, pepper, spices, mustard, horse-radish, tobacco, alcohol, opium, etc.

The constitutional tendency of the living organism is from first to last, upwards; the tendency of stimulation downward. The more sound and vigorous is the organism, the more it can sustain the downward pressure of stimulants while the less sound and vigorous is the body the less able it is to withstand the influence of these. These break in upon the wonderful harmony of the very complicated vital operations, whose only tendency is towards the standard of perfect health, and disconcert life's healthy movements.

But they do more than just occasion an increase in activity. They do further mischief by inflicting a positive injury upon the tissues and organs upon which they act. They wound these parts and time is required to heal the wound. Indeed it is by this goading, pricking, wounding process which irritants inflict upon the cells and tissues of an organ that the organ is excited to increased action or defense. Stimulants and tonics keep the vital machinery constantly goaded up to the height of its power.

The first observable phenomenon in the initial stages of irritation is an exaltation of function in the part affected. Moderate excitement merely exalts the natural sensibilities. If the sense organs are affected sight, hearing, touch, taste and smell may become acute. The uncompensated stimulants are all irritants. They are stimulating in direct ratio to their irritating qualities and are irritating in proportion to their unfitness to serve any need of the body or in proportion to their virulence as a poison. THE STIMULATION THEY AFFORD IS THE EXCITEMENT OF IRRITATION AND NOT THE INVIGORATION AND REVITALIZATION OF NUTRITION. Following the great law of dual effect, all irritation produces its secondary effects. After a time a state of depression occurs, in which function is less vigorous than before the stimulus (irritant) was applied, or function may be temporarily suspended. The overworked and fatigued organ requires a period of rest and repose, in which to restore its substance and recuperate its energies, before it can return to its ordinary duties. During this period of weakness, inaction and prostration the organism is recovering. During the former period of strength, increased action and exaltation of function the organism was being exhausted.

Dr. Robert Walter fully developed a very important principle in his two works, which he stated about as follows: *Under all circumstances, vitality or energy of any character whatever is invariably manifested or noticed by us, as energy, in its expenditure, never in its accumulation.* "What seems to give one strength," he said,

337

"is always making him weak, because the strength exhibited is the patient's power being expended." Jim Corbett sleeping, he frequently said, is no more conscious of his power than a sleeping baby. We see the power of a stick of dynamite only in its expenditure. Man may possess a great amount of potential energy but we do not perceive it until it is being expended. Just as with a storage battery, we do not see the energy. We cannot see the energy accumulating. We can only observe the active expenditure of the energy in doing work.

The energy of stimulation is the energy of the body. The stimulus does not add any power to the body; it only occasions a more rapid expenditure of the power already possessed by the body. In doing so, it exhausts power. Hence, the inevitable after-period of depression. Whether we consider alcohol as a stimulant or a depressant, the following words of Trall, are true in so far as they relate to stimulation and are applicable to all stimulants:—

"***We see how it is that alcohol is an element of force.*** It occasions force to be wasted, that is all. ***If a small draught is taken, only a little force is wasted (not supplied) in defending the system from it, and the individual is but slightly excited; that is, a little feverish. If much is taken, a greater amount of force is necessarily wasted (not supplied), and greater excitement is manifest in stimulation, fever, delirium, madness, etc."—*Alcoholic Controversy*, p. 63.

"The system expends its force to get rid of the alcohol, but never derives any force, great or small, good, bad, or indifferent, from the alcohol."—*Alcoholic Controversy*, p. 64.

"Stimulation does not impart strength; it wastes it. Vital power does not go out of brandy into the patient, but occasions vital power to be exhausted from the patient in expelling the brandy."—*True Temperance Platform*, p. 35.

Whether the stimulation is that of the hot or cold bath, the percussion douche, electricity, massage, vibration or drugs or other *stimulants* and *tonics*, the power which is expended goes out of the patient and not out of these things. The so-called stimulation is excitement, the excitement of irritation and consequent vital resistance. The body resists cold and heat or coffee and strychnine. It does not resist food or air.

Graham truly wrote:—

"All stimulants, I have said, increase the vital action of parts with which they come in contact, and when they are powerful and the quantity considerable, and the organ or part on which they act an important one, such as the stomach, their local effect is sympathetically felt by the whole organic domain, and the whole system is thrown into an increased action by sympathetic excitement or irritation. Substances that act in this manner are called local stimulants. Others are rapidly taken up by the absorbents and diffused throughout the body, exciting every part to increased action by their immediate presence. These are called diffusable stimulants. But while the stimulation produced by these different substances, when the system is accustomed to them, is identified in the mental consciousness with that which is produced by the natural and appropriate stimuli, giving a sense of satisfaction and increased vigor and enjoyment yet the physiological action which they cause is of a very different character. The natural and appropriate stimuli of the system always excites the parts on which they act to the performance of their function, and the stimulation which they produce increases the functional energy of the organ. But the action caused by those foreign substances which are used purely for their stimulating effect, is the action of vital resistance, or what is called vital reaction—a rallying of the vital forces to resist and repel and expel the offending and disturbing cause. This stimulation, therefore, while it lasts, though it increases the feeling of strength, and to some extent the muscular power of voluntary action, yet it never in any case increases the functional energy of any of the organs concerned in assimilation and nutrition, but, on the contrary, always diminishes the functional powers of these organs, and retards their functions and deteriorates their functional results."—*Science of Human Life*, p. 807.

It is quite obvious from what has gone before that this process of stimulation is an exhausting process and that the weaker the organism, or any part of it is, the more reason there is for withholding stimulants. We seem stronger in proportion to our outlay of force, but we are actually growing weaker thereby and the weaker we grow the less force can we afford to expend. We appear wealthy, not by the money that we have in the bank, but by the wealth we display. But the more wealth we display the smaller our bank fund grows and the smaller this grows the less can we afford to display our wealth. The weaker the body is the greater is the necessity for conserving its forces. Carrington rightly observes, *Vitality, Fasting and Nutrition,* p. 42-3.

"The law of action and reaction is one of the most misunderstood laws in the Universe. The weaker the person is, generally speaking, the more he feels he must do for himself; in order to gain strength; what, he does not know exactly, only he must do something—actively! But this activity most obviously means energy expended, and consequent loss by reaction. We cannot force recovery; that truth cannot be too emphatically insisted upon.

"The very fact that he is weak indicates most plainly, in reality, that he must do nothing, and the importance of his doing nothing is exactly proportionate to the extent of his weakness. The delusion that 'something must be done,' in cases of sickness, is the cause of hundreds of thousands of premature deaths. The fear of being obliged to wait passively; the lack of faith in the healing powers of nature, is one of the greatest causes of medical mal-practice of today. We must bear in mind always, that no action can possibly occur without an equal and opposite reaction; that the pendulum of human energy cannot, by any possibility, swing in one direction indefinitely; but must, at some time, turn and swing in the other. Rest must always follow effort, and effort rest; and this law of rythm applies, of course, to the human body, so is it not most obvious that the digestive organs need their periods of rest—just as all our other organs call for rest? And is it not obvious, also, that the only way in which such a rest can be furnished is by fasting? The common sense aspect of this argument should, I think, appeal to every one of my readers."

Upon this same point Graham, after discussing the effects of irritating or stimulating alimentary substances upon the organs of the body, says:—

"And if by any means the organs have been reduced to a state in which they seem to require something more than the natural stimulus of the food, to excite them to the performance of their functions, then are they really so much the less able to bear the action of the pure stimulants, and so much the less qualified to perform their functions with integrity; and the consequence is not only exhaustion, but irritation and debility, and the development of disease."—*Science of Human Life,* p. 298.

The weaker the patient the greater is the need to do nothing, and yet it is precisely at such times that Heteropaths, all cults, seek to do the most. Dr. Jennings tells of a Dr. Shelton who found in Cholera cases that those which responded to calomel recovered while those which did not respond invariably died. He foolishly attributed their recovery to the calomel. Jennings rightly interpreted this experience to mean that those without sufficient vitality to react against calomel did not have enough power to recover, while those who had sufficient power left to reject the calomel had sufficient vitality to recover. But who can say that some of the other cases would not have recovered had no calomel been given them. For, as Jennings said, the calomel "merely acted as a test, showing where there was power to come up, and where there was not; while its whole force was expended in direct hostility to the vital economy, and affected no real good."—*Philosophy of Human Life,* p. 118.

When there is a "pinching scantiness of motive power" and nature is trying by every possible means to conserve energies it is criminal folly to stimulate those energies away. It is in extreme cases of exhaustion and depression, and these are brought on by overstimulation, that the true nature of stimulants is seen. There is no longer any power to respond in the body and the stimulant fails to elicit action. Could better proof be offered that the power of response is in the body, not in the stimulant? Dr. Jennings says, *Tree of Life,* p. 171:—

"Oh if the veil of obscurity that hangs over the whole subject of simulation could be drawn aside for a short period, until the world could get a fair view of the tremendous evils connected with it, it would stand aghast at the appalling spectacle! In virtue of the perpetual and universal sapping of the mainsprings of life, caused by the uncompensated exhaustion of the nervous energies by the action of stimulants, humanity is reduced to, and kept in, a condition in which its three mortal enemies, 'the world, the flesh, and the devil,' find it very easy to subject it to their sway.

"Stimulants might be used to some advantage or satisfaction as tests of vitality in some dubious cases of disease, if the operation did not involve an irretrievable loss, to a proportional extent, of the vitality of essential organs on which the experiment is made, just at the time when it is hazardous to have it diminished."

Stimulants, he declared, increase action, but diminish the power of action. They can arouse action "when there is ralliable power to be called forth" and "in the same proportion, they diminish the power of life" of the organs whose activity they increase. They "*always* leave less of power in any part on which they expend their action, than there was in that part before they acted upon it." "If you stimulate largely, you exhaust largely. If you have a moderate stream of excitation, you have a corresponding steady stream of exhaustion."—*Tree of Life.*

"The action upon the human system of poisonous substances—and all irritants or stimulants that furnish no building material towards its construction or repair, are included in that category—is uniformly and unavoidably deleterious under all ordinary circumstances, in health and in sickness, and more injurious in a diseased or impaired state of the system than in its healthy condition, and in proportion to the feebleness or vitality of the part or parts on which the action of the noxious or poisonous substances is expended."—*Philosophy of Human Life,* p. 239.

Graham rightly wrote:—

"The stimulation produced by these various substances is always necessarily exhausting to the vital properties of the tissues on which they act, just in proportion to its degree and duration; and every stimulus impairs the vital susceptibilities and powers, just in proportion as it is unfitted for the real wants of the vital economy, and unfriendly to the vital interests.

"But whatever may be the real character of the stimulus, every stimulation to which the system is accustomed increases, according to the power and extent of its influence, what is called the tone and the action of the parts on which it is exerted, and while the stimulation lasts, it always increases the feeling of strength and vigor in the system, whether any nourishment be imparted to the system or not.

"Yet by so much as the stimulation exceeds in degree that which is necessary for the full and healthy performance of the function or functions of the organs stimulated, by so much the more does the expenditure of vital power and waste of organized substance exceed for the time the replenishing and renovating economy of the system; and, consequently, the exhaustion and indirect debility which succeed the stimulation are always necessarily commensurate with the excess.***"

"The pure stimulants, therefore, which of themselves afford no nourishment to the system, and only serve to increase the expenditure of vital properties and waste of organized substances by increasing vital action, cause, while their stimulation lasts, a sense of increased strength and vigor; and thus we are led by our feeling to believe that the pure stimulants are really strengthening and in the same manner we are deceived by even those pernicious stimulants which not only exhaust by stimulation, but irritate, debilitate, and impair, by their deleterious qualities.

"The feeling of strength produced by stimulation, therefore, is no proof either that the stimulating substance is nourishing, or that it is salutary, nor even that it is not decidedly baneful."—*Science of Human Life,* p. 353-54.

Any stimulant, (physical, chemical, mechanical, electrical, thermal, or mental), applied to a nerve first increases and later decreases the number of nerve impulses going over that nerve. There is no function without stimuli. Normal stimuli produce normal function. Excess of these reduce function through over-stimulation. If sufficiently long continued, over-stimulation results in exhaustion and suspension or abolition of function. The non-vital stimuli act as irritants and always over-stimulate. Drugless and semi-drugless practitioners are agreed that drug stimulants are ruinous but will not admit that their own methods of stimulation are injurious unless "abused." Abuse! The thing itself is the abuse! The drugless methods are all employed to secure the same results that drugs are used to secure. They are followed by the same depressing reaction and all of them without exception leave the patient weaker.

How often have I seen patients worn out and left completely exhausted by a few minutes of mental treatment! Does not every drugless practitioner know that if he is to continue to secure the same amount of stimulation with electricity, for instance, he must continue to increase the size of the dose, just as the physician has to do with his drugs or the tea drinker must do with her tea? Only the vital or compensated stimuli may be safely used and these only within the immediate needs of the organism.

The Chiropractic thrust, consisting of a quick, forceful thrust of the hand over a spinal center, is a powerful mechanical stimulus to the center or centers involved and is a very effective means of producing enervation. Patients feel better for a few minutes or hours after receiving their so-called adjustment, but there follows the inevitable reactions. Many patients are so irritated by the thrust that they are unable to sleep during the night following the "adjustment."

At the beginning of its short and now closing career, it was the Chiropractic theory and practice to "adjust" each and every so-called subluxation which the Chiropractor imagined he found along the whole course of the spinal column. This was soon found to be too much treatment for the patient. Patients were left weak from over-stimulation. The Chiropractors then divided these imaginary subluxations into *major* or active, and *minor* or inactive subluxations. Without stopping to give a satisfactory explanation of why and how a subluxation could exist without producing that theoretical impingement of the nerves; or how the impingement could exist without interfering with the transmission of nerve impulse; or how the nerve impulse could be interfered with without producing disease; or how a subluxation could be *active* at one time and then become *inactive*; or why one subluxation is *active* and another not; or how an *inactive* subluxation may become *active*, they advised that only *majors* be adjusted and that the *minors* be ignored.

But this was soon found to be too much. It was found necessary to give patients vacations from treatment at frequent intervals to permit them to rest and recuperate. When the author was a student and was being taught all the fallacies of Chiropractic he was told that: If the symptoms are growing worse and the patient is growing weaker this indicates over adjustment.

Upon this point J. Haskel Kritzer, M.D., says in his late book, *Health and Freedom Through Self-Knowledge,"* p. 32:—

"The constant pounding upon the spinal column cannot be considered a constructive practice. The repeated spinal adjustments are productive of over-stimulation, and this in itself causes exhaustion. The patient, remembering the first exhilarating stimulus produced with the spinal treatment, craves its repetition, short-lived as the effect is A habit is thus created for this form of stimulation upon which the individual becomes dependent as does one addicted to narcotic drugs. Who is there to discourage this latest habit-forming artificial stimulation? Surely not the practitioner who is trained not only to treat, but also to sell his course of treatments at so much per."

Four years before the appearance of this book I talked with Dr. Kritzer, who was one of the leading "Natural Therapists," about Chiropractic but he was certain that it was a wonder worker. It is gratifying to see, in this book, that he has joined the ranks of Orthopathy, having sloughed off not only Chiropractic, but all other drugless methods of therapeutics and his faith in homeopathy, as well.

So much for Chiropractic stimulation. It is but one of a great number of methods of mechanical stimulation, either of the spinal centers or of the nerve endings. Naprapathy, Osteopathy, Mechano-therapy, Massage, Neuropathy, Mechanical Physicultopathy, Spondylotherapy, etc., are all means of mechanical stimulation. Like Chiropractic they are each and all wasteful of the nervous energies. Mechanical Physicultopathy frequently employs thermal stimulation (heat and cold) of the spine along with the mechanical means while Spondylopractic employs heat and cold, electricity, vibration, concussion, etc., as well as all the above named mechanical or manual measures to stimulate the spine. These methods of stimulation are not one bit different in their stimulating effects from any other stimulating method. They produce an exaltation of function as their primary effect and a depression of function as their secondary effect. If the stimulation is repeated often enough the depression becomes permanent. In this particular all stimulants are alike. Playing with stimulants is a losing game. The sweetness of the exicitement is not worth the bitter reaction. Like drug stimulants, all the above means of stimulation require a progressive increase in the size of the "dose" if they are to continue to produce their usual amount of stimulation.

That this is true of all electrical stimulation as of all other stimulation (irritation and excitement) will be seen from the following statements contained in Bulletin No. 8, page 1, published by the E. R. V. Corporation, 439 Fort St., Detroit, Mich.:—

"In taking electric measurements to determine the actual potential of a human being or the relative potential difference of one area of the body with another, or one organ as compared with another organ, we have found that certain specific readings can be obtained on a Galvanometer. Tests made under electrical stimulation—this includes any form of known electro-therapeutics—will reveal at once that this potential can be raised considerably, often as high as sixty per cent, but will go back to its original or normal, in most, cases, within ten minute after such stimulation has been given. In fact, it will more likely go below the original existing normal. These are facts. Other experiments have shown and I have just finished observing these in a local hospital and a Chicago institution, that any form of electro-therapeutic treatment will give tremendous reactions, noticeably in the form of haemoglobin counts, urinalysis, observations of heart beat and respiration, in the early stages of treatment; then will come a period when these reactions will diminish to nothing, and if the patient has been cured in the meantime, well and good. If the patient has not been cured, all the medication, electro-therapeutics or manipulation will be useless, for the simple reason, that the patients' system has been stimulated to the zero point of reaction and there is no more capacity left to respond."

In discussing stimulants for the digestive organs Dr. Oswald says:—

"Now, what such 'tonics' can really do for them is this: they goad the system into the transient and abnormal activity incident to the necessity of expelling a virulent poison. With the accomplishment of that purpose the exertion ceases, the ensuing exhaustion is worse than the first by just as much as the *poison-fever* has robbed the system of a larger or smaller share of its little remaining strength. The stimulant has wasted the organic energy which it seamed to revive. 'But,' says the invalid, 'if a repetition of the dose can relieve the second reaction, would the result not be preferable to the languor of the unstimulated system? Wouldn't it be the best plan to let me support my strength by sticking to my patent tonic?'

"Yes, it would be very convenient, especially in times of scarcity, if a starving horse could be supported by the daily application of a patent spur. It would save both oats and oaths. Even a fastidious nag could not help acknowledging the pungency of the goad. But it so happens that spur-fed horses are somewhat short-lived, though at first the diet certainly seems to act like a charm. For a day or two the drug stimulates the activity of the digestive organs as well as the mental faculties, but the subsequent prostration is so intolerable that the patient soon chooses the alternative of another poison-fever. Before long the pleasant phase of the febrile process becomes shorter and the reaction more severe, the jaded system is less able to respond to the goad, and in order to make up for the difference, the dose of the stimulant has to be steadily increased. The invalid becomes a bondsman to the drug store, and hugs the chain that drags him down to the slavery of a confirmed poison habit."—*Nature's Household Remedies*, p. 58-9.

This fact is worthy of special note and is applicable to all stimulants: (1) The period of stimulation grows progressively less, and (2) The depression of the reaction grows progressively longer and more intolerable. The forces of the system are wasted The power of response gradually wanes.

The victims of the stimulant habit mistake irritation for invigoration. It is this deception that leads the dyspeptic to drive away his blues with the fumes of the weed that has caused his sick-headaches. It is analogous to the pot-house habiture who attempts to drown his cares in the source of all his miseries. The depression following the period of irritation is mistaken for a craving for the drug. There is no such thing as a craving for a drug. The pains of the opium addict are the outcries of damaged nerves as they come out out from under the anesthetic influence of the opium. The use

342

of such substances weakens, impairs and damages the nerves. They are soon rendered unable to react to the drug. Bye-and-bye the jaded system fails to respond to the spur. The poison-slave is forced to employ larger and ever larger doses or else resort to other and stronger stimulants.

"No length of practice," says Oswald, "will ever save the poison-slave from the penalties of his sin against Nature. Each full indulgence is followed by a full measure of woeful retributions, while a half-indulgence results in half-depression on the verge of word-weary despondency, or fails to satisfy the lingering thirst after a larger dose of the same stimulant."

More than once in the World's history, infant dragons have been mistaken for harmless lizards. What appeared at first to be harmless, "mild stimulants" have proven themselves to be terrible monsters. Let the stimulant user attempt to give up his stimulant and he will perceive how strongly it holds him in its grip. The chief danger of a relapse is not the attractiveness of intoxication, but the misery of the after-effects, the depressing reaction that follows upon the abnormal excitement, and for severatl weeks, seems daily to gain strength. The apathy of the unstimulated system can become more intolerable than positive pain, and embitter existence till the victim returns to his poison-habit. The violence of the unnatural "craving" is proportioned to the virulence of each poison, and the degree of the original repugnance. The strongest stimulants take the firmest hold upon us.

Instinct strongly resists the incipience of these destructive poison-habits. Dr. Oswald declared that nature has supplied us with the following three infallible tests to enable us to distinguish between a poison-stimulus and a harmless nutritive substance:

"1. The first taste of every poison is either bitter or repulsive.

"2. The persistent obtrusion of the noxious substance changes that aversion into a specific craving.

"3. The more or less pleasurable excitement produced by a gratification of that craving is always followed by a depressing reaction."

Poisons are either repulsive or insipid. Arsenic, sugar-of-lead, and antimony belong to the latter class. Vegetable poisons are either nauseous or intensely bitter. Hasheesh is more unattractive than turpentine. Opium is an acrid caustic. Absenthe (worm-wood-extract) is as bitter as gall. Morphine is so bitter that a trace of its powder can be tasted in the air. It is, all in all, about the most offensive drug derived from the vegetable kingdom. Yet its grip on an addict is almost inescapable. "Alcohol is almost as repulsive as sulphuric acid or permanganate of potassia, and to break its chains requires the effort of a giant." It burns and bites as it goes down the throat of the beginner. Tea, coffee, and cocoa are bitter and repulsive. Cocoa, in particular is very bitter if not combined with sugar. Beer is almost as bad. Tobacco is repugnant. It sickens the young man or woman who uses it for the first time almost immediately. Nausea, vomiting, gripping, dizziness, tremor, fainting, muscular weakness, etc., are quickly produced by nicotine. These poisons all scratch and bite when we first attempt to hug them, but their strangling embrace is difficult to break. There is no such thing as a harmless stimulant. "The incipience of every unnatural appetite is the first step of a progressive disease."

The way to the rum-shop is paved with mild stimulants. Every bottle of medical bitters is apt to get the vendor a permanent customer. Cider and mild ale lead to stronger ale, to larger beer and finally to brandy. The tendency of every stimulant habit is toward a stronger "tonic." Every poison habit is progressive. Dr. Oswald says: "Sooner or later the tonic is sure to pall, while the morbid craving remains, and forces its victims either to increase the quantity of the wonted stimulant, or else resort to a stronger poison. A boy begins with ginger beer, and ends with ginger rum; the medical 'tonic' delusion progresses from male extract to Mumford's Elixir, the coffee-cup leads to the pipe and the pipe to the pot-house. Wherever the nicotine habit has been introduced, the alcohol habit soon follows. The Spanish Moors abstained from all poisons, and for seven centuries remained the teachers of Europe in war as well as science and the arts of peace—free-men in the fullest sense of the world; men whom a powerful foe could at last expel and exterminate, but never subdue.

"The Turks having learned to smoke tobacco, soon learned to eat opium, and have since been taught to eat dust at the feet of the Muscovite. When the Spaniards came to South America they found in the Patagonian highlands a tribe of warlike natives who were entirely ignorant of any stimulating substance, and who have ever since defied the sutlers and soldiers of their neighbors, while the tobacco-fuddled red-skins of the North succumbed to fire-water."—*Vaccination a Crime.*

Dr. Oswald further says: "Claude Bernard, the famous French physiologist, noticed that the opium-vice recruits its female victims chiefly from the ranks of the veteran coffee-drinkers; in Savoy and the adjoining Swiss cantons; *Kirsch-wasser* prepares the way for arsenic; in London and St. Petersburgh many ether drinkers have relinquished high-wines for a more concentrated poison, and in the seaport towns of northern Egypt Persian opium-shops have eclipsed the popularity of the Arabian coffee-houses."—*Vaccination a Crime.*

The farther away from nature we stray the longer and harder is the road back. "Resist the beginnings, crush danger in the bud," is an ancient rule of wisdom which we all do well to observe.

The deceptive power of all stimulants is the same. They appear to give us strength. In reality they take away the strength we have. They appear to increase our capacity to perform work. They really diminish this power. They deteriorate the functional results of the organs they affect. Eggs may be stimulated so that they hatch earlier than normal but the birds or reptiles thus hatched are short lived and the earlier they are forced to be hatched the shorter lived they are. Both the young of plants and animals may be stimulated so that they grow faster or larger than normal, but those so stimulated are short lived and more subject to disease than plants and animals of normal growth. Condiments excite the stomach, but they impair digestion. Sweat cabinets increase sweating but decrease elimination. Salt will cause cows to drink more water and thus give more milk but the milk will be of poor quality. Drinking much water increases urination but decreases elimination. Purgatives and laxatives excite bowel action but build chronic constipation. Heart stimulants impair the heart. When the heart needs rest it is folly to spur it up with stimulants. When one is sick stimulants may hasten the exhaustion of the fund of life as rapidly as the body will respond and delay or prevent recovery, but they cannot add an iota of power to the body nor hasten, by one short second of time, the ultimate recovery. Here I am reminded of Trall's remarks anent the death of Prince Albert:—

"The story comes to us in the English newspapers, that Prince Albert was 'kept up on stimulants' for five or six days. No one suspected any danger. Physicians did not regard the complaint as anything serious. But, all at once, the patient became prostrated. The typhoid set in. His system refused to 'respond' to any further stimulation. Why did his system refuse to respond? Because his vitality had all been stimulated away. His system needed quiet, repose; but he was kept in a feverish commotion, in an inflammatory excitement, in a constant commotion with alcoholic poison—I mean, 'respiratory food'."—*True Healing Art.*

At this point I desire to introduce Trall's explanation of the *tonic or stimulating* effects of drugs as given on pages 16, 17 and 18; vol. 2, of the *Hydropathic Encyclopedia*:—

"There is a class of medicines known as *tonics*, or strengthening medicines. Books on materia medica define them to be such articles as give tone, or tonic contractility to the moving fibres, and at the same time augment the activity of the digestive function. Now among the tonics we find a most incongruous set of materials, as quinine, arsenic, boneset, iron, wormwood, oak bark, quassia, aloes, rhubarb, copper, zinc, etc. All authors agree that if the use of a tonic is long continued, the effect is debility. Here is a paradox. A tonic medicine first *strengthens*, and then *debilitates*. *How* are these results to be accounted for?

"When a drug-medicine of any kind, or a poison of any kind, is taken into the stomach, the organic instincts recognize the presence of a something which is neither food nor drink; something unnatural; something which has no constitutional relation to any want or duty of any part or organ, hence an intruder, an enemy. The vital powers *feel* an attack upon the citadel of life, and prepare to act defensively. The lining membrane of the stomach is aroused to increased action; an unusual quantity of mucous and serum is secreted to protect the coats of the stomach from the poisonous or medicinal agent; but the stomach does not *suffer* alone; the alarm is communicated to other organs, to all parts of the system; and this manifestation of increased vital action, this disturbance of the organism, this commotion of the body, is regarded by the doctors as a tonic effect! How words deceive!

"If but a few of these 'tonic' impressions are made on the stomach, if only a few doses are taken, the vital powers, after enduring the siege, and defending themselves as well as may be, subside into their accustomed quiet, and the exhaustion, being not very great, is not especially noticed. But if these tonic impressions are kept up a long time, if the medicines be long continued, the vital expenditure is so great that the doctors call the evidence of its loss *debility*; and well they may. The organic instincts are finally wearied out, they become torpid, and refuse longer to respond to the impression; the lash ceases to be troublesome. Now it is that the doctor, who wishes to still keep up a tonic impression, who desires to *strengthen the system* yet a little more, brings a new recruit into the field. He administers another tonic, no matter what, if it be a *different* one. It works like a charm! The vital powers, though jaded and half palsied, are not yet dead. A new enemy will startle them again; an unaccustomed impression will again arouse them to resistance. If the first tonic was wormwood, the second may be arsenic, or *vice versa*. After the second tonic has spent its force, or, rather, after the vital powers cease to resist, a third one may be brought to bear; and so on, as long as the patience of the patient or perseverance of the practitioner can endure. Thus do tonics continually strengthen the patient, and leave him weaker in the end.

"A decisive evidence of the correctness of this explanation is found in the fact, that every drug under heaven can be made to operate as a tonic. Mercury, lead, antimony, cod-liver oil, ipecac, gamboge, aqua fortis, or powdered glass—as incongruous a medley as can be conceived—will produce tonic effects, provided the dose is such as not to occasion any decisive evacuant or corrosive operation, by which the article is suddenly evacuated, or the structure altered. Cod-liver oil and ipecac have both had their day of reputation for improving digestion, or fattening the body. Why? Because when taken into the stomach, that organ being the point of attack, the vital powers are disproportionately directed to that organ in defense; and if the doses are frequently repeated, a determination of nervous or vital energy is established toward the digestive function. The digestive organs may thus be temporarily invigorated at the expense of all the rest of the body—a dear-bought method of promoting digestion and fattening the body in the end.

"But why do some poisons or medicines produce vomiting, others sweating, others purging, etc? Simply because they are, by means of those violent or increased efforts of the excrement functions, got rid of. *It is a law of the animal economy, that all injurious agents which gain admission, no matter how, within the domain of vitality, are counteracted, neutralized, or expelled in such manner as will produce the least injury or disturbance to the organism.* (Italics author's). If a very large dose of ipecac, for example, is swallowed, so large as to prove immediately dangerous to life, or seriously destructive to the structural or functional integrity of the stomach, its action is met with such violence of resistance as to produce severe spasmodic contractions of the muscular fibres of the stomach and the abdominal muscles, by which the ordinary peristaltic motion of the alimentary canal is reversed, and vomiting results. If the dose be smaller, a profuse watery secretion is poured out upon it from the mucous and lining membranes of the stomach and bowels to dilute it, and render its presence less harmful, while it is conducted along the alimentary canal by the ordinary peristaltic motion, and expelled from the bowels, and thus we have a cathartic effect. If the dose be still smaller, it is largely diluted with serum, taken up by the absorbents, carried into the mass of blood, and finally thrown off by the skin, this being the manner in which a small quantity can be most easily got rid of, and thus we have a diaphoretic operation. If the dose be even yet smaller, so that no special effort of the organism is made to throw it off at either emunctory, the vital powers meet, decompose, and destroy it in the stomach, for which purpose there is an increased determination of blood and of nervous influence directed to the part, and hence we have its tonic ~~effect. Thus~~

may a single article of the materia medica produce, according to the quantity administered, the various and seemingly opposite operative effects of *vomiting, purging, sweating,* and *strengthening;* while each effect is attended with an absolute waste of vitaly power.

"It is well known, too, that all drugs lose a degree of their potency by repetition; in other words, the vital resistance is gradually overcome or worn out, so that, to produce the same operative effect, the dose must be constantly augmented. Those who find a sufficient stimulus in one glass of brandy per day, frequently find ten required in a few years to produce an equal excitement; those who commence on one cigar daily, generally end with several; and those who commence on one patent pill sufficient to move the bowels, not unfrequently find twenty or thirty an inefficient dose after the vital resistance has been pretty thoroughly subdued.

"When medical books, therefore, tell us that drugs lose their *remedial* effects by long continuance, we are to understand that *vital resistance* is subdued; for so long as the organic instincts act *against* the remedy, so long will the phenomena of resistance occur, which medical reasoners, starting from mistaken premises, call medicinal. It may be remedial, and is, in a certain sense—rendering evil for evil."

"Would you, then, never stimulate?" someone asks. If the principles here laid down are correct, and who will dispute them, there is never a time when stimulation is not hurtful. In the human constitution the sum of unrepaired injuries by stimulation, though small and insignificant in their separate capacity, in a number of years amounts to serious injuries, greatly crippling the vital operations, thus keeping them constantly depressed to a level far below what should be the normal so that they are easily thrown into derangement by fatigue, an unusual meal, exposure, etc. After repeated stimulation has brought the functions of the body to this low state it is worse than folly to attempt to *sustain* or restore these functions on more stimulation— irritation. "The vital forces have no element of laziness in their composition" declared Jennings, "and, of course, do not need even 'a little jogging' to remind them of their duty. ****there can be no hazard in extreme cases, in leaving the disposition of natural force to natural law, for whatever may be the extremity, all that can be done to save life, within the ability of organic power, will be done to the last particle of vitality."—*Philosophy of Human Life,* p. 94-5.

Health is not to be restored or life preserved by measures that impair health and destroy life. How much longer must the Heteropathic professions continue their vast experiment before they find this out?

'Eight hours of sleep," says Dr. Felix Oswald, "are sufficient to restore the energy expended in an ordinary day's work. Extraordinary efforts, emotional exicitement, sensual excesses, or malnutrition (either by insufficient food or dyspeptic habits), induce a general lassitude—a warning that the organism is being overtaxed. Repose and a healthier or more liberal diet will soon restore the functional vigor of the system. But during such periods of their diminished activity the vital powers can be rallied by drastic drugs or tonic beverages—in other words, by poisons. The prostrate vitality rises against a deadly foe, as a weary sleeper would start at the touch of a serpent; and, as danger will momentarily overcome the feeling of fatigue, the organism labors with restless energy till the poison is expelled. This feverish reaction dram-drinkers (patent dram-drinkers especially) mistake for a sign of returning vigor, persistently ignoring the circumstance that the excitement is every time followed by a prostration worse than that preceding it. Feeling the approach of a relapse the stimulator then resorts to his old remedy, thus inducing another sham revival, followed by an increased prostration, and so on; but before long the dose of the stimulant, too, has to be increased, the stimulator becomes a slave to his poison, and passes his life in a round of morbid excitements and morbid exhaustions—the former at last nothing but a feeble flickering-up of the vital flame, the latter soon aggravated by sick-headaches, 'vapors', and hypochondria."—*Physical Education,* p. 247.

The same is true of eating. Those foods and drinks that are most stimulating (exciting), such as tea, coffee, cocoa, chocolate, spices, meat, etc., invariably weaken as a secondary effect. The weakness produced by these corresponds with the strength they appear to give.

It is by such processes that physicians seek to *sustain* the sick. Processes that exhaust the well and build disease in the vigorous are thought to be of value in restoring health and vigor to the sick and weak. The apparent increase in vigor after administration of the stimulant deceives and deludes the ignorant, however well educated they may be. Dr. Oswald rightly observes:—

"In sickness stimulants cannot further the actual recovery by a single hour. There is a strong progressive tendency in our physical constitution; Nature needs no prompter; as soon as the remedial process is finished, the normal functions of the organism will resume their work as spontaneously as the current of a stream resumes its course after the removal of an obstruction."—*Physical Education*, p. 248.

This strong upward tendency in the living body and the naturalness of the healthy condition is our guarantee that where health is possible it will be restored as quickly as is consistent with the welfare of the body. Stimulants can but delay the ultimate recovery of the sick.

Disease, when once established in the system, can only be removed by the constitutional economy of the living body, that is, by the natural functioning of its several organs. Every move of the body, in disease, as in health, is toward the preservation and improvement of life. Every possible means of conserving energy is resorted to in disease. The whole stimulating practice is opposed to this conservation.

Innumerable are the lives that have been snuffed out by the efforts to "sustain" the patient, or "sustain" the heart, with stimulants. Alcohol, strychnine, digitalis and other such stimulatns have many deaths to their credit because of their use to "sustain" life.

A few minutes before Samuel Gompers died, his physician, Dr. W. S. Cockrall, stated to the newspaper men: "The end is near now. It is just artificial life."

Artificial life! How absurd! And yet, how scientific! He meant heart stimulants, "*restoratives*," tonics—poisons that force increased action in an organism that is endeavoring by every possible means to conserve its energies. Artificial life! May the gods preserve us! The alcohol pickeled brains of the boot-legging Allopaths will not!

"Artificial life" is a short cut to death. It consists in the vigorous application of a long-shank spur, to the horse-of-life, in order to drive him faster than his remaining powers justify. The forces of life are rapidly consumed—consumed, not in carrying on the original work of cure, but in defending the body against the powerful poisons that have been sent into its domain. Artificial life is the approved plan of exhausting natural life. There is too much of this accursed effort to run the body on stimulation, at the expense of its precious powers, and not enough willingness to step back and let the living organism run its own self and regulate its own affairs. Physicians are too wise! They know too well how the body should be run, and with what it should be run! Their boasted science is so much superior to Nature! A visit to the grave yard will convince the most skeptical!

Just before Pope Leo XIII died, his physician, Dr. Lapponi, said:—

"He is being kept alive by stimulants." "During the last 23 hours he has had two injections of camphorated oil, three of caffeine, and two of salt water, besides drinking stimulants."

Such ignorance is inexcusable in a physician. Any man who makes any pretense at science, as all HETEROPATHIC physicians do, should know that stimulants do not give power to the body. They only force the body to expend the power it has in reserve with greater rapidity and thus bring about exhaustion and death sooner. If stimulants can keep a man alive he should live as long as the stimulants hold out. The more he is stimulated the more alive he should be. But the reverse of this is true. The more he is stimulated, the sooner comes the end. Man cannot be kept alive by stimulants or "artificial life." If he could be so kept alive, no one should ever die. No greater delusion was ever entertained. Stimulation *per se* is the same, by whatever means accomplished.

An enervated body needs rest, not the goad. Recuperation of power, not the dissipation of its energies, is its greatest need. It is capable of regulating its own internal affairs and conducting these in the manner that best serves its present needs.

But the physicians will not permit. If it isn't functioning to suit them they force it to do so—not by correcting the causes of its "abnormal" action, but by stimulating and inhibiting its functions.

Drs. Jennings, Graham, Trall, Dewey, Walter, Oswald, Densmore, Tilden and others thundered the message to the world that the body needs rest and not interference; that cause should be corrected and no attempt made to force an appearance of health; but the work of stimulating the life out of patients goes merrily on. The voices of these men were drowned in a paeon of strident yells from the camps of the stimulant users.

CONDITIONS OF CURE
Chapter XXVII

"IN the tragedy of errors, called the history of the human race," wrote Dr. Oswald, "ignorance has often done as much mischief as sin." In the treatment of human ills, ignorance and short-sightedness have done far more mischief than sin. No greater tragedy of errors is conceivable than that presented by Medical Practice and Theory and by Medical History.

In forgoing chapters it has been amply demonstrated that the constructive forces of the body strive ceaselessly and unerringly in the direction of perfect health. What is commonly called disease, was shown to be, in reality, a beneficial process, or remedical and curative action. Toxemia, resulting from lowered functional power (enervation), which is, in turn, due to habits of living that weaken and poison the body was shown to be the condition that makes disease necessary. Cure has been shown to be the prerogative of living matter and of nothing else. It remains, therefore, for us to inquire: What are the conditions essential to a speedy consumation of the work of cure?

Before going into details about these conditions I deem it well to give in a general way the conclusions of the earlier Hygienists upon this matter. The following words of Jennings' are of interest to us in this connection,—*Philosophy of Human Life,* p. 39-40:—

"From what has been said, the attentive reader will infer that the fundamental principle by which I was governed in practice—a principle directly antipode to the one in common use—was to give free and full scope to the action of the law of the vital economy, irrespective of immediate consequences, no matter how appalling or alarming the developments or symptoms might be: nothing would induce me to interfere with the law and operations of nature, further than to remove opposing obstacles, when such were discovered to be present, and their removal was practicable, and supply wants.

"If a man was in a fit, I would let him lie in a fit until he was brought out of it by due course of law.

"The general result of this 'let-alone' principle, in comparison with those of the perturbating one in common use, in any and all of its multitudinous forms, were such as to convince any sober-minded and common sense man, of the superiority of their claim to soundness, over that of the later. DISEASES WERE MORE UNIFORM AND REGULAR IN THEIR PROGRESS, AND SHORTER IN DUATION; RECOVERIES WERE PROPORTIONATELY GREATER IN NUMBER, AND MORE PERMANENT AND ENDURING IN THE END. SUDDEN AND RE-MARKABLE CURES WERE A MATTER OF NOTORIETY, and the wonder was often expressed how such astonishing results could be compassed by such apparently trivial means. It came to be well known that the weapons which I used were few in number and of small dimensions, but it was conjectured that they made up in power what they lacked in number and size, and especially that their peculiar efficiency consisted in the skillful direction of them to the very seat and centre of disease." (caps. mine.)

Dr. Trall agreed with Jennings when he said of the power of cure:—

"****We must never forget that nature is the true physician. The restorative power is inherent in the living organism. ALL THAT THE TRUE HEALING ART CAN DO IS TO SUPPLY FAVORABLE CONDITIONS, REMOVE EX-TRANEOUS MATERIALS, AND REGULATE HYGIENIC INFLUENCES, and thus place the system as fully as possible under organic law."—*Hydro. Enc.,* vol. 2, p. 6 (Caps. mine.)

Again emphasizing that all the true "healer" can do in caring for the sick is to supply the best possible conditions for carrying on the curative processes, he says:—

"All morbid actions are evidences of the remedial efforts of nature to overcome morbid conditions or expel morbid materials. All that any truly phylosophical system

349

of medication can do, or should attempt to do, is to place the organism under the best possible circumstances for the favorable operation of these efforts. We may thwart, embarrass, interrupt, or suppress them, as is usually the case with the allopathic practice, or we may direct, modify, intensify, and accelerate them, as is the legitimate province of hydropathic practice."—*Hydro. Enc.*, vol. 2, p. 64.

It is plainly evident in the writings of Graham that what he calls the systems *"renovating economy"* does all the curing that is done. Here, we can only present a few quotations giving his views. He says, *Lectures on the Science of Human Life*, p. 191.

"Besides supplying the ordinary wants of the body by the general function of nutrition, the vital economy possesses the power, to a certain extent, of repairing the injuries which are done to it by physical violence. If a bone be broken, or a muscle or nerve be wounded, and if the system be in a proper state of health, the vital economy immediately sets about healing the breach. The blood which flows from the wounded vessels, by a law of the economy, coagulates in the breach, for the double purpose of stanching the wound and of forming a matrix for the regeneration fo the parts. Very soon minute vessels shoot out from the living parts into the coagulum of the blood, and immediately commence their operations, and deposit bony matter where it is required to unite a fractured bone, and nerve substance to heal a wounded nerve, etc. But the vital economy seems not to possess the power of reproducing the true muscle, and therefore where any fleshy part has been wounded, its breach is repaired by a gelatinous substance which gradually becomes hard, and sometimes assumes something of a fibrous appearance. It however so perfectly unites the divided muscles as to restore its functional power.

"In this wonderful process of healing, the little vessels employed in furnishing the matter for the several structures seem to know precisely when to commence and where to end their labors; and unless disturbed and driven to irregular operations by irritating causes, they never leave their labor incomplete, nor go beyond the proper bounds. But under the constant abuses of the body, when the nerves of organic life are continually tortured, and the vital economy generally disturbed, by the unhealthy habits of the individual, not only in the process of healing a wounded part, but in the ordinary functions of nutrition, substances will be misplaced or imperfectly elaborated, and dieased structures will be the restult."

Again, p. 420-24:—

"In relation to disease, and the true principles and means of cure, the almost universal and lamentable ignorance prevails among mankind. Few, probably, ever attempt to define their own notions of the subject, but are content to go through life with the most vague and indistinct impressions. Yet if we are to take the actions of men as true expressions of their ideas, we should unhesitatingly say, that human beings almost universally consider health and disease as things absolutely and entirely independent of their own voluntary conduct, and of their ability to control. They regard diseases as substances or things which enter their bodies with so little connection with their own voluntary actions and habits, that nothing which they can do can prevent disease, nor vary the time nor violence of its attack: and, according to their education, they believe it to be the effect of chance or of fate, or a direct and special dispensation of some overruling Power or Powers. The consequence is, that they either submit to disease, as an element of their irresistable destiny, or seek for remedies which will kill it, or expel it from their bodies, *as a substance or a thing independent of the condition and action of their organs.* This latter notion is probably far the most prevalent. People generally consult their physicians as those who are skillful to prescribe remedies that will kill disease; and these remedies they expect to act either as an antidote to a poison, or as an alkali to an acid, or in some other way, with little or no reference to the condition of their organs, and to their dietetic habits. Many, indeed, seem to think that their physician can take disease out of them and put health into them, by the direct application of remedies, and that there is in the remedies themselves, when skillfully chosen and applied, a health-giving potency which, of its own intrinsic virtue, directly and immediately, imparts health to the body.

"This erroneous notion, as a matter of course, leads people to place their dependence on the sovereign virtue of remedies, and consequently to undervalue the highest qualifications of the well-educated and truly scientific physician, and to place equal or even greater confidence in the ignorant and blustering quack who impudently pretends to have discovered a true and infallible remedy for every disease. The result of all this error is, in the first place, mankind do not believe that their own dietetic and other voluntary habits and actions have much, if anything, to do with the preservation of health and the prevention of disease; in the second place, when diseased, they expect to be cured by the sovereign power of medicine alone, and do not believe that any particular diet can of itself be of any great importance in preventing or promoting their restoration to health; in the third place, relying wholly on the intrinsic virtue of remedies, they conceive that medicine is quite as potent from the hands of one man as another, and are ever ready to run after those who are the loudest and most confident in their pretensions, and this opens the door for unbounded empiricism and quackery, and for the immense evils which flow from blind and indiscriminate drugging.

"All this mischief arises mainly from a want of correct knowledge of the nature of health, and the general principles of the philosophy of disease.****.

"Pure healthy chyme is produced exclusively by the healthy function of the alimentary canal, and the alimentary canal can perform this function healthfully only while itself is in a healthy and undisturbed condition. Pure healthy chyle can only be produced by the healthy function of the lacteals. Pure healthy blood can only be produced by the healthy function of the lacteals, lungs, and other organs concerned in haematosis, or the formation of blood. Perfectly healthy bile can only be produced by the healthy function of the liver; and so on, of all the other fluids and humors of the whole system. Now then, suppose the chyme, or chyle, or blood or bile or any other fluid or humor of the body to be unhealthy and impure; is it possible for any physician, or any other human being in the universe, to apply such a remedy as will of its own intrinsic virtues, directly and immediately impart health and purity to any of these substances? Most certainly not. There is no possible way in nature of producing these effects, but by the healthy function of the organs constituted for that purpose. If the bile is unhealthy, no medicine in the universe can make the bile healthy; and while the function of the liver is perfectly healthy, the bile cannot be unhealthy. If the blood is impure, no medicine in the universe can, by its own intrinsic virtues, directly and immediately impart purity to it. There is no possible way in nature by which it can be purified, but by the healthy function of the appropriate organs of the body.

"If, then, by any means the blood becomes impure, the healthy functions of the appropriate organs will very soon purify it. But whatever may be the quality and potency of the medicines used to purify it, so long as the functions of these appropriate organs are unhealthy, the blood will and must remain impure; and this is true of all the fluids and humors of the system." (italics mine).

Again, *Lectures on the Science of Human Life*, p. 436:—

"Whether we embrace the scheme of humoral pathology or either of the other two which have been named, we must admit that, as a general fact, organic irritation, disturbing the functions and deteriorating the functional results, and inducing a morbid condition of the solids, leading to acute and chronic inflammation, general fever, local disease, change of structure, etc., is the ordinary source of our diseases, and these irritations are produced by the dietetic use of substances unfriendly to vitality and to the physiological interests of our bodies, and by the improper qualities and quantities and conditions of our food, and by many other means and circumstances pertaining to our dietetic and other voluntary habits and actions. But, by whatever cause induced, disease, when once established in the system, can only be removed by the constitutional economy of the living body, by the healthy functions of the several organs. Yet so long as irritation is kept up, the healthy functions of the organs cannot be restored."

"If a body has vitality enough to live under wrong conditions, it has vitality enough to get well under right conditions."—Wm. Howard Hay, M.D., a reformed Old School physician and surgeon.

There is no truth in nature more positive than that the normal condition of man is one of health. That all the organs and functions of the human body are designed and adapted to produce this result, appears to be a proposition so self-evident that to argue it would seem to be a work of supererogation. Yet man has lived so long in violation of the laws of his being, and as the inevitable consequence, has suffered disease so long that he has come to forget, or lose sight of the fact that the natural condition of all organized beings is one of health and not of disease; that instead of the sickly, deformed creature he is, with both mind and body dwarfted in conformity to the false conditions under which he lives, he might be and should be a healthy and well developed being, in the enjoyment of all the resulting consequences of such a condition.

Those who have never attempted to present health truth to mankind in general are hardly aware of the prejudices to be combatted, the ignorance to be removed, before mankind will be brought to see that it is far better, from every point of view, to live in a state of health than in a state of disease—in a state of happiness than in one of misery and suffering. Upon no subject is aggitation more necessary than on this. Line upon line, precept upon precept, and volume upon volume are needed to arouse and convince the suffering millions of the grand truth that health, not disease, is their birth-right—a birth-right which they continually sell for a mess of indulgence.

Notwithstanding the constant evidence of our senses that nature is capable of, and does maintain the organism in health during its existence, it is very difficult for some to believe that she has any power to restore lost functions or heal an organic lesion without some artificial spur or aid. Something positive and decided must be done to meet adequately the emergency. The old school physician is never easy unless he is putting something into his patients or abstracting something from them. As some one has wittingly remarked, the old school physician believes in cutting out things, lopping off things, rubbing on things, pouring down things, and squirting in things. Operations are performed and medicines given to impress, most powerfully, the vital domain with the idea that there is the most absolute and stringet necessity therefor —while, perhaps, a little discretion would have done more service by letting alone. Nature is constantly and ceaselessly working for life and health and any interference of a decided character may be hazardous.

Among Heteropaths, there are many who, although professing implicit faith in the power of nature to accomplish her work, nevertheless, manifest an almost total lack of faith by their insistence that something be done for the patient. That admirable American Hygienist, Dr. Oswald, wrote, *Nature's Household Remedies*, p. 15:—

"Diseases plead for *desistance*, rather than for *assistance*, and the discovery of the cause is the discovery of the remedy. For there is a strong upward and healthward tendency in the constitution of every living organism. Nature's revenge is but an enforced condition of peace. Pain, discomfort, and even the premature loss of organic vigor, are the attendant symptoms of a reconstructive process, and their permanence is a presumptive proof that, in spite of such admonitions, that process is a struggle against a permanent obstacle or against a constantly precated frustration of its efforts."

Cure may properly be said to be the natural and spontaneous return to normal condition and function after the purposes of abnormal function have been accomplished. The return to normal function, after the occasion for abnormal function is removed, does not require to be aided or forced. It is as natural as the return of water to its natural channel after the obstructions have been removed from the channel.

The disposition of natural forces may safely be left to natural law. The conduct of the forces of life under all circumstances and conditions of life, always and of necessity will be lawful and orderly. The forces of life can no more violate the laws of life than the force of gravity can violate the laws of gravity or than the forces of chemistry can violate the laws of matter and chemistry. Every action and operation of the living body in health or in disease is, and must be, in strictest harmony with the laws of life. Were it otherwise, did chaos and disorder reign in the vital or organic realm, life, health and disease would be as uncertain and fortutious as the medical professions all conceive them to be.

There could be no science of life (biology), or science of function (physiology), or science of cause (aetiology), or science of disease (pathology). Where chaos and uncertainty reign science is impossible. When the medical professions learn that law and order reign in the living realm, the search for "cures" will cease and a study of causes will begin. It is probably too much to except this to occur in the lifetime of the present generation.

Therapeutic methods are all of the same nature,—that is, they are all methods of driving nature with a whip of scorpions, on the idea that the recuperative power of the body does not know how to free the body of the pathoferic matter that is back of the disease. God's great scheme of human healthiness and endurance is regarded as a failure, and practitioners of all schools are agreed that the great thing to be done, in all cases of disease, is to "arouse the prostrated vital energies as quickly as possible."

The antagonizing precepts taught by the various schools are, however, seen to neutralize each other in theory, while the results in practice are quite identical, so as scarce to indicate a preference, except that we would choose the comparatively harmless methods of the drugless schools, rather than the more harmful drug methods. None of these methods are, however, quite satisfactory to the thinking community. They are destined to pass away and be forgotten.

The sick seek to be cured. The term cure not only implies a reinstatement of health in an organism that is suffering from disease, but, in its common acception, it also has reference to the means whereby this is accomplished. Ordinarily cures are supposed to be wrought by some external aid. As has been said: "The man is doctored as he is booted and coated; and physicked, as he is fed, in the confident assurance that he is fitted and burnished for new service in either case." The sick would scarcely be said to be cured, however perfect the recovery, without the aid of some therapeutic measure. Hence, cure has reference to an external rather than to an internal resource. It is the operation or the effect of something external. The term, then, will convey different ideas to different persons, depending on their understanding of what the act intrinsically consists in.

Living things only are the subject of these effects, and it is to the different estimates, relatively, that are attached to the vital or recuperative power, and the part that treatment plays, that serves as a basis of the different views on this subject. Heteropaths consider disease as a destructive principle, or even an entity, that will inevitably consumate its work unless it is met by some neutralizing or counteracting agent. These consider vitality as little more than an onlooker at the show, until it is either vanquished or accepts the victory wrought in its behalf. Others reluctantly award some credit to the vital forces, when stimulated or goaded by measures capable of drawing out its actions defensively. There are but few of us who place no dependence on any other means of recuperation, save those that are all efficient in continuing vital changes in the healthy state.

Among all the many hundreds of theories and practices of medicine, drug and drugless, which have passed in view, and presented special claims to superior merit, there has not been one but that lived and acted on the assumption that all desirable ends in cases of disease are effected by therapeutics or treatment, and they have scarcely bestowed a modicum of reliance upon the inherent vital capacities. It has been assumed that those symptoms which we call disease are, necessarily and invariably, evidences of a destructive process which must be counteracted before they destroy the life of the patient.

Many substances that are known to be inimical to health and life were thought to be also antagonistic to disease; and that, on special occasions, they might even be special vivifying means, working upon local parts a curative act which is conceived to be different from the ordinary nutritive and reproductive processes. The modern Hygienic or Orthopathic practitioner regards these assumptions as utterly false and untenable. This school seeks to bring those liable to suffer from disease to a true knowledge of the causes of their miseries, and finds a cure for these in the discipline and correction of faulty and perverted voluntary habits of everyday life. We refuse to admit, because it is untrustworthy and ambiguous, the evidence offered in favor of the various therapeutic systems.

Life and its variable phenomena, rather than therapeutic methods and their uses, should furnish the proper field of our inquiry. From such a study we acquire a knowledge of how nature acts under different circumstances. We will then know what life ordinarily does, and how it will act under constraint and cumpulsion, and what are the PROPER CONDITIONS FOR ITS ASCENDENCY OVER MORE MA-TERIAL, CRUDE AND CHEMICAL FORCES.

We can never know what the vital principle or life is, but we may observe the circumstances which attend it, and what it does, its invariable conditions, its laws; and on these we must base our actions in reference to it, in sickness as in health.

The medical profession having, hitherto, arrogated to itself all knowledge having any important relation to health, saying, in effect, we and we alone, are the con-servators of the bodies and health of men, has witheld the little knowledge it possessed from the people. However useful so important a general diffusion of such knowledge as relates to our very existence, as the means of influencing and developing the forces concerned therein, might be considered; yet it was to remain the behoof of the learned dignitaries of this elect and holy profession—too sacred or too occult for the common understanding. Their prescriptions being supposed to be of a character that defies the scrutiny of popular inquiry, demanded a confidence almost unqualified. The public was asked to place the same faith in the physician—who concealed his prescriptions in corruptions of a dead language—as they were supposed to impose in their god. The patient knew enough if he could open his mouth and swallow the prescription without demur or refusal.

No inquiry was instituted to determine whether a person ought or ought not to be sick under given circumstances. That he ought to keep from getting sicker while he is trying to get well was never dreamed of. The enchantment of the magic dose was —*nolens volens*—to charm him into a condition of fresh vigor and manliness; and as recovery in the great majority of cases succeeds an "attack" of disease; and as a remedy, or a supposed remedy, was always given, the inference continued to be drawn that there was a useful connection between them; both physician and patient laboring for ages under a delusion from not understanding fully enough the true relation of such things.

Undoubtedly this idea of the value of medical specifics has operated very disasterously, indirectly inviting the cause of disease by the promise of immunity it holds out in the ideas of medical absolution. The causes of disease are disregarded so long as people think they can dodge the result under the shield of medicine, and just in proportion as freedom from peril is offered is the inducement to sever the lines of law whereby organic existence is bounded.

At present both physicians and patients are ever ignorant of the quality of the medical service rendered; a kind oblivion, except in case of the most obvious blunder, steps in and enshrouds from observation the interference. *Good nature, while her forces remain in the ascendency, is ever working to perpetuate organized existence in her best possible manner.* She gradually overcomes those conditions that conflict with her aim, whether spontaneously or artificially induced, thus the sick as well their advisors, constantly labor under the delusion that it is some potency of the prescription that effects the desired object; while in reality, its only merit is that of COINCIDENCE IN TIME. *A mere coincidence is mistaken for cause, hence arises the popular credulity in reference to medical means—a magnified importance having been for ages attached to measures which have no use or importance.* Hence, also, the ever-readiness with which the public resign themselves to the physicians. It is no matter whether he be stupid or clever—the grossest emperic or a philosopher—he generally soon discovers that his "bread and butter" come of qualifications quite different from this latter; and his inclinations take the direction of his interest.

All the importance that the matter of the management of health and disease by medicines and treatments obtains, comes from a non-recognition of these principles,— from a mistake in regard to the essential nature of the action induced in vital objects by medicines and therapeutic measures. It should be known that any benefit accruing to health must come through the ordinary physiological acts. Medicines and therapeutic measures possess no power to antagonize or neutralize the cause of disease or to assist the organism in its work—they cannot add power to the organism—but can only excite to a morbid extent the physiological functions; and it is by these in sickness that the blood is restored, as in health it is maintained in its pristine qualities. In short, recuperation and restored health are never the effects of drugs and treatments, but of the organic force, and the conditions that usually maintain it. It is asserted that good effects sometimes, at least, follow the use of drugs and other methods of treatment, and we shall be called upon to show how this can never happen. The record of experience, which is appealed to, can substantiate nothing, for it takes no account of the vital force, or of the nature of disease itself, and assumes that the effect of the drug or treatment is additional to the work of the vital power, whereas, it only changes it. That this is true, we have amply demonstrated elsewhere.

In her *Notes on Nursing,* (page 9), Florence Nightingale gives evidence of Ortho-pathic leanings and reveals that she was frequently called upon to answer the objections of those who could not give up their faith in "cures," and who insisted on DOING SOMETHING in disease. She says:—

"Another and the commonest exclamation which will be instantly made is—would you do nothing, then, in cholera, fever, etc.?—so deep-rooted and universal is the conviction that to give medicine is to be doing something, or rather everything; to give air, warmth, cleanliness, etc., is to do nothing."

The Hygienic practice is commonly referred to, even today, as the do-nothing treatment. We have expanded it into "*doing-nothing-intelligently*" for the reason that it requires more skill and intelligence to "*Do Nothing*" in the Orthopathic sense than to "do something" in the medical sense. Orthopathy is a let-alone plan only in so far as disease and the symptoms of disease are concerned. It gives every attention to hygiene. This is its "aids to nature." It removes, as far as possible, all pathoferic influences. It does not try to remove disease nor the symptoms of disease. Miss Nightingale replied to the above objections: "in these and many other similar diseases the exact value of particular remedies is by no means ascertained, while there is universal experience as to the extreme importance of careful nursing (hygiene) in determining the issue of disease."

The name of Miss Nightingale is honored today by a nursing profession that is trained in Heteropathic schools and which lacks the keen insight into disease and the wholesome doubt of the value of "remedies" possessed by this English girl. There is more wisdom in her *Notes on Nursing* than in the entire nurses training course of today.

Professional men are moulded by the educational system through which they acquire their training. If the teachings of their system are fundamentally wrong, as is the case with medical teachings, the victims of such education find it hard to step out of the matrix, in which they were forced to crystalize, into another world of thought. The doctor who has been taught that disease is an evil that must be fought against, that he must treat and suppress symptoms, as these arise, instead of correcting and removing causes, finds it exceedingly difficult to get away from these teachings, especially so, since they have been ground into him from childhood.

"There are but two medical systems in existence," said Trall ". . . the Drug Medical System and the Hygienic Medical System. One employs *poisons* as the proper and natural remedies for disease; the other employs normal or hygienic materials and agencies. There are several branches or sects of the Drug Medical System— the Allopathic, Homeopathic, Eclectic, Physio-medical, etc. But they are all essentially one and the same. They all differ in certain secondary and unimportant problems and theories; but they all agree in primary premises. They are all reduceable to the fundamental proposition of 'curing one disease by producing another.' They are all based on the principle of inducing a drug disease to cure a primary disease. It is true that Eclecticism and Physio-Medicalism do not recognize this principle; but it is true nevertheless.

"Drug medication, no matter in what disguise nor under what name it is pre-scribed, consists in employing, as remedies for disease, those things which produce disease in well persons. Its materia medica is simply a list of drugs, chemicals, dye-stuffs—in a word, *poisons.* They may be vegetable, animal or mineral, and may be called 'apothecary stuff' or medicines; but they are, neverthelss, *poisons.* They may come to us in the shape of acids, alkalies, salts, oxides, earths, roots, barks, seeds, leaves, flowers, gums, resins, secretions, excretions, etc., but all are subversive of organic structures; all are incompatible with vital functions; all are antagonistic to living matter; all produce disease when brought in contact in any manner with the living domain: *all are poisons.*

"On the contrary, Hygienic Medication consists in employing, as remedial agents for sick persons, the same materials and influences which preserve health in well persons. It rejects all poisons.

"****It is a prevalent opinion that the advocates of this system accept the philosophy of the Allopathic System, but reject its remedies, employing water, diet, etc., as substitutes for drug medicines.

"The true system of the Healing Art—Hygienic Medication—rejects not only the drugs, medicines or poisons of the popular system, but also repudiates the philosophy or theories on which their employment is predicated. It is in direct antagonism with the Drug System, both in theory and practice. It does not propose to employ air, light, temperature, water, etc., as substitutes for drugs, or because they are better or safer than drugs. It rejects drugs because they are intrinsically bad, and employs hygienic agencies because they are intrinsically good. I would reject drugs if there were no other remedial agents in the universe, because, if I could not do good, I would 'cease to do evil.' I would not poison a person because he is sick. No physician has ever yet given the world a reason that would bear the ordeal of a moments scientific examination, why a sick person should be poisoned more than should a well person; and I do not believe the world will endure until he finds such a reason. The medical profession may prosecute this inquiry another three thousand years, and destroy other hundreds of millions of the human race in experiments with drugs and doses, but they will never arrive any nearer to a solution of the problem. They will never be able to give a satisfactory answer to the question, for none exists."—*True Healing Art.*

The relation of drugs, serums, vaccines, etc., to the living tissues is one of antagonism. Take one of them separately and it is a poison. Give a patient a whole drug store and it is one mass of poison. Trall truly wrote:—

"Says Dr. Bigelow (*Nature in Disease*, p. 17); 'The effects of remedies are so mixed up with the phenomena of disease, that the mind has difficulty in separating them.' Indeed it has. It never can separate them. The 'effects of remedies' are the 'phenomena of disease,' and nothing else.

"And what are the remedies which God and Nature have provided? Drugs, poisons, chemicals, banes, of every name and kind! *Banes, did I say?* Has not every medical school its favorite bane? Allopathy regards arsenic—*rat's bane*—as a very good tonic. Homeopathy prescribes nux vomica—*dog's bane*— as an admirable nervine. Eclecticism selects hyoscamus—*hen bane*—as a proper sedative. And Physio-Medicalism considers eryngero—*flea bane*—as an excellent febrifuge. Professor Pain is right. We do indeed 'cure one disease by producing another.'

"But the provings; aye the provings! How do medical men prove that these medicines are remedies for sick folks? In precisely the same way that Toxicologists prove that they are poisons for well folks.

"When these poisons are given to well persons they produce more or less of nausea, vomiting, purging, pain, heat, swelling, griping, vertigo, spasms, stupor, coma, delirium and death. When they are given to sick persons they produce the same manifestations of disease, modified, more or less, by the condition of the patient and the circumstances of the prior disease.

"Was there ever any reasoning in the world like unto medical reasoning? If the medical man with good intentions *administers* one of these drug poisons, or a hundred of them, and the patient dies, he dies because the medicine can't save him. But if a malfactor with murderous disposition gives the same *medicine* to a fellow-being, and the fellow-being dies, he dies because the *poison* killed him! Does the motive of the one who administers the drug alter its relation to vitality?"—*True Healing Art.*

When Dr. Trall stated that there were but two medical systems in the world—the Drug Medical System and the Hygienic Medical System—the present day group of medical systems that belong to neither of these two classifications, had not arisen. In 1908, Herward Carrington asserted:—

"To begin with, then, I must state that there are, broadly speaking, two and only two schools of healing in the world; the hygienic, on the one hand, and every other school, sect, or system, on the other. No matter what the physician may be—allopath, homeopath, osteopath, eclectic, faith-curist, mind curist, Christian Scientist, or what not, he is not a hygienist, in that he does not know the real cause and cure of disease. The theory or the philosophy of disease which the hygienist defends is totally opposed to all other medical systems, being directly opposite to them in theory."—Vitality, Fasting and Nutrition, p. 4.

This list may now be enlarged to include chiropractic, naprapathy, physio-therapy, and any other system of drugless therapeutics which may now exist, or which may arise in the future. We have never claimed that hygienic agencies were to be the sole reliance in every conceivable emergency of life, as the following words from Trall will show:—

"The hygienic agencies—absurdly called 'non-natural' (by the medical profession of Trall's day), in medical books—comprise the whole and ample materia medica of the true hydropath. They are air, light, water, food, temperature, exercise, sleep, clothing, and the passions. These agencies, variously modified and intensified, I believe are capable of producing all the really remedial effects in all diseases which the whole pharmacopoeia of allopathy, with its thousand drugs and destructives, can produce, and without any of the evil or injurious results always attendant upon the operation of the latter; while to sustain the vital machinery in its most vigorous and enduring conditions, in other words preserve health, we have but to employ them according to established and invariable laws.

"In claiming for these agencies by which every part and organ of every living animal and vegetable in existence is nourished, built up, sustained, and finally changed and decomposed, by which the integrity of every structure and function is maintained during life, and resolved into its primitive elements and conditions on the cessation of the life principle, a complete and perfect materia medica, I mean as far as regards functional derangement, which, indeed constitutes ninety-nine-hundreths of the diseases of society. Mechanical injuries, displacements of parts, organic lesions, etc., coming appropriately under the management of the surgeon, may and often do require mechanical agencies of some sort."—Hydropathic Encyclopedia, vol. 1, pp. 2-95.

We are punished by our sins, not for them and when the fires of retributive justice flare up there are no asbestos jackets turned out by drug vendors or serum squirters that can prevent our pelts from being singed. Sickness and suffering are the legitimate and necessary effect of their producing causes. They are consequent upon breaking of the laws of life. They cannot be escaped.

Almost the whole of the practice of medicine is an effort to enable man to escape the inevitable and necessary results of his transgressions of the laws of life. In the days of our fathers disease was regarded as a dispensation of Divine Providence. God was chastizing man. He was wreaking vengeance upon sinners. Our fathers, though professing to believe that God's chastisements were just, did not hesitate to try to cheat Him out of His vengence. They tried to drug and dose away His chastizements. What an impious crowd they were to attempt to arrest, by medicine, a dispensation of an all-wise Providence!

Like them, we attempt to drug and dose away the effects of violated law. We have ceased to regard disease as a chastizement. To use it is a misfortune to be escaped by pus punching and serum squirting. Law and order do not reign in the field of health and disease. All is chance and accident. Effects are not the results of causes and causes do not produce their effects. Or, if they do, by the theurgic and thaumaturgic powers of serums and vaccines, we may set aside the law of cause and effect.

All of Nature's chastizements are remedial in character and need not end in disaster. Nature spanks us only to correct us and corrects us that we may be saved from worse folly and greater suffering. As soon as we cease our quacking schemes of palliation and learn to interpret the voice of nature health will be ours.

Disease is a cry for peace not for aid. Every disease is a plea for desistance, not for assistance. Pain is not a plea for pain killers but for rest and desistance. Discomfort does not call for sedatives or tonics, but for desistance. Nausea and vomiting are not pleas for anti-emetics, demulcents and digestives but for abstinence from food. Loss of appetite is not a call for tonics and digestives but a "closed for repairs" sign hung out by the body.

If you roast your shins too near a glowing fire the toasting nerves cry out for a lower temperature and not for linaments or pain killers. Desist! · Desist! This is the cry of nature. She does not need your puny "aid." She only asks that you cease your foolish interference. Physicians of all schools insist that nature cures and that they only "aid nature." Some of them have some rather curious and damaging ways of aiding her, however. Too often they assist her out altogether and the patient succumbs to the "aid." ·

Pain is not a cry for aid but for desistance. If you tread on tacks the pain is not a call for linaments and salves but for the removal of the tacks. Keep off the tacks, the forces of the body will do the rest. Pain in the stomach following a meal is not a call for pepsin or Bell-ans but for rest—for abstinence from food. Nature but cries out for you to cease abusing your stomach. The natural forces of repair and recuperation will take care of the stomach when you cease to abuse it. Indeed these forces are continuously at work in an effort to counteract and overcome the effects of the abuse you heap upon your stomach or any other part or parts of your body. No doctor and no drug can do this work, but Nature can if you cease the abuse.

Pain and discomfort speedily disappear without any injury being inflicted upon the body, if their causes are corrected and removed. The avidity with which the public grabs up every proffered mode of postponing and arresting pain, these methods usually consisting of lethean dosing, evinces the fear of pain that civilized man, particularly the more effete portions of civilized peoples, has developed. This practice of never ending palliation is all based on the assumption that pain is actually lessened or obliterated by such proceedures. This assumption is not only false, but it is true, on the other hand, that such methods prolong and intensify the pain and retard, or even prevent, recovery. Everything that interferes with the natural processes and functions of the body hinders them in their curative work.

Medical practice, including that of all schools of medicine, is a fruitless routine of palliatives and methods of meddling with the senses and the functions of the body, all of which methods leave an aftermath of complications and sequelae, which are worse than the disease for which the palliatives were given, and all of which are far more difficult to overcome and eradicate than the original malady.

Pain is not the disease nor its cause. It is a symptom. Palliatives that "relieve" pain do so by depressing and paralyzing the nerves of feeling, and not by controlling the antecedents of the disease. However, much skill may be employed in removing consequences, nothing permanent, EXCEPT HARM, is secured unless the antecedents are corrected or removed. So long as the producing factors and influences are permitted to continue, these will keep up the diseased state and reproduce the pain as rapidly as the "relief" wears off. To conceal your condition by sand-bagging your senses is utter nonsense and positively harmful. Every method or measure that is directed at the removal of symptoms and not at the removal of causes is an evil.

A small cut, a bruise, a nail in the foot, a lame back, sore muscles, a sore throat, a cold, and other minor ailments, are small when compared to a disease like pneumonia. Many will readily grant that nature is fully adequate to the cure of such small things, but contend she must have aid in dealing with a pneumonia. There can, however, be no doubt that the process of cure is the same in either case. Not only is this true, but if nature is not able, unaided, to cure pneumonia, no case would ever recover, for it is admitted by the highest authorities in medicine, that they have no cure for this disease, and it is doubted by many of these if the death rate in this disease is any lower than it was a thousand years ago. It is admitted that the death rate in pneumonia has increased since 1900.

Then there is pulmonary tuberculosis, which assuredly nature cannot cure without help. But it is asserted on post mortem evdience that almost everyone in civilized life has this disease at some time during their existence, get well without ever knowing they had it, and "die of some other disease." This assertion is based on the finding of lung lesions, in the dead, that have healed up. Of course, there are other causes for lung lesions than tuberculosis, and no one is justified in assuming that all such lesions found are due to this disease, but it is very probable that many of them are caused by tuberculosis. Not only this, but many who do have the disease and who know they have it, recover, and recover without some "cure" for no "cure" for the disease is known. Either nature cures it or it isn't cured. And she cures it by means of fresh air, exercise, proper food, out-door living, sunshine, rest and sleep, and abstinence from injurious habits—in short, by hygienic measures.

Nature does not employ food as a "cure," but to nourish the body and to carry on her usual work of secretion, excretion, and de-toxification. She does not employ water and air as cures, but uses them in the same way and for the same purposes that she uses them in health. Exercise is not used to cure disease any more than it is used to cure health; nor are rest and sleep. Sunlight is an important and necessary factor in metabolism or nutrition in health and disease. It is not a "cure" in the accepted meaning of the term. These forces, elements, agents and factors are necessaries of life, both in health and disease, and are not in any proper sense to be regarded as therapeutic agents. They belong exclusively to the field of natural hygiene.

Orthopathists differentiate between natural hygiene, which consists of the use of those natural conditions upon which active life depends; and, that pseudo-hygiene promulgated by the sons of Chiron, which consists chiefly in a germ chase. Natural hygiene, for instance, demands ordinary cleanliness, while medical hygiene demands sterility. Sterility is secured by extreme heat, anti-septics, germicides, etc. Natural hygiene has proven adequate to the needs of plant and animal life in all ages of the world, in all climates and at all seasons. Medical hygiene has not proven to be worth a whoop; indeed, it has often worked incalculable harm.

Therapeutics is defined as "that branch of medical science concerned with the application of remedies and the treatment of disease." A therapeutist is "one versed in therapeutics." Hygiene, on the other hand is the science of health, or, more fully; that branch of biological science that deals with the natural factors and influences essential to the healthful and continued activity, growth, development and reproduction of living beings. Natural hygiene does not necessitate the destruction of germ life nor the pollution of the blood stream with pus and foreign proteins in order to maintain life and health. Natural hygiene is simply those natural conditions upon which life and health depend. And these conditions never cease to be necessary. Well or sick the living organism is always dependent upon these conditions and they cannot be substituted by some therapeutic method—some "cure."

The living organism cannot make use of elements and factors in disease that it cannot use in health. The laws of life do not change during disease. The needs of life may be modified somewhat, just as they are often modified in health, but they do not change. The laboring man needs more food while at labor than he does during a vacation. His food needs are modified, but not changed. He cannot substitute something else for food. So, the sick man needs less food than the well man. He may require a fast, but even then he is not subsisting without food. He is simply utilizing the food stored in his body. When this gives out, if he does not consume more food he soon starves to death. He cannot substitute anything else for food.

Man's normal instincts are a reliable guide in the matter of eating or fasting, but under present conditions few men reach maturity with normal instincts, or if they do the doctors will seldom permit them to follow their instincts. The doctor usually has a "scientific (?) theory" to sustain as well as a reputation and a fortune to make. What matters the welfare of the patient in the face of this trinity of "interests." Ever since Pluto prevailed upon Jupiter to aim a thunderbolt at the head of that Parvenue, Aesculapius, because the latter was interferring with the immigration to hades and cutting down the income from the ferry boat over the Styx, the doctors have been sacrificing the instincts of their patients upon the alter of the unholy trinity of scientific theory, reputation and fortune. Yes! Even earlier than this; when I-em-Hetep became "Master of Secrets" and "Consoler of the Afflicted," the physician was soothing pain with the juice of the poppy instead of heeding the warning voice of instinct.

In repairing a house the carpenter uses the same materials, tools and methods that were employed in its construction. No man attempts to repair a house built of lumber, out of brick and mortar. He employs a saw and hammer and other tools for working with wood and not a trowel and other tools for working with brick and mortar. Carpenters are employed to repair wooden structures and masons to repair stone structures. Any other methods and materials of repair would not be tolerated by an intelligent owner of a house.

The process of repair in houses is the same as the process of construction. So it is in all other structures, in all machines, etc. We do not even think that it could be otherwise. We use less intelligence in dealing with the human body. For food we substitute poisonous drugs. For rest we use stimulation; for cleanliness we substitute antiseptic-sterility; in the place of sunlight we employ electric lights of all colors and hues; pure water is rejected for coffee, tea, soda fountain slops or mineral waters. No man expects his house to be repaired instantly but he wants instantaneous cures. He knows that if the workmen are rushed they do not do as good or as neat work and his house will not be substantial or beautiful; but he wants the curative process forced forward at a rapid rate. He knows that the slow growth of the oak or hickory is more enduring than the rapid growth of the mushroom, but he thinks he can force rapid healing and still have an enduring structure.

The human body is composed of cells. These require, if they are to continue to live, grow and reproduce, proper nutrition, adequate drainage, a suitable temperature, and protection from violence. The organs of the body are capable of replacing, by growth and reproduction, such as they have been observed to undergo for the scientist, in the test tube, all worn out and broken down cells, while the body is capable of removing and expelling the injured or dead cells. The stability and integrity of structure and function, displayed by the living organism, is maintained by the continual formation of new cells and cell products to supplant the old and outworn ones. It is by their powers of assimilation and self-maintenance that they maintain their condition in the face of the changes to which they are subjected by external forces.

What the vital or organic force is we may never know, but we do know that it is not independent of certain conditions. The necessary elementary combination of the vital principle may be present and yet not manifest life. This dormant state of life, as seen in the impregnated germ of the egg before incubation or in the seed before germination, is not to be mistaken for death. The manifestations of life begin only under the influence of certain necessary conditions, such as warmth, air, moisture, nutriment, etc., and these conditions never cease to be necessary for the continued manifestation of life. Whether life is passive or active depends upon the conditions under which it operates.

The ova of animals and seed of plants remain in a state of "germ" only so long as they are maintained perfectly quiescent and beyond the influence of the external factors essential to their development. They remain capable of development and maintain their creative force, but this force is latent or dormant. It passes from passivity to activity only under certain essential conditions. The ova of some animals will, if withdrawn from the influence of the atmosphere and warmth, retain their latent capability of development for a long period. Thus the productive powers of the ova of many insects are preserved throughout the winter. The same is true of the germinating power of seeds. Under favorable conditions this power is preserved in the seeds of many plants for many years. As soon, however, as these are subjected to the external influences necessary to call this inherent power into activity, the germ, if still capable of development, becomes developed; if not still capable of development, putrefaction ensues.

If those conditions that called the passive life of the seed or ovum into activity are withdrawn, development and growth cease and either speedy death ensues, or else the plant or animal falls into a state of suspended animation. These form the necessary materials and influences with which growth and repair or maintainence as well as elimination are carried on.

I might easily expand this subject into a volume and discuss many more parts of it, but to do so would be to neglect the purpose of this chapter. It is enough here that we see that life is dependent upont certain external influences and conditions, or vital stimuli, as they have been called—heat, light, air, water, food—and that under the influence and by the use of these the organic being is developed from the germ and by the use of these same forces, influences and materials, it carries on its processes and functions, repairs and maintains its parts, defends and reproduces itself.

After the young bird or reptile is hatched or after the young mammal is born, they require exercise or voluntary muscular activity, rest and sleep. After birth, also, their minds become active, and it is then the mental influence begins to affect function. The young bird, starting life with a normal organism and supplied with light, air, water, food, warmth, exercise, rest and sleep, mental poise and protection from violence, will develop into a sturdy, healthy, well formed representative of its type. The young infant, starting life under these same conditions, supplied with these same external factors and refraining from indulgencies in harmful habits, such as animals do not indulge in, will likewise develop into a sturdy, healthy, well formed human being.

The essential conditions of life are, therefore, seen to be very simple. They are usually within easy reach of the rudest savage, though often out of reach of his boasted civilized brother. If there is a lack of any of these essentials of life or an over abundance of any of them, or if harmful habits are permitted to interfere with the processes of life, disease is the result.

Now, when we see that organisms are self-evolving depending only upon a few simple conditions; that they are self-maintaining and self-repairing, depending upon these same few simple conditions and that the normal or natural condition of all organisms is health, with disease, which is also natural, following upon a disturbance of these same few natural conditions; it would seem the most reasonable and natural thing in the world for us to look for the disturbing factors and correct these and then let the body return to health. This is the very opposite to that which is usually attempted and is the very opposite to what the reader is going to do after he reads this. The usual practice is to try by some "remedy" or "cure" or "therapeutic" method or device, to force the organism to act normally in spite of the disturbing conditions, and without correcting these. Organs and functions are stimulated or inhibited, as, in the opinion of the doctor, they should be and little or no attention is given to finding and correcting the conditions that have impaired the life functions. The stimulating or inhibiting method employed may be chemical, mechanical, thermal, electrical or mental; the results are the same in kind.

Just as you can't sober a man up by letting him drink, or rest a fatigued man with work, so you cannot therapeutics a man into health while the pathoferic conditions or influences remain uncorrected. After these are corrected the so-called therapeutics are not needed; at no time are they useful. The organism can make use of those natural elements and influences that are used daily in producing and maintaining it in health, and no other. The amount of food or rest or exercise or water or air or sunshine, etc., needed may vary from time to time, depending on the general condition or work of the body but, beyond this there is no difference in the needs of the body. It cures itself.

Just as the carpenter, in repairing a house, has to tear away the old worn out or rotten material before he can proceed with the work of putting in the new material, so, in the human body, before repairs in a damaged or destroyed portion can be made, the worn out and destroyed parts must be removed. In the living body the process of wear and tear is continuous, so the process of removal of waste and renewal and repair of structure is also continuous. In disease, this same process of removal of waste and repair, that is employed in health, is employed to repair damages. The same materials are used in disease as in health. In the very constitution of things it could not be otherwise than this.

Curative or therapeutic agents and materials are neither needed nor usable by the sick body. Health building or hygienic agents alone are needed or usable. The process we call disease is itself the process of cure—it is the process of purification and readjustment and to cure it is to kill or maim the organism. Cure does not reside in any external thing, power or agent, nor in the doctor or nurse. It is inherent in living matter as was amply demonstrated in a former chapter. Food is not a cure in disease any more than in health—it does not cure disease anymore than it cures health. Health is that state of the living organism in which all its functions and processes are carried on in an easy and harmonious manner for the preservation of life and maintenance of functional and structural integrity. Food is one of the essential elements for the successful performance of this effort. Disease is that state of the living organism in which all its processes and functions are carried on in a less easy and less harmonious manner for the same preservation of life and maintenance of functional and structural integrity. Food is one of the essential elements for the successful performance of this effort. Health is the normal conduct of living beings, under normal conditions to maintain normal conditions, disease is the abnormal conduct of the living functions under abnormal conditions to restore normal conditions.

The success of the effort to restore normal conditions, like the success of the effort to maintain normal conditions, depends to a great extent upon the factors influencing those conditions. Any influence that impairs the forces of life and brings about the abnormal conditions which necessitate disease (unusual vital action) for its correction, will, if not corrected, impede, or perhaps, prevent recovery. Any influences that produce disease in the well person, if brought to bear upon the sick will impede or prevent recovery. The less pathoferic any influence, the less it impedes or prevents recovery, and, therefore, the greater the percentage of recoveries that will be made under it.

Here is a principle, then, we may apply to therapeutics and if the results of these as recorded in medical history confirm it, we can be certain that it does make a difference in the results what methods of treating the sick are employed. And we shall see that it does make a vast difference in the death rate as well as in the number of chronic cases, what methods are employed. In the light, however, of what has gone before, we would say that the death rate is less under some methods than under others, not because they cure more, but because they kill less. To illustrate my meaning, let me say that more cases of typhoid fever recover under hydrotherapy than did under the old method of bleeding, purging, puking, stuffing, and giving brandy, opium, antimony, mercury, with no water and no fresh air. And this is true, not because hydrotherapy cures typhoid fever, but because it kills less patients than the old method.

Suppose, while we are dealing with typhoid we look at a few facts in relation to the results secured under two different methods of treatment and determine once for all if it makes any difference in results whether the methods employed are beneficial, or harmful, or merely indifferent.

The records of the Board of Health, New York (1876 to 1885) show 7,712 cases of typhoid, with 184 deaths or 42 deaths out of every 100 cases. The mortality from this disease in the city hospitals from 1878 to 1885 averaged 24.66 per cent, or a trifle less than 25 deaths out of every 100 cases. In 1861 the death rate from this disease in Germany is given at as 21 per cent. This rate continued under medical treatment. The water cure people were, at this time, treating typhoid with a death rate of from 4 to 5 per cent. This was noticed by Dr. Brandt, a German regular who was losing the regular 21 per cent of his cases. He therefore adopted the water cure with the result that he also lost only about 4 to 6 per cent of his typhoid cases.

Liebermeister, Brandt, Ziemsen and others a few years later showed that the typhoid mortality rate in Germany had been reduced to 7 per cent by the general adoption of hydrotherapy. The basis of this was 19,017 carefully gathered cases of typhoid fever. Later Brandt obtained from twenty-three German and French sources, aggregating 5,573 cases, statistics showing that the method advocated by him in 1881 had reduced the mortality rate in typhoid to four per cent. It was claimed that there were many badly managed cases among these, so they were eliminated leaving 1,223 cases treated up to 1887 by Juergensen, Vogl and Brandt of which only 12 died, or one per cent. It was also claimed that not one of these 12 deaths occurred in any case that came under treatment before the fifth day of the disease. Brandt himself treated one-fourth of these 1,223 cases.

362

These figures came from University clinics and Military hospitals and reveal a drop in the death rate in typhoid from 25 per cent to 42 per cent under the old drug plan to 4 per cent or less under the water cure. Is it any wonder, then, that the German medical profession was unable to stay the rising tide of water as it gushed forth from the fountains of Preissnitz, Rausse, Hahn, Kneipp, Bilz, Kuhne and the few medical men who also adopted it? With such a difference, too, in the results of such treatment, can we not overlook the mistake of these men in attributing to water curative powers which it does not possess?

The results in other diseases were about the same. In fact, the results of this change of methods were often so great in other diseases as to eclipse the results in typhoid. By far, the greater portion of those who sought relief from the water-cure establishments were old chronic cases that had been under medical treatment for years and had been, in a majority of cases, pronounced incurable. It was in "curing" such cases as these that the water-cure first obtained its reputation.

It may be argued that water did cure those cases, or, at least, that it aided the cure. Such an argument is illogical in the light of the facts that have gone before and the principles that have been developed in previous chapters. However, since I do not expect the average drugless physician any more than the average drug giver to reason logically, for they always reason from appearances in utter neglect of underlying principles, I will pause here for a minute to answer this argument. Perhaps the best answer is to be found in the experiments of Dr. Magendie, the justly famous French physiologist, which he performed at an earlier date. These have been mentioned before but will bear repetition here. He divided his typhoid-fever patients into two classes. To one class he prescribed according to the medical practice of his day. Of the patients thus treated he lost the usual proportion, or about one-fourth. To the other class he gave no medicine at all depending entirely upon hygiene and nursing. Of this class he lost none. Nor did he select his cases. He lost none in this latter class whether he got them before or after the fifth day of the disease. Is there any wonder, then, that he said in a lecture before his medical class: "Gentlemen, medicine is a great humbug?"

If 100 per cent of typhoid cases recover without any treatment of any kind and 5 per cent die under water cure treatment and 25 per cent to 40 per cent die under the old drug treatment, is it not right to say that drugs kill 25 per cent to 40 per cent and water kills 5 per cent?

I do not believe we can escape this conclusion, even, if we reason as the average physician reasons. He reasons that the methods employed are responsible for the results —that if a patient is treated in such and such a manner and recovers, the treatment cured him. *Results prove it.* The logic in the reverse direction is equally as good. If a patient is treated by these same methods and dies, the treatment killed him. *Results prove it.* One position is as logical as the other and the latter one is in strict accord with the facts.

Let us, then, develop more specifically the conditions of cure. In doing this I shall break them up into four general groups, the first three of which were given by Dr. Walter, in *Life's Great Law,* and then subdivide these as the subject seems to demand. They follow:—

1. "THE REMOVAL OF THE OCCASIONS OF THE DISEASE." Dr. Walter correctly observed that vital power is the cause of disease, cause being defined as the power by which a thing is, while agents and conditions that are usually called causes, he called occasions or conditions of disease. It should be obvious to all that if we persist in supplying the conditions of disease, the disease will most surely persist, even though its form may be changed or the symptoms suppressed, by treatment.

By virtue of the living organism's inherent power of self-repair and self-maintenance, all the healing that is ever done is accomplished when the causes of the damage are corrected or removed.

As an example, let us consider the common accident happening to those engaged in certain trades—the mashing of a finger or thumb. It results in a painful bruise, with inflammation, discoloration and an effusion of blood under the surface. The tissues are mangled and broken and many of the cells die, while many of the red blood corpuscles are killed. But this condition does not remain forever. In just a few days the work of repair has been accomplished. The tissues are repaired, the dead cells are absorbed and carried away, the inflammation subsides, the pain ceases and the matter is forgotten. This work of cure and repair is all accomplished by the processes and functions of the organism and is carried out in a skillful and admirable manner. No drugs, no serums, no adjustments, electrical currents, baths, packs, etc. are needed. None could help. No one but a fool would, after mashing his finger, bandage it up in linament or ointment or use some form of drugless treatment, and resume mashing his finger and expect the finger ever to heal. It can never recover until the mashing is ceased. When this is done it will speedily and quickly heal without treatment.

This simple fact is applicable to all the disorders to which our system is susceptible. Take, for instanec, the man who, by gross dietetic habits, or by indulgence in alcohol, or in some other way has weakened his digestive powers so that he is no longer able to digest his food. He can no more recover from this condition through treatment, drug or drugless, while continuing the abuse than he can fly. Yet this is the very thing he will attempt to do, if he is an average man, and the healers of all schools save the Nature Cure or Orthopathic, encourage him in it. Mr. Average man goes down to the corner drug store, buys a bottle of Dr. Dopem's Syrup Pepsin, shakes it well before taking and goes right on in the same old manner. He does not correct the habits of life that are responsible for his condition. He expects the drugs, or, if he employs some drugless practitioner, the metaphysical formula or the adjustment, to cure him in spite of his pathoferic habits.

He may succeed in palliating his condition for a time but real cure has never been accomplished in this way. Nature demands that cause be removed first, and then, she can do her own curing. If the individual gives up the abuse of his digestive organs they will recover without treatment. If he persists in his evil practices, no amount of treatment, whatever its nature, can save him from the consequences. All that nature asks, or can receive, from human skill in disease conditions, is the removal of disturbing causes, after which, she will of her own accord, as naturally as a stone returns to earth, return to health. Repair of tissue, elimination of toxins and recuperation of health are specialties of the vital power working through the organs and functions of a living organism. Given an opportunity, this work is done well. Success often comes in spite of obstructive and destructive treatment.

Therefore, we are safe in concluding that disease is not only due in the first place, to disturbing causes, but that it is perpetuated by the continuance of such causes. We do not deny that when such morbid elements have brought about a change of structure in the organism, this, while it remains, will, in the absence of pathoferic causes, keep up the abnormal action to a greater or less extent, but we may set it down, as a general rule, that in chronic disease where degenerative changes have not advanced too far for vital redemption, the disease action will not continue long after the complete removal of the primary cause. Hence, chronic disease is in almost every case, perpetuated from day to day and from year to year by the continued action of the disturbing influence. Chronic disease represents chronic provocation.

Any attempt to cure a disease without removing the pathoferic influence is rank folly. Take, for instance, the prevailing methods by which it is sought to purify the blood. Some method is employed to whip up the activities of the eliminating organs. It is like the attempt to dip a fountain dry without cutting off the water supply. One dips and dips until exhausted only to find that as much water exists in the fountain as before. Likewise, when the eliminating organs are made to work overtime by some drug or drugless method, and the source of the impurities is not cut off, these organs are soon exhausted and the blood stream is as foul as before. Such methods may whip up the eliminating and other organs and produce a temporary semblance of health, but the exhaustion following such treatment soon permits the victim to become worse than before.

Breaking this requirement of cure up into two subdivisions we must:—

(a) CORRECT ALL ENERVATING PRACTICES AND INFLUENCES. This is a necessity both in *primary* and *secondary* diseases, although nature herself corrects as many of these as relate to the individual himself, in the primary *diseases*.

Let us notice these a bit further. Why should enervating practices and influences be corrected? Because these are the remote causes of the trouble. These have brought on the enervation responsible for the lowering of organic function. So long as these are continued the enervation must continue. Thep prevent recuperation. So long as enervation lasts elimination and drainage will be faulty. Recovery, real lasting recovery, is impossible under such conditions.

How are such habits and influences corrected? By stopping them. Suppose the patient is addicted to the use of stimulants, correct such a habit by withholding the stimulants. Suppose he is being forced to expend his nervous energy resisting cold. He is chilled. Correct such influence by supplying him with warmth. If it is an acute disease the patient will be forced to remain in bed, he cannot be spending his nights in revelry but the chronic sufferer may be doing this very thing. It must be stopped.

(b) STOP THE ABSORPTION OF ANY AND ALL POISONS FROM WITHOUT. Diseases are due to poisons and so long as these are entering the body from any source they will be added to the poisons already present and thus add to and complicate the disease. Drugs thus add to and complicate the disease. Drugs, serums and vaccines are equal offenders, in this respect, with other poisons, of whatever nature. These add to the toxemia further poisoning the body and building complications. Toxemia is the condition immediately responsible for the disease. This is the condition the body is seeking to throw off, eliminate. This can be accomplished much sooner, much easier if we stop adding to the toxins already in the system.

How is this done? By stopping their intake. Suppose the patient is in the habit of absorbing alcoholic drinks or opium, or is using drugs of some nature for his trouble. Stop their use immediately. Perhaps there is a pent up wound. Clean it out and supply proper drainage. Or there is gastro-intestinal putrefaction. This is a common and also the most abundant source of toxic absorption. In fact every case of disease with which we deal, if not due to accident, has this as a contributory cause.

Immediate steps should be taken to cleanse the alimentary canal. All food but water should be stopped. Refer to chapter on fasting.

2. "THE SUPPLYING OF THE CONDITIONS FOR HEALTH." In other words supply any element or condition required by nature for the comfort of the patient, or that is needed by the vital forces in the work of cure. The elements of an unbounded success are wrapped up in the Orthopathic doctrine of health by healthful living and hygienic measures are entitled to be applied in the care of the sick just as surely as to the maintenance or even the recovery of health. If health is to be restored the conditions of health must be supplied.

Health by healthful living is the only correct practice and applies to the sick as truly as to the well. It is the true plan of regaining as well as of maintaining health. A mode of living, not a plan of treatment is the road to health. Both the power and instinct of repair are inherent in the living organism and these will restore all lesions and heal all diseases, provided only that the conditions of health are supplied.

After pointing out that the elements of nutrition—warmth, moisture, food, exercise, etc,—are the requirements of health, growth and maintenance, Dr. Densmore says:—

"This is a universal law in organic life, as applicable to a grass plot or a tree as to the organism of an animal. If a grass-plot has sunshine, warmth, moisture, and fertility (or food), there is health and growth. If food or moisture or warmth be taken away, there is sickness; and if continued, there is death. No medicine is needed to secure a restoration of health and vigor to the plant that has thus been made ill; all that is necessary is to supply any or all of the lacking elements of nutrition—light, warmth, moisture, or food.

"It is a universal law of organic life, be it vegetable or animal, that all tendencies are toward health. It is as natural to be well as it is to be born.

Note the grass-plot before instanced. It may be ever so brown from the summer sun and drought, or scarcity of fertility; if disorganization be not already set in, if there yet be life, all that is needed to restore the beautiful green color and vigorous growth to the grass is to supply it with whatever elements of nutrition it has been deprived of— sunshine, warmth, rain, or fertility—and it at once begins to mend; in a few weeks green blades have take the place of seared ones, and in a short time there is often no trace of the previous lack of vigor.

365

"As for the grass-plot, it is quite universally known that growth and vigor always follow upon a supply of the necessary conditions— sunshine, warmth, moisture, and food. If from the outset the plant has had these necessaries, an unvarying vigor results; if the gardener perceives a failing color in the plant, or any other sign of disease, he knows that some of the necessary conditions of grass life are lacking. If this inquiry be extended to an examination of the more complex forms of life, it will be found that the same law obtains. The fishes of the sea, the birds of the air, and the wild animals of the wood are quite usually found in perfect health and vigour. When the fisherman or the hunter finds an exception to this rule, he knows at once that some of the normal conditions of animal life has been wanting; there has been a lack (in the absence of poison or injury from violence) of food, or water or light, or warmth.

"It will be seen after the most searching scrutiny from whatever point of view, that a tendency toward an abounding health and vigour is inseparable from life; and, moreover, whenever and wherever the normal conditions of healthy life have been interfered with, and weakness, lassitude, or any of the symptoms of ill-health appear, as soon as the conditions natural to the organism are restored, a movement toward health is always sure to follow.

"The law of cure may be defined as the unfailing tendency on the part of the living organism toward health; and since disease; as above defined, is but the expression and result of a disturbance of the conditions natural to life, the only useful office of the physician is to restore those conditions; and there will be seen to follow, as a result of the law of cure, the disappearance of disease and the establishment of Health."—How Nature Cures, p. 4-6-7-8.

How different from this is the usual practice! The physician is the creature of his education, and his treatment is sure not only not to follow hygienic methods but to rely upon drugs, for, he feels called upon to interfere with the working of nature. He builds more and more complications as his treatment continues. The impropriety of calling such a harmful force into the household should be plainly evident.

A "change of symptoms," says Dr. Walter, "is what is usually sought and generally obtained, whether the patient gets well or not. Medical treatment consists in doctoring symptoms. The physician hears little but a detail of symptoms. The patient talks of little else to the doctor; it is the one thing that the doctor is expected to remove. And most physicians become expert in doing it, even though hardly two will be found who will prescribe the same medicines unless, indeed, we may except the homeopath."—Life's Great Law, p. 177.

The Orthopathic way is to ignore the symptoms and give attention to the hygienic needs of the patient. These are as follows:—

FOOD: Feed in accordance with the demands of the body for and its ability to digest and assimilate food. This rule applies to chronic disease and to the period of convalescence following an acute disease. No feeding is to be done during an acute process. Stuffing the chronic sufferer, as is often done, is an evil and prevents recovery.

FASTING: Partake of no food so long as acute symptoms are present and for twenty-four to forty-eight hours thereafter. So long as these symptoms continue digestive power is lacking. Secretion is at a standstill. To feed under such conditions only adds to the sufferings of the patient. In cases where there has been much inflammation and possible necrosis of the digestive tract do not feed until healing has occurred.

QUIET: Absolute quiet should be secured as far as this is possible. When an animal becomes sick it seeks a quiet, secluded, sheltered spot and lies down. It takes no food and but little water. Rest, quiet, fasting and a little water, as instinct demands, are its remedies. Noise is enervating. It irritates and annoys. It disturbs rest and sleep and hinders recuperation—no one should be permitted in the sick room except those who are attending to the patient. Loud talking, heavy walking, etc., should be avoided.

POISE: Mental poise is one of the greatest aids to recovery. Fear, anxiety, self-pity, etc., are all destructive and hinder recovery. The attendants and relatives should also remain poised. Neither by word, look or deed should they show anxiety or apprehension to the patient. *Poise is essential in both acute and chronic diseases.* The sick room should not be converted into a visiting rendezvous, where people congregate and discuss cases of sickness and recount the sufferings of themselves or of someone else.

WARMTH: *Do not permit yourself to become chilled.* Chilling checks elimination and adds to the discomfort. The extremeties especially, and the feet in particular must be prevented from chilling. In low states of disease the whole body must be safeguarded. If fever is present there is little danger of chilling, except in the coldest weather. On the contrary, a cool draught of air playing over the body is comforting and restful. Hot bricks or bottles to the feet are usually sufficient to prevent chilling.

PHYSICAL COMFORT: *The sick person should be made physically as comfortable as possible.* Florence Nightingale said: "In watching disease, both in private houses and in public hospitals, the thing which strikes the experienced observer most forcibly is this, that the symptoms or the sufferings generally considered to be inevitable and incident to the disease are very often not symptoms of the disease at all, but of something qiute different—of the want of fresh air, or of light, or of warmth or of quiet, or of cleanliness, etc., **** when you have done away with all that pain and suffering, which in patients are the symptoms not of their disease, but of the absence of one or all of the above-mentioned processes, we shall then know what are the symptoms of and the sufferings inseparable from the disease."

The patient should be in a quiet, well lighted, well aired room; on a hard, comfortable mattress, covered not too heavily (heavy covers are uncomfortable and enervating), and kept warm. The bed should be changed as often as cleanliness demands and the linen kept straight. Blankets are better than quilts or comforts for covering for two reasons. First, they can be washed; and second, being porous, they permit the escape of the emenations from the patient's body.

AIR: *Keep the windows open.* The room in which the sick are housed should be well ventilated from the outside. Air coming in from another room or from a hall is not good. Often these other rooms are kept closed except at such times. Hallways are often long, dark and foul. The air in the sick room should be as pure as possible. It should not come from an insanitary court yard, or chicken yard, or cow lot. The purest air of the great outdoors is none too pure. The patient should not be forced to breathe over and over again the excretions from his own lungs and body, nor from the lungs of another. Gas stoves and oil stoves should be kept out of the sick room. FRESH AIR IS THE GREATEST NEED.

Smoking in the sick room should be prohibited. Neither the patient nor anyone else should be permitted to smoke. The patient should also be placed in a room where the rugs, curtains, wall-paper, closets, etc., of which, have not been saturated with tobacco smoke from long-continuance of the vulgar habit of smoking in the house. Medical men commonly permit their sick patients to smoke. They believe in "cure," however, and know of no reason why they should stop, "nerve-leaks" and cut off all sources of poisoning. Trall truly declared: "Many an infant has been killed outright in the cradle by the tobacco smoke with which a thoughtless father has filled an unventilated room."

WATER: *Drink water as often as demanded by natural, unstimulated thirst.* Water need not be taken beyond the instinctive demands of the body. Drinking copiously of water on the theory that it increases elimination is a delusion. Excessive water drinking is harmful.

Few people ever heard of "water intoxication." This is because it is difficult to produce. Thirst normally regulates the intake of water to the body's needs. Unless it is consumed greatly in excess the kidneys and skin excrete the surplus. However, by inducing an unquenchable thirst so that an individual was kept drinking water, he developed "marked headache, nausea, a staggering gait, unsteadiness of muscle and inability to stand or walk, which lasted for a few hours."

Cats, rabbits and guinea pigs, forced to drink of water, "an ounce per pound of body weight every hour," were "also sent on a dangerous water jag." In spite of the excess water drinking, the amount absorbed was definitely limited. Blood pressure was increased. "The convulsions of water poisoning are cerebral in origin and of extreme violence at times, usually lasting from one to ten or fifteen minutes.**** All the symptoms of uremia can be experimentally induced by excessive water."

Water does not "flush" the system as is claimed. It does not increase elimination. of toxins and solids. More urine or more sweat, measured as to volume, is excreted, but it is "more water." Thirst indicates when water is required.

SUNLIGHT: *A well lighted room is essential to the comfort and most rapid progress of the sick.* Nothing more effectively purifies and "sweetens" the atmosphere of a room than sunlight. It also has a comforting, cheering effect upon the mind of the patient. It does not harm the eyes, not even in measles. Sunlight is a stimulant and should not play too strongly on the acute patient. Nature indicates that a slightly shaded place is best.

Sunlight is an indespensible factor in plant and animal nutrition. Some chronic diseases like rickets, anemia, tuberculosis, scrofula, etc., do not get well without sunshine. It is in chronic diseases that the sun-bath is of such great importance.

CLEANLINESS: *The patient, his clothes, his bed, the room and everything that comes in contact with the patient, or the patient's environment should be scrupulously clean.* This has no reference to sterilization, antiseptics, listerism, etc. The patient may be sponged with plain luke-warm water as often as necessary. His hands and face may be washed in plain water. The eyes, nose and mouth should be washed in plain water, or, at most, a little lemon juice may be added to the water. Soaps, antiseptics, mouth washes, gargles, etc., are unnecessary and often harmful. If the mouth and throat are to be cleaned, dilute lemon juice, or dilute pineapple juice are preferable, as cleansing agents, to drugs. The same is true in cleansing the other orifices of the body, eyes, nose, arms, vagina, etc.—or in cleaning a wound.

The patient's clothes and the bed linen should be changed as often as cleanliness demands. Slop jars, bed pans, etc., should not be left sitting under the bed. Empty and clean them immediately after using and set them out of the room. Sunshine and a constant stream of fresh air will insure atmospheric cleanliness.

EXERCISE: *No exercise should be indulged in during an acute disease. During convalescence exercise should be mild and graduated. In chronic disease, exercise within the powers of the patient is indespensible.* Nature plainly indicates that rest and not exercise is the need in acute disease. In chronic disease exercise adapted to the individual needs should be taken daily where strength will permit, and gradually increased in both vigor and amount as the strength of the sufferer increases.

3. "THE ACCUMULATION OR RECUPERATION OF THE VITAL OR HEALING POWER." This can only be accomplished by giving the organism an oppotrunity to recuperate its vitality. Two factors are concerned:—

- (a) Correction of all influences that occasion the waste of power. This was discussed under *a* of No. 1.

(b) Supplying the body and mind with rest, relaxation and sleep in order to recuperation. This was fully covered in the chapter and rest but will be briefly discussed at this point.

Jennings wrote:—

"The great object to be steadily aimed at in all cases of sickness, is to favor the renovating process which is in constant progression within. *Rest, quiet, is the great remedy.* Let there be no unnecessary expenditure of vital funds, either through mental exercise, or any undue exercise of the bodily functions. When there is a disposition to sleep, let it be indulged. And as there is no medicine to be given by the hour, sleep may be protracted to any length, unless it is laborious, then a slight jog, or a little change of position, or a swallow of water, will start it in its regular train again."— *Tree of Life,* p. 187.

If enervation is to be overcome and normal function re-established recuperation is essential. Recuperation occurs only during rest. There is a sense in which a change is rest but it not true rest. A man may change from one form of activity to another and keep this up continuously without stopping until he "rests" himself into exhaustion. True rest is secured only by reducing function and by stopping temporarily all function that can be stopped without harm.

This is accomplished by all of the following:—

(1) By stopping the habits and indulgencies that increase function (stimulating habits).

(2) By ceasing physical effort.

(3) By ceasing mental effort.

(4) By reducing physiological effort. Physiological effort is reduced by correcting those habits that stimulate function, by stopping mental and physical effort and by either stopping the food intake entirely or by at least reducing it to a minimum.

Rest and sleep conserve energy and permit recuperation. Work—mental, emotional, physical and physiological—expends energy. Tonics and stimulants increase function causing an increased expenditure of energy.

It is said that to compel a man to maintain the erect position, even during sleep, produces the most painful death that the genius of torture can devise. It rapidly exhausts. It completely exhausts the heart which must continue to pump the blood against gravity. The recumbent position, in which the blood circulates pretty nearly on a level, is, therefore, a wonderful relief to the over-burdened heart. This relief was thought by Dr. Walter to be the most valuable part of sleep. It was largely to secure this relief that he sent his patients to bed to rest.

Of course the withdrawal of stimulation and the cessation of physical activity and control of the passions and emotions afford the heart as well as the rest of the body an opportunity for rest. But there is another means of resting the heart and the other organs of the body which was much insisted upon by Walter.

The heart is the great central organ of circulation. The blood moves in a circle, returning to the heart and being pumped out again. The more food one consumes the greater is the work of the heart and other organs of the body. The less food consumed the less the heart must work. By reducing the amount of food consumed, or by fasting the heart is given a rest. Heart-failure often follows a hearty meal. Dr. Walter said:—

"Fifty years ago the term 'heart-failure' was unknown; bleeding and purging had been so constantly relieving the blood of its nutritive materials, and relieving the heart of its burdens that death seldom occurred from failure of the heart's action; today the term is a common one, due, as the reader will surely see, to the theory that food is nutrition, and, therefore, the blood must be loaded and the heart burdened with material which the tissues cannot appropriate. Stuffing and stimulating patients during the progress of acute diseases, even of those who are in good health, beyond their power to appropriate the food, is, we believe, he chief reason for the heart-failures of today."—*Life's Great Law*, p. 204-5.

But to reduce the food intake is to materially rest every other organ and function in the body. Man needs food with which to build his body, but the power to build is of greater importance. Reduced nutrition in spite of the habitual consumption of large quantities of food is an ever-present fact in our existence. Increased nutrition following upon a reduction of food is becoming equally as common as people learn the facts of life. Rest of the organs of the body, through reducing the food consumed, recuperates power and improves nutrition.

4. TIME, IS THE NEXT GREAT REQUISITE IN ALL DISEASES. This is demanded by the physicians of all schools. Some have claimed they could cure instantly or almost instantly and we shall discuss these claims here.

Dr. Richard C. Cabot asks:—

"If nature, assisted by the proper mental and emotional moods, is capable of curing an ulcer in three or four weeks, why isn't it possible for the same force to heal a similar ulcer in a few minutes, when the curative processes have been speeded up abnormally by the subject's passing through an intense religious experience?"

To put this question a little differently. If nature, assisted by warmth and moisture, is capable of hatching a chicken in three weeks, why isn't it possible for the same force to hatch a similar chicken in a few minutes when the evolutionary processes have been speeded abnormally up by passing through an intense stimulating experience?

Dr. Cabot's question is absurd. It assumes that instantaneous healing is a possibility and wholly ignores all the facts of pathology and tissue regeneration now known. Cure is an evolution in reverse and no more takes place instantaneously, than a chicken can be hatched instantaneously.

I am well aware that many apparent cures of long standing chronic conditions have occurred. Emil Coue registered a few such when he exploited American credulity a few years ago. Daddy Flynn did the same thing before he died. Many others have done likewise. Most of these apparent cures are not cures at all and only last a few days or a few hours.

In those that were permanent, there was, back of each of them weeks, months and years during which the silent creative processes of the organism had been doing their curative work. The really essential work of cure had been accomplished before the miracle monger came along.

Dr. Tilden well declared, A Stuffed Club, June 1913, "Disease is an evolution; it is not an infection; it is not a subtle entity that gains entrance into a healthy body and destroys health and life.**** Disease in its development obeys the same laws that govern gestation, growth, education, crystalization, ossification, fossilization, etc."

Health is subject to and controlled by the same laws. Health must be evolved, as Dr. Dewey well said: "Cure is an evolutoin in reverse." The evolution of health requires time. Disease is a development—cure must be a development. As well expect to cure disease instantaneously, or even in a few days, as to expect to hatch chickens in a few minutes.

A common mistake is to regard disease as cured and health restored when the symptoms have ceased. In reality the patient is in just the same condition he was just prior to their appearance. It is still a long way back to full health. There is much road that must again be traversed before one arrives at the health which he enjoyed before he began the evolution of his sufferings. Man regards the appearance of symptoms as the beginning of disease and their disappearance as its end; and each new appearance of symptoms of disease as a new disease, instead of merely new incidents in one general and continuous condition. So long as these mistaken notions of disease are entertained he will be the prey of fakers and exploiters who will profit off his ignorance.

Time is an indespensible element in all cures. If the necessary time has not elapsed before the employment of the "cure," it must elapse during the "cure." This is because nature does her work slowly not rapidly—instantaneously. Forces that have been slowly gathered may be suddenly loosed and rend a mountain but no sudden losing of force could grow and mature a tree. In the animal organism forces that have been slowly and silently accumulating for years may be suddenly loosed, either spontaneously or in response to some external influence but time is assuredly required for their accumulation.

An excellent example, showing the necessity for time, is the childhood affliction of Selma Lagerlof, winner of the Nobel Price in literature, an account of which was published a few years ago in the New York Times. When a child she developed "hip disease" and lost the use of her limbs. After a year of such illness she was taken to the baths in Stromstad in the hope of effecting a cure. The account does not state how long she remained at Stromstad but it does say that the baths did her little good.

Sometime later, upon hearing that the husband of a family friend—a sea captain —was returning home and bringing with him a bird of paradise, she wanted to go and see the bird. The family visited the ship in the harbor. The sailors carried the helpless child up the narrow gangway, the rest of the family following, and left her alone on the high deck. At first she was afraid at being left alone, but seeing the cabin boy she asked him where the bird was. He replied: "In the captain's cabin; come down these steps; I'll show you the way."

She followed him down the steps and into the captain's cabin. In a few minutes her alarmed parents, followed by all the others, including the captain, rushed in and found her kneeling upon the table gazing at the mounted bird. "How did you get here?" came simultaneously from the lips of the wonder struck and amazed crowd. It was not until then that she realized that she had walked unaided down the stairway and into the cabin. She was then asked to come down off the table and let them see if she could walk. Slowly she crawled down from the table onto a chair and from the chair onto the floor and proved that she could both stand and walk.

No reasoning person would contend that the same circumstances would have enabled her to walk a year or six months before. The process of reparation in the domain of life, like growth and development, is slow, silent, gradual and almost imperceptible so that the return to firm and vigorous health requires weeks, months or even years, and is influenced favorably or unfavorably by every circumstance and habit of life.

Remedial efforts are always going on in the organism when it is in any way morbidly affected. This is true even in those cases where the morbid influence is unknown to the individual and its effects are still so slight as to be unnoticed by him. When these morbid influences are greater than the organism can overcome their effects pile up until a formidable condition develops. The efforts of the organism are disproportionately manifest in one or more parts of the body or at one or more of eliminating organs and we call this, disease. That the living organism, by virtue of its own inherent powers, does purge itself of impurities and repair its damages is no longer a matter of doubt. That its curative efforts are sometimes disproportionately directed to one or more organs of the body and is accompanied with more or less systemic commotion is equally as certain.

But no remedial effort, however vigorous and powerful, is capable of producing an instantaneous cure. Take a look at the condition of the average sick body and you can readily see that such is impossible. There is more or less vital and nervous depletion with a consequent functional impairment of all the organs of the body; the blood and tissues are saturated with toxins; there is more or less destruction of tissue in all parts of the body, more in some parts than others; some parts of the body are engorged, congested, inflamed, while other parts are anemic; perhaps in some parts there are deposits, while some organs are more impaired than others; secretion and excretion are greatly impaired, perhaps in some instances almost wholly suspended; digestion is impaired, there is constipation or diarrhea, a sluggish circulation. In many cases there is some form of degeneration of one or more organs or the degeneration is more or less general; there may be degeneration of some of the nerves or a sclerosis in the spine; hardening (sclerosis) of the arteries and liver, perhaps, even, the formation of scar tissue in the brain.

It is not possible for this condition to be overcome instantly. It requires time for the body to heal a broken bone or a flesh wound and no one would pretend that his method could bring about an instantaneous healing of these. Just so it requires time to clean out such a condition as we have described above and return to normal and usually it requires more time to do so than to heal a broken bone or a flesh wound. No organism can cleanse itself of its morbid matter instantly, nor can it repair its damaged tissues or regenerate its atrophied and degenerated parts instantly. Hypertrophied parts cannot be instantly reduced to their normal size. Normal secretion and excretion are not instantly re-established nor is recuperation of vital force accomplished instantly.

It does not matter what the conditions are, time is a required element. Those mind cures, faith cures, etc., that appear to be instantaneous and that are permanent can occur only in those patients where the actual work of cure is already accomplished. The really essential part of the cure is accomplished before the "healer" comes along. Cases that are "cured" temporarily are cases in which nature has not completed her work of cure while those cases that the healer fails on are cases where the work of cure has not advanced very far, or perhaps, they are cases in which the destruction of vital parts has advanced too far for vital redemption—in which the functioning tissue has been replaced by connective or other tissue. Instantaneous cures, are only apparently so. The process of recovery from the effects of years of wrong living, is no instantaneous process, but a gradual evolution back to normal health. And truly it is "influenced favorably or adversely by every circumstance and habit of life," as Dr. Trall has so admirably shown in the following quotation:—

"I may here, perhaps, make a remark, en passant, of some practical importance. It is with all schools of medicine as it is with each individual practitioner of the healing art—the less faith they have in medicine, the more they have in Hygiene; hence those who prescribe little or no medicine, are invaribly and necessarily more attentive to Hygienic conditions—to good nursing—which always was, and ever will be all that is really good, useful, or curative in medication. Such physicians are more careful to supply the vital organism with whatever of air, light, temperature, food, water, exercise, or rest, etc., it needs in its struggle for health, and to remove all vitiating influences—

371

all poisons, impurities, miasms, or disturbing influences of any kind. And this is Hygienic Medication; this is the True Healing Art. Nor God nor Nature has provided any other; nor can the Supreme Architect permit any other without reversing all the laws of the universe, and annulling everyone of His attributes, as I expect to make clear in due time."—*True Healing Art.*

THE HYGIENE OF HEALTH
CHAPTER XXVIII

HYGIENE is that branch of biology that relates to the preservation and restoration of health. Bionomy is the science of the laws of living functions; or that branch of biology which treats of habits and adaptation. Orthobionomics is a word I have coined to designate the correct adaptation of life and environment to each other.

The hygiene of health and the hygiene of disease is one. However, for convenience, we divide it into *Preventive Hygiene*, or the *hygiene of healthful maintenance*, and *Remedial Hygiene*, or the *hygiene of health restoration*.

By *Preventive Hygiene* is meant the intelligent employment of hygienic principles, forces and agencies for the maintenance of functional and structural integrity.

By *Remedial Hygiene* is understood the intelligent employment of hygienic principles, forces and agencies for the restoration of sound health.

"There must be a way to live exactly right, which, if a man does, he will grow into health," said a young school-teacher to himself some years ago. He was beginning to despair of his life because every doctor to whom he went diagnosed his case differently and proceeded to make him much worse than ever. Then began a long series of experiments upon his own body, and years of study of the subjects that relate to health and disease. That man, young Robert Walter, later became one of the leaders in the nature cure or hygienic movement. Like many others who have turned to hygiene he was forced to study the matter out for himself because physicians are interested in disease and not in living. .

A soap-box lecturer was once entertaining a crowd on Broadway in New York City. He told the following story:—

"The superintendent of an institution for the feeble-minded sent an inmate into the basement to mop up the water from a faucet that accidently had been left running. Later in the day the man was found mopping with the water still running full blast. 'You darned idiot, why don't you turn off the faucet,' shouted the superintendent. The simpleton grinned and replied: 'Nobody's paying me to turn 'er off. I'm gettin two bits an hour to mop 'er up."

When the roar that greeted this jibe at the medical profession had subsided, the speaker continued: "The land is flooded with sickness which flows from ignorance of nature's laws. Proper instruction would shut off disease at its source, but if doctors turned off the tap, they would put themselves out of a job."

Nobody pays the medical profession to "turn 'er off," they get "two bits an hour to mop 'er up."

Physiology, alone, can teach us how man must live in order to secure the best health and attain to the greatest age of which the human constitution is capable. The fact that there are individuals now living a hundred years old, proves that the human constitution is capable of sustaining life a hundred years at least, and perhaps much longer, if the mode of life is, in all respects, correct. Here we shall probably be met with the very ancient and utterly absurd doctrine, that there are different constitutions, and therefore, that what may be true of one, cannot truly be affirmed of all. What is one man's elixir is another man's bane. We freely admit that, in the present state of mankind, some individuals have more vital energy and constitutional power to resist the causes of disease and death than others have, and therefore, what will break down the constitution and destroy the life of some individuals, may be borne by others a much longer time without any striking manifestations of immediate injury. Some can withstand more abuse than others. It is also true that, in the present state of man, some individuals have strongly marked idiosyncrasies or peculiarities; but these are far more rare and of a much less important character than is generally supposed, and in no instance do they constitute the slightest exception to the general laws of life, nor in any degree interfere with, or militate against, the correct principles of a general regimen. Indeed, such peculiarities, though really constitutional, may in almost every case be overcome entirely by a correct regime. "I have frequently," says Graham, "seen the most strongly marked cases completely subdued by such means. It is an incontrovertible truth, therefore, that so far as the general laws of life and the application of the general principles of regimen are considered, the human constitution is ONE; and there are no constitutional differences in the human race which will not readily yield to a correct regimen, and by thus yielding improve the condition of the individual affected; and consequently, there are no constitutional differences in the human race which stand in the way of adopting one general regimen to the whole family of man; but, on the contrary, it is most strictly true that, so far as the general laws of life and the application of general principles of regimen are considered, what may be truly affirmed of one man may be truly affirmed of all, and what is best for one is best for all; and therefore, all general reasonings concerning the human constitution, are equally applicable to each and every member of the human family, in all ages of the world, and in all conditions of the race, and in all the various circumstances of the individual."

All of which simply means that what is truly a healthful life for Mr. Smith is equally healthful for Mr. Jones. But it does not follow that because Smith, with a much more powerful constitution than Jones, resists the influence of a disease building regimen longer than Jones, that what is Smith's meat is Jones' poison. It only shows that due to the differences in their constitutional strength, not to any differences in their constitutional nature, it requires more poison to kill Smith than to kill Jones. But the essential point which Mr. Graham, and so far as we are aware, all subsequent writers on this subject, overlooked is that, we are not trying to fit an unhealthful regime to Jones and get him to live as long as Smith under the same unhealthful regime; but we are attempting to fit a regime that is essentially healthful to all—we would remove, as far as possible, the causes of disease that the constitutional powers of both men are forced to resist. We seek to accomplish this in a strictly natural way for as Graham pointed out, artificial means are all harmful.

It would be impossible for two men with equally excellent constitutions, to reach an equally advanced age, with habits of life exactly opposite, without a very marked and apparent difference in condition and appearance of both body and mind. *It is not possible for two men of equally excellent constitutions to start out in life and follow such equally opposite courses and arrive at the same goal.*

That a life just lived as it happened, filled with numerous and various excesses, would enable a man to reach the hundred mark in as good mental and physical condition as another would be in, at the same age, who had led a temperate and well ordered life, is absurd on the face of it. To believe such is to believe that life is subject to no law, that man is at the mercy of fortuitous circumstances or a capricious Providence; that hygiene and sanitation are valueless, inebriety is as good as temperance, gluttony as salubrious as moderation, sensuality as healthful as virtue, impurity and nastiness as beneficial as purity and cleanliness, chaos as approved as order. Are we to believe that there are no rules of health—no laws governing life? Or, are we to believe that, if such laws do exist, they are not binding, and that we may voluntarily set them aside when we will? Are the laws governing health any less real than those governing mathematics or chemistry. Do acts have no consequences in the realm of life?

Anyone, with common intelligence, can readily discern that, if health and rigid hygiene do not prevent disease, then, man is left a helpless victim of chance, a ready prey to the "devouring monsters," and must remain so until he discovers some effective barrier against the inroads of germs and worse. If a body pulsating with vitality and full of pure blood, is no guarantee against disease, so long, as, by hygienic living, it is maintained in this state, then health and hygiene are failures and man is indeed the helpless victim of circumstances beyond his control. If he possesses good health, it is simply due to his good fortune and not to his good behavior.

Those who hold to such a doctrine may laugh at the laws of life, and violate them continually, and, then if they possess a sound, vigorous constitution, they may abuse themselves a long time before the effects of those abuses show. But none but the fool can believe that even the most rugged constitution can be abused indefinitely without hurt.

In the preceding chapters the following facts have been shown:—

1. By virtue of the body's inherent and automatic powers of self-renewal, self-renovation and self-regeneration and its undeviating tendency to fullness of life, it is capable of a much longer existence and a much higher existence than men and women now live.

2. Disease, degeneracy and death come as the immediate result of poisoning and starvation of the cells of the body, as a consequence of a combination of forces and influences which are largely under individual control and usually self-inflicted.

These facts serve to confirm the old statement that "man does not die; he kills himself." Men and women are dying far short of the age they are capable of attaining because they are engaged in committing slow suicide.

Given a normal organism, at birth, and a proper mode of living afterward, together with absence from injurious influences, and every baby born into this world will grow into a strong, healthy man or woman. Those same simple conditions that are the sources of the development of plant, animal and man from germ to maturity are the constant sources of the maintenance of these organisms after maturity is reached. Those same influences that impair or prevent development in the growing child or youth also impair the powers of life in adults.

Whether you have a good organism at birth will depend partly upon heredity and partly upon the nutrition you received from your mother. What that organism will become after birth, that is, whether it will reach up to its highest potentiality, or fall far short of its inherent possibilities, will depend upon how you live. Of course there will be social factors that are not subject to individual control that may mar your life to a certain extent, but for the most part you and your parents and teachers will determine your life.

You cannot change your heredity. You cannot change your past. You cannot make society over. But you can work for the betterment of these things for the future. Civilization has many influences in it that are inimical to health and life. But these are not inherent in it and may be eradicated. We can build for a better future and assure our children and grandchildren better conditions to grow up under. The standard of living can be raised; the conditions of life can be improved not merely for the fortunate few, but for all.

So prone is man to look upon the conditions under which he is born and reared as natural and to look upon those things which the majority of mankind do as an average as the best for us to do as a whole that few are inclined to question the wisdom of the conventional standards of health and living, with a view to ascertaining if these best serve the physiological and psychological welfare of the individual and the race, but take it for granted that they do so. There is a happy delusion, a very convenient substitute for thought, that our present customs and standards represent the boiled down results of thousands of years of race experience and that they should not be tampered with. If it can be shown, historically, that a particular custom is old, this suffices to establish its value in the minds of many. Nothing could be farther from the truth.

Laboring under the delusions above noted, the physician or health advisor who insists that his patients abandon certain of their pet vices and health destroying practices and indulgences, is justly considered severe. The practitioner, however, if he is to be held responsible for the health and life of his patient, must necessarily be firm and insist upon obedience to natural law. The laws of nature are sharply defined, their penalties inexorable, if not always swift, and as an interpreter of her decrees, the hygienist, under present thought, at least, cannot seem otherwise than severe. However, it is not the hygienist but nature that is severe. This being true, it behooves the health seeker to strive to understand God's rational order, that he may render an intelligent obedience to laws which cannot be broken, but, upon which, we only break ourselves, in the attempt.

When we come to consider the means best suited to maintain life and health, youth, strength and beauty, it is obvious that THE HIGHEST POSSIBLE STANDARD MUST BE ACCEPTED. How, then shall we live?

1. CULTIVATE POISE AND CHEER. Do not attempt to see the world through the rose-colored glasses of a sentimental Pollyana but learn to take joy and

375

sorrow, good fortune and misfortune with the same calmness and equitableness. Avoid worry, fear, anxiety, excitement, jealousy, anger, self-pity, etc. Control your temper, passions, and emotions.

2. EXERCISE DAILY. Daily physical exercise, preferably in the fresh air and sunshine, and, as often as possible, in the form of play, is essential to both mental and physical health. Avoid the strenuous life, however. Do not make the Rooseveltian mistake and imagine that a strenuous physical life can offset gluttony.

3. SECURE PLENTY OF REST AND SLEEP EACH DAY: Learn to retire early. Learn to relax and "let go." Earn your sleep by honest work and avoid stimulants and sleep will come easily and naturally. Do not turn the night into day. Time is never wasted that is spent in recuperation.

Sleep may be defined as the periodical suspension of all the functions of external relation. Profound or quiet sleep is the complete suspension of the functions of the mind and special senses and is attended with entire unconsciousness. Normal sleep is dreamless. Dreaming implies imperfect rest. In default of this oblivion, sleep is only partial. It is not perfect nervous repose. It indicates some disturbing cause, some source of irritation and worry, such as gastric irritation. No person who suffers severly from indigestion but is also troubled with much dreaming, and, more or less, wakefulness. Irritants, stimulants, fear, apprehension, worry, grief, etc., interfere with sleep and prevent prefect repose, rest, recuperation.

The amount of sleep required will vary with the varying habits and occupations of individuals. Those who are the most active will require most sleep. Meat eaters, as in the animal kingdom, require more sleep than vegetarians. Mental workers require more sleep than physical workers. Those who dissipate much must sleep much. The sick require more sleep than the well. The accepted rule of eight hours in twenty-four is probably not enough, for as Trall says: "The statute of nature appears to read: Retire soon after dark, and arise with the first rays of morning light; and this is equally applicable to all climates and all seasons, at least in all parts of the globe proper for human habitation, for in the cold season, when the nights are longer, more sleep is required." When man learned to turn the night into day he forsook this natural rule.

4. KEEP CLEAN: This refers to both body and mind. Keep clean clothes, clean beds, clean houses. Keep the mind clean. Avoid lustful thoughts and desires. Do not become covetous, deceitful or corrupt. Nature penalizes you for all these things with hardening of the arteries and a shortened life.

Keep your body clean but do not indulge in too frequent and prolonged bathing. Do not soak yourself. Keep in mind that man is neither fish nor amphibian. He is a land mammal and his body was originally self-cleansing. Bathing is an artificial proceedure made necessary by clothing and civilization. Trall says: "Were human beings in all other respects to adapt themselves to the laws of their organization, and were they in all their voluntary habits in relation to eating, drinking, clothing, exercise, and temperature, to conform strictly to the laws of hygiene, I do not know that there would be any physiological necessity or utility in bathing at all." Page agrees with this saying: "The less clothing one wears, the less essential a daily bath becomes, and the less time necessary to devote to it. At the same time there is an increased ability to withstand exposure to wet or cold, whether of the bath, an involuntary ducking, or however caused."

A daily friction bath is sufficient for many. No one except those who sweat much or who work in occupations that make them dirty, requires a daily water bath. In these cases the water should be lukewarm or slightly cool. Hot and cold bathing should be avoided. Unless the nature of the "dirt" on the body demands soap for its removal, this is best avoided. Soap should form no part of the average bath.

5. BREATHE FRESH PURE AIR: Keep your windows open. Have your living room, bed room, office or workshop well ventilated. Get out of doors as much as possible. If you live in the city take advantage of every opportunity to get into the country.

6. SECURE AS MUCH SUNSHINE AS POSSIBLE: This means that your nude body, or as much of it as circumstances will permit, should be exposed to the direct rays of the sun. To merely sit by the window, or take a walk in the sunshine heavily clad, or clad in dark clothing will be of no benefit in so far as the sunshine is

concerned. Get your sun-baths in the morning or evening when it is not excessively hot.

7. EAT MODERATELY OF WHOLESOME FOODS: What are wholesome foods? All true foods that are fresh, pure, unadulterated and that have not been processed, refined, and cooked until their food value is largely destroyed, are wholesome foods. All foods that, in the process of refining, manufacturing, pickling, canning, preserving, and cooking, etc., have been deprived of their mineral elements and vitamins or that have been adulterated and poisoned by bleaching, coloring, flavoring, seasoning and by preservatives, are more or less unwholesome. All foods that have been raised in defective soil, hot houses, or on manure-fed lands or on lands fed with packing-house fertilizers, or that are raised out of the sunlight, are more or less unwholesome. All foods that have begun to undergo decomposition are unwholesome.

Man may eat unwholesome foods all his life, thanks to his wonderful powers of self-immunization and adaptation, and enjoy what ordinarily passes for health. "Excess in moderately unwholesome viands," says Oswald, "has to be carried to a monstrous degree before the after-dinner torpor turns into a malignant disease; the stomach**** seems to acquire a knack of assimilating a modicum of the ingesta and voiding the rest like so much unnutritious stuff."

However, the rule that applies to unnatural habits in general also applies, and very forcibly, to chronic dietetic abuses—namely: The further we have strayed from nature the longer, wearier and more painful will be the road to reform. Dr. Oswald paints a vivid pen picture of the trials of the dyspeptics in his *Household Remedies,* p. 54-58.

"To the alcholic stimulants of the ancients we have added tea, coffee, tobacco, absinthe, chloral, opium, and pungent spices. Every year increases the number of our elaborately unwholesome-made dishes, and decreases our devotion to the field-sports that helped our forefathers to digest their boar-steaks. We have no time to masticate our food; we bolt it, and grumble if we can not bolt it smoking hot. The competition of our domestic and public kitchens temps us to eat three full meals a day, and two of them at a time when the exigencies of our business-routine leave us no leisure for digestion. At night, when the opportunity for that leisure arrives, we counteract the efforts of the digestive apparatus by hot stove-fires and stifling bedrooms. Since the beginning of the commercial-epicurean age of the nineteenth century the votaries of fashion have persistently vied in compelling their stomachs to dispose of the largest possible amount of the most indigestible food under the least favorable circumstances.

"That persistence has at last exhausted the self-regulating resources of our digestive organs. But even after such provocations the stomach does not strike work without repeated warnings. The first omen of the wrath to come is the *morning languor,* the hollow-eyed lassitude which proves that the arduous labor of the assimilative organs has made the night the most fatiguing part of the twenty-four hours. The expression of the face becomes haggard and sallow. The tongue feels gritty, the palate parched, in spite of the restless activity of the salivary glands, which every now and then try to respond to the appeals of the distressed stomach. Gastric acidity betrays itself by many disagreeable symptoms; loss of appetite, however, marks a later stage of the malady. For years the infinite patience of Nature labors every night to undo the mischief of every day, and before noon the surfeited organs again report ready for duty. Habitual excess in eating and drinking sometimes begets an unnatural appetency that enables the glutten to indulge his *penchant* to the last, only with this difference, that the relish for special kinds of food has changed into a vague craving for *repletion,* just as the fondness for a special stimulant is apt to turn into a chronic poison-hunger. This craving after engorgement forms a distinctive symptom of *plethoric dyspepsia,* but even in the first stage of asthenic or nervous dyspepsia the hankering after food is not hunger proper, but a nervous uneasiness, suggesting the idea that a good meal would, somehow supply the means of relief. The first full meal, however, entails penalties which the sufferer would gladly exchange for the less positive discomfort of the morning. Instinct fails to keep its promise, as a proof that Nature has been supplanted by a deceptive second nature. Headache, heart-burn, eructations, humming in the ears, nausea, vertigo, and gastric spasms, make the after-dinner hour "the saddest of the sad twenty-four!": a dull mist of discontent broods over the whole afternoon, and yields only to tea and lamp-light. The patient begins to fret under the weight of his affliction, but still declines to remove the cause. To out-door exercise he objects, not on general principles, but on some special plea or other. He has to husband his strength. The raw March wind would turn his cough into a chronic catarrh. The warm weather would spoil his appetite and aggravate his vertigo. The truth is that of the large quantum of comestibles ingested only a small modicum is *digested*, and that the system begins to weaken under the influence of indirect starvation. Business routine prevents the dyspeptic from changing his meal times. He cannot reduce the number of his meals; people have to conform to the arrangements of their boarding-house. The stomach needs something strengthening between breakfast and supper. The truth is, that the exertions of the digestive organs alternate with occasional reactions, entailing a nervous depression which can be (temporarily) relieved by the stimulus of a fresh engorgement. Business reasons may really prevent a reduction of working hours, and domestic duties a change of climate or of occupation. The daily engorgement in the meanwhile goes on as before.

"Nature then resorts to more emphatic protests. Sleep comes in the form of a dull torpor that would make a nightmare a pleasant change of programme. The digestive laboratory seems to have lost the discretion of its automatic contrivances; the process of assimilation, in all its details, obtrudes itself upon the cognizance of the sensorium, and urges the co-operation of the voluntary muscles. Contortions and pressing manipulations have to force each morsel through the gastric apparatus; the lining of the stomach has become sentient, and shirks its work like a blistered palate. Special tidbits can be traced through the whole course of their abdominal adventures. Undigested green peas roll on like buckshot shot from the smelting-pan of a shot-tower. A grilled partridge crawls along like a reluctant crab, clawing and biting at each step. Nausea and headache strive to relieve themselves in spasmodic eructations. Vertigoes, like fainting-fits, eclipse the eyesight for minutes together. Constipation, often combined with a morbid appetite, suggests distressful speculations on the possible outcome of the accumulating ingesta. The overfed organism is under-nourished to a degree that reveals itself in the rapid emaciation of the patient. The general derangement of the nervous system reacts on the mental faculties, and impairs their efficacy even for the most ordinary business purposes, till the invalid at last realizes the necessity of reform. He tries to reduce the number of his meals; but the lengthened intervals drag as heavily as the toper's time between drinks. He hopes to appease his stomach by a change of diet, but finds that the resolution has come too late; the gastric mutiny has become indiscriminate, and protests as savagely against a Graham biscuit as against a broiled pork sausage. He tries pedestrianism, but finds the remedy worse than the evil. The enemy has cut off his means of retreat; the necessitous system has no strength to spare for such purposes as an effort of the motive organs. But nine out of ten dyspeptics resort to the drug-store. They get a bottle of "tonic bitters." They try Dr. Quack's 'Dysepepsia Elixir.' They try a 'blue pill'—in the hope of rousing Nature, as it were, to a sense of her proper duty.

"Now, what such 'tonics' can really do for them is this: they goad the system into the transient and abnormal activity incident to the necessity of expelling a virulent poison. With the accomplishment of that purpose the exertion ceases, and the ensuing exhaustion is worse than the first by just as much as the *poison-fever* has robbed the system of a larger or smaller share of its little remaining strength. The stimulant has wasted the organic energy which it seemed to revive."

8. BE MODERATE IN WEARING CLOTHES: It may be stated that, as a general rule, the less clothes one wears the healthier he will be. The materials should be light, porous and white or of light colors. Dark or black clothing should be avoided like snakes. No tight bands, belts, corsets, garters, etc., should be allowed to interfere with the circulation nor cramp up the organs of the body. Shoe heels shauld be absent or, at most, very low. Shoes should fit the feet and the feet not made to fit the shoes. Some day sandals and a string of beads will be our chief articles of clothing.

We may present the case for and against clothes in the words of Graham, *Science of Human Life*, p. 637-9:—

"It is entirely certain that no kind of clothing is strictly natural to man;*** all the physiological and psychological properties, powers, and interests of the human constitution would be better sustained, as a permanent fact, from generation to generation, by entire nudity, than by the use of any kind of clothing. Strictly speaking, therefore, all clothing is, in itself considered, in some measure an evil. In passing into climates much cooler than that to which he is constitutionally adapted, however, man finds it necessary to employ clothing to a greater or less extent, for the purpose of preserving the proper temperature of his body. In such a situation therefore, clothing becomes a *necessary evil*; and in so far as man suffers cold without it, it is a comparative good; that is, it prevents a greater evil than it causes. Nevertheless it cannot serve to adapt man so perfectly to such a situation as to make it equally conductive to the highest well being of the human constitution with his natural climate without clothing, it remains true, as a general proposition, that clothing is in some measure detrimental to the physiological interests of the human body.**** Clothing, then, is an evil so far as it prevents a free circulation of pure air over the whole surface of the body, or in any manner relaxes and debilitates the skin; and increases its susceptibility to be unhealthily affected by changes of weather and by the action of morbific agents; it is an evil in so far as, by compression or otherwise, it prevents the free action of the chest and lungs, or in any manner or measure restricts respiration; it is an evil in so far as it interferes in any degree with the digestive organs; it is an evil in so far as it prevents the most perfect freedom of voluntary action, and ease and grace of motion and attitude, or prevents the full development of any part of the system, or serves, by the substitution of artificial means for natural powers, to relax and debilitate the muscles, or render the tendons, ligaments, cartilages, and boxes, less healthy and powerful, or in any measure to abridge the control of the will over any organ of voluntary motion; it is an evil in so far as it tends to increase the peculiar sensibility of any organ of animal instinct, and to augment the power of that instinct on the intellectual and moral faculties; it is an evil so far as it serves to enfeeble the intellectual faculties, and render the mind sluggish and sensual; and it is an evil so far as it serves to excite an unchaste imagination, and cause the sexes to act towards each other more from the impulse of animal feeling than from the dictate of sound reason."

Mr Graham quotes one Rev. Grout as saying in 1168:—

"The Zulus depend on the products of the soil for subsistence, and go entirely naked. Licentiousness is wholly unknown among them. I have been among them for three years, seen them on all occasions, have many a time seen hundreds of males and females huddled together in perfect nakedness, but never once saw the least manifestation of licentious feeling, and they are as remarkable for their intellectual activity and aptitude as for their chastity."

This is the general testimony of missionaries, explorers and scientists and accords with just what we should, on general principles, expect. Prudery and shame for the body came after and not before man began to wear clothes.

Man will not be ready to discard clothes for at least another decade and in the meantime he should clothe himself as lightly and sensibly as possible. Overclothing weakens the body. It lowers resistance to heat and cold and impairs the power of adaptation to weather changes. It deprives the body of the sun and air and keeps the excretions of the skin locked up against the body. You are literally wallowing in your own excretions.

9. HAVE AN INTEREST IN LIFE: A purposeless life is marked for early dissolution. A purposeless life is not worthy of preservation. That man or woman who has no purpose in life is driven about from place to place; from discontent to despair.

10. GET MARRIED: Build a home. Rear a family. Statistics show that married people live longer on the average than single people.

Dr. George Robertson of the Edinburgh Royal College of Physicians recently stated that "Young men between 25 and 35 who remain bachelors die four years sooner than married men." He added that they also "Run three times the risk of becoming insane." It is not, of course, fair to charge all this apparent evil of "single blessedness" to the single life. We can only correctly interpret such figures when we understand why these men remained single. All normal, healthy men marry, or, at least, desire to.

It is safe to assume that a great majority of those who remain single from choice are lacking in virility and are diseased perhaps in many ways. The thing that prevented them from marrying may also have been the thing that caused their early death or that caused so much insanity among them. *Statistics give results, not causes.*

Childless couples die before those with children. A childless marriage is usually more unhappy than where there are children. Home and children stabilize life.

Avoid contraceptives of all kinds. They are all harmful and all lead to sex glutteny. They are partly responsible for so much cancer of the womb in women. Don't build your married life on lust.

11. AVOID ALL POISON HABITS: Coffee, tea, cocoa, chocolate, tobacco, alcohol, opium, heroin, soda fountain slops and other drugs. These all weaken, poison and destroy the body.

12. AVOID SEXUAL EXCESS: All sexual relations,—"petting," mental self-abuse, self-abuse and all indulgences—drain the nervous system of much of its powers. Conserve these powers.

13. AVOID ALL EXCESSES: Build your life on the conservation of energy, not upon its dissipation. Don't waste your forces in useless and needless expenditures. Be moderate and temperate in all things. If you waste your forces you impair your functions and build toxemia and impaired nutrition.

We are living in an age of thrills and excitement. These things have been commercialized and organized on a large scale. They are habit-forming and progressive in their tendency. They build a very unstable nervous system and wreck one's health. Life without some thrill and excitement would be monotonous, but the pursuit of these things as an end in itself is an unmitigated evil. One invariably goes to excess and as satiety is derived from one form, craves and seeks a more thrilling and more exciting form.

14. DO NOT BECOME ONE-SIDED IN YOUR MANNER OF LIVING: You cannot remain or become well and strong through exercise alone, or through diet alone, or rest and sleep alone. Fresh air and sunshine alone are not enough. Do not imagine that by breathing alone you can reach the heights. All these things are good, but life is more than exercise, or food and drink; more than thought, or rest and sleep. It is all these and more. Life must be lived as a whole.

Do not get the idea that you are an exception to laws of life. There are no exceptions. The laws that govern life, health, growth, development, disease and death in your body are the same laws that govern these same processes in the bodies of your neighbors. Physiological laws and processes are the same in Jones as in Smith. Both Jones and his neighbors are injured by the same harmful indulgencies, practices, habits, agents and influences. Both are helped by the same factors. Paste this in your hat. YOU ARE NO EXCEPTION.

We must learn to view life as a struggle between self-control and self-indulgence and must come to realize that self-control alone leads to strength and happiness. Self-indulgence leads to misery and destruction. The late Eblert Hubbard well said: "The rewards of life are for service, its penalties for self-indulgence."

There is absolutely no need for any action or habit that impairs life and produces weakness and disease. But people are so enslaved by their habits, so bent on the pleasures of the moment, so lacking in self-control that they cannot free themselves. Self-control is the world's greatest need. Self-discipline is the only saving force. Our pleasure-mad and over-stimulated age is almost wholly lacking in self-control.

Many will say: "I would rather live as I now do and only live ten years than to live as you have outlined and live a hundred." They do not realize that this is the despairing cry of a slave. These people are hopelessly enslaved by their bad habits and thoroughly perverted in both mind and body. Mind and body alike are dominated by their habits. They are beyond redemption. They will declare they derive more satisfaction from their pipe or cigar than from anything else in life. Or they cry out. "Please don't take my harem away." It is but a waste of time to reason with such. One is always defeated in an argument with their appetites and morbid desires and perverted instincts.

Their cry is "We live but once. Let us enjoy life while we are here." We believe in enjoying life, real life, life in the highest and fullest sense, not life on the low groveling plane they mean. What they should say is: "We live but once, let us make it short and snappy."

If these people would only die at the end of their ten fast and merry years, little objection could be offered to their foolish "philosophy" and worse practices. But many of them do not do this. Instead, they hang on year after year, going from doctor to doctor and from institution to institution in search of a cure for the effects of the very abuses of their bodies from which they think they derive so much pleasure and satisfaction. They desire to be SAVED IN THEIR SINS—not FROM THEM. The "satisfaction" they derive from their pipe, or their gluttery or their alcohol or from their harem is a poor satisfaction. It is a poor substitute for the higher joys of real health based on wholesome living. If you would live longer; live simply, live wholesomely, live right.

A few words anent the hygiene of pregnancy and the hygiene of infancy are required before we close this chapter.

Pregnancy is a strictly normal, natural condition, it is not a disease, and those abnormal symptoms that are usually listed as symptoms of pregnancy are not symptoms of pregnancy at all. Likewise, when pregnancy is given as a cause or a predisposing cause of disease those who give it do so either ignorantly or thoughtlessly. Pregnancy actually serves to benefit the body and many women have lost their ills through this alone.

Live a normal life as outlined above and pregnancy will take care of itself. Throw away all foolish fears of marking your baby. This is an impossible thing, a mere superstition. Avoid all sexual relations during this period and during lactation.

Parturition is not a surgical operation. It is not a wound, accident, infection or other abnormal condition. If you have lived as you should and were normal at the beginning of pregnancy, an easy, sometimes painless and rapid delivery will be experienced and a rapid recuperation follow. There will be no necessity for remaining on your back for days, as is the common practice.

Babies should be nursed at their mother's breast, whenever possible for as long as possible. Three to four years should be the normal length of the period of lactation, and not four to five weeks as one so often sees today.

Babies should be fed as directed in the chapter on diet. They should be kept clean, let alone as much as possible and dressed lightly, if at all. A daily sun-bath should be given them. Even Dr. Tilden, who objects to the sun-bath for the almost childish reason (or vanity) that he does not want his skin brown like a Mexican, but prefers it pale like a corpse, advocates sun-baths for infants and children.

Babies should be placed on their stomachs from the day of birth. In this way they develop their backs, necks, arms and legs much more rapidly than when lying on their back. This is Dr. Page's method and is the best exercise of which I know for infants.

Place them on a hard bed, give them plenty of fresh air, do not bundle them up, keep stays, swaddling bands, caps, etc., off of them and give them a chance to kick and grow. Never put flannels on a child. Cotton, linen or silk will answer far better. Nudity is better still.

Do not be afraid that they will "Catch Cold." A child that is properly cared for could no more have a cold than it could fly. You could freeze it to death, but you could not cause it to have a cold by exposure. Do not think from this, however, that you should expose the child unduly. Forget the old superstitions about night air.

THE HYGIENE OF ACUTE DISEASE

Chapter XXIX

WE are suffering from a frightful incubus of so-called science that murders millions with its almost incredible ignorance. For "Medical Science" we have a "science" which is fighting nature with every resource at its command. Science is the knowledge of a body of ascertained facts (ascertained by observation and subsequent demonstration), and their causes, organized and classified according to their natural relationships. The terms "science" and "scientific" are employed today in such a loose, haphazard and indiscriminate manner, and people have become so thoroughly hypnotized by the term, that it becomes frequently necessary to discuss the question, "what is science?" Medicine is not, was never, and can never be, a science. When the problems of health, disease and living have been reduced to a science, medicine will quickly cease to exist.

When the essential nature and purpose, the rationale, of acute disease is fully understood, it will no longer be treated. Its symptoms will no longer be suppressed, subdued, changed, or combatted. To again quote Jennings:—

"The vital economy has but one great and absorbing object before it and in the prosecution of that object, it is not easily diverted to the right hand or to the left. When difficulties thicken in its pathway, its forces are all put in requisition, disposed and used to the best advantage for surmounting the difficulties, and it is instructive as well as astonishing to witness the amount of obstacles that human nature will often overcome and still hold on her way, even under apparently, an almost exhausted state of the vital energies."—*Philosophy of Human Life*, p. 219.

The Orthopath is legitimately absolved from all warfare against "disease." For in his view there is nothing against which to battle. For as Dr. Jennings declares:—

"For the recovery of his charge he looks to the operation of internal vital machinery most perfectly adapted to the purpose,—and controlled by laws that need and admit of no improvement. While faithfully serving in the capacity of handmaid to nature, in the arrangement and constant adaptation of external circumstances to the natural renovating efforts, he expects occasionally to witness fearful and agonizing convulsions and disturbances of the motory portions of the vital mechanism, or great deviation of some kind from the natural state. But instead of regarding these changes and these irregular actions as subversive in their nature and tendency, he considers them as directly the opposite of this, and as truly essential to the reparation and replenishment of a damaged living body, as thunder storms are for the purification of the atmosphere. And a principal source of his anxiety and vigilance is to guard the delicate nervous, apparatus whose function is to transmit intelligence and power, and control motion—from the presence and action of anything that has a tendency to impair its perceptive faculty, agileness and force.

"It is immaterial, therefore, to the Orthopathist, so far as his direct interference is concerned in what shape disease makes its appearance, and with what severity; or what changes it undergoes. His business is to guard and take proper care of the exterior of the body, furnish a little 'bread and water' as it may be called for, secure a quiet and equable state of mind, and leave nature full scope and freedom in the discharge of her own appropriate duties. If death should peer forth in pale and ghastly visage, and show its icy hand as if to clutch away the remnant of humanity, it would be out of order for our Orthopathist to attempt to repel it by the employment of any of the troops of Admiral Mercury, King Alcohol, General Diffusive Stimuli, Subordinate or Local Irritants, or any other contraband force. He should fall back submissively upon the extreme resources of nature, as his *dernier resort*, and if these fail, the final catastrophe is sealed."—*Philosophy of Human Life*, p. 267.

The Orthopathic practice is a let-alone practice. Prof. O. S. Fowler declared: "The Let-Alone Cure is but the outgrowth of the Will-Cure. How many millions have grown worse by doctoring till they had no more means or hope, given up, did nothing, waited to die, (in these cases not *willing* to get well. Author's note.) kept on living to their wonderment, and finally got well. What a pity! Not their getting well, but keeping themselves sick so long by so expensive a practice."

Orthopathy recognizes no therapeutics of acute disease. It only recognizes the hygiene of acute disease. Seeing in the acute process the PROCESS OF CURE, it does not seek to cure disease, CURE THE CURE, but seeks merely to supply the body with the best hygienic conditions to the end that it may carry forward its curative work with the least possible hinderance. Knowing no power of cure except that inherent in living matter, orthopathy does not seek for curative agencies and influencies outside the body. Knowing that every action of the living body in disease as in health must be in harmony with the laws of life, true to the highest interests of the body and therefore RIGHT, it does not seek to suppress or control symptoms.

Dr. Jennings replied to a physician who had asked him in what respects he (Jennings) differed from many physicians of that day who employed but few drugs in these words.—*Medical Reform,* p. 306.

"We differ in two fundamental particulars:—

"*First,* the general principles on which we form our indications of treatment are directly opposite to each other. You hold that disease is wrong action; I maintain that it is right action.

"*Second,* to be consistent, the general rule for practices based upon your general principle must be break up diseased action. On my general principle, let diseased action alone."

Again:—

" 'That is all very well,' said a good friend, 'in mild disease, but when disease becomes violent, if there is nothing done to check it, it will overcome the powers of life.' This friend admitted that disease was not a some *thing,* emphasizing the word *thing.* It must be a *some*-thing or a *no*-thing; and Orthopathists are content to let *nothing* take care of itself. But just here is the tug of war; the pivot on which the question of medicine or on medicine hinges. Admitting that mild diseases do not of themselves afford a basis for a system of medication, the question arises, 'does the extension or aggravation of symptoms change the *nature* of disease?' "—*Tree of Life.* p. 187-8.

Let there be no overlooking of the main point—THE ESSENTIAL NATURE OF DISEASE. Is the tendency of vitality—for there is no other agency concerned —in the aggregate of movements called disease, right or wrong? This is fundamental Either ORTHOPATHY is right, or else, HETEROPATHY is right.

If the *right action* theory is correct, then the let-alone plan is right and the name attached to the group of symptoms present is of no consequence. The let-alone plan may be adopted from the outset. There need be no waiting for developments, no anxiety, lest we are treating for typhoid fever and the patient is developing menengitis. We may safely carry out the following advise of Jennings:—

"Don't stop to inquire what disease is about to be developed, whether pneumonia or measles. In Old School times—and I suppose those times are not quite 'already past'—physicians were sometimes puzzled to distinguish between these diseases, for often in their incipiency they are easily confounded, and when they were bleeding, blistering, and dosing to break up and keep back a pneumonia, and at length discovered it was a case of measles, they would immediately desist from their break-up efforts, and let the measles come out and develop themselves. Orthopathy has, no trouble or perplexity of this kind. ALL DISEASES ARE 'SELF-LIMITED' AND MAY BE PERMITTED TO MAKE A FULL DISPLAY OF THEMSELVES. WHETHER THE SYMPTOMS RUN HIGH OR LOW, LET THEM RUN TILL THEY HAVE HAD THEIR RUN OUT. 'THE HARDER THE BATTLE, THE SOONER OVER' AND THE LESS IT IS INTERFERED WITH, THE LESS THERE WILL BE OF IT, AND THE MORE LIKELY IT WILL BE TO END WELL. There can be no wrong action, for whatever action there is, is controlled by an immutable righteous law, which insures its tendency toward recovery, whether it reaches that point or not."—*The Tree of Life,* p. 186. (Cap. Mine).

Under this plan of treatment, too, there need be no waiting for developments, as it can be instituted from the very beginning of any case. The physician is called to see a patient presenting symptoms like these: rapid pulse, high temperature, loss of appetite, prostration, etc. What is the disease? It may be the beginning of pneumonia, typhoid fever, measles, spinal menengitis or any other acute febrile condition. He must await developments. The symptoms are not far enough advanced to enable him to make a differential diagnosis. His theory and practice calls for a specific treatment for each separate symptom complex. But he can't tell what the symptom complex is going to be. He can only give "expectant" treatment and await developments. Under Nature Cure treatment, this is not necessary. It is not even necessary for the disease to ever reach a stage where a special name can be given it. While the Allopath or Homeopath waits for such developments, the Orthopath is doing his best work.

Acute diseases are self-limiting. Their tendency is towards recovery and the patient will recover without treatment. In fact they are always better off without treatment than when they are subjected to the meddlesome interferenc that is usually given and which passes under the name of therapeutics.

In treating an acute disease, the first rule to learn is: DON'T DO IT. The disease, it must be remembered, is a vital process in self-defense. It is not to be treated, but permitted to run its natural course.

An acute disease is a more or less violent reaction against disease influence. It is usually sudden in its onset and does not last long. Pain and increased temperature are usually present, with a loss of appetite, a sense of weakness or exhaustion, etc. Except in mild cases, the person so affected is forced to go to bed and cease all other activities. This is a wise provision of nature to conserve energy. It is not to be supposed that the sick person has any less vitality or nerve energy when the acute symptoms set in than he had ten minutes or a half hour previous when he may have been ploughing, cutting wood, digging ditches or some similar work that requires strength and energy. But there is every reason to think that the energy that is used under ordinary conditions for the performance of such work has been withdrawn from these channels and is now being used in the effort to throw off the Pathoferic matter. Were this not true how could an organism already greatly enervated marshal enough energy to accomplish the extra work it is undertaking in acute disease?

If the work of house cleaning is to be successful, it is essential that the undivided attention of the organism be devoted to the curing process. For this reason, all activities that can be dispensed with temporarily and that have no direct bearing on the task of purification are stopped. The digestive process is temporarily suspended, little or no digestive juices are secreted, the appetite is cut off, the patient is forced to rest.

This brings us, then, to our first rule of practice in acute disease: The primary requirement is rest: Physical rest. Mental rest. Physiological rest.

PHYSICAL REST—is secured by putting the patient to bed and making him comfortable A comfortable bed should be arranged and kept clean. All bedding should be as hard, and all bed-clothing should be as light, as a due regard for comfort will allow. Soft beds that permit the patient to sink down into them are exceedingly debilitating and uncomfortable. Heavy covers weigh down upon the sick person and make him uncomfortable. They prevent rest. And, as Jennings truly declares, "in passing through a grave renovating process, rest, rest, REST, is the remedy."

No organ, however small and comparatively insignificant, is ever permitted to utter a note of protest or complaint until all the resources of power are low and the present stock of power consistently available to that organ is nearly exhausted. If an essential organ has been impaired or injured by any means whatsoever, it is proportionately the more important that early and careful heed be given to the saving of power at the first evidence of impairment, and it is especially urgent that the body should be carefully guarded against further injury in any and all of its parts, until its present damaged condition is thoroughly repaired and recovered from.

Where much, and perhaps everything, depends on the economical and undisturbed expenditure of a few feeble vital forces, no disturbing causes should be admitted and as the orthopathic care of the sick is founded on the fact that the tendency of the movements of life, in disease, all and singular, is to save life as far as this may be threatened; and especially to avert threatened danger to any of its organs, the first object to be aimed at in the conduct of any case is to shut down all unnecessary wastes-gates, that is, to place the body as far as this may be possible, under those conditions in which there shall be no unnecessary expenditure of its powers, in order that the organs that are called upon to accomplish the essential work of cure, but may otherwise be deficient in power, may receive added force.

384

Give the *Law of Distribution* full scope in apportioning power to the various organs, and dispensing the powers of life as necessity demands. Let it withhold power from one organ or set of organs, and appropriate it to others, as the ultimate and highest good of the whole organism may require.

The first death to occur in the author's practice was that of a man, nearing sixty years of age, who had pneumonia. There had been a rapid decline of symptoms. At the end of five days there were no fever, pains in chest, coughing, or other acute symptoms. I instructed him to remain in bed and remain perfectly quiet until one week later, when I would call again. Instead of following my instructions, he felt so good that he got up on the second day and sat up for over an hour. He talked much and tired himself greatly. Upon walking to his bed to lie down again, he "felt something break and fall" in his lungs. In a few hours thereafter he was in a coma from which he revived for a few hours, after it had lasted twenty-four hours, then lapsed back into the coma and in another twenty-four hours was dead. I am certain that had he remained quietly in bed, as instructed, until his lungs had fully repaired themselves and resolution was complete, he would be alive to this day. But he had been misled by reading the fallacious and often fatal advice to be up and around when you feel like it, because to remain in bed is to "give up to disease," and to be active stimulates the vital processes.

When it becomes plainly evident that the vital forces are to be severely tasked and tested in a curative, renovating, and defensive process, there should be no unnecessary delay in placing the body and mind under conditions and circumstances in which the forces of life can carry forward their work with the least possible interruption or loss of power. The mind should be set at ease, the body made comfortable, the conditions of recovery supplied, and no means employed to control the operations of the body or the symptoms of the renovating process. As fast as the *Law of Limitation* is enforced, and activity becomes tedious or wearisome, the body should be yielded up, and not the slightest obstacle placed in the way of the operation of any of the laws and forces of the vital economy. No fallacious theories about food or exercise adding to your powers and helping you "throw off" the disease should be permitted to cause you to continue active and to continue eating. Mental, physical and physiological rest are needed and the quicker these are secured, the more rapidly will be your recovery, and the less will be your suffering.

The evidences of a developing disease are indications that vitality is low, and its expenditure should be cautiously guarded. Nature never permits a single fiber of the body to deviate in its action from the normal state, or to suffer pain, so long as she can prevent it consistently with the general welfare of the body. Where there is much or continued complaining by parts of the body every waste-gate should be closed in order to conserve power.

If appetite and the desire to be about continue, it is permissible to eat lightly and to be lightly active, however, a quicker recovery will be made and a more comfortable sickness will be experienced if one ceases even these. "Keep still," says Dr. Jennings, "Rest, *rest*, REST, is the grand panacea."

If your body is in a disabled condition, and you are about to undergo a renovating process, or if it is already in operation, avoid exposure to all sources of additional damage to the body, at least until you are restored to a healthy condition. Exposure to cold, extreme heat, fatigue, excitement, grief, shock, physical violence or injury, etc., all lessen the chances of recovery. Many of the fatal cases of disease that are daily reported, are rendered so by the additional burdens imposed upon the powers of life, which a little prudent foresight might easily have prevented.

In many cases, the vital operations are kept so incessantly harassed by drugs, serums, operations, and treatments of various kinds, that they are kept so busy defending the body against these, they are not able to repair the original damage, or eliminate the cause of the original trouble.

Nothing should be permitted to interfere with a full and free operation of the laws of life, and the full development of disease. How extensive these developments may need to be we have no means of knowing, accurately, until the process is completed. Therefore, the appropriation and distribution of the vital forces that may be made in the particular circumstances, should be freely submitted too. "If this carries

a man," says Jennings, "into a pleurisy, let him have a pleurisy; if it brings on typhus fever, bilious fever, or yellow fever, let him have that fever; if it plunges him into a deep lung affection, threatening confirmed consumption, let it have free course and push him as far in that direction as it will, for safety lies only in that direction; if it throws him into a fit, let him remain in the fit, until he is released from it 'by law.' Remember the words of Napoleon. 'We are a machine made to live. We are organized for that purpose; such is our nature. *Do not counteract the living principle.* Let it alone; leave it the liberty of defending itself—it will do better than your drugs'."
—*Medical Reform*, p. 326-27.

Bodily warmth is essential to physical comfort and rest. If the sick person becomes chilled, and unless in high fever, he chills easier than a normal person, he is made uncomfortable, and elimination is checked. "Keep the feet warm is a prescription of universal application," said Dr. Walter. "By keeping the feet warm, the whole surface is correspondingly warmed, and the circle of circulation enlarged, and the labor of the heart correspondingly reduced."

Whatever its saving to the heart, if the body is kept warm, its energies are conserved and the processes of elimination are not interfered with. By keeping warm, however, is not meant to roast in an electric cabinet, or stew and boil in a hot bath. A comfortable warmth of the body maintained by a moderate amount of clothing and supplimented by a hot water bottle, or a jug of hot water, or an electric pad to the feet, is sufficient.

The patient should be made comfortable at all times. All his needs should be attended to carefully and gently. He should not be pampered or petted. Petting and pampering patients builds the sick habit. It produces self-pity and causes the patient to magnify his troubles. Firmness is essential, while care should be confined to the essentials.

MENTAL REST—It is of first importance that the mind be at rest. The sick man or woman should have perfect confidence in the power of nature to accomplish the work begun. The alarm and anxious concern of relatives, friends, and neighbors, must be met as resolutely as possible. It would be well if every individual could give the whole subject of disease a careful and thorough examination while he or she is yet well, and make up the mind then what course shall be pursued when ill. Sickness is not the time to examine the merits of the clashing and conflicting theories and practices now in vogue. Strive to get and habitually maintain a correct idea of disease so that when you become sick, if you are foolish enough to do so, your mind may be allowed to rest at ease in the perfect confidence that all that can be done to good purpose will be done by due course of law.

Where this has not been done those who have the care of the sick in their hands should take heed of every word, act or appearance, that may tend to shake the confidence of the sick person. Anxious faces, forlorn looks, and manifest fear are quickly discerned by the sick person and these weigh heavily upon him or her. Try to be cheerful and optimistic in the sick room. Your own confidence will help to buoy up the confidence of the sick person.

Mental rest is best secured by assuring the patient that he is in no danger and removing from his environment any mentally distractive object or sound. Especially should visitors be excluded from the room. The sick room is too often a visiting rendezvous where friends and relations congregate and talk. They recite all the ugly details of how Mr. or Mrs. so-and-so had this or that disease, how he or she suffered, how long he remained sick and how he or she died. Such talk is not calculated to create a peaceful, restful state of mind in the patient. Besides, the noise itself is distracting to a sick man. The habit of the "mental healer" of spending from a half hour to hours at the bedside of a patient chattering to him a lot of mummery which he neither understands nor appreciates, should never be permitted. It tires the patient and leaves him much weakened.

In his *Hygienic Handbook*, Trall roundly condemned the habit of making the sick room a visiting rendezvous where friends, neighbors and relatives congregate and talk, often, far into the night. In his *Water-Cure for the Million*, (p. 31-2), he says:—

"The usual custom and manner of watching with the sick is very reprehensible. If any persons in the world need quiet and undisturbed repose, it is those who are laboring under fevers and other acute disease. But with a light burning in the room, and one or more persons sitting by, and reading, talking, or whispering, this is impossible. The room should be darkened, and the attendant should quietly sit or lie in the same or in an adjoining room, so as to be within call if anything is wanted. In an extreme case, the attendant can frequently step lightly to the bedside, to see if the patient is doing well; but all noise, and all light should be excluded, except on emergencies. It is a common practice with watchers to awaken the patient whenever he inclines to sleep *too soundly*. But this is unnecessary, because when the respiration becomes laborous, the patient will awaken, spontaneously. Under the drug-medical dispensation, the custom is to stuff the patient, night and day, with victuals, drink or medicines, every hour or oftener, so that any considerable repose is out of the question. But, fortunately for mankind, the Hygienic system regards sleep as more valuable than the whole of them."

Stuffing the patient with food, drink and medicine, at all hours or half-hours of the day and night, not only disturbs rest and sleep by frequently awakening them to take these things, but these things keep the system in a state of excitement, add to the discomfort and suffering of the sick person, and make rest and sleep almost impossible. Most of the sufferings of the acutely sick, are due to the treatment and care they receive.

Brilliant light disturbs rest. The sick room should be both light and airy but not brilliantly lighted. The habit of keeping a light burning all night in the sick room is a bad practice and one to be avoided. It is sun-light alone that is of value to the sick. They should not be denied this, but at night, the dark room is conducive to sleep. The blinds need not be drawn during the day. I have always insisted that the sun-light be permitted free access to the sick room. Even in measles, where light is commonly regarded as very injurious to the eyes; I have insisted on open windows and raised shades and I have yet to see a single case in which any damage was done to the eyes. Indeed, I am convinced that the opposite and prevailing course will, and frequently does, injure the eyes.

Sleep is the highest form of rest. During sleep, all the reparative and recuperative processes go on most efficiently. The sick should be permitted to sleep as much as possible and should not be awakened for any reason whatsoever, except, of course, where cleanliness demands it. But sleep should not be confounded with the stupor that follows the use of narcotic drugs.

Noise disturbs rest and sleep. It is irritating to the sick person, much more so than to the well. All noise should be eliminated as far as possible and the sick person should make every effort to relax his or her mind, acquire poise, and be disturbed as little as possible by the remaining noise. Absolute quiet is essential in low stages of disease. Even the little noise caused by walking across the floor is irritating and should be avoided as much as possible. No one should be allowed in the room save the nurse, and no talking to the patient should be permitted.

PHYSIOLOGICAL REST—Is secured partly by the two preceeding rests—physical and mental rest—and by stopping the food intake. A certain amount of functional activity is essential to the continuance of life. Suspended animation is, no doubt, a fact in Nature, but it cannot continue for very long without ending in death. Aside from this essential activity, the activity of our physiological economy is largely determined by our food intake. To stop the food intake takes a heavy load off the internal economy. The work of digesting and assimilating food and of discarding the waste and refuse portions all ceases. The heart and lungs have less work to perform. The liver and kidneys are given a rest. In fact, the whole physiology is given a rest. The energy usually employed in digesting and assimilating food is now used for eliminating or neutralizing the toxic matter that is forcing the reaction.

There is no danger of starving to death. The human body can go for weeks and months with only water and air. Food that is eaten in acute disease does not nourish anyway. The more the patient eats, the worse he becomes so that the danger lies really on the other side.

All food should be withheld from the patient who is suffering from an acute disease until all acute symptoms subside. As long as there is any pain, fever of inflammation or other troubles, to give food is to add to the trouble. This is, then, rule two: IN ALL ACUTE DISEASE, DON'T FEED.

All the water may be allowed that the patient desires. There is no need, however, of forcing the patient to drink large quantities of water on the absurd theory that it increases the elimination of poisons.

The following quotation from Trall is to the point in this connection:—

"Food should not be taken at all until the violence of the fever is materially abated, and then very small quantities of the simpliest food only should be permitted, as gruel, with a little toasted bread or cracker, boiled rice, mealy potatoes, baked apples, etc. There is not a more mischievous or more irrational error abroad in relation to the treatment of fever than the almost universal practice of stuffing the patient continually with stimulating animal slops, under the name of 'mild nourishing diet,' beef tea, mutton broth, chicken soup, panada, etc. The fever will always starve out before the patient is injured by abstinence, at least under hydropathic treatment, and the appetite will always return when the system is capable of assimilating food."—Hydropathic Encyclopedia, vol. 2, p. 84.

In speaking of the treatment of smallpox, Dr. Shew declared, Hydropathic Family Physician, p. 429:—

"Most fever-patients are allowed to eat too much. Some may be allowed too little; but this must be the exception to the rule. In all severe fevers, the system absolutely refuses all nourishment; that is, it is not digested or made into blood. Hence all nutriment, in such cases, is worse than useless, since if it does not go to nourish the system, it must only prove a source of irritation and harm. If the disease is severe, then it would be best as long as the fever lasts, to give no nourishment whatever. In mild cases it would of course be otherwise, although it would harm no one to fast a few days, but would, on the contrary, do them good. When nourishment is given, it should be of some bland and anti-feverish kind. Good and well-ripened fruit in its season would be especially useful, taken always at the time of a regular meal."

Dr. Jennings wrote:—

"The great, extensive, and complicated nutritive apparatus, that requires a large amount of force to convert raw material into a living structure, is put at rest, that the forces saved thereby may be transferred to the recuperative machinery within their respective limits, so that there is no call for food, and none should be offered until the crisis is passed, or a point reached where some nutritive labor can be performed, and there is a natural call for nutriment. ****And food has no more to do with the production of vitality, than the timber, planks, bolts and canvas for the ship have in supplying ship-carpenters and sailors. In the mass of diseases—such as simple, continued, or remittent fever, scarlet fever, measles, mild bilious fevers—and most of the disorders that are termed febrile, that require a few days to do up their recuperative work in the proper course of treatment to be pursued, is exceedingly plain and simple. So long as there is no call for nutriment, a cup of cool water is all that is needed for the inner man."—Tree of Life, p. 187-7.

Dr. Tilden sagely observes:—

"Given any one of these so-called diseases, from a cold to smallpox, and the only logical treatment is to stop food, wash out the bowels with enemas, and rest. A physic irritates, enervates and further checks elimination; to feed adds to the decomposition in the stomach and bowels. Such treatment builds disease; and if the patient is old or very young, the remaining resistance may be overcome by a continuation of the same treatment and death result. Nothing but rest, rest from everything, restores nerve energy and establishes secretion and elimination. Forcing remedies act the opposite. Every illness is an effort at house-cleaning, and all the aid that nature needs is to be left alone.

"This is hard to believe for a profession spooked on the idea of cure. Toxemia is the only disease. Enervation checks the elimination of toxin. At every opportunity vicarious elimination takes place. An indigestion creates irritation of the stomach, and elimination of toxin takes place through the mucous membrane of the stomach. This is called catarrh of the stomach. Cold air irritates a sensitized mucous membrane of the throat and nose, Catarrh follows. Every toxemic crisis is brought about in the same way. Rest cures; food and drugs add to the so-called disease."—Philosophy of Health. Aug. 1924.

Again he says:—

"Rest, with all that the word implies, cannot be preached too strongly. It does not mean to stay in bed and eat and take drugs. Food and drugs stimulate, which is opposed to rest. Mental poise is restful, and must go with physical rest. So strong is the ingrained belief in food, that there will be readers who will insist that patients in the state in which young Coolidge is should be in bed. (This was written while young Calvin Coolidge was ill and his spectacular physicians were making their spectacular efforts to save him. Author.) No; if feeding is all that is necessary, such invalidism would not evolve. Such patients are taxed to death by food. A limited amount of properly selected food at the right period of such lives, would forestall such catastrophes; but when profound enervation and Toxemia are once evolved, there is but one way out of the trouble—but one treatment—namely, a wise, scientific letting-alone. This must be started before an insignificant accident like a friction blister starts an infection conflagration. A half-extinguished match has fallen in the wrong place many times, as history has recorded."—*Philosophy of Health*, Aug. 1924.

AIR: A plentiful supply of oxygen is one of the prime necessities of life, at all times. Deprive a man of all oxygen and death results in a few minutes. The need of oxygen is more urgent in disease than at other times, except, of course, when under violent exertion. The sick person cannot breathe without air. The sick-room should be well ventilated both day and night with the purest air obtainable, coming directly from the outside, and not from an adjoining room or hall or from a foul courtyard.

WATER: All the water may be given that thirst demands. One may rely implicitly upon instinct in this regard. Those who doubt the competency of man's natural instincts often insist on copious water drinking, even in the absence of any natural demand for such. This practice is not only not necessary, but it is decidedly harmful. Water should be as pure as can be obtained and may be given warm or cool, as relished most by the patient.

CLEANLINESS: It is difficult to over-estimate the importance of cleanliness. Not merely the patient, but his clothing, bed, room, the air he breathes, and his surroundings should be kept clean.

Cellars, yards, cess-pools, out-houses, garbage cans, slop-jars, dead and decomposing animal and vegetable matters, pools of stagnant water, hog-pens, cow-pens, stables, near the house, are prolific sources of disease. An environment reeking with the emanations from these is not fit for well or sick.

The sick person should be gently sponged with warm water once daily, or more often, if cleanliness demands it. The eyes, nose, mouth, throat, anus, opening of the vagina under the prepuce, should all receive particular care. Plain warm water will do to cleanse these, but if the need for something else is felt, dilute lemon juice is preferable to soap or antiseptics. This may be used as an eye wash, a mouth wash, or as a gargle for the throat, and for cleansing the surface of open sores.

In diphtheria, the patient should be placed face down, with the head a little lower than the body, to cause the throat to drain outward and the excretions to be spit out:—

Dr. Tilden says:—

"In pseudomembranous inflammation, (diphtheria, membranous croup) of the throat, everything should be done to avoid breaking or loosening up the membrane; for the more it is interrupted, the greater the local poisoning, and the more toxins there will be swallowed to be neutralized by the stomachic secretions.

"Positively nothing is to be put into the child's mouth; not a drop of water, for swallowing must be avoided. The act of swallowing breaks the membranous protection. The old treatment of gargling and swabbing, was barbarous and, for intelligent people, criminal.

"Thirst must be controlled by frequent small enemas of water. Nourishment is not life-saving, as many think, but positively disease and death-provoking.**** From the foregoing explanation, it is obvious how dangerous is the old-time practice of swabbing and gargling the throat. No wonder the mortality was great, and no wonder the anti-toxin treatment has proved such a success. Its success, however, has been of a negative character—on the order of the lesser evil. If the anti-toxin has any influence—if it is not inert—it certainly must make a change in the nervous system; and this change must be reconciled and an equilibrium or readjustment take place, before a normal healing process can be resumed.'—*Impaired Health*, vol. 1, 271.

In cases where there is infectious matter, as in erysipelas, etc., care should be exercised not to carry the infection to another part of the body.

THE BOWELS: The bowels are usually points of great concern to doctors, nurses, patients, relatives and friends. Pills, powders, enemas, suppositories, etc., are frequently resorted to, to force these to act. Indeed, it is no uncommon thing to see the bowel goaded with cathartics or flushed with water, even when it is already moving freely and frequently. So deeply ingrained is the belief that we must DO SOMETHING, anything, so long as something is done, the physician and patient and all concerned, are not satisfied unless the body is being excited and stimulated.

A sound, vigorous body, with pure sensibilities, neither needs nor courts any kind or degree of unnatural excitation, but disdains and resists it in toto; and an impaired body and sensibilities, needs it no more, disdains it no less, and is less able to bear its devastating effect. "Stimulants," says Jennings, "act on the principle of the spur, 'increase action, but diminish the power of that action,' *always* leave less of power in any part on which they expend their action than there was in that part before they acted upon it." (*Tree of Life*, p. 198.) Shall we, then, exhaust the power of the bowels, and consequently, of the whole system, by forced labor, or shall we allow them to rest and recuperate?

Says Dr. Tilden:—

"There is a continual tendency in the minds of those who give thought to medical subjects (professional and lay) to think of bowel evacuation and elimination as identical. Consequently, when enervation has brought elimination to almost nil, doctors and patients use eliminating remedies. (?); and when the bowels are forced to move, the bladder to empty, the skin to act, etc., etc., they think elimination has been established. Not so—only voiding what has already been excreted. This is an old medical error of confusing excretion or elimination with evacuation or voiding, and much suffering and many deaths have been caused by the practice of forcing the bowels to move. Irritating drugs act in the opposite way from what is desired. They may force voiding, but always check excretion or elimination, and build Toxemia."— *Philosophy of Health*, Aug. 1924.

Dr. Page observed:—

"Tanner had no movement during his fast; Griscomb's experience was similar, and Connolly, the consumptive, who fasted for forty-three days, had no movement for three weeks, and then the temporary looseness was occasioned by profuse water-drinking, which in his case, proved curative."—*The Natural Cure*, p. 112.

Dr. Tilden records the case of a man suffering with appendicitis or something else, whose bowels moved on the nineteenth day. They moved twice that day—two very large movements of fecal matter, pus and blood, with a "dreadfully offensive" odor. Dr. Tilden gives it as his experience that in such cases it "usually requires from fourteen to twenty-eight days" for the bowels to move.

In discussing a case of typhus fever, which he cared for and in which there was no bowel action for a period of three weeks, Jennings says:—

"The special object in noticing this case, is to call attention to one feature of the disease, to wit: the suspension of the peristaltic, or natural downward motion of the bowel, for the long period of three weeks.**** Some of the friends of Mr. G. felt a concern for the quiet state of the bowels, and for *this concern*, I prescribed some pills which I knew 'would do no hurt, if they did no good.' For myself, I had no fear about the bowels, and should have had none if they had been kept at rest three weeks longer, if there had been no other sign of danger."—*Philosophy of Human Life*, p. 176-7.

I know of no more reason for forcing bowel action than for forcing heart action or lung action. Bowel action is automatic, and, except in cases of obstruction, may be confidently expected to do all the work that is really essential and to conserve all the energy possible by failure to act, when there is no urgent necessity for them to act. Even in obstruction, they usually succeed in sending the feces back the way it came and get rid of it.

Purgatives, laxatives and enemas, are sources of excruciating pain in cases of appendicitis, inflammation of the colon, etc., and are frequent causes of a break in nature's defense, resulting in a rupture of the bowel wall or a rupture of the appendix into the abdominal cavity instead of into the colon.

"Doctor," once said an anxious captain to Dr. Jennings, "my wife can't breathe much longer unless you do something for her." "Captain," replied the doctor, "Your wife can't stop breathing if she tries." Then he proceeded to administer some colored water and some "powders" composed of corn starch. After a short time, the lady's difficulty in breathing was relieved and she recovered, thanks to the potent "medicines" which she had received.

A fact, unknown, to physicians and laymen alike, is that all the functions of the body are performed with as much promptness, regularity, and efficiency as, under existing circumstances, is compatible with the safety and highest welfare of the body. In "disease" and in "health," that is, so long as life lasts, every organ and tissue of the body is at its post, ready and disposed to perform its particular functions, to the full extent of its abilities. They do good work when they have the power to do so, and when lacking in power to produce a perfect work, must do the best they can.

There are many ways of forcing increased action in debilitated organs for a brief period, providing there is enough power in reserve to produce the action, but these things always and necessarily, diminish the power of that action and do so in precisely the degree to which they accelerate the action. The increase of action is occasioned by the extra expenditure of power called out, not supplied, by the compulsory process, and therefore the quantity of power is diminished by this amount. The power is wanted for other purposes and will be used more judiciously and advantageously by the undisturbed law of appropriation, and distribution of the living system.

These facts apply equally to the bowel as to the heart or lungs or liver. We may depend on the body to regulate its own internal conduct to its own best interests.

PAIN: The relief of pain is an unmitigated evil. Most of the work of physicians consists in relieving pain and discomfort and almost invariably they "relieve" these with agents and by means that themselves produce more pain and discomfort than they "relieve." So true is it, that all drugs produce, as their secondary effects, the exact opposite to their primary effects, that Dr. Jennings suggested that drugs should be classified according to their secondary effects. Tonics should be called debilitators, pain-killers should be pain-producers, etc.

Pain is merely a symptom. Symptoms are such only and not cause. The office of pain is beneficial, protective. It may serve as a diagnostic guide, if it is not suppressed. Its suppression does not remove cause, but does retard or actually prevent recovery. "Grin and bear it," is the best advice ever given a patient in relation to pain or discomfort.

FEVER: Nothing better than a high fever can come to the sick person. The higher the fever, the quicker the recovery. No effort should be made to suppress, reduce or control fever. There is no reason to fear fever. The idea that two, three, four or more degrees of fever destroys the tissues of the body is arrant nonsense. A temperature of a hundred and four or a hundred and six certainly is not the fierce burning process some would have us believe it to be.

"Let the manner of its (animal heat) production be what it may. ****it must be under the control of vitality, ****it never rises more than seven, eight, or nine degrees above the healthy standard**** this may be uncomfortable, but can do no serious mischief. ****There is no wrong action."—Medical Reform, p. 132-3-4.

DELIRIUM AND CONVULSIONS: These are symptoms, right actions, and should not be suppressed. Their causes or occasions may kill, but these never do. So long as the occasion for these is present, they should be present. Their suppression by depressing the nervous system is injurious in the extreme.

COLLAPSE: This is a frequent phenomenon under the sustaining plan of treatment. It is an exceedingly rare thing under orthopathic care and is confined almost exclusively to old people. Collapse, under the methods in vogue, usually means death. This is so because the method of treating collapse is simply an increase of the methods that have produced it. If these methods are abandoned, recoveries are frequent.

If relatives, friends, nurses and physicians, upon whom the responsibilities for care of the case rest, can exercise the needed patience and not become panicky, recovery is reasonably certain in most cases. If the air of the room is kept pure, the temperature of the patient warm and equable, absolute quiet maintained, and the patient left alone, with only a little water touched to the lips and mouth at intervals, and some permitted to be swallowed when there is power of deglutition, resuscitation will occur.

However, if the usual mad-cap endeavors to save life are resorted to, if heart stimulants, respiratory stimulants, and various other perturbating measures are employed, there will be a sudden flaring up of the powers of life, as though the patient is improving and these powers will be exhausted in this final flare, and death will end the scene.

Dr. Jennings once suffered with a case of acute pleurisy. He has left us the following observations of his experiences, during this illness, which observations Dr. Oswald declared "deserve to be framed in every hygienic sanitarium." I desire to introduce these at this place.

"In January, 1840, the eighth month of my residence in a Western state, my general health began to decline. My appetite and strength gradually failed me; exercise became irksome, attended with great lassitude and a sense of soreness over the whole system, which at length made my couch and a recumbent posture desirable. While sitting up one evening, in preparation for the night's repose, I had a chill and a heavy rigor pass over me, shaking my whole frame, and making my teeth chatter, which continued for two or three minutes. As the chill subsided, a pain commenced in the top of my left shoulder, soon became agonizing, and after some ten or twelve minutes, gradually descended by the shoulder blade until it became fixed and exceedingly distressing in my left side, and whence, like a dense cloud, it spread through all the middle region of the chest, and in a short period, I was in a confirmed, acute inflammatory pleurisy. For twelve hours breathing was at best laborious, and painful, confining me to nearly an erect position in bed; but the distress occasioned by efforts at coughing was indescribable.

"The confidence of my wife in the 'let-alone' treatment, which had been strengthening through a number of years, and had carried her unflinchingly through a number of serious indispositions, on this occasion, faltered, and she begged me to send for a physician to bleed me or do something to give at least temporary relief; for, said she, 'you cannot live so.' In my own mind there was not the least vestige of misgiving respecting the course pursed.

"In view of the constitutional defect in the pulmonary department of my system, and the nature and severity of the symptoms, it appeared to me very doubtful whether the powers of life would be able to accomplish what they had undertaken and put me again upon my feet. But I felt perfectly satisfied that whatever could be done to good purpose would be done, by 'due course of law.' ****My mind, therefore, was perfectly at ease in trusting Nature's work in Nature's hands. There was no danger in the symptoms, let them run as high as they would. They constituted no part of the real difficulty, but grew out of it. The general movement which made them necessary, was aiming directly at the removal of that difficulty. INSTEAD, THEREFORE, OF BEING TROUBLED WITH SUCH SYMPTOMS, MY CONVICTION WAS VERY STRONG THAT I COULD LIVE BETTER WITH THEM THAN WITHOUT THEM, (caps. mine, author).

"In the morning, ten or twelve hours from the beginning of the cold chill, there was some mitigation of suffering, which continued till afternoon, when there was a slight exacerbation of symptoms; but the heaviest part of the work was accomplished within the first twenty-four hours. From that time, there was a gradual declension of painful symptoms, till the fifth day, when debility and expectoration constituted the bulk of the disease.

"Full bleeding at the commencement of the disease, followed by the other 'break-up' means usually employed in such affections, would have given me immediate relief and, by continuing to ply active means (for there would have been no stopping of it, short of stopping the action of the heart), the strongest, most distressing, and critical part of the disease might have been pushed forward to the fifth day; and I might even then possibly have recovered. But, granting that my life would have been spared, I suffered much less on the whole, under the 'let-alone' treatment than I should have done under a perturbating one, besides having the curative process conducted with more regularity, made shorter, and done up more effectually."—*Medical Reform*, p. 312.

COMPLICATIONS: A little boy became sick. A doctor was called. He said appendicitis and advised an operation. The boy was taken to the hospital. At the hospital, he was said to be suffering with typhoid fever. He was given an injection of serum. His brother removed him from the hospital the same day he was admitted. The author was called. He advised fasting and rest. The boy's condition grew better. After five days, the first doctor called again. He said the boy had a "touch of typhoid" and could not recover without food and drugs. He left two prescriptions. The brother tore these into bits. At the hospital when the brother took the sick child, the doctor in charge tried to impress him with the seriousness of the boy's condition. The brother replied: "He will be serious if I leave him here for you to feed and drug."

The brother was right. Feeding and drugging convert simple acute diseases, that should be well in two or three days to a week, into serious difficulties that last for weeks or months, and end in death or chronic disease. Drugs and feeding build complications. The boy only had a "touch of typhoid" because he did not receive typical text-book treatment. It takes typical text-book treatment to convert a simple fever into a typical text-book case of typhoid fever.

No disease can present all the symptoms attributed to it in standard text-books of medicine unless treated as outlined in these same text-books. Doctors build most of the pathology they spend years in studying. Feeding and drugging are the greatest sources of suffering and death in disease. An acute disease should be a comfortable illness. And it would be if the patient was given warmth, quiet, rest, air and water, and all feeding and drugging omitted. Death except in old age, would be extremely rare, and the length of human life would go upward with a bound.

If these suggestions are followed faithfully, and no drugs or serums are given the patient will be out of bed in a few days. Cases of typhoid fever, pneumonia, etc., which usually run three to four weeks or even longer, need not last more than seven or eight days to two weeks, providing these suggestions are followed from the very onset of the disease: In fact, these diseases will never develop into typical cases under this plan.

CONVALESCENCE: Is a period in which care must be exercised if the patient is to fare well. The body has just emerged from a severe fight. It is weak from the expenditure of much energy. There has been more or less destruction of tissue. The patient is in no condition to return to normal activities until he has thoroughly recuperated from his illness. A premature return to duties may easily prove disasterous.

The destroyed tissues must be repaired. The used up nerve force or vital force, must be recuperated. This requires time, although it takes place under proper conditions fairly rapidly. It is possible to hasten or retard the recuperation and reparation.

Over exertion, a return to the old destructive habits, over-eating, exposure to extremes of temperature, etc., may not only hinder recovery, but may actually work injury. On the other hand, recuperation may be hastened somewhat by proper attention being given to rest, sleep, exercise, diet, one's air supply and sunshine.

Rest is essential to recuperation of vital force. This we have already learned. Now consider the condition of the convalescing patient. He has already greatly enervated, else he would not have been toxemic and would not have become sick. He has just gone through a hard trying struggle which has left him much weaker than before. Rest must be enforced now, in order to recuperate.

Sleep, we have already learned, is the highest form of rest. If the patient can sleep much, this will hasten the recuperation. He should lie down at intervals during the day and attempt to sleep. No sitting up until late hours at night should ever be permitted. He should retire early.

During the process of disease there was more or less destruction of tissue. This must all be repaired before the organism is ready to resume normal operations. This requires some time and necessitates rest. Tissue repair is only accomplished during rest and reaches its maximum point of efficiency during sleep. Thus we have an added reason for rest and sleep.

By the foregoing, is not meant that the patient should lie in bed or sit in an invalid's chair and rest and sleep twenty-four hours out of every day? On the contrary, we insist that a small amount of mild exercise be taken daily and that the amount taken be gradually increased.

Life and health demand a certain amount of exercise. Even plants must have exercise if they are to do well. Plants get their exercise in a passive form, that is, the wind as the operator, gives them passive exercise.

There are times when exercise would be highly injurious, but outside of these, a certain amount of exercise is essential to good health and strength. So in convalescense, the patient who exercises judiciously will recover faster than the one who does not. He must not attempt a hundred-yard dash or enter a weight-lifting contest by any means. His exercise should be moderate, and of short duration. He should not exercise until tired or exhausted. As he grows stronger, he can exercise more strenuously, and exercise longer.

Walking is the favorite form of exercise. For my part, I could never see why it should be better than other forms as long as they are not carried to excess. The safe rule is moderation. Take the exercise you derive most pleasure from.

Feeding in convalescence is a very important item. The digestive organs are still weak, their secretions are not normal so that they are by no means fitted to handle a "square" meal. Great care must be exercised in breaking the fast which the patient has been on.

If the disease has been of such a nature that there is likely to be any ulcerations or open sores in the intestinal tract time should be given for these to heal before food is given, and this applies especially to the feeding of solid foods. A small piece of solid food may easily become lodged in the ulcer, and produce irritation, set up fermentation, and cause infection.

Again, if food is given before the stomach, intestine, or bowel are thoroughly healed, the movements of these organs as they convey the food along, is likely to produce mechanical injury to the unhealed parts. A safe plan is not to be in too much of a hurry to feed.

To resume feeding, fruit juices or vegetables juices may be used. Here again should moderation be the watchword. Don't try to rush matters. *Nature does her work slowly, but well.*

After a day or two, small amounts of other foods may be added. The amount eaten should be gradually increased. Don't hurry.

Let the food be of simple wholesome nature. It should consist chiefly of fresh fruits and green vegetables. Starch foods, protein foods and fatty foods, should be used very sparingly. Some proteins are needed for repairs, but one does not have to eat these in large quantities.

Air and sunshine are as essential during convalescence as at other times. It would be well to spend as much time outdoors as possible. A hammock or chair under a tree makes an ideal resting place. Don't stay in the sun too much at first. Sleep with windows open so that fresh air can be yours at all times. The body needs plenty of oxygen in its work of reparation.

Don't allow yourself to become angry or excited. Don't indulge in card games or other such games that may excite and tire you. Keep out of exciting or distracting arguments. Keep away from exciting shows. Treat yourself decent and a quick return to normal will be yours. Your system will then be all the better for the house cleaning.

This is all very simple, so simple, indeed, that it doesn't seem possible that it will do the work. But if the reader has read and understood the foregoing chapters, he will readily understand how it is possible. In fact, he can easily see that this is the only logical way of treating the patient.

HYGIENE OF CHRONIC DISEASE

Chapter XXX

THE seomewhat unique principle is maintained by *Orthopathy*, that the first condition of successful restoration of health is a philosophical comprehension, by the sick person, of the cause or causes of the malady. All cure is self-cure and every sick person must cure himself or herself. The sick person must learn to distinguish between effects and their antecedents in order that he may not waste time, and perhaps irreparably injure his health, trying to remove or suppress effects by measures that do not correct or remove their antecedents. Dr. G. H. Taylor has so admirably expressed these facts in his *Pelvic and Hernial Therapeutics,* (1885) that we shall reproduce what he says.

"Morbid phenomena, especially those usually designated chronic disease, are regarded in one of two general ways. As these modes of estimating often lead to differing, even to opposing remedies for what is essentially the same morbid condition, it becomes important that the proper distinctions between these modes should be made.

"One way of estimating disease is that adopted by the patient and by sympathizing friends, and doubtless influences the physician to a large extent. This estimate is based upon subjective facts—what the patient feels, sees, and experiences. It includes his consciousness of defect of power and excess of sensibility, and the accompanying exterior manifestations.

"Remedies are therefore sought in accordance with these conceptions, and include prominently whatever means may be capable of mitigating, or even abolishing, disagreeable sensations, or at least the consciousness thereof, often with little reference to the source from which those feelings spring.

"The invalid, unfortunately for his own true interests, is disinclined to discriminate between the two distinct ideas of suffering and of disease. He blends the two as one. This leads to the radical mistake of trying to cure the one by causing suspension of the other. He seems to think that pain is causing him injury, instead of referring it to the morbid action from which the pain is derived. It is not the pain, —which is doubtless on the whole advantageous,—but its causes, which demands correction.

"It is therefore with difficulty that the invalid learns that while this and other subjective manifestations are undoubted verities, they alone are untrustworthy indications as to remedies because incomplete indications of disease. The facts of pathology are far more extended, and all, not a part, are required as a basis for any proper remedial prescription. Too close reliance on sensory indications inevitably leads to therapeutic difficulties. These consist in the mistakes of trying to remedy mere effects in place of removing their causes.

"Another consequence of undue regard to the subjective indications of disease, is the premature arrest of diagnostic inquiry. Further investigation, as the tracing of effects to their causes, is discouraged; the idea of philosophical relationships of seen and unseen facts is repressed, and the advantages to therapeutics of such inquiries become unavailable. The physician is guided by only a limited number of subordinate facts, which, being isolated from their true connection, are untrustworthy.

"A still further difficulty, usually indirectly expressed arising from the above stated sources of misconception, is the tendency in the popular mind to associate, in idea, defects of the vital organism with those of non-vital objects. Diseased manifestations are thought to be like something broken, requiring local repair by trained and dextrous hands. The remedy must accord with the immediate, patent, and obtrusive difficulty, as a broken implement is mended. Medical science is limited to the record of experience in correcting local faults of the organism and insufficiently correlates with science in its wider aspect.

"The defects of this mode of regarding chronic disease, and the practical therapeutic errors to which it inevitably leads, will be shown in succeeding chapters in connection with such affections as those pertaining to the pelvis and adjacent parts. These errors are so surprising, and so easily detectable that it is a wonder that the

395

medical profession, trained to great acuteness in pathological observation, should not have long ago insisted on their correction.

"The other mode of estimating chronic disease in reference to remedies, regards its ordinary manifestatoins as only symptoms, products, and evidences of antecedent causes, without which such manifestations would be impossible. It therefore assumes that however distant and obscure these causes, they are the primary objects of medical interest, and of remedial attention. The actual departure from health is a *process* rather than a *product*. The objective phenomena are a cumulative record of transitional defects and errors. The physician points out and corrects these, and the consequences, however manifested, cease perforce. Nothing exists, not even local disease, after the withdrawal or cessation of the processes whereby it exists.

"This is the physiological method. This method regards health and disease as flowing from essentially identical sources, the difference consisting solely in the degrees of perfection attained by the inchoate activities at the ultimate sources of vital power. Remedies are therefore concerned in the control of precesses, rather than in obscuring the effects and products of these processes. The processes of physiology embrace the whole career of matter entering the organism, onward to its final exit. During this transit it is subjected to a series of changes, and a variety of differentiations in physica! quality and form, for the sole ultimate purpose of evolving force or energy. The processes of physiology are minute, involving not merely the tissues of every part, but the ultimate molecules, and constituent elements, beyond the powers of ordinary observation; these may, but often do not, make an impression on the consciousness or sensibilities

"In the diseased state (indicated in medical science by the word pathology) there is the same career of the same matter, but under conditions less favorable for the attainment of perfected results. The changes due have in some stage of the career been imperfectly attained. In some local part, or by some inferior physical change, the progressing matters have failed to yield energy and *therefore*, and coincidently, failed to attain the chemical form necessary for exit. The product, both of energy and of substance, depends on processes in the respective organic instruments devoted to these purposes. Pathology, therefore has its potential existence in transitional acts, rather than in the form which the consequences of the imperfection of these acts assume. The distinction should always be made between the effects, consequences, and products of imperfect physiological processes, and the processes from which these evidences proceed. It is the former of which we are chiefly cognizant, because more exposed to observation; they are exterior and objective, and often present a cumulative mass. The latter are interior, elusive, and known by comparison and by the reasoning faculties.

"These considerations unmistakably imply a wide distinction between the inward, invisible and intangible form of disease, irrespective of the sensation, and the consequences thereof as exhibited in objective phenomena. The one is continuously contributing, by the changes occurring in successive particles of substance, to produce and maintain the other; the relation of cause and effect being precisely the same as that recognized as resulting in health. Pathology therefore exists less in formed product than in its forming. The impressions of consciousness may or may not exist, according to the nature and location of the imperfect process, and are always to be classed with the objective phenomena, or formed products, so far as relates to therapeutics. It is therefore a profound mistake to merge together as an undistinguishable whole two considerations so radically distinct as cause and effect, antecedent and consequent, process and product, in pathology; and such confusion of separate and different things inevitably introduces into practical therapeutics the gravest inconsistencies and mistakes.

"The adequate comprehension of disease therefore considers it in the two aspects above presented. These for convenience may be styled the antecedent and the resultant *factors*, meaning the defective processes, and the cumulative products.

"The susceptibility of the two distinct parts of pathological phenomena to separate consideration arises from the nature of vital processes, of which disease is but a form. These processes are progressive, and never concluded as long as life lasts. It probably extends throughout all the forms and variations of these processes, which receive distinct names, according to subordinate peculiarities. The evidence of this statement is derived from a variety of sources.

"Prophylactics, or the means of prevention of diseases, emphatically recognizes an antecedent principle and antecedent action. The malarial infections, zymotic and incubative affections generally, are confessed demonstrations of the same principle; and the same is legitimately inferred of acute affections having abscure sources though no less positive manifestations, but whose processes and products are so blended as regards time, that the distinction has less practical therapeutic value.

"The failure to recognize the distinction above pointed out as to antecedent and resultant parts or factors of diseases, opens the way for the perversion of therapeutics from its greater to its lesser uses. Remedies addressed to the resultant, or consequent object, are necessarily only palliative, and in general can have no effect on the contributive factors. The abatement of pain, one of the consequences of the morbid, or unperfected process, easily becomes the primary, instead of an incidental purpose. The sufferer is countenanced in his delusion that pain is something synonymous with disease, and that the latter disappears with it. Besides, a practical error of still more serious import is committed. The advantages of pain as a pathological guide are lost. Another and very disadvantageous consequence arises from medicating the sources of sensibility, which should not be the therapeutic purpose. These sensory powers are inevitably perverted by the constant use of remedies adapted to diminish pain, without paying attention to its causes. The nervous system is therefore liable ultimately to become an overwhelming factor, additional to the primary ones.

"The relations of the antecedents to the resultants in pathology are necessarily those of equality, because effects must proceed from adequate and therefore an equal cause: but this fact does not imply interchangeability, but the contrary. The latter always depends on the former, and not the former on the latter. Remove the morbid processes by converting them into healthful processes, that is, into perfected morphological and chemical activities, and the morbid effects, however conspicuous, cease to exist. No radical curative effect is attainable, if therapeutic attention be limited to the resultant factors; such medication may be palliative, but is devoid of direct control of antecedent processes. However deftly the consequences be removed nothing permanent is secured: the continuance of the producing factor is sure to reinstate the morbid result, however concealed, altered, or obscured to the senses.

"An intelligent appreciation of the distinctions above made, appears to be necessary to prevent medical practice from degenerating, as it is manifestly inclined, into a fruitless routine of palliative procedures. Methods of toying with the senses, and ways of disconnecting imperfect results from the elementary processes on which these results depend: devices in short for concealing these results mistakenly regarded as the disease, whether the manifestation be interior in the form of pain, or exterior in some outward tangible indication, as in the pelvis, or at the hernial border, assume unwarranted importance. The antecedents and the consequences, which are entirely distinct considerations become inextricably mingled in therapeutics and remedies adapted to radical cure, in the sense of correcting the primary departure from true physiological action, become impossible.

"One of the leading obstacles to the recognition, and therefore the remedying of the primary factors of disease instead of the resultant factors, cannot be too strongly insisted upon; one that imperils and often negatives the value of medical science. This practice is based on the presumption that the fact of pain is actually diminished by this class of so-called remedies. This is an assumption that is manifestly improbable; but, on the other hand there is much evidence showing that symptoms relating to the seat of consciousness may thus be easily deferred, and possibly their location changed, yet the amount of pain, taking time into consideration, is actually often very greatly increased by the method invoked to stifle it. These statements are necessarily confined in their application to chronic affections; for it is readily conceded that in acute affections nature is at work, repairing defects, and gaining ground by intensifying compensative processes, in spite of the temporary interference of medicaments when these have no relation whatever to reparation."

In overcoming any disease condition the problem is not so much one of overcoming the disease directly, as it is of attacking and overcoming the popular misconception regarding its essential nature. The mind of the patient and the minds of the patient's relatives and friends have first to be freed of the perverted views and erroneous theories of disease that have been and are being fostered by the medical profession.

The very expression "Cure" as used today is misleading and wrong. It is understood to require the expenditure of time, attention and energy on the part of the healer, attendants and patients upon a subject that should require no attention whatever. Disease should not exist at all and healing should be unnecessary. However, all real cure is self-cure and cannot be accomplished by outside agencies and skill.

The fact that millions of men and women are engaged in an effort to patch up the remainder of their fellow men and women is actually humiliating. In this particular we are lowered below the beasts of the fields and fowls of the air. In spite of all our boasted wisdom and science, in spite of our boasted superiority, we are not equal to the animals of the forest and plains in health and hardihood.

Man is capable of possessing a higher degree of health and vigor than any other animal on the face of the earth—yet he actually possesses far less than any other. Man alone requires, or THINKS HE REQUIRES to be in the shops for repairs. Man alone, except those animals he has enslaved, supports doctors, nurses, attendants and costly hospitals.

"Cure of Disease!" exclaimed Trall. "What a world of delusion in that expression! It has always been the fundamental error of the medical profession. It forever misleads the public mind. The phrase is founded on a false conception of the nature of disease. Instead of trying to cure diseases, we should seek to remove their causes. Diseases never can be and never should be cured while their causes exist. It is on the fallacy of curing disease that the doctors are drugging the world to death."
—*The Hygienic System.*

Some people possess an undying faith in the doctor and his methods. They possess more faith in the doctor than the religious man is supposed to have in his God. The doctor can do everything to them short of killing them and they trust him still. If there is any survival after death they probably retain their faith in the doctor and his methods even after these have killed him. Such faith is beyond all understanding: If faith had any curative power such patients should not long remain sick.

If they lose their faith in one doctor or in one system of "healing" it is only to transfer their allegiance to another doctor or to another system. They go from doctor to doctor, from institution to institution, from system to system but they never lose faith. They never get well because they never reform their lives. They are in search of cures and cures they will find if they have to die in the attempt.

About five years ago a prominent "Natural Therapist" triumphantly exclaimed:—

"My soul now rests in peace. My life-work is completed. I have witnessed the fulfilment of my heart's desire—the conquest of disease."

A year later this same man declared:—

"We are constantly testing new methods and we shall continue to incorporate in our system everything that gives positive results in the treatment of human ailments."

Today, five years after he made his first statement, the wonder-working machine that he had seen conquer disease is a thing of history. It has come and gone. Its heyday of popularity is over. Its day of miraculous accomplishment is passed. It has been "modified," and "improved" over and over again. Its inventor is dead. The man who made the above statement is dead. Other machines and apparatuses have come and gone. They enjoyed their day and followed it to oblivion.

"Natural Therapeutics," now obsolescent, was a Heteropathic system identical with Naturopathy. "Physiological Therapeutics" were of the same order. They each attempted to cure disease and each possessed many methods of "cure."

Dr. Walsh maintains in his "Cures; The story of the Cures that Fail," that in proper conditions of confidence literally anything will cure a large number of cases. This attributes the cure to the mental effects of the "remedy" and ignores, completely, the self-curative powers of the body. If his contention were true the more cases that were cured by some vaunted "cure" the greater would grow the confidence imposed in its curative virtues. The greater the confidence in the "cure" the more cures it would make and thus, the longer it was used the more effective it would become. A vicious circle would thus be established that would be self-perpetrating. A remedy, once popular would have little chance of ever losing its place in the confidence imposed in its powers. This is, however, contrary to what the history of the cures that failed (after they had literally "cured" their thousands and tens of thousands) reveal. Their period of popularity is usually brief. Dr. Walsh will have as much difficulty in trying to explain this fact in the light of his theory as he will in explaining how these same cures also "cured" infants, animals and plants. I do not believe the success of the "cures" in the cases of infants, animals, and plants can be explained with Dr. Walsh's assumption as a basis. It will either have to be admitted that the methods did possess some curative power at the time they were used, even if they did not possess it later, or else the self-curative powers of the organism will have to be recognized and given full credit. I do not deem it necessary that I here restate the Orthopathic position in the matter. I leave the matter up to the candid and thoughtful reader now, who, after having carefully weighted the evidence, should be able to decide whether or not our position is the correct one.

The effort to beat the laws of nature, to cheat cause out of its effect, by the use of remedies or medicines is so childishly absurd and so inherently impossible that man should long ago have realized his folly in persistently attempting such a thing. Any real and permanent cure (of an abnormal condition of the body) must be the result of a constitutional reconstruction within the body itself and this can only be brqught about by the forces of nature that are concerned in growth, development, repair and maintenence of the animal and vegetable world. No form of artificial treatment (therapeutics) embodies these principles.

Every form of artificial treatment is sympotomatic and is in no wise directed at cause. To treat a patient merely symptomatically is most decidedly wrong. Symptoms are such only and not causes, and to direct attention to effects and ignore causes is like the effort to rid a swampy region of mosquitoes by swatting individual mosquitoes instead of draining the swamps. It is only patch work.

Dr. Walter has left us the following bit of wisdom, which, if rightly understood and heeded will free man from both ill-health and the cure mongers.

"Men try everything and fail to get well. Let them stop trying for a while and they will get better results. 'Not try but trust' is often as important to health as to religion. What most people want is more rest and less worry. Drowning men catch at straws but it is the catching at straws that drowns them. The drowning of people is almost invariably due to their struggles to save themselves. If they would lie quietly on the water, with nose elevated, they could float and breathe for hours; instead of which they plunge and roll and struggle, until, exhausted, they give up the contest and sink to rise no more. In the matter of health in our day, it were folly to be wise. Nearly all thought, all doctrine and all practice is opposed to good health. About all theories of disease are exactly wrong."—*Vital Science*, p. 177.

"Be still, and know that I am God." Be still. Cease to resist. Cease trying to overcome evil with evil. "Cease to do evil and learn to do good." "Be not overcome of evil, but overcome evil with good." "Go and sin no more." This is good Orthopathy as well as good religion. Man fights disease (which he conceives to be evil) with methods that are evil, while, at the same time, continuing the evils that are responsible for his disease. He has not and does not, "cease to do evil and learn to do good." The Orthopathic doctrine of Health by healthful living and cure by the same means, by learning to "go and sin no more," has never appealed to many. But it is as certain as anything that so long as he sows "to the flesh" he must continue to reap corruption.

Chronic diseases are usually considered to be incurable and we are sorry to have to say that they are usually not cured. Despite the noise that is made by many drugless institutions and by certain drugless practitioners about their wonderful success in dealing with chronic disease they do not accomplish as many wonders as their talk and writing would lead one to suppose.

This is equally as true of other systems of treatment. Chiropractors have in recent years been making a lot of noise about their wonderful cures of chronic diseases. Naprapaths, likewise, publish a list of wonders they have performed.

Now the truth about the whole matter is that these men never mention those cases in which they fail. And their failures are many. Again, many of their boasted cures are not cures at all. It often happens that a patient is pronounced cured, he writes an "unsolicited" testimonial at the request of the one who treated him, and in a week or a month is as bad as ever. These facts are not given to the public. When they talk, they tell of their successes or apparent successes, not of their failures. These things are all equally as true of those who "heal" by "mind power," "Divine power," etc.

The drugless professions are as much given to fads in treatment as the drugging professions. The whole human race indulges in fads, therefore the drugless "healers," being partly human, are afflicted with much of this human weakness. Only a few years back, hydrotherapy and mechanotherapy held the day. Water cure institutions filled our land. These were followed by osteopathy, this by such things as the vibrator, the beautfiul "violet ray," spondylotherapy. Then Chiropractic took the field. Chiropractic gave way to a conglomeration of all kinds of methods. These conglomerationists call themselves mixers and are usually mixed.

They have developed hosts of methods of treating ailments and invented myriads of instruments and appliances to do the work with. The office of a "mixer" reminds one of a store room or junk shop—sometimes we can see a resemblance in them of a Curio Shop. It seems that their inventive possibilities are never to be exhausted.

Medical men usually admit that they cannot cure chronic diseases, however sure they may be that they can cure the acute or self-limited forms. The drugless branches of Heteropathy, however, insist that they can cure chronic diseases. One psuedo-nature cure sanitarium that was formerly located in Chicago and which claimed to achieve remarkable results in the chronic forms of disease, used to give patients the following routine treatment each day. The patients were made to get out of bed at six o'clock in the morning. They then went into the basement where the treatment rooms were located and were given the cold blitz-gus, a high pressure stream of cold water, over their bodies, and particularly along the spinal column. From this they passed into the massage room where they received from twenty to thirty minutes of maulings and poundings and were shipped into another room for another twenty minutes of Sweedish movements. After this, an Osteopath played with the spine of each one for another ten minutes and they were sent up to dress for breakfast.. They were ready to go back to bed, of course, but instead of this, they were taken in the middle of the forenoon out of doors and given several minutes of exercise. In the evening, before retiring, each patient was given a cold sitz bath or a cold pack. Such treatment kept them in a state of vital depletion and "crises" were of frequent development.

The development of chronic disease has already been discussed considerably in previous chapters. We will content ourselves with but a brief recapitulation as this time.

Disease is vital action (in self-defense), abnormal because of abnormal conditions, and is occasioned by anything which is sufficiently disliked by the organism to war against it. If the organism is unable to overcome and destroy the condition or occasion for the fight, it is forced to either accommodate itself to the condition or perish.

The initial fight against any disease influence is an acute reaction (crisis) against it. If the acute effort fails to accomplish its purpose the organism attempts to accommodate itself to the condition and carry on the battle less vigorously and over a longer period of time. This gives us chronic disease.

Chronic disease, is therefore, usually the result of the same conditions that produce acute disease, with the added element of accommodation. The failure of the organism to overcome the disease influence by acute eliminative efforts is usually due to the suppressive methods used by the physician. Every abnormal symptom is suppressed as quickly as it arises. If, after one is suppressed, another appears, it is as quickly suppressed. This often results in the death of the patient. Here we cannot refrain from quoting the remark of Dr. Trall in reference to the death of General Taylor. He said: "When I heard of blackberries as among the causes of General Taylor's death, I thought of blue-pills, and gray powders, and green tinctures, and red lotions, and brown mixtures."—*True Healing Art.*

These same colored pills, powers, tinctures, lotions and mixtures are as effectively suppressing acute symptoms, and producing chronic disease or death today as they did in the days of Dr. Trall, only we have more of them and have serums, vaccines, anti-toxins, etc., to help them. The increase in Chronic disease keeps pace with our increasing means for suppressing acute forms.

The organism would, in most cases, be able to throw off the disease influence by the efforts it puts forth in chronic disease were it not that the condition that makes it necessary is kept alive by the prior habits. The chronic sufferer keeps up his enervating habits and weakening indulgencies. This, of course, perpetuates his condition and results ultimatly in more and greater trouble and varied forms of trouble. Every new phase in the development of chronic disease is prepared for by its precedents. The continuity of the process is nowhere broken. When a new stage "begins" which appears to be a new and distinct disease, or which presents a new and different form, it has been gradually prepared for beneath the surface of events. It is a serious blunder to single out each link in a series or chain of successive or concomitant developments and give to each of these a different name and ascribe them to different causes. They originate out of the same antecedents.

Elimination is accomplished by the body itself (if it is given an opportunity), but cannot be forced. But if the organs of elimination are given more work than they are able to perform the toxemia must continue to increase. If out-put does not equal income there is bound to be an accumulation of the residue within the system. If the patient is piling into his system by way of food, drink, tobacco, etc., more than the organs of elimination can send out, how is the patient to recover? If there is gastro-intestinal putrefaction resulting in the absorption of more toxic material than these organs can handle it must be stopped before recovery, can take place. Physiological rest will accomplish this.

As this process of toxin accumulation continues it reaches a point where life is endangered. The organism then institutes a crisis and eliminates it through other channels. Or perhaps there is exposure to cold or rain, or an unusual meal and a crisis is forced. These crises, however, do not result in health but succeed only in reducing the toxemia to the toleration point, after which the acute symptoms again subside. We then have a short period of what commonly passes for health during which there is more toxin accumulation followed by another crisis. This merry-go-round of toxin accumulation, followed by a crisis; then more toxin accumulation and another crisis keeps up until death puts a period to our existence.

Under hygienic conditions, as the body's powers are gradually raised the amount of toxic material it will tolerate is gradually lessened. As the body grows stronger, and the vital powers increase, the effort to become master increases. The organism often develops acute efforts to throw off the enslaving toxins. Thus we have the appearance of the healing crisis, in the recovery from chronic conditions. Often times, too, the body is able to eliminate the toxins without resorting to crises.

Chronic disease is a subdued effort at cure, resulting either from suppression of acute disease or from long continued indulgence in its causes. Chronic disease represents chronic provocation. It is kept alive from day to day, from year to year by continuance of the causes which have produced it.

The essential thing to remember is that there is an inherent tendency in the organism towards health and that a return to health will always follow the removal of the conditions and influences that are interfering with health, providing, of course, that some irreparable damage has not been done. Cure is accomplished by the forces and functions of the organism itself and not by so-called therapeutic methods. The office of the hygienist is to furnish the conditions that are required by the organism to enable it to accomplish its work of cure with the least amount of hindrance. Weakening and enervating influences can and should be removed. And these are the true methods of aiding Nature. Surgery is sometimes essential, especially in cases of accidents.

Orthopaths maintain that there are no incurable diseases, although there are incurable cases, which simply means that all cases are curable if causes are corrected in time, but all cases are incurable if allowed to advance too far. Degeneration may reach a point where regeneration is impossible, but until that point is reached any condition is curable. Curable by the body's own processes and functions. There are no therapeutic devices or agents, except in the sense that therapeutcis is the application of agencies for the suppression of symptoms. And it is just this more often than otherwise.

To show just what we mean by this let us take a look at the present practice of endocrinoloy. The facts and theories upon which the practice is based are contained in the following propositions:—

1 The endocrine glands secrete substances that are essential to normal metabolism and function.

2 Through some derangement of a gland, either functional or structural, the gland's secretion is either of poor quality, or is insufficient or excessive in amount, and produces certain functional and structural derangements in the body, depending upon the gland deranged and the nature of its derangement.

3 By means of various chemical, mechanical, or electrical agencies, or by food, etc., and by glandular extracts from animals the endocrine secertions may be modified or normalized. The action of the gland is either stimulated or inhibited.

The agent most commonly used for these purposes is powdered glands from animals.

The weak link in this chain lies in the fact that it does not go deep enough. It treats the deranged gland as though it were the primary cause. No attention is given to the reason for the glandular derangement.

The question is a pertinent one: Why are the glands deranged? Can the reason for their derangement be found and removed? The practice of stimulating or inhibiting the glandular derangement cannot give more than temporary relief.

As long as the cause or occasion for the glandular derangement is present the derangement will persist. If the interfering element be removed the gland will again become normal in its activities, providing it has not been irreparably damaged. And this is one reason we object to stimulating or inhibiting them, it hastens their destruction and at the same time leaves cause untouched, so that the glands reach a point where a return to normal is impossible. An intelligent practice will not allow degenerative changes to reach such a point.

Treatment of this nature may and often does produce temporary relief. However, no method or system of treatment can be properly judged by its immediate effect. A dose of opium, a cup of coffee, may produce an immediate feeling of well being, the eating of an orange may not produce such an effect. But if we look into the future and note the ultimate results we can easily decide which is the best. Our test must ever be the condition of the patient six months or a year after treatment.

Any method that attempts to overcome the effects of indulgence, uncleanliness, lack of self-control, sensuality, gluttony, inebriety, intemperance, etc., without correcting these can only end in failure. Nature has no plan of vicarious atonement. She demands obedience to her laws and exacts her penalties for every infraction of these.

All attemps to beat Nature only show the foolish things that a false theory will lead man to do. She cannot be beaetn. We may easily move off and beat our board or rent bills. We may beat our grocery bills, etc., but we cant' beat Nature. She will not be denied. We may move to California, Colorado, we may travel to Europe, but we cannot escape Nature. She goes right along with us wherever we go.

Cures are attributed to various lauded methods of treatment. Now there can be no denying that recovery does often take place under all methods, but there can be some doubts about the curative power of the method. The organism is, as we have shown, a self-curative thing and is capable of putting up a winning fight against great odds.

If the treatment employed must always account for the recovery then experience can easily be made to show that all the millions of absurd and even harmful practices that man has employed in the treatment of disease possessed remarkable healing powers. Again, if the thing done must always account for the results obtained, isn't it just as logical to say when a patient dies: "The patient was sick, he was treated in this way and died, therefore the treatment killed him," as it is to say: "The patient was sick, he was treated in this manner and recovered, therefore the treatment cured him?"

Health comes through healthful living and for this there are no substitutes. There can be no substitutes.

I cannot refrain from repeating a story told the class by Professor John W. Sargent, D.P., N.D., then with "The International Health Resort," and "The International College of Drugless Physicians" (Chicago). He stated that he once had a patient under his care in the institution who, being rich and used to being petted, pampered and fussed over, complained that he was not getting enough treatment. To his complaint Dr. Sargent replied: "Why man treatment won't cure you. If it would we would hire three shifts and give you treatment for twenty-four hours a day." The gentleman saw the point and became content with the treatment he was receiving and soon recovered. That treatment won't cure is a truth that is yet to be learned by both the public and the healing professions.

The requirements for recovery from chronic disease do not differ essentially from those required in acute disease. The condition that is forcing the trouble must in all cases be removed. This means that both the immediate and remote occasions for the abnormal action must be removed. Thus our first prescription must be a proscription of those habits and indulgences that are enervating and weakening the patient. A real recovery cannot take place until the enervation is overcome. Stimulating methods may palliate for a time, but palliation is not cure.

Vital recuperation cannot take place as long as the enervating habits are continued. Vital recuperation will be retarded by stimulating methods of treatment. Such recuperation will be hastened by a period of rest. By rest we mean mental, physical and physiological rest.

Nature demands that the disturbing elements be removed. Give the organism an opportunity to cleanse itself and it will eliminate its wastes and free itself of toxins, providing, of course, it has the necessary vitality to do so. If it hasn't sufficient vitality we cannot supply it with this precious force and all our attempts at forcing it to work, by stimulating its activities only weaken it and hasten the end. Such practices only enervate the patient and render the organism less able to return to normal.

The essentials of cure are:—
1 Stop all enervating habits.
2 Stop the absorption of all poisons from the outside.
3 Give the organism an opportunity to recuperate its dissipated force.
4 Supply any element or condition that is required for the comfort of the patient.

"We have found," says Dr. Walter, *Exact Science of Health*, p. 237. "it to be invariable that what makes the man sick is the thing which he never wants to relinquish. Evil habits make for themselves such a place in the organism that it is almost impossible to live without them, and so the patient is willing to do almost anything in order to recover, except the thing which he must do. This would seem to be the chief reason why we have had the greatest success with the most desperate cases. Such a patient is willing at length to submit, and do what is necessary, but the rule is with patients who are only playing sick, to follow your prescriptions as long as they are agreeable, and for the rest evade all requirements."

People will not abandon their pet vices and cherished indulgences until they have reached that point of desperation where they are willing to do anything, even torture themselves, if only they may return to comfort. Those who are not very sick, those who still have hope of cure by methods that do not require correction of cause, are unwilling to forego the injurious habits to which they are enslaved. But Graham truly declared:—

"In chronic diseases, all practice which is not based upon a careful and thorough investigation of the causes, as well as the symptoms of the case, is in fact nothing but downright quackery, and far more frequently does harm than good. For in such practice, the causes of the disease, existing in the dietetic and other voluntary habits of the patient, ARE SUFFERED TO REMAIN AND CONSTANTLY EXERT THEIR MORBIFIC INFLUENCE BY WHICH THE DISEASE WAS ORIGINALLY INDUCED, AND CONTINUES TO BE PERPETUATED. (Caps. mine. Author). Nay, indeed, those very causes are frequently employed as remedial agents to remove the diseases which they have originated and are perpetuating. Thus I have in multitudes of instances seen people who have been severely afflicted for years, by diseases which were principally induced by the habitual use of alcoholic and narcotic substances, and which had been kept alive by the continued use of those substances as medicine; and all that was necessary to remove the diseases and restore the sufferers to health, was to take away their medicine. Again, I have seen instances in which individuals had suffered under the most cruel affections of the heart and head and other parts, and submitted to medical treatment for years without the least relief. Yet on taking away their tea and coffee, which were the principle originating and perpetuating causes of their sufferings, they were soon restored to perfect health. But the practitioner had wholly overlooked or entirely disregarded these causes, and suffered them to keep alive the symptoms which they were combatting with their medicine, and by their medicine rendering their patients only the more morbidly susceptible to the effects of these morbific causes, and I have seen hundreds of miserable dyspeptics who had suffered almost everything for years; scores of those whose symptoms strongly indicated pulmonary consumption, and sometimes apparently in its advanced stage; many who had been for years afflicted with epileptic and other kinds of fits and spasmodic affections, or with cruel asthma, or sick headache; in short, I have seen nearly every form of chronic disease with which the human body is afflicted in civilized life, after resisting almost every kind of medical treatment for years, yield in a very short time to a correct diet and well regulated general regimen. And why was all this? Because, in almost every case, the disease had been originated and perpetuated by dietetic errors; and the practitioners had been unsuccessful, because with all their administration of medicine, they had suffered these dietetic errors to remain undisturbed, unquestioned —nay, perhaps even recommended."—*Science of Human Life*, p. 437.

So long as man believes in cures and immunizers he will continue to search for these things and ignore the real causes of his trouble. How do men expect to cure the effects of coffee drinking while they continue drinking coffee? How do they expect to cure these effects of coffee drinking by drinking more coffee? Such expectations are not worthy reasoning beings, whether it is coffee, alcohol, sexual abuses, gluttony or other evil habits.

Graham truly declared:—

"It ought, furthermore to be understood that ALL MEDICINE AS SUCH, IS IN ITSELF AN EVIL; that its own direct effect on the living body is in all cases, without exception, unfriendly to life; and the action of all medicine, as such, in every case, to a greater or less extent wears out life, impairs the constitution and abbreviates the period of human existence. To throw an immense quantity of medicine into the diseased body, and accidentally kill or cure, as the event may happen to be, requires but little science or skill; and extensive experience has taught us that it may be done as well by the acknowledge quack as by the licensed physician: but to understand all the properties, powers, laws, and relations of the living body, so well as to be able to stand by it in the moment of disease, and, as it were, to look through it at a glance, and detect its morbid affections and actions, and ascertain its morbific causes, and to know how to guide and regulate the energies of life in accordance with its own laws, in such a manner as to remove obstructions, relieve oppressions, subdue diseased actions, and restore health, with little or no medicine, but principly or entirely by a regimen wisely adapted to the case, evinces the most profound skill; and such qualifi- cations are essential to the character of the truly enlightened and philanthropic physician: and such physicians truly deserve the support and respect and admiration and love of every member of society, as standing among the highest benefactors of the human family."—*Science of Human Life*, p. 425.

Again:—

"We see, therefore, that the essential elements of health are the healthy condition and functions of the organs of the body; and these elements are preserved by a strict conformity to the laws of constitution and relation established in our nature, and they are destroyed or impaired by every infraction of those laws. And such are the sympathies of the system, that not only are the organs immediately acted on by disturb- ing and morbific causes themselves affected and their function deranged and diseased by such causes, but other organs also, sympathizing with those immediately acted on by those causes, partake of their irritations, and by these sympathetic irritations, are often made themselves the seats of local disease; and when disease is thus once induced, even slight habitual disturbances and irritations from dietetic errors and other causes are sufficient to keep it up for many years, till it terminates perhaps in death.

"We see, also, that no physician, nor any other human being in the universe, can come to us when we are diseased, and by any exercise of skill or the application of any remedy, directly and immediately impart to us any health, or remove from us any disease. But the truly enlightenend, scientific, and skillful physician, is generally, able to discover the nature of our disease, and to ascertain what disturbing causes must be removed, and what means must be employed in order to the restoration of healthy action and condition of every organ and part, and thus, by assisting nature's own renovating and healing economy, relieve the system from disease, and enable it to return to health.***

"All that nature asks, or can receive, from human skill, in such a condition, therefore, is the removal of disturbing causes; and she will, of her own accord, as naturally as a stone falls to the earth, return to health, unless the vital constitution has received an irreparable injury.—*Science of Human Life,* p. 424-5.

Lastly:—

"The only aid, therefore, that human skill and science can afford the diseased body in recovering health, is, with strict regard to the physiological properties and laws of the system, to assist it, so far as possible, in throwing off oppressions, removing obstructions and all irritating causes, and in subduing irritations, and restoring healthy action and function. And in order to do this, it is requisite, in the first place, that the physician should well understand the physiological powers and laws of the body; in the second place, that he should understand the nature of the disease; and in the third place, as a general rule, that he should fully and clearly ascertain the cause of the disease. For, as Hippocrates justly observes, the man who attempts to cure a disorder without knowing the cause, is like a blind man or one groping in the dark,—he is as likely to do harm as good."—*Science of Human Life,* p. 436.

Let me caution you against alarm from the immediate and apparently depressing effects which are unavoidable when one suddenly gives up any long-continued violation of physical law. There is not the slightest danger to health and life in the total, final and sudden abandonment of all wrong doing, of whatever kind, complexity or degree, and no danger in leaving the system to pass through the subsequent renovation and recover itself from the effects of any cause or causes, however depressing, painful or difficult this renovating process may be.

It is in vain to look for gradual emancipation from confirmed habits and transgressions. Tobacco, coffee, tea, alcohol, opium, etc., keep alive the craving for their use. Those who attempt to "taper off" usually end up in failure to break their bondage and free themselves.

The morbid desire for these substances is kept alive by the least indulgence in them. There is no safety for the user until the morbid irritability of the nervous system is overcome and normal *sensibility* is restored. The least quantity that the organic instincts can appreciate is sufficient to forever prolong the morbid condition of the nervous system; and, until the nervous system is restored to a normal state, the user is not safe for an instant. Until then the smell of tobacco, for instance, sight of a cigar or even the thought or mention of tobacco may revive the morbid craving with almost irresistable force. The habit will be overcome with greater ease and much less suffering if broken off at once.

The blood is poisoned even by small amounts of these substances. Take alcohol as an instance. If one attempts to "taper off" on its use, and while continuing its use, daily uses a little less, he is still daily taking into his system the poison and is being injured even by these amounts. Absolute abstinence from the start will lessen the suffering incident to overcoming the practice.

Sexual excitation and gratification are of the same character. The more the sex function is excited and gratified, the more it demands of these. "The artificial and varied repetition of sexual excitation," says Forel, "by means of objects which provoke it, increases the sexual appetite." When habitual mental and mechanical excitation of the sexual organs have produced in them a morbid condition which demands frequent "gratification" every repetition of the excitation serves to perpetuate the condition.

What is true of tobacco, alcohol, sex, etc., is equally true of other excitants or irritants, such as condiments,—salt, pepper, spices,—opium, cathartics, mechanical irritants, etc.

As soon as the sources of irritation and waste of organic power are corrected and removed, so that there is no longer any need of power to combat the irritation and the power usually wasted in various dissipations is conserved, there follows a reduced determination of nervous energies to these points and an increased amount of energy is devoted to the more important work of cleansing and repairing the damaged organism. The organs of elimination are reinforced to enable them to eliminate what Jennings called "the arrearages of expurgation that have accumulated in consequence of their having been overtaxed."

Make up your mind to abandon these things once and for all—not one at a time, not by some miscalled transition program, but abruptly, and all at once. Have it over with. Go through the pain, discomfort and depression all at once and be sure that you will suffer less than by the tapering off method. Your recovery will be more rapid, more sure and more satisfactory.

"What would be the result" asks Jennings "of a sudden and universal cessation of hostilities against the vital economy, throughout the length and bredth of the land? Imagination would fail to draw a picture equal to the reality.

"Nature would hold a jubilee."

The *Law of Limitation* would immediately withdraw all forces from the former points of attack and begin the work of renovating the system. A depressed, irritable, languid people with frequent cases of *delirium tremens*, many aching heads, and shaking limbs would be the immediate result. But the ultimate outcome would be a happy issue. Improved health and strength, clearer minds and more cheerful dispositions would result

MENTAL INFLUENCES: The mind should be poised, worry, anxiety, grief, anger, jealousy, self-pity, irritableness, etc., should be avoided as far as possible. Fears of all kinds should be put out of the mind. Hope, faith, confidence, cheer and courage should dominate the mind of the recovering sick man or woman. Relatives, friends, and all those around the sick should offer all the encouragement possible. This they often fail to do. On the contrary these often do all they can, although, not wilfully, to prevent recovery.

Nothing can so effectively illustrate the self-reliant vitality and inherent truthfulness of the hygienic practice than the manner in which it daily and hourly triumphs over great obstacles. We are forced to meet and overcome the ingrown prejudices, blind adherence to age-long traditions, morbid feelings and artificial appetences, not alone of our patients, but also of their relatives, friends and former physicians. The impertinent intermeddlings of the patient's friends, the insolent machinations of their have-been and would-be physicians, the dogged and persistent opposition of members of their families, renders the problem of caring for a sick person by the hygienic method a delicate and trying one.

This ignorant opposition and malicious meddling on the part of relatives, friends and physicians is more effective when the patients are in their home than when they are in a hygienic institution. Sometimes it is a drugged-to-death wife, at other times a drugged-to-death husband who is anxious to try the hygienic system, but who finds it impossible to do so at home because of unreasoning interference and determined meddling. I have seen patients who were so harrassed and annoyed by members of their family because such patients dared attempt to get well through hygiene, after drugs had failed, that they were made worse, and, often such patients do not get better until they get away from home and the hurtful psychology of friend and relative.

The technically professional part of our practice is the easiest part. Our most difficult work is that of overcoming and counteracting the traditions and habits of society, the ignorance and perjudices of the patient, the feelings and opinions of friends and relatives and insolent machinations of physicians. It often seems that every one around the patient is doing all in his or her power to prevent recovery. So true is this that I often think that the first thing a sick man or woman should do who is going to attempt to get well hygienically, at home, is to get a good club and empty the house of everyone except himself or herself.

"Fasting will kill you." "You are too thin now." "You are not strong enough to fast." "You will never come out of it alive." "I should be afraid to risk it." "Fasting is good in some cases, but—but, very dangerous in others." "Your stomach will get so it cannot take food." These and similar encouraging exclamations and dogmatic statements are offered by relatives, friends and physicians, to cheer up those sick men and women, who disparing of help from poisonous pills, plasters, powders and potions and from knives and saws, are about to embark on a hygienic ship for a voyage to the land of health. Well meaning, but misguided and unthinking members of one's own family are frequently guilty of such discouraging and disheartening suggestions. I have heard them fall repeatedly from the lips of those who pretend a knowledge of psychology and who should know the evil wrought by such suggestions.

"Your doctor is starving you to death!" "You are looking terribly bad!" "There is no color in your cheeks and you are losing weight!" "This diet may be alright for some cases, but you need plenty of good nourishing food." "You need to be built up."

If you were sick and on an eliminating diet and your system was being cleaned out, and due to lack of its accustomed stimulation your body did look bad, and some one hurled a barrage like the above at you, wouldn't it depress you and actually make you worse? And if it came from your whole family and all your friends day in and day out would you expect to get well? If you knew you were on the right track and felt your relatives and friends were either ignorant or stubborn or both and you became irritated or angry at their opposition to what you were doing, and fought back, would you expect to be able to digest your food?

If you quarreled with them and then cried and finally became hysterical would you not expect to have headaches, pains and gas in the abdomen, weakness and other throubles? Just these things, I have seen in many cases. Only those of strong wills and strong convictions can pass through such a barrage of evil influences as frequently come from family, friends and physicians, and recover in spite of the efforts of these to prevent recovery. A man's enemies are of his own household. His best friends are often his worst foes.

CLEANLINESS:—This is essential both locally and generally. To effect this, simple bathing in plain water at a moderate temperature is sufficient. Hot and cold baths should never be resorted to. The nearer the temperature of the water approaches that of the body the less of an excitant it is, the less it shocks the body and the less energy is wasted in resisting it. Luke warm or slightly cool baths, as often as needed, may be employed. One does not always require a daily bath.

Stay in the water only so long as is required to cleanse the body. Do not soak yourself. Get out as quickly as possible and dry off with a coarse towel. Vigorously rub the body with this.

Years ago the author fell victim to the cold bathing fad. Each morning he had his cold bath, even breaking the ice and going in on more than one occasion. Such a bath is a powerful stimulant, if one does not remain in the water too long, and has sufficient reactive power. But by so much as it stimulates at first it also depresses later. It is an enervating practice with not the shadow of an excuse for existence. I would strongly caution everyone against such foolish practices.

"The end of the day," says Dr. Owald, "is the best time for a sponge bath; a sponge and a coarse towel have often cured insomnia when diacodium failed. A bucketful of tepid water will do for ordinary purposes; daily cold shower-baths in winter time are as preposterous as hot drinks in the dog-days. Russian baths and ice water cures owe their repute to the same popular delusion that ascribes miraculous virtues to nauseating drugs—the mistrust of our natural instincts, culminating in the idea that all natural things must be injurious to man, and that the efficacy of a remedy depends on the degree of its repulsiveness. Ninety-nine boys in a hundred would rather take the bitterest medicine than a cold bath in mid-winter. If we leave children and

407

animals to the guidance of their instincts they will become amphibious in the dog-days, and quench their thirst at the coldest spring without fear of injurious consequences; but in winter time even wild beasts avoid emersion with an instinctive dread. A Canadian bear will make a wide circuit or pick his way over the floes, rather than swim a lake in cold weather. Baptist missionaries do not report many revivals before June. Warm springs, on the other hand, attract all birds and beasts that stay with us in winter time; the hot spas of Rockport, Arkansas, are visited nightly by raccoons and foxes in spite of all torch-light hunts; and Haxthausen tells us that in hard winters the thermae of Pactigorsk, in the eastern Caucasus, attracts dear and wild hogs from the distant Rerek Valley. I know the claims of the hydropathic school, and the arguments pro and con, but the main points of the controversy still hinge upon the issue between Nature's testimony and Dr. Priessnitz's."—*Physical Eductaion*, p. 100-1.

THE FRICTION BATH: This consists in going over the body with the hands, or with a towel or a flesh brush, or the friction mittens and thorougly rubbing every part of it. It is an excellent means of cleansing and invigorating the skin. Care should be used not to rub hard enough to injure and peel the skin. This should be taken daily.

THE SUN BATH: Some diseases like anemia, rickets, tuberculosis, leukemia, scrofula, psoriasis, etc., do not get well without sunlight. It is of distinct value in all chronic conditions. A daily sun bath should be had whenever possible.

THE AIR BATH: Just what effect the air has on the skin, and nerves in the skin is not well known but it is known to benefit these. A daily air bath should be had. This may be had at the same time the sun bath is taken. The friction bath may also accompany these.

EXERCISE: Many cases of chronic disease are largely due to a lack of physical exercise. Thousands have regained their health by doing little more than taking up systematic physical exercise.

In all cases of chronic disease where no condition of the joints, muscles, heart, lungs, kidneys, or elsewhere, contraindicate it, daily physical exercise should be indulged. This should be mild at first and should be increased both in amount and vigor as returning strength permits.

In diseases of the heart, hardening of the arteries, advanced diseases of the lungs, inflammation and tuberculosis of the joints, and similar conditions, exercise must be indulged in very cautiously and moderately.

In dropsical conditions, advanced Bright's disease, etc., it is usually advisable to take no exercise at all, until the condition is greatly improved. Inflamed and tuberculous joints should not be exercised. They should be given perfect rest.

REST: "Rest and replenishment of power," says Jennings, "is the first step in the ascending pathological transit; removal of useless matter by the decomposing function, with its activity and force increased by resting, constitutes the second step, and the third consists in a repair of breaches. These three steps form the first grand division in the ascending pathological transition, the removal of *structural* derangement, or cure of organic disease. The next grand step in the ascending pathological work consists in the re-establishment of regular or natural *functional* action."—*Philosophy of Human Life*, p. 102.

Neither functional nor structural derangement can be remedied except by the reinforcement of appropriate power and this can only come when all the waste-gates are closed and recuperation through rest is secured.

The path of professional duty in plain. Point out the importance of strict regard to economy in the expenditure of organic funds, that they may be brought so far within the income and accumulate, that nature may be able to liquidate her debts, and get above board again, before she is thrown into other and more embarrassing straits.

In most cases of chronic disease, a prolonged period in bed, say from three to six weeks, and longer in many cases, constitutes the speediest means of recovery. The individual should go to bed, reconcile himself to it and remain there as long as is necessary for full recuperation.

Some mild exercise, unless this is contraindicated, should be taken each day or twice each day during the period in bed.

The mind should be set at ease so that mental rest is secured.

Where it is not possible to get away from one's work and rest, as above described, one should cut down his daily mental, physical and physiological activities, as far as this is possible, and secure as much rest and sleep each day as circumstances will permit. Go to bed at the earliest possible hour. Remain in bed as late in the morning as possible. Rest during the day if this can be arranged. Where this can be done it is well to lie down for a half hour to two hours and rest and sleep, if possible, in the afternoon.

Amusement, excitement, stimulation, late hours, etc., should all be avoided in every possible way. The conservation of energy in every way this can be done is desirable. The more one can rest the more rapid and more satisfactory will be his recovery.

SLEEP: Invalids and chronic sufferers generally do not get enough sleep. The importance of sound, quiet and sufficient sleep cannot be overestimated. It is during sleep chiefly that structures are repaired. Recuperation reaches its maximum of efficiency during sleep.

The rule for invalids and chronic sufferers is: RETIRE EARLY AND REMAIN IN BED AS LONG AS YOU CAN SLEEP QUIETLY.

The bedding should be as hard, and the bed-clothing as light as a due regard for comfort will permit. A hot jug to the feet will assure warmth if the weather is cold. If one is chilled he does not sleep.

Heavy meals, indigestible and stimulating foods, stimulating beverages, as tea, coffee, cocoa, chocolate, alcohol, soda fountain drinks, etc., and all drugs should be avoided, as these prevent sound, restful sleep. If sleep is inclined to be restless, vapory and dreamy during the nights, the evening meal may be omitted.

Do not sleep on pillows. Avoid all crooked bodily positions. Relax the body and mind as fully as possible . If sleep does not come immediately do not fuss and fume over it. Worry will keep you awake. Do not roll and toss in bed. This will exhaust you. Lie still and rest. Do not get up and walk the floor. Relax and rest, you'll go to sleep much quicker. Don't try to go to sleep. The effort will keep you awake. Don't resort to any kind of sleep producers or any sleep inducing procedures, however harmless these may appear to be.

Have your bed room well ventilated. Flood it with sunshine during the day. Whenever possible sleep out doors.

SLEEPLESSNESS: This, declares Page, "is often referred to as a cause of insanity, but it would be much nearer the truth to say that insanity causes sleeplessness

"To attack insomnia as a disease instead of a symptom, is sure to result in discomfiture, in the great majority of cases and is in every instance unsound in principle.*** A man is wakeful at night because under his present physical condition he ought to be—just as in diarrhea, the looseness is doing its work of cure.*** Let him know that sleeplessness is an analogue of pain, and he will, or may, bear it philosophically, and thus tend to its removal.

"But, thinking all the while that it is sleep only that he needs, his sleeplessness distresses him, causes him to be more and more alarmed, and, consequently, has the effect to postpone the oblivion so devoutly prayed for, but so little earned. To *deserve* sleep is to have it."—*The Natural Cure*, pp. 133-4-5.

One should lie down after a half-hour of quiet and freedom from exciting mental exercise and then, when he draws the covers over him, it should be with a sublime indifference as to whether he shall or shall not fall asleep immediately. Resort to no sleep producers. Those efforts at subduing the senses, such as attempts to shut out external impressions by closing the eyes, stopping the ears and lowering the sensibilities generally, are frequently the causes of persistent wakefulness. Efforts to go to sleep by repeating metaphysical formulas are fruitless and often keep one awake. Any exercise of the higher mental faculties will tend to keep one awake. One remains awake because he tries to go to sleep. To *endeavour* to go to sleep is a mistake.

Narcotics or sleeping-draughts do not produce sleep, but stupor. Their use is both irrational and injurious, and if long continued, fatal. They produce a worse form of sleeplessness than that for which they are given.

Go to bed, relax, let go—do not roll and toss on the bed, do not get up and walk the floor, do not worry and fret—and calmly await sleep. Let your eyelids finally droop in sleep because you are truly sleepy. Every effort to force sleep keeps you awake and prevents both mind and body from resting.

Cut out your coffee, tobacco and other stimulants and earn your sleep. Then, and not until then, will you have normal sleep.

CRISES: Even the strongest Heteropath will usually concede that when the symptoms of a disease are obviously improving, the action is *right action*—but when the symptoms appear to be growing worse, he will insist that the action is *wrong action*. He conceives disease as a "pulling down" process. A woman who was under Dr. Jennings' care for a chronic affection of the lungs developed several crises—"there would be a gradual improvement in the general symptoms for two or three months, and then a sudden falling back of them, attended by spitting of blood, pain and soreness about the chest, with diminution of appetite and strength, and depression of spirits"—said to him on one occasion: "I am satisfied that on the whole I am gaining, and were it not for these running down turns, I should feel very much encouraged." The doctor replied:—

"You greatly misconceive of these things to which you give the appelation of 'running down.' They are *running up* turns.' A feeble team in ascending a long hill finds it necessary to stop and rest a little occasionally to recruit its strength. You gain more in those days when you feel the worse, so far as acquisition or treasuring up of your vital energy is concerned than you do in three weeks when you feel the best. The machine exhausts its power, runs down its weight and these are the winding up spells.

"It costs comparatively little to sustain the vital operations when you feel the worst, and it is simply because there is but little energy expended on the complaining parts that they do thus complain. The income of power continues the same now that is was under the free distribution of it, and while the law of limitation is in force, and you have, consequently, no muscular power to exercise with, be contented to keep still."—*Medical Reform*, p. 341.

Do not expect nature to go forward in a steady, uniform and undeviating course. In difficult cases, and cases of low vitality, she must have her resting spells. During these periods the symptoms will appear from the Heteropathic view, unfavorable. Appetite will fag. The pulse will grow weak. The patient will feel weak, tired, depressed. Sores will look bad, the breath will become foul. There will be an increase in all or most of the symptoms. Acute symptoms may develop. The invalid, that previously seemed to be improving, now seems to be growing worse.

These crises are to be handled just as all acute conditions are handled. Above all the invalid should avoid becoming discouraged or frightened when these appear. Welcome them and rejoice in the improved health which follows them.

FITS: "Instead of fits tending to the destruction of life, they tend to its preservation; and indeed, are as absolutely necessary, in some cases, for the eking out of life, as the repairs of a ship, every day thumped against the rocks, are for its salvation. No man ever died by a fit; and when a man dies in a fit his life is prolonged somewhat by it."—*Medical Reform*, p. 145.

THE BOWELS: These are usually a source of much worry and annoyance, due to the persistent propaganda kept up by those who have constipation cures for sale. Dire consequences are pictured as sure to follow if one does not have one or more bowel movements daily. Constipation, or intestinal stasis, as it is now known, is not the real source of evil. It is an effect.

"Intestinal stasis" is the reaction from overaction. Or, to put this more simply, it is a period of rest of the bowels following overwork of the bowels, or of the body as a whole. As soon as they have had sufficient rest for recuperation, the bowels, will act if there is need for action. Hysterical, impatient dupes of the medical bund grab a pill or a bottle as soon as their bowels fail to act, and give them the lash.

The drugs, being powerful irritants, occasion rapid, forceful contractions of the muscles of the stomach, intestines and colon, and the pouring out of large quantities of secretions to wash away the irritant drug. The dupes of such practices secure the bowel action they desire, but at frightful cost. There is now greater need for rest than before the drug was taken. There is now less of the normal lubricants of the intestine and bowel than before. There must, of necessity, be a longer period of rest. following such violent activity. But the rest is not allowed. Another dose of the drug is taken, resulting in another period of overwork, necessitating more rest. This process keeps up, until chronic constipation results and, if it goes on, permanent weakness, and ultimately, atrophy of the muscles and glands of these organs, with a thickening and hardening of their lining membranes and derangement of secretion.

There are many ways of forcing increased action in debilitated organs, for a brief period, providing there is enough power in reserve to supply the action, but these things always and necessarily diminish the power of that action and do so in precisely the degree to which they accelerate the action. The increase of action is occasioned by the extra expenditure of power called out, not supplied, by the compulsory process, and therefore this quantity of power is diminished by this amount. This is a needless and criminal waste. For the power is wanted for other purposes and will be used more judiciously and advantageously by the undisturbed law of appropriation and distribution of the living system.

Few people realize how much time and money they really spend trying to cover up evidences of their ill health instead of improving their health. If they are constipated, they blame the constipation for their ill health instead of blaming the impairment of their health for the constipation. This leads them to try to improve their health by using cathartics and laxatives to force their bowels to act, instead of overcoming their constipation by improving their health. Constipation is an effect, a symptom—they regard is as a cause.

If they have a filthy mouth, they regard this as the cause of their ill health, instead of the ill health as the cause of the filthy mouth. A healthy mouth is a clean mouth. A healthy breath is a sweet breath. All of the orifices and cavities of man's body are sweet and clean so long as they are in a state of health. None of the excretions of man's body are offensive if he is truly healthy. If the sweat from your body smells offensively it is an evidence of disease. If your breath is offensive instead of being sweet, you are sick. If your mouth is dirty, you are diseased.

But don't persist in your habit of getting the cart before the horse. An unclean mouth is not the cause of disease. It is an effect—a symptom. You don't improve your health by scrubbing your teeth, rinsing your mouth, and gargling your throat These remedy nothing. Good health is the best mouth wash, the best tooth brush, the best laxative, and the best deodorant. Get Health First and all these things will be added unto you.

Every organ in man's body acts automatically and to its own and the body's best interests. Every opening or cavity of the body which opens upon the outside world is self-cleansing. The eyes are self-cleansing. The nose, mouth, ears, bowels, vagina, etc., are each and all self-cleansing. The normal secretions of all the cavities and orifices of the body are antiseptic and the normal condition of all these cavities and orifices is aseptic.

A healthy mouth is a clean mouth. A healthy alimentary canal is a clean canal. It is health that produces a clean canal, and not a clean canal that produces health These organs are supplied with an adequate means of cleansing themselves, and it is astonishing with what promptness and thoroughness they do their work when they have sufficient power. When enervation has impaired secretion and nutrition, so that there is a depravation of the secretions of the intestine and bowel, then these cavities may become septic. Bacterial decomposition sets in and poisons are generated.

Whether these poisons will be absorbed or not will depend on a number of things. Absorption may occur in the small intestine where resistance is not great. but the colon is largely an *excreting* and not a *secreting* organ and much absorption can only occur when it is forced by obstruction. It can never occur if motive power is abundant, for the decomposing food will be sent out of the system too quickly for this. We should work for good health, and then all the organs and functions of the body will take care of themselves.

Bowel action is automatic like the pulsations of the heart and the rythmic motions of the chest in breathing. If the power of motions is present and there is need of a movement a movement there will be. If there is need of a rest due to deficiency of power the bowels will rest. They may be goaded to action by drugs, enemas, rectal dilators, spinal stimulation, etc., but this only makes their condition worse. The best plan is to let them alone and permit them to attend to their own business.

"But doctor, aren't you going to do anything to make my bowels move?" asked a young lady of me once.

I replied: "your bowels do not require to be made to move any more than your heart needs to be made to beat or your lungs to breathe. The trouble with your bowels now is that they have been made to move too much, already."

This lady whose age was about twenty, had taken laxatives and cathartics every day of her life from infancy. We let her wait upon nature. On the thirteenth day her bowels moved, and in a few days they were moving twice a day on two meals a day. This has continued for two years, even continuing throughout the entire length of one pregnancy.

Two movements a day on two meals a day is normal. These movements should not require more than five to ten seconds to completely empty the bowels and should be accompanied with a distinctly pleasurable sensation. They should be absolutely free of all odor. No effort is required in normal bowel action. No straining and grunting is necessary. The movement is so easy and so quickly over that one hardly realizes he has had a bowel movement.

I have let numbers of cases run from ten to fourteen days in order to let their bowels move spontaneously. This they always do and after they once begin to move they continue to do so. Never once have I seen any harm result from this procedure. Indeed in every case there has been a steady improvement in health. As instances, one case that went thirteen days made the following improvements—temperature which had been 101° F., became normal, tongue cleared up, fetid breath became normal, rapid heart became normal, strength returned so that the patient could get out of bed and headaches ceased. All of this before the bowels moved. Another case, one that required fourteen days of waiting before the bowels moved made the following improvements—pimples that covered his face healed up, yellowish cast to white portions of the eyes cleared up and he grew stronger. A diabetic patient who had been running .4% to .2% sugar in the urine under medical care and who showed .3% upon beginning my instructions, showed no sugar from the seventh day on and grew stronger during the time.

Dr. Page says: "Tanner had no movement during his fast (40 days); Griscomb's experience was similar, and Connolly, the consumptive who fasted forty-three days, had no movement for three weeks."

Dr. Page, who opposed the employment of laxatives, cathartics, enamas, laxative foods etc, for the purpose of "curing constipation," saying that if there has been no action for two, three or even four days, it need occasion no alarm, and the novice will be surprised to see how natural a movement will finally reward his or her patience in awaiting her call, instead of badgering her into unusual activity, declares:—

"A good rule for many who suffer tortures of mind because of constipation would be: mind your own business and let your bowels mind theirs. Strive not to *have* movements, but rather to *deserve* them. That is, attend to the general health by living hygienically, and the bowels will, if given *regular opportunity*, move when there is anything to move for."

Again:—

"In common life, it is rare indeed that constipation is the result of a deficient diet, although it often arises from lack of nourishment consequent upon excess, or an unwholesome variety of food, or both. Usually it may be regarded as the 'reaction' from over-action. The not uncommon experience, in regular order, is this: Excess in diet, diarrhea, constipation, physic or enema, purgation, worse constipation, more physic and so on. The term reaction here means simply that the organs involved having been irritated by undigested food, and having by means of increased action cleared away the obstructions, now seek restoration by the most natural method, as the name itself implies—rest. What are commonly called diseases are in reality cures; and the common practice with drug doctors, of controlling the symptoms is like answering the cries of a drowning man with a knock on the head."—*The Natural Cure*, p. 112.

It is well known that the effects of all laxative and cathartic drugs "wear out." The size of the dose must frequently be increased and the drug must occasionally be exchanged for a different one. But it is not generally understood that laxative foods also "wear out." One must eat more and more of them; even then they will finally cease to occasion action. Eating quantities of "roughage" or "bulk" will not cure constipation. *Of more importance than the thing to be moved (the bulk) is the motive power—the power of movement.* Constipation is due to enervation and will end when this is corrected and its causes removed. Keep in mind that *it is good health that insures daily movements and not daily movements that insure good health.*

We might just as well attempt to escape the law of dual effect as to try to escape the secondary effect of forcing bowel action with laxative foods. As Page truly says:—

"Next to the mistake of resorting to drugs in these cases, is the quite common one of swallowing special kinds of food for the same purpose, and there is some question as to which of the two evils is the least. An excessive quantity of rye mush, wheaten grits, or oat groats, with a generous dressing of butter, syrup, milk, or honey to wash it down in abnormal haste, will often purge the bowels like the most drastic poison."—*The Natural Cure*, p. 114.

Olive oil, wheat bran, agar agar, etc., taken for the same purpose are no better than drugs.

Dr. Gibson has admirably expressed this same thought in his "*Facts and Fancies in "Health Foods.*" He says:—

"To most dietitians the main object of diet seems to be to prepare such food-mixtures as increase intestinal peristalsis. This, however is a misconception of the real value of diet. As there are two ways of increasing the activity of your horse, so there are two ways of stimulating a sluggish bowel: by whipping or feeding. The one is irritation, the other nutrition; and to stimulate a system into a physiological heightening of its activities, without impairing a corresponding amount of nourishment is no less ridiculous than the notion that a worn-out horse can be strenghtened by a freely applied whip.

"Peristalsis is due to a wave of nervous energy, arising in the semilunar ganglia and solar plexus, from which center the ensuing momentum is dispensed throughout the intestinal coil. The process resembles the mechanical movement of a watch in which the wheels receive their impulse from the movement generated in the static, high-tensioned power of the coiled-up mainspring. And, futhermore, just as in the case of a weakened mainspring, the watch may occasionally be made to move up to the correct time by an appropriate manipulation of its hands and wheels, so intestinal peristalsis may be temporarily regulated by mechanical or chemical irritation, due to coarse, indigestible food-stuff, while in reality not a single momentum of vital energy may have been added to the nerve life of the organism."

With equal truth the doctor might have added that the stimulation of intestinal peristalsis actually robs the organism of part of its "nerve life." For, as he truly observes on another page: "an agent which has the power to move the bowels yet does not possess the vital elements necessary for the regeneration of the weakened nerve power, in place of adding energy to the organism becomes a positive loss to its reserves."

WATER DRINKING: Thirst should be the guide in this matter. Drink only when thirsty and drink enough to satisfy thirst. But be sure it is true thirst and not merely irritation from salt, condiments and the like. Much damage is done to invalids by excessive water drinking taken with a view of increasing elimination.

FASTING: In chronic disease a fast is not always essential. Indeed, it is seldom necessary. Recovery may be brought about in most cases merely by limiting the diet as previously indicated. However this will require more time than if a fast is employed. A short fast of from three to ten days, and longer in many csaes, will be found beneficial in practically every case. Indeed, it is possible in most cases to continue the fast until all or nearly all the symptoms of the disease have disappeared and health is re-established. This has been done in thousands of cases.

DIET: Graham declares: "The question is, how to remove all irritations from the system, and restore each part to healthy action and condition. But almost all the articles of medicine, not excepting those called tonics, are either directly or indirectly irritating or debilitating in their effects on the living body, and therefore should be avoided as far as possible. Many of the articles of diet ordinarily used in civilized life are also decidedly irritating and pernicious; and many of the modes of preparing food, are sources of irritation to the system. In fact, when the body is seriously diseased, even the necessary functions of alimentation, under the very best regimen, are, to a considerable extent, the sources of irritation; and where it is possible to sustain life without nutrition, entire and protracted fasting would be the very best means in many cases of removing disease and restoring health. I have seen wonderful effects result from experiments of this kind."—*Science of Human Life.*

After controverting the opinion that fleshiness and the muscular power of the body are to be considered as criteria of the excellence of any regimen prescribed for the chronic invalid, and pointing out that to eat increases the pain, inflammation, discomfort, fever and irritableness of the system, and does so in proportion to the amount of food eaten and in direct ratio to its supposed nutritive qualities, and that to fast or to consume non-irritating, non-stimulating foods and drinks in moderation reduces the "violence" of the disease and renders recovery more certain, he says, (p. 441):—

"Nevertheless, the chronic invalid himself, and generally his friends, and sometimes also his physician, seem to think that fleshiness and muscular strength are the things mainly to be desired and sought for, and that any prescribed regimen is more or less correct and salutary in proportion as it is conducive to these ends. Whereas if they were properly enlightened, they would know that THE MORE THEY NOURISH A BODY WHILE DISEASED ACTION IS KEPT UP IN IT, THE MORE THEY INCREASE THE DISEASE. THE GRAND, PRIMARY OBJECT TO BE AIMED AT BY THE INVALID, IS TO OVERCOME AND REMOVE DISEASED ACTION AND CONDITION, AND RESTORE ALL PARTS TO HEALTH, and THEN nourish the body with a view to fleshiness and strength, AS FAST AS THE FEEBLEST PARTS OF THE SYSTEM WILL BEAR WITHOUT BREAKING DOWN AGAIN. (Capitals mine. Author.) And the regimen best adapted to remove the diseased action and condition, more frequently than otherwise, causes a diminution of flesh and muscular strength (Please note, it is only muscular strength that is diminished. Author's note.), while the disease remains, in regulating the general function of nutrition to the ability of the diseased part. But when the diseased action ceases, and healthy action takes place, the same regimen perhaps will increase the flesh and strength as rapidly as the highest welfare of the constitution will admit." This latter increase in weight and strength on the same regimen would not be possible if the previous loss of fless and strength on it represented an actual loss of vital power. Yet every experienced orthopath knows that what Graham here says is true. The common practice of suffing the chronic sufferer, like a harvest hand is evil. It is even bad for the harvest hand, but is much worse for the invalid. Graham disposed of this practice as follows:—

"In regulating the diet of chronic patients, however, it should always be remembered that the extensiveness and suddeness of any change should correspond with the physiological and pathological condition, and circumstances of the individual; and most especially should it be remembered that the DISEASED ORGAN OR PART SHOULD BE MADE THE STANDARD OF THE ABILITY OF THE SYSTEM. If the boiler of a steam engine is powerful enough in some parts to bear a pressure of fifty pounds to the square inch, while in some other parts it can only bear ten pounds to the square inch, we know that it would not do for the engineer to make the strongest parts of the boiler the standard of its general ability or power, and to attempt to raise a pressure of forty pounds to the square inch, because some parts can bear fifty pounds; for in such an attempt he would surely burst the boiler at its weakest parts. He must therefore make the weakest parts the standard of the general power of the boiler, and only raise such a pressure of steam as those parts can safely bear. SO HE

WHO HAS DISEASED LUNGS OR LIVER OR ANY OTHER PART, WHILE AT THE SAME TIME HE HAS A VIGOROUS STOMACH, MUST NOT REGULATE THE QUALITY AND QUANTITY OF HIS FOOD BY THE ABILITY OF HIS STOMACH, BUT BY THE ABILITY OF THE DISEASED PART. This rule is of the utmost importance to the invalid, and one which cannot be disregarded with impunity, and yet it is continually and almost universally violated. Few things are more common than to find individuals who are laboring under severe chronic disease, indulging in very improper qualities and quantities of food, and other dietetic errors, and still strongly contending for the propriety of their habits and practices, on the ground that 'their stomachs never trouble, them.' Alas! They know not that the stomach is the principle source of all their troubles; yet by adopting a correct regimen, and strictly adhering to it for a short time, they would experience such a mitigation of their sufferings, if not such a restoration to health, as would fully convince them of THE SERIOUS IMPROPRIETY OF MAKING A COMPARATIVELY VIGOROUS STOMACH THE STANDARD OF THE PHYSIOLOGICAL ABILITY OF A SYSTEM OTHERWISE DISEASED." (Capitals mine. Author.)—*Science of Human Life*, p. 440.

It is often a difficult task to feed an invalid with a diseased or depraved stomach. A really healthy stomach knows when it has had enough and is fully satisfied with this amount. Its powers of discrimination are strong, the speediness with which it resents any and all injurious or irritating substances, remarkable. It is able to digest any food it may be called upon to digest, and so long as it is treated with fair consideration will never let you know that you have a stomach.

Dr. Jennings rightly said that when "nervous power is supplied in full measur to the ready, obedient workmen; the gastric juice is poured forth abundantly and of good quality, and the important work of digestion is done up in the best manner, and in the shortest time. In this case there is a double guaranty against the unfortunate. occurrence of a fermentative or putrefactive change in the food, which would send forth sharp, irritating gases, accompanied with sour belchings, acrid eructations, heart burns, gastric pains, and a hoast of other dyspeptic difficulties."—*Philosophy of Human Life*, p. 51.

The human stomach is possessed of remarkable powers of adaptation, being able, if supplied with sufficient nerve force, to digest any nutritious substance in any climate, season, altitude, and under almost any circumstance of life; is capable of performing a large amount of labor; is content with a very small allowance of food, or will patiently abstain entirely from all food for a long time, when circumstances render this necessary or unavoidable; or it will receive and digest, at one meal, a full twenty-four hours supply for the body; or will receive and digest food in small amounts at frequent intervals. The sound stomach, receiving a full tide of nervous energy is a willing and long-suffering servant of the body.

An unsound stomach, that is, one long abused and maltreated by being kept under the perpetual excitement of irritation and stimulation, and by being habitually overworked, will present more and different morbid aspects at different times than it is possible to adequately portray. Its blood vessels become dilated and distended, and, as he abuse continues its coats become thickened and hardened, or, as sometimes occurs, softened. Its glands are impaired. It becomes limited in its digestive power and dietitic-range.

It is unfortunate that, in such a state, the very means that have been employed to bring on this state are the ones that offer the most speedy means of relief. They temporarily mitigate the pain and discomfort only to augment these in the future. The unfortunate victims of their own follies are thus almost irresistably lured on in the increasing repetition of their mistakes. Just as opium relieves the pains it causes only to make them worse, and just as coffee relieves the headache it causes only to fasten the headache upon the victim, so the glutteny of the gourmand will relieve the stomach disorders it causes, only to perpetuate these.

The more stimulating and irritating one's food has been, the more distress and discomfort he experiences during the fast. There may be nausea, vomiting, a gnawing sensation in the stomach, depression, headache, nervousness, etc., all due to the withdrawal of the accustomed stimulation or excitement.

It should be understood that the sick person should give careful attention to the rules and regulations for eating and combining. In fact, it is more necessary for him to do so than for the healthy individual. The healthy person with good digestion may disregard all the rules of diet perhaps for years, without any apparent harm but the sick man with weakened digestion suffers perceptibly following every transgression.

We often hear the young and healthy say "I eat what I please, I do as I like. Nothing hurts me." Our many years of experience in handling the sick and treating all forms of disease have revealed to us the fact that there was a time in the life of nearly every chronic sufferer when he too did and said the same thing. In fact, it often seems that the only trouble they find with their diseased state is that they can no longer eat and do as they once did without suffering. Apparently, the only reason they desire to get well is that they hope to return to the old "flesh pots." It does not seem ever to have entered their minds that their past conduct is responsible for their present woes.

You dear reader, if you now hold to the idea that you may abuse your rugged health and powerful constitution with impunity, should disabuse your mind of this at once. You may be able to digest pig-iron, as you say, but you'll be better off in every way if you do not force yourself to do so. "Don't be a fool just because you happen to know how."

Extreme moderation is required in feeding the sick. If elimination is to proceed with the greatest speed it is necessary that the amount of food eaten be considerably less than that required by the body in health.

All stimulating and irritating foods should be excluded from the diet. All foods that undergo fermentation very readily should be withheld. No denatured foods,— white flour, polished rice, white sugar, degerminated, demineralized corn flour, canned, pickled, embalmed foods, jams, jellies, preserves, pastries, so-called breakfast foods, etc., —should be consumed. All foods eaten should be wholesome, natural foods. Condiments of every nature should be tabooed.

Such dried fruits as apples, peaches, pears, apricots, fancy dates, figs and raisins are bleeched with sulphurous acid: Crystalized fruit peels, citron, walnuts and almonds are also subjected to this same whitening process. These should never be used, well or sick. The sulphurous acid disturbs metabolism, destroys the blood corpuscles and other cells and over-works the kidneys.

Commercial apple jam and other jams are made up of sulphurated skins and cores. "Chops" as these are called are composed of about 10% fruit, 10% juice. The rest of the jam is composed of about 10% sugar and 70% glucose. The whole is held together and given a jelly like consistency by phosporic acid. Amrath, a coal tar dye, gives it a bright strawberry color while it is prevented from decomposing by benzoate of soda. The government allows one-tenth of one percent of benzoate of soda to be used and requires that it be stated on the lable. It is usually indicated in very fine print. Sulphuric acid is present in almost all commercial syrups and molasses. The syrups have little food value and are harmful in many ways.

The so-called breakfast foods have been refined too much and subjected to such intense heat that their food value is practically all lost.

It can easily be seen that the use of such foods by either the well or sick cannot result in anything else but harm. We have not yet discovered a way to prepare foods, to add to them and subtract from them, that will make them better than they are as Nature gives them to us. Our preparations usually only impair their nutritional value. Until such a method is found it is the part of wisdom for us to stick to the natural foods.

Having decided upon the kind of foods that must be fed the sick—wholesome natural foods, rich in the organic salts and lacking in proteins and carbohydrates— let us now begin our feeding.

It is usually beneficial to begin the treatment of a case of chronic disease with a fast. As fasting will be considered in a separate chapter, we will limit our remarks at this place. The duration of the fast must be determined by the condition and progress of the patient. Usually, such fasts are not necessarily long.

The purpose of the fast are manifold. Almost every case of chronic disease is accompanied by a foul gastro-intestinal tract. No health is possible so long as this condition remains. Fasting enables us to get rid of such a condition in the shortest possible time.

It is sometimes found beneficial to precede such a fast with a few days of fresh fruits or raw vegetables. These increase peristalsis and aid in cleansing the intestines and bowels. After the alimentary canal is once thoroughly cleansed and is given a complete rest it will be in a condition to care for the foods eaten in a thoroughly normal manner, whereas before such was not possible.

The length of time that one should fast depends upon the individual's condition. No two cases are alike. A long fast should never be undertaken by any one unacquainted with fasting and ignorant of how to properly conduct it unless under the care of a competent hygienist experienced in handling fasts. Few medical men are capable, because of lack of knowledge and experience with fasting, of conducting a fast. Fasts are always best taken in an institution away from the petty annoyances of friends and relatives.

Feeding after the fast must depend on the individual case. Breaking the fast is a very important matter for if this is not done rightly all the benefits of the fast may be lost. For instructions about how to break the fast see the chapter on fasting.

After the fast is properly broken the best method of feeding the patient consists in placing him or her on a very frugal, cleansing diet of fresh fruits and fresh green leafy vegetables. The patient's weight is purposely kept down by the diet to insure perfect elimination and to insure the absorption of any exudates, deposits, tumerous growth, etc., which were not fully absorbed during the fast.

An acid fruit diet may be employed following a fast of only a few days. This diet may be continued for several days depending on the condition of the patient. Obviously a diet of this kind cannot be employed for more than a few days following an extended fast. Oranges, lemons, grapefruit and acid grapes are the fruits most commonly used. For the conduct of such a diet see chapter on Feeding.

In certain chronic diseases we are brought face to face with the paradoxical proposition that there is but little that can be done and there is much which can be done to restore health.

In liver abscess, fatty degeneration of liver, in cirrhosis (hardening) of the liver, in waxy liver, in cancer of the liver, in cyst of the liver, in ascites, what is there to be done? In Chronic Bright's disease, in degeneration of the kidneys, waxy kidneys, advanced pyelitis, hydronephrois (water on the kidneys) cystic kidneys, tumors and cancers of the kidneys, what can be done? In diabetes, hardening of the arteries, atrophy of the spinal segments, organic heart disease, advanced tuberculosis, etc., what is there that we can do? In arthritis, where the joints are deformed and ankylosed what can be done for such conditions? Other such conditions as these, or rather, the same conditions in other organs, might be named but always with the same question mark after them.

The destroyed parenchyma of the various organs cannot be replaced. The hepatic cells of the liver, renal cells of the kidneys, the destroyed tubules of the kidneys, the islands of Langerhans of the pancreas, the neurons of the spinal cord—these cannot be replaced. The degeneration has reached a stage where regeneration is no longer possible. The hardening cannot be overcome? The overgrowth of connective tissue cannot be removed. Hardened arteries cannot be "softened." The tumor or cancer cannot be cured, except, perhaps, in its earlier stages—and its existence is seldom known in such stages.

In most cases of ascites, what can be done beyond draining off the accumulated fluid at frequent intervals as it continues to accumulate, until the patient dies.

In such cases we deal with seemingly hopeless conditions; conditions which have developed gradually, insiduously, and perhaps with little or no direct warning. This should emphasize the necessity for right living at all times. The mere fact that an individual feels well, looks well, and is able to work and eat is no sufficient proof that his mode of living is not harming him. Indeed he may be on the brink of the grave and imagine himself to be in good health.

As hopeless as such cases appear, and as little as it may appear can be done for them, there is much, very much indeed that we can do and should do. "Cure" will depend on the amount of functioning tissue left. If enough remains to perform the necessary functions of life, and the sufferer will learn to live within the functioning powers of these tissues, he may enjoy good health for many years and the progress of the degenerative condition be stayed. The reader will recall what we learned, in the chapter on *Physiological Compensation*, about the reserve powers of all the organs of man's body. Much of the liver or kidney or pancreas may be destroyed and yet the remaining cells be equal to the work entailed upon them by a normal life or by a life carefully lived. One whole kidney may be removed and, if the other is sound, life and health may continue.

Although the irreparable damages to the organs of the body cannot be undone, if these conditions are discovered early enough, there is much that may be done to stay the further progress of degeneration and decay and to make it possible to live in comfort and a fair degree of health.

The hardening process will be stopt if its causes are corrected. If the causes of degeneration are corrected and removed the process will end. The blood pressure may be lowered to a safe standard and maintained there. The growth of the tumor may be stayed, and, in some cases, materially reduced in size. In liver abscess, the fistula through which it discharges may be caused to heal more rapidly. Comfort may be established and maintained. Life and usefulness may be prolonged. The mode of living may be so ordered and regulated that no undue strain is placed upon the remaining tissues of the impaired organs. If this is done and the invalid will continue to live carefully, that is within his physiological abilities, he may live many years in fair health.

But the true lesson to be derived from the above facts is one of *prevention*, not one of *restoration*. These conditions are all preventable by a correct mode of life. Remember the laws of thy being from thy youth up and you will develop no such conditions. You will have no such problems to meet.

THE CARE OF WOUNDS

Chapter XXXI

IT required thousands of years of torturing the wounds of sufferers with almost every substance in the three kingdoms of nature before surgeons finally discovered that there is no *healing virtue* in any "remedy" and that the healing of a wound is not the result of any application, but is the work of *nature*, that is, of a restorative principle identical with the principle of life, and by which each organ and tissue, is, to a certain extent, enabled to repair the damages it sustains. In vain would the surgeon set the ends of a broken bone in a case of fracture, except for the power of the bone to reunite itself; or to reduce a dislocation, if the torn ligaments were not able to heal themselves. In vain would he bring together the severed edges of a wound if the power of healing possessed by these did not exist in them. These things they now know, although they did not always know them.

They have not yet learned that there is no *healing strengthening*, or *helping virtue* in any "remedy" used in disease and that the healing of internal as well as external injuries is not the result of "drug action" or "serum action" but of the inherent restorative principle which is identical with life and which enables each organ to repair its own damages.

The general public still believes in *healing* salves, ointments, bsalms, etc., which will heal wounds and open sores. The medical profession still believes in healing remedies which will heal internal injuries. Wounds heal of themselves—so also do diseases.

In the recuperative process, a certain series of changes must necessarily take place in the damaged part, before it can be restored to soundness, and these changes require time. It was an easy matter for those who did not know of these changes, nor of how and by what they were made, to attribute the healing of a wound or bruise to whatever happened to be used on it. The *remedy* was applied, the wound healed—ergo! the remedy healed the wound! The child had diphtheria, antitoxin was given, the child recovered. Ergo! antitoxin saved the child's life.

In proportion to the soundness and general health and vigor of the system, will be the facility with which the individual organs will recover themselves from local injury and disability, and others hold on to their integrity and activity in spite of the crippled state of ther neighbors.

It is a fact, evidenced by every day occurrences, that wounds or broken bones heal without great difficulty, no matter into whose hands they fall. Bones and wounds often heal under circumstances that would seem to render healing impossible. On the other hand, cases are occasionally met with when neither broken bones, bruises or wounds will heal no matter how and by whom managed. The external conditions may be ever so favorable, yet instead of healing, suppuration occurs. In such cases the internal condition of the body is exceedingly foul and its energies at low ebb.

Although the forces of life are not easily overpowered and crushed beyond the possibility of final recovery, even while prostrate and staggering under hostile influences, except when the scales are just balancing between life and death, it may make all the difference between life and death, whether the care and treatment is such as to *favor* the natural upward tendency of life, or and obstruct that tendency. The examples given below will make this clear.

A physician in Philadelphia once infected his chin while dressing a case of diabetic gangrene. His mouth and chin swelled and he was forced to remain in bed for weeks. He was unable to take food, due to the swollen mouth and tongue, and this, as he says saved his life. "Had the infection been on my leg, so I could have taken food," he said to me, "I would have died." However, a time came when he was told that he must take food, and when he replied that he could not, his wife was requested to take him from the hospital. At this time there were nine sinuses on his chin discharging pus. He went to Florida and took daily sun baths and made a rapid recovery.

A prize fighter had a broken leg which refused to heal. He went to Florida and took daily sun baths for three months. The bone healed rapidly and his health was better than for some time previous to his southern journey.

419

A young boy severely injured and lascerated his foot by riding, while on horse-back, against the corner of a porch. He was placed on fruit diet. Healing was proceeding rapidly, with a minimum amount of pain and inflammation. He refused to "starve" himself and returned to the conventional diet. In two days pain and inflammation were much greater and pus began to form. A return to the fruit diet soon arrested the greater trouble.

A soldier who had an operation performed on his chest and which had refused to heal but which had discharged pus for three years, during which time his health had grown *better* and *worse* "by turns," was placed upon a fast. He grew rapidly better and the wound healed up entirely while he was yet fasting.

A young man who had gonorrhea, was placed on a five days' fast, and then for another five days on unsweetened grapefruit. The discharge had practically ceased. He was given other foods. Then circumstances took him away from his diet and for three days he ate the conventional diet. At the end of this time the gonorrhea was worse than it had been at any previous time. Another five days on grapefruit resulted in a complete cure.

It is well known that wounds heal more readily and quickly in the well than in the sick, in children than in adults, in "savages" than in the "civilized," and in wild animals, quickest of all. The more vigorous and healthful an animal the more rapidly and satisfactorily he recovers from wounds of all kinds.

Graham wrote: "Captain Cook, the celebrated navigator tells us that when he first visited the New Zealanders, he found them enjoying perfect and uninterrupted health. On all the visits he made to their towns, where old and young men and women crowded about the voyagers, they never observed a single person who appeared to have any bodily complaint; nor among the numbers that were seen naked, was once perceived the slightest eruption of the skin, nor the least mark which indicated that such eruptions had formerly existed. Another proof of the health of this people was the facility with which the wounds they at any time received healed up. In a man who had been shot with a musket ball through the fleshy part of his arm 'his wound seemed so well digested and in so fair a way to be healed,' says Captain Cook, 'that if I had not known that no application had been made to it, I would have inquired with very interested curiosity after the culinary herbs and surgical art of the country. An additional evidence of the healthiness of the New Zealanders is in the great number of old men found among them. Many of them appeared to be very ancient, and yet none of them were decrepit, although they were not equal to the young in muscular strength, they did not come in the least behind them in regard to cheerfulness and vivacity.'

"This statement is strikingly corroborated by the testimony of Mr. William Bryant, a respectable merchant of Philadelphia, who, in the year 1809, went with a company of a hundred and twenty men, under the United States Government, beyond the Rocky Mountains, to conduct to their far western homes the Indian Chiefs who were brought to the seat of government by Lewis and Clark. Mr. Bryant states that the company carried their provisions of food, tobacco, and spirits with them, until they had exhausted them in the western wilds, where they were far beyond the reach of any supplies. From that time, during their whole stay of about two years among the Indians, the company subsisted entirely as the Indians did, on the flesh of the wild buffalo and other game, with such esculent fruits and roots as the forest afforded, and water. They had no alcoholic nor narcotic substances, nor any other pure stimulant to use, not even salt with their flesh meat, which at first they burnt a little to destroy its fresh and natural taste; but they soon learned to relish their flesh-meat very highly without salt, even when slightly cooked. Most of the men belonging to the company were, when they left the United States more or less disordered in their health and afflicted with chronic ailments. They were all restored to health, and became, like the Indians among whom they dwelt, remarkably robust and active. Their wounds healed in the same manner as stated by Captain Cook of the New Zealanders. One of the company had the fleshy part of his leg torn off by a bear. The Indians stripped some bark from a tree for a bandage, and did the wound up with a little bear's oil, and it healed with astonishing rapidity, apparently without inflammation, and entirely without pain."

420

Large and severe wounds call for the services of a surgeon, but the little wounds anyone is liable to sustain may be cared for by the one who receives them. Whether it is a contusion, puncture or cut the rapidity and ease with which it will heal will depend more upon internal conditions than upon external circumstances and every legitimate hygienic measure should be employed to improve the internal condition.

Whether a cut is large or small the external circumstances required are the same. These are (1) drainage, (2) cleanliness, and (3) rest.

Cleanliness may be properly included under drainage or *vice versa*. However, by cleanliness we shall here mean protecting the wound from contamination from without and by drainage, protecting it from contamination from within by permitting secretions to drain instead of allowing them to become pent-up. Shallow cuts hardly involve any problem of drainage. Deeper cuts, those that penetrate through the skin, will drain well if permitted to do so. However, where the severed edges are drawn together and sewed, or held together by adhesive tape, unless an opening is left for drainage trouble will occur.

Rest simply means that the injured part should not be used in such a way that it involves motion in the wound. This delays healing.

A young lady once consulted me about a "sore finger." I looked at the finger and asked her a question or two and this is the story I received. About three weeks previous she had cut or scratched the finger (it was the index finger of her right hand) near the point, but the cut was so slight that she was not aware of it until it began to get sore. She suffered with a *dependence complex*, such as is being fostered by nearly all schools of healing of today, and being unable to do anything without first consulting a doctor, she rushed off to see her family physician about the matter. He gave her a drug, the name of which has escaped my memory, and advised her to apply this, keeping the finger tied up, and bathe it frequently in alcohol. She carried out his instructions all too faithfully during those three weeks with the following results:—

1. The sore on the finger had not only refused to heal but had grown larger.

2. The skin on the whole finger, and even down onto the back of the hand was dead, dry, hard, cracked open, and all sensation lacking—all this being due chiefly to the alcohol.

3. The joints of the finger were stiff, the one nearest the cut being almost immovable. She could not bend this finger in closing her hand.

I explained to her that the alcohol had destroyed the skin of her finger and that it had done likewise to all new tissue that formed in the sore, and had by destroying surrounding tissues, not only prevented healing but had enlarged the sore. I also explained that the other drug had added its full share of anti-healing influence.

"What shall I do" she asked. To this I replied: take off all that bandaging, wash off all these drugs and keep them and all other drugs away from it, keep it clean using plain water, and don't bind it up. It will heal quicker if exposed to the sun and air. She then wanted to know if she should not wash it with some antiseptic. I said: "No, any antiseptic that will destroy a few harmless germs that get into it, will also kill the new cells forming there and retard healing." With a few manipulations of the finger, I soon restored part of the movement to the joints of her finger and explained to her how to exercise the finger, for complete restoration of movement.

The sore then healed in three days, the skin destroyed by the alcohol began to peel off and a new skin formed. Now why did I not treat her finger? Because I have no means whereby I can heal a wound or a sore or abcess, and I have no means whereby I can grow a new skin. The living organism has a monopoly on both these processes and refuses to share with anything or anyone its power of self-repair and self-cure. The only thing I can do is to stand guard and prevent anything being done that prevents recovery.

SHOCK: Injuries are attended with what is known as shock. As a general rule the shock is proportionate to the extent of the injury, though this is not always so. Often seemingly trivial injuries produce an almost fatal shock. In these cases there is a faltering in both the fundamental and expressed powers of one organ after another, in more or less rapid succession, not from so-called sympathetic association, or because one organ has learned that its neighbor is in peril and gives down under strenuous efforts to render aid, but the whole system, or its most vital parts, is bankrupt of power and its structures impaired, so that it is but able to keep up a semblance of health in the absence of added or new disturbing and impairing causes, and as soon as a little extra burden is added, so that a little more power is demanded to keep the machinery of life in regular motion, derangement follows. The whole organism is involved in the destruction, and the best that its several organs can do is to stick to their posts of duty, and hold out as long as they can with what power they have, for no reinforcement can be raised, sufficient to check the derangement, and restore health. It should be obvious that in such cases every effort to conserve vitality should be made and no stimulation of any kind employed. Quiet, warmth and rest—mental ,physical and physiological—are the remedies. The head should be lowered and the feet slightly elevated.

I have seen a man grow pale, weak, trembly, and then faint after which he vomited, all as a result of running a small sliver under one of his finger nails. So trivial an accident does not cause so much shock to one in good health.

The symptoms of shock are cold, clammy skin, face very pale and pinched, widely dilated and staring eyes, rapid and irregular pulse, and, even in severe injuries, little or no pain. Some of the mental faculties are usually retained.

ULCERS: A wound arises from some external source; an ulcer has its cause within the body. A wound is always *idiopathic*; an ulcer is always *symptomatic*. The tendency of the wound is to heal because its cause is removed. The cause acted but momentarily. An ulcer persists and often enlarges, because its cause persists and often increases. The healing of an ulcer therefore depends primarily upon the removal and correction of the internal condition of which it is but a symptom. This done and the ulcer quickly heals. Beyond this it should merely be kept clean.

The bites and stings of insects, rodents, etc., are to be ignored or "treated" as any other wound should be cared for. The dangers from such things are *nil*. It is popularly supposed that to be bitten by a spider is to suffer greatly, perhaps to die; to be bitten by a dog, cat, rat or other animal is to be in great danger of developing rabies or hydrophobia. These are merely popular superstitions fostered by the medical profession and serum manufactuerrs for their financial gain. Rabies-phobia (not hydrophobia) correctly expresses the state of mind that it is sought to keep the public in with regard to such things. Rabies is as myth. There is no such thing. Septic infection may occur, however, if one is bitten by an animal that has just been eating a rotting carcass. The same is true if one is scratched by such an animal.

There formerly existed, and remnants of it still persist, a superstition that the horned toad (which is really a lizzard), if bothered, would throw "blood" upon one and that this was extremely virulent. The toad was supposed to emit this "blood" through holes in his horns and to be able to eject it some distance, even twenty feet. He was a good marksman, aiming always at his tormentor's eyes and seldom missing. A good shot meant death to the one so poisoned. There was not a word of truth in it. They never emit anything resembling blood, nor any other substance which I have ever seen. They are not poisonous in any way and their horns are not hollow. As a boy, in Texas, the author has caught many of these animals and played with them for hours at a time. Catching snakes, insects, bees, birds, oppossum's, squirrels, etc., was a favorite boyhood pastime of the author's and he was frequently stung and bitten, although never bitten by any of the many snakes of various kinds which he has caught and played with for hours. Such bites and stings are simply more or less painful and cause a little swelling and inflammation, sometimes a little enlargement of the neighboring lymph glands; but cause no harm.

On our western deserts lives the Gila monster, which is, I believe, the only poisonous lizzard known. Its bite is popularly supposed to be sure death. However, experiments conducted in one of our western universities showed that its venom was of sufficient virulence and amount to kill a rat but not a dog or a man. It causes pain, inflammation, perhaps some fever, etc., but not death. Deaths that have been attributed to this cause were due either to fear or to the heroic attempts to save life.

The tarantula is a large spider that lives in the south-west and in Mexico and in Southern Europe. They are often reported to be as large around as a saucer, however, since I have never seen one that approached anywhere near this size, I think that fear and that part of a man's make up that gives rise to the "fish story" are the things that magnify the size of these spiders. Similarly, their reputed abilities as broad jumpers, (I have heard stories of them jumping all the way across a large room) is fiction. They can jump, but not so far. Their chief occupation in jumping, however is out of your way, not toward you. Paul Ginswold Howes, writing in *Nature Magazine*, (March 1926), under the suggestive title "Our Friends the Spiders," says:—

"The spiders are nearly all harmless or nearly so. They do everything in their power to avoid contact with man in an aggressive manner. They come about our homes for the flies and other insects that are also attracted there, and it is in this manner that they are continually working for our benefit. Even the dread tarantula of South America is among the spiders that are beneficial and I have seen them in camps remaining hidden during the day and venturing forth by night to prey upon the gigantic roaches that infest the houses. They grow to an enormous size, but the people in these countries do not often kill them because of their predatory habits and peaceful nature. In British Guiana I have lived in a shack containing a dozen or more tarantulas which never disturbed me as long as I treated them in a like manner.

"The bite of the tarantula, as far as its deadly quality is concerned, is greatly over-estimated. In some few cases where the person has been weak, or in a run-down and non-resistant condition, it is possible that death may have occurred, from it. In the cases that I have seen and have suffered personally, it resulted in nothing more than a swollen member, accompanied by some fever, which passed off rapidly, leaving no ill effects."

The sting of the scorpion is simply painful for a short time like that of the ant, wasp or bee, and soon over. I have never yet felt the necessity of doing anything about the matter when I have been stung by scorpions, bees, ants, wasps, etc. Afer all is said and done there is no danger to life in anything of this kind except in the bite of poisonous snakes. Here in the United States we have three poisonous snakes, only two of which are virulent enough to endanger life. The water moccason, is but slightly poisonous. The rattle snake, of which we have fifteen varieties, and the copperhead are our only dangerous snakes, and the dangers from these have been greatly exaggerated. Statistics show that only about two to seven percent of such bites prove fatal and there is every reason for believing that most of these fatalities would not have occurred except for a treatment that was more death dealing than the snake bite. The enormous doses of whiskey which are poured into the vicitms because of the ignorant idea that alcohol antidotes the snake poison is responsible for most of these deaths. People do not know that the death rate from snake-bite is so very low, and they know still less about the body's powers of self-cure. They, therefore, attribute recovery to the alcohol, although the alcohol actually tends to defeat the end desired. Its use is pernicious. The depressing effects of alcohol is exactly the same as the depressant effect of the snake venom itself. "Therefore," says Chas. Stuart Moody, M.D., "the man who recovers from a rattlesnake wound after drinking a large quantity of whiskey does so in spite of his remedy, not with its aid."—*Backwoods Surgery and Medicine*.

Dr. Moody says that "such information as may be contained in this chapter is not the result of conjecture and guesswork, but is derived from over twenty-five years study of reptilian zoology, many years investigation in the laboratory, during which time an extended series of experiments were carried out, and twelve years actual practice in which all the methods that have been suggested from time to time have been thoroughly tested," and for this reason I shall quote much of what he says on the subject.

"While rattlesnakes are dangerous, their bite is not nearly so fatal as is popularly supposed. This fact has at least two important reasons, viz., season and the habits of life of the snake. In the extreme South and in midsummer the venom attains its highest state of virulence. Then, the person fairly struck by a large rattler is in extreme danger, provided the second factor in the equation does not intrude, that is, the habits of life.

"All venomous snakes, and more especially rattlesnakes, are sluggish. They do not move rapidly or over great distances. Their lethal power is given them as a means of procuring food and when once the snake strikes he expends practically all the ammunition in his arsenal. It requires hours and perhaps days to renew the supply, during which time the serpent is defenseless. Should the human victim happen along at such a time and be bitten it is quite probable that he would not receive a fatal dose of the poison.

"The manner in which the rattlesnake inflicts his wound is worthy of some study. In the first place, it may be assumed as axiomatic that the snake cannot strike farther than his own length and seldom even that. Stories of rattlesnakes lifting themselves from the ground bodily and hurling themselves through the air are purely imaginative. Nor can the snake strike unless coiled. It does not follow that he must be in complete coil, but he must have at least a few kinks in his spine before he can deliver a blow; then he can only strike the length of the kinks.

"If permitted he will assume full coil before striking and when undisturbed he lies in that position. The maneuver of assuming full coil takes longer than is generally thought. Writers who assert that the snake can throw himself into full coil instantly are far fram the truth. In fact it takes, on an average, something like five seconds for him to get his length in position to deliver his most powerful blow. My experiments have developed another interesting fact, that the snake cannot strike an object held directly over his head. It must be held at an angle.

"How deep will the needle-sharp fangs penetrate? That depends too, upon conditions. A large snake, striking from full coil, will naturally drive his fangs much deeper than another smaller, striking from a less advantageous position. Upon the bare flesh the snake will sink his fangs to their full extent. His blow however, is often delivered with a raking motion and the wound inflicted resembles the scratch of a briar.

"Certain articles of dress are less permeable than others. Rubber, even thin rubber, is well nigh impenetrable. Soft, closely woven cloth is also resistent. In experiments I have placed blotting paper behind two thicknesses of heavy flannel and only in rare instances have I found the virus staining the paper. This fact will serve to inform the reader that the ordinary protection of the lower limbs will be adequate to shield the wearer in a rattlesnake country.

"The chances of being bitten even in a country abounding in snakes, are really quite insignificant. The rattler is the most inoffensive gentleman of my serpentine acquaintance. He is perfectly willing, if you will permit him, to lie all day basking in the sun upon some convenient rock and never molest the passer in the least. If he has sufficient warning he will slip quietly out of your path and give you the right of way. He only strikes when in his reptilian mind he deems himself insulted or in danger.

"An extended discussion of the chemistry of serpent venoms would be manifestly out of place at this time. We owe practically all our knowledge upon the subject to the painstaking efforts of two men, S. Weir Mitchell and Prof. Reichert. These gentlemen gave to the world almost simultaneously the result of their labors. The lethal principle of all serpent venoms consists of two elements, a venom peptone and venom globulin.

"These elements are albuminoid in character, and it is interesting to note that they act no differently from the pure albuminoses of digestion. One element has the power to destroy the fibrin ferment in the blood the other acts as a paralyzant upon motor and sensory nerve trunks.

"Time has no effect apparently upon the poisonous quality of these venoms. After twenty years' preservation in glycerine Dr. Mitchell found the virus as active as ever, and it is known that arrows steeped in rattlesnake venom retain their power for many years. Heat in varying degress, or a sudden violent application of it, will destroy the poisonous property, as will also absolute alcohol.

"The action of the virus on the animal economy is interesting and worthy of study. When taken into the circulation the symptoms are quite characteristic and not easily mistaken, even by the man of no scientific training. This is well, as the wound itself is insignificant and might be overlooked. In fact, I have known many persons to be bitten and not know it until the symptoms apprised them of the fact.

"A stinging, burning pain radiates from the wound and the wound itself becomes inflamed and angry. Swelling comes on, the heart action is immediately accelerated, and the respiration hurried. In a short time, as the virus penetrates deeper into the systemic circulation, the heart and respiratory symptoms change, the heart slows down, the respiration decreases, the face becomes dusky and anxious, covered with profuse perspiration, and the mind grows dull. Blindness, due to the effect upon the optic nerves, takes place.

"The patient staggers as he walks, and soon unless relief comes, he will become totally paralyzed. Spots of blood appear just beneath the skin and especially upon the limb bitten. If the amount of the virus is sufficient to produce death, all the above symptoms are soon followed by tetanic convulsions and lockjaw. If, however, the dose is not sufficient to produce death, they gradually subside, leaving the patient much debilitated and subject to poisoned blood states that manifest themselves in the form of skin eruptions and ulcers.

"The reader will appreciate that in the above has been pictured an extreme case. Nothing like nearly all cases bitten present even half the symptoms described. Statistics reveal that only something like 12 per cent of all persons bitten by the New World venomous serpents die from their wounds.

"Before passing to a consideration of the means for combating a poison let us pause for a time and glance at the probabilities of being struck even in a country where venomous serpents abound. The 'rim rock' of the Columbia River in Washington and Oregon is an ideal place for rattlesnakes and they abound there in profusion.

"Children run barefoot all summer among the basaltic rocks, and but few of them are bitten. Haymakers fork them up with haycocks, haversters find them beneath the bundles of bound grain, still it is rare to hear of an accident. Among the 'brakes' of the Clearwater, in Idaho the great 'timber' rattler dwells. The Indians never molest him; yet during my nine years' sojourn among them only seven cases appeared, and two of these were very young children.

"Still, people are bitten, and the location of the wound has much to do with the chances of recovery. About 60 per cent. of all persons wounded are struck on the lower limbs, thirty-five on the hand or arm, and five on the trunk and face. Of these, wounds on the lower limbs are the least dangerous and those on the trunk and face, being near large nerve and arterial vessels, most so. The more remote from the general circulation, the less danger from the wound.

"The treatment of a rattlesnake wound resolves itself into the application of a few very simple rules. In the first place a person wounded by a snake usually does the very thing he should not do that is, goes tearing off at top speed for the nearest human habitation, thereby increasing the circulation and disseminating the virus through the system more rapidly. The man should sit calmly down and bind his handkerchief around the limb (if it is a limb) break off a stout twig and insert beneath the handkerchief, producing a rude tourniquet, and twist until circulation is effectually shut off.

"With a sharp knife make an X incision over the wound, taking care to penetrate deeper than the fangs have done. If he has good teeth and no canker in his mouth, he may now suck the original wound. It is quite difficult to get any virus back through an opening not greater in calibre than a fine needle.

"If all this is done without delay, the chances are that the patient will suffer no great inconvenience from his experience. If he chances to have handy a stick of silver nitrate he can cauterize the wound thoroughly. Failing that, a brand from the fire will serve. After a time he may release his tourniquet somewhat and permit a portion of the retained blood to enter the circulation; the system is capable of taking care of a great deal of poison if it is allowed to flow into the blood gradually."

There is reason to doubt the wisdom of the employment of the tourniquet. By obstructing the circulation it causes the blood to accumulate below the point of constriction and the blood cells, due to lack of oxygen are greatly injured and some of them die. There is a great probability that in many cases the injury to the body caused by throwing a lot of dead blood into the circulation is as great as that caused by the snake bite itself. For this reason, if the tourniquet is used at all, it should be for a very brief time and it should be removed as soon as one is reasonbly sure he has extracted or destroyed all or most of the venom. The employment of permanganate of potassium as an antedote and of strychnia as a "heart stimulant" can only be productive of injury. Ammonia applied locally is of no value.

All serpent venoms act chemically in the same manner but some are more virulent than others. No antidote to these is known—that is, nothing is known that can be taken into the body which will antidote, them. Dr. Moody says: "Very few Indian tribes have any suggestion of a remedy for rattlesnake poison. The Moquis probably have, though if so no white man has ever been able to extract the secret from them. It is known that during the Moqui Snake Dance MANY INDIANS ARE BITTEN AND NONE OF THEM DIE. It might be inferred then that they do possess an effective antidote."

I consider this inferrence far fetched and unnecessary. The "effective antidote" is good health. Within the last few years an anti-venom serum has been developed and is being exploited. Much front page publicity is given to each case of snake-bite treated by it and there are many spectacular cross-country runs in autos and trains to carry the precious "life-saving" serum to the bitten individual. In every case recovery is attributed to the serum and the popular superstition that rattlesnake bite is invaribly deadly is inferrentially upheld in the interest of the serum. All serums build their reputations on the self-curative, self-reparative, self-immunizing and self-defensive powers of the body. They are all injurious and not one of them of the slightest value.

THE PLACE OF ART

CHAPTER XXXII

WITH the onrush of reform that began with the 18th century, the heroic dosings and copious bleedings of the duly ordained and law-entrenched scientific school fell gradually, more and more, into popular disfavor, and despite every effort to keep the people in ignorance and subjection, and the "quacks" in jail, medicine has been slowly dying for a hundred years. Medical men had always held that the people know enough, if they could close their eyes, open their mouths and swallow whatever the learned Aesculapians might prescribe, without question, demure, or hesitation, and with all the faith in their doctors that a saint has in his god. The reformers reversed all this. They taught the people and the people "heard them gladly."

Of course, all great reformations have been beset by a lot of parasites whose object, ostensibly, is to take care of and preserve from ruin, the NEW IDEA. These "friends" are afraid of "extremes," declaring, "Truth lies between extremes." This is a poor sophism, all of the force of which lies in its ready adaptation to those who seek first and last their own success and mostly at the expense of truth. These beset the reform schools and protected and improved them so well that what real truth they had found was soon forgotten and buried beneath the debris of a multitude of new forms, inventions, devices, appartuses, and methods. As was previously true in medicine, and is yet, so in the reform schools; theory has risen upon theory, and hypothesis upon hypothesis, till amid the rubbish that has accumulated, one may search for years without discovering one well established fact.

Many had so much respect for the universal opinions of mankind that they dared not go on with the reform, but rather turned back a ways. Respect for the universal opinions of mankind is a rather indolent manner of disposing of new truths and side-tracking them for a more propitious day. But it has been done, and, if today we reproach those who have so acted for their methods, they point to their apparent results and say, "But more get well than die under our treatment." And this only proves that the majority of constitutions are strong enough to withstand a great deal of non-sense and abuse, and that it is the rule rather than the exception for the sick organism to succeed in its curative efforts.

Art cannot be made to do the work of the body nor to aid the body in its work, except in a limited way, in a very limited sphere, and even here it is almost always an evil and not a benefit. To quote Graham on this, he says:

"It is a general physiological law of organized bodies, to which there is no exception, that all artificial means to effect that which the living body has natural faculties and powers to accomplish, always and inevitably impair and tend to destroy the physiological powers designed to perform the function or to produce the effect. Thus, as we have seen, every artificial means substituted for the natural and proper use of the teeth in mastication inevitably injures those organs and always tends to destroy their power to perform the functions for which they were intended. And thus, every artificial means employed for the regulation of the temperature of the body always and inevitably diminishes the natural power to regulate its own temperature. If our feet are cold, for instance, and we, by walking, dancing, or other exercise of the lower limbs, increase in a natural and healthy manner the calorific function of the feet, and thus restore them to a comfortable temperature, we invigorate all the physiological interests of the body; but if instead of this, we warm our feet by a fire, we necessarily weaken all the physiological powers of the parts, and consequently diminish the calorific function of the feet, or their natural power to generate animal heat and regulate their own temperature, and thereby render them more liable to suffer from cold. All this is true of every other member or part of the system, and also accurately illustrates the effects of all other artificial means on the physiological powers of the body."—*Science of Human Life*, pp. 513.

Some hold that if we give a man a drink of water, this is a treatment. All right,

427

if giving a thirsty man a drink of water is treatment, we believe in treatment.. But we would like to know what we treat. We would never give a man a large quantity of water to drink daily on the absurd idea that, by this means, we may flush the kidneys. We remember our physiology better than this. And, what do we treat if said thirsty man is not sick? Healthy men get thirsty too, and drink water.

It is just here that we draw a sharp line of demarkation between therapeutics and hyigene and it is about this line that the "fight" is being waged. Hygiene is required by the well and sick alike. Therapeutics is an extra-natural factor that is supposed to be a super-added requirement of the sick. It is generally admitted that the well do not need therapeutics—these are for the sick. But a sick organism, and a well organism, is the same, their laws and processes are the same, their needs are the same.

Dr. George Starr White, a leading advocate of Pseudo-Nature Cure, once wrote:

"The true Physician must understand that sanitation and Natural living and right thinking are the only preventives of disease. Right thinking and right living will prevent disease and will cure any disease that is curable."

Now, I do not believe, for a minute, that Dr. White meant any such thing as he here says. But I do believe his words are true, every one of them. I can see no reason for speaking of sanitation and right thinking as though they were separate from right living. To me, right living or natural living includes both of these and much more. There is too much loose talk by those who want to say something that will take with the crowd, and who do not know what to say. I have heard and read hundreds of times that right living will cure every curable disease, and I have found that not one out of every ten million who parrot this statement, ever believe any such thing. They do not even understand what they are saying. They all have their little pet systems of therapeutics that must be super-added to right living. Yes, MUST BE ADDED, or else, there's no money in it.

Dr. White further stated:

"The True Physician must understand all the modern methods of healing and must be able to choose the good from the bad. There is some good in all NATURAL systems, but there is nothing good in any UNNATURAL system."

I thought so! I knew there must be some kind of a healing system to go along with natural living. There is only one NATURAL system of healing and that is locked up in the living organism. It isn't in any machine or apparatus or manipulation or bath.

I know what is meant by "all NATURAL systems." He means drugless and semi-drugless methods—machine shop practices and health producing machines. By "UNNATURAL systems" is meant drugs, serums, vaccines, etc. Oh, yes! The other fellow has horns and a forked tail and cloven hoofs; we wear the golden crowns, white robes and harp upon our golden harps. It must be so, for, we ourselves, admit it.

Now I am going to deny that there is no good in any unnatural system. Surgery is unnatural, but it is often necessary and beneficial.

What! I, a no-treatment advocate, admit that surgery is often necessary and beneficial! Yes, I admit it, and if the Hottentots and child minds that have been spitting at the no-treatment advocates had exercised as much of that spirit of investigation in regard to our position as they want the medical men to exercise toward them and their position(s), they would have understood more and gnashed their teeth less.

Surgery is necessary and beneficial in wounds, hemorrhages, fractures, and other accidents. Surgery is good when some organ of the body has become so far destroyed and rotted, due to treatment, that it is no longer redeemable and becomes a menace to the life of the body as a whole.

Surgery is good in some deformities, and for some time yet, will be good in complicated and most "normal" child-births. Dental surgery is often necessary. Not only is surgery, in such cases, good, but until the drugless man is fully prepared to perform such surgical work he is only a piece of a physician. He is not fit to trust the care of patients to.

Imagine a drugless man attending a partruent woman and caring for the tear that almost always occurs, even in "normal births." Imagine one of them trying to set a compound fracture or trying to care for a man with a deep knife wound received in a fight. He would be about as helpless as a one legged man at a kicking match. Drugless men will get legal recognition and supercede the drugging professions when they are trained in all the requirements of a complete physician. Until then, they deserve less than they now have.

How many drugless men could reduce a dislocated femur? Not one in a thousand. This is a muss for a profession to be in that aspires to become the physicians of the world. When in school I was taught the Le Grange method of reducing dislocations. This method is said to come from France, and the instructor who taught it to me was a bit doubtful of its efficacy. I, too, have grave doubts of its servicibility. So far as I am aware, this is the only system of reducing dislocations taught to drugless men (except Osteopaths), and most of these schools teach none. Enough time is wasted in these schools on such worthless subjects as iridiagnosis, Basic diagnosis, electrotherapy, colored light entertainment, etc., to, if devoted to instructing the student in essential things, turn out much better qualified men. Any method of reducing a dislocation is an unnatural one, but needful at times.

Then there are certain deformities and conditions of diminished and abolished movement that can be overcome by mechanical—I mean manual—methods. It can't be done with diet and thinking. Some of them can be overcome with exercise, but not all.

When adhesions have formed in the urethra (stricture), there is but one way to overcome these, and this is by forcibly breaking them up. Of course, they need never form, but then the whole world is not Orthopathic yet. There are still plenty of allopaths who can turn out more strictures and similar conditions in other parts of the body than the orthopaths can ever hope to overcome. Nothing more than the sound should ever be employed in breaking up a stricture.

· Adhesions in the abdomen are seldom the cause of trouble. There are few people who do not have one or more. They are the result of inflammation, and almost everyone in modern life has suffered at some time with enough internal inflammation to produce an adhesion. They are not always permanent. They are almost never troublesome. They are often accused of causing trouble, but even in these cases, the trouble is present only at times, while the adhesion is constant. They are blamed for the trouble because the doctor knows not the cause. Bear in mind that every abdominal and pelvic operation leaves adhesions, and every operation for adhesion leaves more adhesions than it finds. Unless an adhesion is in the lumen of a hollow organ or otherwise obstructs a duct, or passage, it causes no trouble and should not be interfered with.

The exceptions to the rule of non-intervention are found wholly in the realm of surgery, and in the realm of constructive surgery at that. Strangulated hernia should be relieved by any kind and amount of means necessary for the accomplishment—using always as both the cheapest and most effective, the mildest means that will secure the end. A defective tooth may be pulled. The Orthopath does not violate his fundamental principles in ligating a severed artery, cleaning and stitching and shielding a wound, reducing a luxation, setting a fractured bone, and in manipulating a deformity.

Jennings says of strangulation:

"I have succeeded in reducing a number of bad cases of strangulated hernia by the following treatment:—Have the patient laid quietly in a warm bed; a large, quite large, soft and warm poultice compress applied over the tumor; the foot of the bedstead moderately elevated, and as much warm water thrown into the lower portion of the bowels as can be borne without pain and uneasiness.

"After these means have been in operation an hour or two, it will generally be found that the hernia is self-reduced, or may be put back with very little tact. Nothing but moderate force by handling, and that skillfully applied, should ever be used for the reduction of hernia; for unskillful pressure or much violence****would conduce to adhesive inflammation, and thereby render reduction without an operation impossible."
—*Medical Reform*, pp. 366-7.

A few facts about hernia will help to clear the atmosphere about this trouble. First, it is due to weakness. No amount of strain will produce a hernia in a normal individual. Operations for hernia are seldom successful. They temporarily close the opening, a thing they do not always succeed in doing, but by reason of the very fact that they do not overcome the weakness that was the cause of the hernia, but do produce more weakness, most of them recur. The operation is always attended with great danger, death frequently resulting, and this danger increases as age advances.

Hernia tends to spontaneous recovery, as Dr. Taylor pointed out, and most, if not all cases would recover if causes were corrected. Recovery in most cases may be positively assured by corrective exercises. Dr. Taylor was the first to work this matter out and his *Pelvic and Hernial Therapeutics* is devoted largely to this particular subject. Exercises for this condition are best taken on a slanting table with the head down and feet elevated. These cannot be given here, but I must add that they are equally as effective in remedying visceroptosis, uterine displacements, etc., doing what surgery and braces, belts, stays, rings, etc., can never do.

These things are not natural, but they are often useful in the conditions named and I have no objection to their use for the purposes mentioned. I would use them myself in such conditions. But beyond this, the artificial procedures are not only valueless, but positively harmful. By this, I mean that any mtehod that is employed to cure disease is to be condemned. Manual or mechanical methods that are employed to stimulate or inhibit organic functions waste nerve energy and interfere with the processes of cure and their interference is in direct proportion to their stimulating or inhibiting influence.

Question this all you will, offer all the silly objections to it your mind can formulate, talk about results "are what, really count," until you have Coued yourself into believing your Auto-suggestions, the facts will not down; they refuse to bow to "any system built on prejudice, superstition or self-interest" for such a system is "wrong and cannot endure." And, those of us who know that such systems are wrong, are in full accord with Dr. White, when he says: "You cannot extemporize with evil. If you know a thing or a system is wrong, try to remedy it. Do not try to condone it, for in so doing, you act as a partner to the wrong. A system is either right or wrong—just or unjust."

Those who are trying to build a bridge across the chasm that exists between Nature Cure and the popular medical system by a fabrication of falsehood are doomed to disappointment. Truth can never be served by fallacy. She will build her own bridges and lay their foundations in solid rock not in the shifting sands of fads, fakes, freaks, frauds, fallacies and foolishness. People cannot be taught the truth by filling their heads full of fallacies and telling them these fallacies represent the latest demonstrations of "science." Tell them the truth, and the bridge is built.

I deem it wise at this place to offer some criticisms of surgical practice, in order that the reader may be the better able to distinguish between truth and error in the surgical fads of today. It has become the custom to operate upon the sick, and even the healthy, upon the slightest provocation, or upon no provocation at all. There are a number of reasons for this all of which enter more or less into each operation performed. I do not, here, intend to deal at any length with these reasons, but shall content myself with a short statement of each one:

SPECIALISM: The specialist is predisposed to see the need for his services in each case that comes to him. The surgeon quite naturally sees the need for his services often, where, even from the orthodox view-point, no such need exists.

AMBITION: Surgeons, as a rule, are not exempt from the ambitions that motivate other men. A surgeon quite naturally desires to make a name for himself. To do this requires skill. The development of surgical skill, like that of musical skill, requires practice. He must be continually operating if he is to develop the skill and acquire the reputation he desires.

ECONOMIC FACTORS: Surgeons desire wealth as much as do brick masons or merchants. They must meet their living expenses, keep up a dignified appearance before the world and, if possible, lay up some for the future. This they must make largely out of their work, and operations bring in large fees.

IGNORANCE: Men who only know one side of the surgical question and who know the wrong side at that, often sincerely believe that an operation is the surest, quickest and perhaps the safest means of "curing" a disease. Looking at disease from the Heteropathic viewpoint and having no adequate conception of the community value of organs, they do not hesitate to cut, slash and mutilate the body.

COMMERCIALISM: I prefer to consider this as separate and distinct from economic factors. No man should be condemned for his desire to pay his food bill, but he should be condemned for his desire to corner the food market. The surgeon, whose sole aim is the acquision of money and who does not hesitate to operate and sacrifice healthy organs as well as diseased ones and even the lives of his patients, to secure that money, is a menace to the public. He is a criminal of the lowest type. The country is full of this type of surgeon and the evil results of his practices.

Sir Berkely Moynihan, the famous English surgeon, says in his work on Abdominal Operations:

"Surgery today is being practiced by too many light-hearted and incompetent surgeons, who have neither sought in due service to acquire a mastery of their craft, nor have they learned, from the experience gained by long association in hospital work, when an operation should be done, when left undone, how made safe, how made to fall lightly upon a patient already afflicted, it may be, by mental no less than by physical distress."

Dr. LeRoy Long, a leading American Surgeon, stated in an address before the American College of Surgeons at their 1925 meeting that:

"In this country, there are 30,000 untrained men performing surgical operations. Many of them are operating small hospitals. Without training and without the necessary intellectual equipment, they must depend upon some other means to secure patients, and most of them resort to fee-splitting. In the very nature of the situation, patients are not properly examined, but they are operated upon. They are operated upon when no operation at all is indicated. They are operated upon when they are moribund, or when they are suffering from some hopelessly incurable malady, because a fee is in sight. They are operated upon as 'emergency cases, to keep them from going to some place where they would have an opportunity to be properly examined; but where they would be beyond the reach of the grasping fingers of the fee-splitter."

J. F. Baldwin, M.D., F.A.C.S., one of the leading surgeons of this country, who says of Dr. Long's statement, that "no experienced and observing surgeon will question the truth of this statement," also says:

"Were the practice of fee-splitting limited to young and impecunious physicians, and steadfastly opposed by the men of supposedly high standing, the condition would not be so disheartening, but it is certainly depressing to find so many physicians of ample means, of large practice, and supposedly of high professional, religious and social standing, demanding without a blush, their 'pound of flesh.'

"With competition between fee-splitting operators, the poorest operator will necessarily offer the highest commission; one case is known in which such an operator offered 90% of the fee."

We are told on good authority that many operations are performed when the surgeon himself sees no need for the operation, simply because he does not wish to offend the physician who brought him the patient. He depends upon the physician, with whom he splits the fees, for patietns. The physician wants the fee. If the surgeon refuses to operate, he loses the patronage of this physician. So he operates!

These are a few of the most apparent reasons for the widespread use of surgery. These things, one or all of them, consciously or unconsciously, influence the surgeon and frequently the physician in advising an operation. I shall now briefly state a few of the most important objections to surgery:

UNNECESSARY: Granting that operations are often necessary, not more than five per cent of the operations now performed fall into this class. Outside of what we denominate constructive surgery, it is extremely doubtful if any operation is ever necessary or beneficial.

HARMFUL: Every structure and function in the body is intimately correlated with other structures and functions and closely connected with them. No organ is an independent isonomy, but forms an integral and necessary part of the body. Its removal, as is often done by the surgeon, permanently and irremediably cripples the body.

The ruinous effects upon the nervous system, particularly of major operations, is almost immeasurable. As Dr. Lindlahr used to say, it is like cutting into the brain.

DANGEROUS: The dangers of operations are manifold. First there are the dangers from the anesthetic. All anesthetics depress the nervous centers, and often they depress the cardiac or respiratory, or other centers to such an extent that death results immediately. This is true of local, as of general anesthetics. Even a local anesthetic applied to a tooth or tonsil may, and frequently does, result in death. Deaths from this cause are far more frequent than the public has any idea of, and it is doubtful if as many as ten per cent. of such deaths are reported as such. Where death does not occur, the injury is often more or less permanent.

Next there is the danger of shock. This may result in death or in such a lowering of the powers of life that, under the prevailing mode of treatment, the patient dies in a few hours or a day; or else it may simply result in a lasting impairment of health of the individual.

Hemorrhage constitutes another source of danger in operations. The removal of so apparently an insignificant organ as a tonsil or adenoid may be followed by a fatal hemorrhage. Fatalities of this kind are far more frequent than is commonly supposed and but seldom reported as being due to this cause.

The dangers of infection always attend an operation, however small. The mere cutting of a corn may be followed by an infection which, under the prevailing mode of treatment, may easily result in death. Thrombosis may, and frequently does arise and cause death.

A child is taken to the hospital in the morning to have its tonsils removed. In the afternoon of the same day it is brought home dead. A man in average health goes to the hospital in the morning to have a hemorroid removed. In the evening of the same day he is brought home in a coffin. A man has hernia for many years, but it does not bother him and he gives no thought to it. Finally, his friends persuade him to have it "fixed" by an operation. He has the operation performed and dies as a result. These are not mere suppositions but are actual cases. Nor are they isolated examples. They may be duplicated thousands of times. They occur in every community. No great publicity is given to them and the public, so used to taking its medicine on faith, gives no though to the matter.

DESTRUCTIVE: Apart from these unavoidable evils of surgery there are other and more fundamental objections to it. It is a confession of ignorance. When a physician admits that he does not know anything more to do for a sick man than to cut out one or more of his organs, he simply parades his ignorance. The destruction of an organ is not its cure. If the destruction of one organ is the logical method of treating its affections, then surely the destruction of another organ is also the logical method of handling it. If tonsilectomy is the cure for tonsilitis, then why not cardiectomy for carditis, phrenectomy for phrenitis, etc.? If the removal of the tonsil is the cure for hypertrophy of the tonsil then why not remove the heart to cure cardiac hypertrophy? Why not remove the stomach to cure enteritis or enteric fever (typhoid), if the removal of the appendix is the cure for appendicitis? The larynx should be removed for laryngitis, the pharynx for pharyngitis, etc. It is easy to sacrifice an organ, but the loser must always suffer as a consequence. No one ever had tonsils or appendix removed without paying dearly for their loss. The operation is not cure—it makes cure forever impossible. It leaves permanent and lasting effects upon the body and mind that can never be eradicated.

IT DOES NOT RESTORE HEALTH: The removal of a diseased organ is not the correction or removal of the causes of the organic affection. To cut out affected tonsils does not correct the causes of the tonsilar trouble. On the contrary, it adds to these . It is no unusual thing to see a patient have his or her tonsils and adenoids removed, then a few weeks or months later, a few teeth pulled, then later the appendix comes out and still later the gall bladder and finally, the patient is told he is incurable, or, else, that there is nothing wrong except hysteria. (Hysteria is what you have when the doctor can't find your trouble.) As fast as one organ is removed, another becomes affected because nothing is done to correct or remove cause. Instead of amputating the patients bad habits, they cut out an organ, then another, and so on, so long as the patient or his money lasts.

Blood transfusion is a procedure which lends itself very readily to commercial exploitation and to much spectacular grandstand play. There is plenty of money to be made from it but no benefit to be derived therefrom. Its use is always followed by shock and disagreeable reactions in varying degrees. These manifest as fever, malaise, nausea, vomiting, chilly sensations, actual chills, muscular pains, dyspnea, cyanosis, urticaria and headache. The fever ranges from 2 to 12 degrees. Hemolysis (destruction of red blood cells), is practically certain to follow and this is often great enough to prove fatal. Anaphylaxis following transfusions, also, is a frequent cause of death.

THE PASSING OF THE PLAGUES
CHAPTER XXXIII

THE story of the "Plagues" that raged in much of the World in Ancient and Medieval times and even in parts of it in these Modern days is most interesting and instructive, although, at the same time, very saddening. They carry, or should carry, for us a lesson of the greatest importance. As Trall puts it:

"The history of the plague, like that of the cholera, is a tremendous lesson, whose true moral is hygiene, unfortunately, however, but little understood, and still less heeded. Wherever and whenever it has raged, the place and the people were buried, as it were, in their own filthiness, and rioting in the grossest sensuality. The narrow streets, dirty houses, unventilated apartments, and gross food of the inhabitants, with drunkeness and debauchery, have ever been the inviting causes of this pestilence in all the cities of the Old World where it has ravaged and desolated. Athens, Rome, London, which were formerly more than at present, the world's greatest centers if luxury and licentiousness, have been repeatedly scouged with this prince of pestilences. Since the habits of the civilized world have become more cleanly, yet more debilitating, we have internal dyspepsias instead of external carbuncles, and the cholera instead of the plague."—*Hydropathic Encyclopedia*, Vol. 2., pp., 107.

We do not believe that "plagues" are any more than more virulent types of disease due to the same causes except these causes are increased or intensified. We do well, in this study, to keep in mind that the "plauge spots" are fitlh spots and that until within recent years the medical profession has opposed cleaning up these "plague spots." A few instances must suffice.

In the year 1760, the King of Spain issued a public decree, to free Madrid from the abominable custom of throwing the ordure out of the windows into the streets. He ordered, by proclamation, that the proprietor of every house should build a proper receptible, and that sinks, drains and common sewers, should be made at public expense.

"Every class," proceeds the narrator, "devised some objection against it; but the physicians bid the fairest to interest the King in the preservation of the ancient privileges of his people, for they remonstrated that if the filth was not thrown into the streets as usual, a fatal sickness would probably ensue, because the putrescent particles of the air, which such filth attracted, would then be imbibed by the human body."

In August 1853, a yellow fever epidemic raged in New Orleans. The death rate reached nearly 200 a day. The Crescent, writing of the epidemic said:

"Dr. McFarlane, the old war-horse of physicians, who has had great experience for the last thirty years, has addressed a letter to the Mayor through the Delta, of this morning, in which he boldly asserts that, 'so far from believing that the filth and impurities in our streets, yards and suburbs, have anything to do with the creation of a yellow fever atmosphere, I believe that, to a certain extent, they are calculated to retard its formation'."

Yellow fever vanished from New Orleans, Cuba and Panama when these were cleaned up. The medical profession still refuses to admit that cleanliness did the work. They insist that it is all because they or the Sanitary engineers did the St. Patrick act with the mosquitoes. There are still as many mosquitoes in these places as there are in Jersey. I have never been able to figure out how they succeeded in getting just the right mosquitoes to leave, and the harmless ones to remain.

It is amusing to recall medical opposition to the early use of the bath tub. When it was introduced into this country, the medical profession denounced it as the "obnoxious toy from England," and passed resolutions and called on the government to prohibit its use because it would bring on "phthisis, rheumatic fever, inflammation of the lungs and a whole category of zymotic diseases." In 1842 the Philadelphia doctors placed before the Common Council of the city a proposal to prohibit by law the use of bath tubs between November 1st and March 15th. In Boston, likewise, the medical society secured the passage of an ordinance in 1845, making bathing unlawful "except upon medical prescription." The doctors violently opposed the railroad and the rapid travel thereon as extremely dangerous to public health, even going so far as to advocate a ten foot fence on each side of the track.

The march of time has repeatedly proven that medical wisdom is not always public wisdom, and that medicine is prone to condemn new ideas, only to adopt and advocate those same ideas after others have established their merit.

Trall cried out: "O· for a Moses among the doctors· When Moses, in olden time, led the reckless and sensual Israelites a forty years' journey through the wilderness, how strict and inexorable were his Hygienic injunctions· How careful was that admirable physiologist in directing all the minutia of the sanitary conditions of his people. And that no source of pestilence should be tolerated, he would not allow any nuisance, or impurity even, to defile the camp ground. Fortunately for his people, he had no quinine to 'neutralize malaria,' no arsenic to cure fevers; and so he was obliged to prevent them. Had Moses been as ignorant or as regardless of Hygiene as our modern medical men, civil or military, before he could have led the Isrealities a quarter of a forty years' journey, they would all have perished of the pestilences so prevalent among modern armies."—*True Healing Art.*

Again he says: "And Florence Nightingale! Is that name new or strange in this place? For what purpose did that noble and heroic English girl, overflowing with patriotic emotion, and full of sympathy for suffering humanity, as only woman can be, pitch her tent and make her ambush and abiding place amid the wailing of the wounded, the groans of the dying, and the stench and contagion of camps and hospitals? Alas! She must needs go to the Crimea to teach the British surgeons health; to instruct the graduates of the first medical schools in the world the simplest maxims of plain, unsophisticated common sense; to show to medical men of learned lore, and scholastic honor, and high-sounding titles, and large experience, and many degrees, that invalids cannot breathe without air; that personal cleanliness is esstial to the successful management of disease; that water, and light, and equable temperature, and rest, are requisite to correct morbid excretions, restore normal secretions, purify the vital current, and destroy the ever-engendering miasms and infections of such places.

"The British surgeons could amputate limbs admirably, dress wounds skillfully; bleed dexterously, mercurialize strongly; narcotize effectually; give quinine hugely, and administer arsenic powerfully; but they could not purify—and purification was the one thing needful in most cases."—*True Healing Art.*

Sir Frederic Treves, renowned English surgeon, in his "The Elephant Man and Other Reminiscences," in speaking of the London Hospitals at the time he began his career, says:

"There was no object in being clean. Indeed cleanliness was out of place. It was considered to be finicking and affected. An executioner might as well manicure his nails before chopping off a head. The surgeon operated in a slaughter-house, suggesting frock coat of black cloth. It was stiff with blood and the filth of years. The more sodden it was, the more forcibly did it bear evidence of the surgeon's prowess. I, of course, commenced my surgical career in such a coat, of which, I was quite proud. Wounds were dressed with 'charpie' soaked in oil. Both oil and dressings were frankly and exultingly septic. 'Charpie' was a species of cotton waste obtained from cast linen. It would probably now be discarded by a motor mechanic as being too dirty for use on a car. I remember a whole ward as being decimated by hospital gangrene. The modern student has no knowledge of this disease. He has never seen it, and thank heaven, he never will. People often say how wonderful it was that surgical patients lived in those days. As a matter of fact, they did not live, or at least, only a few of them."

Trall was right. And the voice of the Nightingale went unheeded for years to come. Trall, Graham, Shew and others, lifted their voices in this country in a plea for cleanliness, but the medical profession drowned their voices in a paeon of strident yells—"quack! imposter! ignorant pertender!"

Sepsis was the prevailing condition in hospital wards in those days. Practically all major wounds suppurated. Pus was the most common subject of conversation, because it was the most prominent feature in the surgeon's work and was classified according to degrees of vileness. What wonder then that the hospital was anathema!

People hated them and looked upon them primarily as places where patients died—an attitude that was not far wrong.

Miss Nightingale tells us of the air patients, received in homes and hospitals, *Notes on Nursing*, pp. 12. "It may come from a corridor, into which other wards are ventilated, from a hall, always unaired, always full of fumes of gas, dinner, of various kinds of mustiness; from an underground kitchen sink, wash-house, water-closet, or even, as I myself have had sorrowful experience, from open sewers loaded with filth, and with this the patient's room or ward is aired, as it is called—poisoned, it should rather be said ****Again, a thing I have often seen both in private houses and institutions. A room remains uninhabited; the fire-place is carefully fastened up with a board; the windows are never opened probably the shutters are always kept shut; perhaps some kind of stores are kept in the room; no breath of fresh air can possibly enter into that room, nor can any ray of sun. The air is as stagnant, musty and corrupt as it can by possibility be made. It is quite ripe to breed small-pox, scarlet-fever, diptheria, or anything else you please.

"Yet the nursery, ward, or sick room adjoining, will positively be aired (?) by having the door opened into that room. Or children will be put into that room, without previous preparation, to sleep."

Where such conditions prevailed in the hospitals, as described by Miss Nightingale, and Sir Frederick, and the same or worse conditions prevailed in the homes, even of the well-to-do, disease and death were rife. Miss Nightingale again says, Pages 26-7:

"I have known whole houses and hospitals smell of the sink. I have met just as strong a stream of sewer air coming up the back staircase of a grand London house from the sink, as I have ever met at Scutari; and I have seen the rooms in that house all ventilated by the open doors, and the passages all unventilated by the closed windows, in order that as much of the sewer air as possible might be conducted into and retained in the bed-rooms. It is wonderful.

"Another great evil in house construction is carrying drains underneath the house. Such drains are never safe. All house drains should begin and end outside the walls. Many people will readily admit, as a theory, the importance of these things. But how few are there who can intelligently trace disease in their households to such causes! Is it not a fact, that when scarlet fever, measles, or small-pox appear among the children, the very first thought which occurs is, 'where' the children can have 'caught' the disease? And the parents immediately run over in their minds all the families with whom they may have been. They never think of looking at home for the source of the mischief. If a neighbor's child is seized with small-pox, the first question which occurs is whether it had been vaccinated. No one would undervalue vaccination; but it becomes of doubtful benefit to society when it leads people to look abroad for the source of evils which exist at home.

"Without cleanliness, within and without your house, ventilation is comparatively useless. In certain foul districts of London, poor people used to object to open their windows and doors because of the foul smells that came in. Rich people like to have their stables and dunghill near their houses. But does it ever occur to them that with many arrangements of this kind it would be safer to keep the windows shut than open? You cannot have the air of the house pure with dung-heaps under the windows. They are common all over London. And yet people are surprised that their children, brought up in large 'well-aired' nurseries and bed-rooms suffer from childrens' epidemics. If they studied Nature's laws in the matter of children's health, they would not be so surprised."

Miss Nightingale tells us also that houses were dark, poorly ventilated, if at all, carpets dirty, walls covered with paper of years standing, furniture uncleaned, dung-heaps in the basements, and sewers and drains emptying their foulness into the whole house.

"A dark house is always an unhealthy house, always an ill-aired house, always a dirty house," she declares. "Want of light stops growth, and promotes scrofula, rickets, etc., among the children.

"People lose their health in a dark house, and if they get ill, they cannot get well in it again. More will be said about this further on."

436

In explaining why in the homes of the people "all the servants" were sick or there "is always sickness in our house," she refers to "cases of hospital pyaemia, quit as severe in handsome private houses as in any of the worst hospitals, and from the same cause," and says, pp. 30:

"I will tell you what was the cause of this hospital pyaemia being in that large-private house. It was that the sewer air from an ill-placed sink was carefully conducted into all the rooms by sedulously opening all the doors, and closing all the passage windows. It was that the slops were emptied into the foot pans!—it was that the utensils were never properly rinsed; ****it was that the chamber crockery was rinsed with dirty water; ****it was that the beds were never properly shaken, aired, picked to pieces, or changed. It was that the carpets and curtains were always musty;—it was that the furniture was always dusty;—it was that the papered walls were saturated with dirt;—it was that the floors were never cleaned;—it was that the uninhabited rooms were never sunned, or cleaned, or aired;—it was that the cupboards were always reservoirs of foul air;—it was that the windows were always tight shut up at night;—it was that no window was ever systematically opened even in the day, or that the right window was not opened.

"A person gasping for air might open a window for himself. But the servants were not taught to open the windows, to shut the doors; or they opened the windows upon a dank well between high walls, not upon the airier court; or they opened the room doors into the unaired halls and passages, by way of airing the rooms. Now all this is not fancy, but fact. In that handsome house I have known in one summer three cases of hospital pyaemia, one of phlebitis, two of consumptive cough; all the immediate products of foul air. When, in temperate climates, a house is more unhealthy in summer than in winter, it is a certain sign of something wrong."

Whenever such conditions have passed away, health has improved and epidemics have ceased. Sickness and death have always been more prevalent among the poor. Wherever these have had better housing, better food and better working conditions, their health has improved. The labor unions and other forces which have aided in bettering the condition of the working classes, have done more to prevent disease than all the doctors of all schools of "healing" that ever lived. A brief glimpse at a few of the plagues of the past will help us to understand how and why they passed.

In 1347-49 an epidemic of the Black Death swept over Europe. The Historian tells us: "In many places almost all the people fell victim to the scourge. Some villages were left without an inhabitant. Many monastries were almost emptied. In the Mediterranean and the Baltic ships were seen drifting about without a soul on board. Crops rotted unharvested in the fields; herds and flocks wandered about unattended. It is estimated that from one-third to one-half the population of Europe perished. Hecker, an historian of the pestilance, estimates the total number of victims at twenty-five millions. It was the most awful calamity that ever befell the human race."

This same historian says: "Its virulence without doubt" was "greatly increased by the unsanitary conditions of the crowded towns and the wretched mode of living of the poorer classes."

The Black Death disappeared from Europe many years ago. It retreated, as did the English sweat, typhus fever, cholera and small-pox, before the rising tide of hygiene and sanitation. No vaccine or serum conquered these diseases. No blood contamination caused them to disappear.

Montgomery's English History says: "The next year a terrible plague occurred in London (1665) which spread throughout the Kingdom. All who could fled from the city. Hundreds of houses were left vacant, while on hundreds more a cross marked on the door in red chalk, with the words 'Lord have mercy on us' written underneath told where the work of death was going on. This pestilence swept off over a hundred thousand victims within six months.

This plague finally ceased, as all epidemics do when all who were in a condition to succumb had the disease. It was not checked by the early enforcement of vaccination orders from the Board of Health (?).

Montgomery continues: "The death-cart had hardly ceased to go it rounds, when a fire (1666) broke out****By it the City of London proper was reduced to ruins, little more being left than a fringe of houses on the northeast****Great as the calamity was, yet from a sanitary point of view, it did immense good. Nothing short of fire could have effectively cleansed the London of that day, and so put a stop to the period-ical ravages of the plague. By sweeping away miles of narrow streets crowded with miserable buildings black with the encrusted filth of ages, the conflagration in the end proved friendly to health and life."

If the cleansing of London by fire put a stop to the periodical ravages of the plague, and if the "unsanitary conditions of the crowded towns and wretched mode of living of the poorer classes" increased the virulence of the plague, doesn't it seem probable that the revival of sanitation and hygiene and the work of the various labor organizations in raising the standard of living among the workers are also responsible for the disappearance of other epidemic diseases, including small-pox?

Did Bubonic Plague, English Sweat, Cholera, Typhus Fever, etc., retreat before the rising tide of hygiene and sanitation, or did they just "die out" of their own accord? Did yellow fever disappear from New Orleans, Cuba and Panama, because of improved hygiene and sanitation or did it just "die out" of its own accord? Epidemic cholera was once prevalent in America. Health Boards every bit as ignorant as those that attempt to prevent small-pox by contaminating the blood of the populace with pus from a cow, attempted to prevent cholera by prohibiting the transportation into the cities of fruits and vegetables. It required a Sylvester Graham to demonstrate that more fruits and vegetables and better hygiene and less meat, eggs, milk, white bread, wine, etc., would prevent cholera. Cholera is no more in this country. Did it just "die out" of its own accord, or did hygiene and sanitation have anything to do with its disappearance? It was banished without the aid of vaccine or serum.

In 1924 an epidemic of cholera raged in Shanghai, China. In one section of the city it was estimated that more than a thousand died daily from the disease. The news reports stated that "Foreigners living in well governed concession districts under modern sanitary conditions have suffered comparatively little." Of 20,000 foreigners, only two succumbed.

What of the Chinese. There are 1,500,000 people closely jammed into the city. The native sections are densely crowded and insanitary. The heaviest mortality occured in congested industrial centers and beggar villages where the people live in filthy hovels. The foreigners have better food, better houses, bath tubs, plumbing, sewers and less crowded quarters. Their standard of living is higher. This and no vaccine or serum saved them from cholera just as it eliminated cholera and typhus from America.

Catlin tells us, *Shut Your Mouth*, pp. 35: "The Brute creations are everywhere free from cholera and yellow fever, and I am living witness that the Asiatic cholera of 1831, was everywhere arrested on the United States frontier, when in its progress it reached the savage tribes living in their primitive conditions; having been a traveler on those frontiers during its ravages in those regions."

Dr. Chas. Phillips Emerson, M.D. says in his "*Essentials of Medicine.*" (Pp. 322):

"Typhus fever called also 'hospital fever,' or 'camp fever,' 'spotted fever,' 'jail fever' and 'ship fever,' formerly, one of the great epidemics of the world, has during the past great war been the worst of scourges for the half-starved peoples of Serbia, Russia and other inland nations. It occurs wherever starving human beings are over-crowded amid filty surroundings, and wherever there were war, famine and misery."

Typhus fever is prevented by good food, clean beds, well ventilated, well aired houses, baths, etc.,—in a word hygiene and sanitation. This disease was again epidemic in certain regions of Europe following the world war, when Hygiene and sanitation had broken down in these regions and the people were left hungry, shattered, and poverty-stricken.

Anti-vaccinationists are frequently accused of thinking that smallpox "just died out" of its own volition. We are frequently reminded that smallpox has almost wholly vanished since the beginning of the use of vaccination and asked to explain why this is so if vaccination did not banish the disease. It is my purpose here, to show from the facts of history, why smallpox disappeared.

A health commissioner in New York State recently stated to a friend of mine that if he could not prevent smallpox by vaccination he would not know what else to do to prevent it. This is the type of man who heads the health boards of this land. If they cannot prevent disease by polluting our blood they cannot concieve of anything they can do to assure freedom from epidemic diseases. A knowledge of the facts of history would have prevented such a confession of ignorance. Even wild animals know better, as will be seen from the following quotation from Robert S. Parks Walter:

"As the good old horse wades into a stream, he ducks his head for a draft of fresh water, but before permitting any to pass down his throat he fiirst uses his mobile lips, throwing the water in all directions in order to clear off from the surface dust or floating germs. The horse is one of the many animals that is very clean in his habits, and if fed regularly, never gormandizes or becomes intemperate in his eating or drinking.

"And then there is the humble toad. This little creature is very particular that nothing is taken into his stomach but what is wholesome. In feeding toads, I have never yet been able to induce one to eat a dead insect, even freshly killed. The toad utilizes this principle in protecting its own body from injury and possible death. If we take a cat, a dog, or other animal, and force it to paw or claw the toad, it immediately inflates its own body and then feigns death. The swelling of the body is purposely accomplished to make a morsel of itself that no animal of a certain size can swallow, and the feigning of death will usually result in abandonment by enemies after they pronounce the toad 'dead.'

"The spider is another creature that has for its standard rule in selecting things fit to eat 'life.' Things must be very active to convince the spider that it is a fit morsel for food. If a dead insect is dropped into a spider's web, the little owner will politely clip the web and toss the unwelcome food to the ground below. Like the toad, the spider recognizes the fact that activity seems to be the world-wide password, for when his own life is threatened he rolls up into a ball, drops to the ground, and plays off dead.

"Animals, whether large or small, adhere closely to sanitary principles, and as strongly in some instances as members of the human family do. The birds are very careful about their baths; the old cat not only cleanses her body daily, but washes the kittens as well. But of all the animals, the rabbit is, perhaps, the most sanitary. They are careful about cleansing every part of their bodies. Even insects may often be observed taking their daily ablutions. On a sleeping car one night I sat up until nearly midnight. Late in the evening a katydid lit on the window outside, and the light from the car shone directly on its body. It remained on the window-pane for thirty minutes, and during that time went over its entire body, giving it a thorough rubbing with saliva. The speed of the train apparently did not interfere in the least with its action. When the body was cleansed, it flew away into darkness. The American mantis, which is so common to the lawns in the United States, may be observed to take frequent sponge baths, as the katydids do.

"Even the goat is a sanitary creature. Kids brought up on bottles often refuse to take milk from a bottle if the nipple and bottle have not been thoroughly cleaned. The sanitary idea is so pronounced throughout nature, that animals, with few exceptions, strive toward eating pure and wholesome food, keeping their bodies from dirt and selecting good sites for their nests and dens. When an animal's den becomes unsanitary, it is not long until it is either deserted or cleaned. Even birds construct new nests every year. Birds are unwilling to take any chances on filth, decay or disease." *Literary Digest*, Sept. 25, 1926.

In ancient times diseases resembling small-pox raged in Africa and Asia, but they failed to gain a foothold in the health-worshipping nations in Southern Europe. During the long period of Pagan civilization, neither Greece nor Rome, nor any of their European colonies suffered an epidemic that could possibly be mistaken for variola. From B.C. 800 to A.D. 450 the records of memorable events are almost complete, but no instances of small-pox epidemics are recorded.

Their populations were trained in athletics, rational dietetics and public and private hygiene. Every larger town had free municipal baths, while no prudish notions about the body prevented the free access of the sun and air to their skins. They had their own ideas of how their dieties maintained their health, but it is safe to say that the mere suggestion of compulsory blood contamination as a means of preventing disease would have sent the budding young Jenner to a madhouse. By hygiene and sanitation, alone, a population of some 120,000,000 eager traders and restless adventurers coming in unavoidable contact with small-pox in Africa and Asia avoided the disease for nearly fifteen hundred years.

When Rome fell and Oriental darkness and superstition crept over Europe small-pox came along with these. In the midnight hours of the Millenium of madness, the thousand years' reign of anti-naturalism, the unsanitary conditions of Europe sunk below anything in the era of primitive barbarism. We may justly charge many of the effiminate nations of pagan antiquity with mere neglect of hygiene but it remained for Christian Europe of the Middle Ages to publicly commend and even enforce neglect of hygiene and sanitation as a public duty and moral and spiritual necessity. It remained for world-renouncing fanatics of that age to welcome disease as a sign of divine favor and glory in decrepitude and deformity. Never before did men outside the medical profession deliberately work to bring about the physical degeneracy of the human race.

The *thermae*, built by the Romans wherever they went, were destroyed. Bathing was denounced as a sin. Any attention to the body's welfare was regarded as detracting from man's spiritual welfare. The sanitary conditions in European towns became frightful Montgomery's English History says of the English cities: "The streets of London and other cities were rarely more than twelve to fifteen feet wide. They were neither paved nor lighted. Pools of stagnant water and heaps of refuse abounded. There was no sewage. The only scavengers were the crows."

Hillocks of garbage accummulated in the narrow streets and were removed only when they began to obstruct traffic to an unendurable degree. Dead dogs and cats, rotten vegetables and fruits, human and animal excreta, slops and refuse from the kitchen all were thrown into the cities streets.

Cities were surrounded with high walls and moats of stagnant water, thus preventing expansion and enforcing crowded slum-like conditions. The ill-ventilated rookeries were crowded from attic to sub-cellar. Three generations of poor mechanics were often herded in one room; this frequently a basement room receiving light through holes in the walls. These holes, at the beginning of the cold season, were apt to be stopped with stable litter.

These people had no bath tubs, almost never washed and then but superficially. They had no underclothes and wore the same clothes night and day. Five and six or more slept in a bed and smelled to high heaven. They were all equipped with instruments for scratching their filthy backs, while the old adage "You scratch my back and I'll scratch yours" was put to practical application frequently.

Houses had but one window. The tax on *Purtes et Fenetics* (tax on doors and windows) in France and Italy and other European nations caused the French, Italians and others to sleep in rooms without windows. They put in imitation windows (on which there was no tax) and left their homes without ventilation. It is said that some of these old imitation windows are still to be seen in Europe. Often there was only a hole in the roof for smoke to escape. The houses were low. Leaves, boughs, straw, etc., laid on the ground which formed the floor, were "rarely changed" and "became horribly filthy, and were a prolific cause of sickness," according to Montgomery's history.

In the days of Ben Johnson and Shakespear, the stench in the theatres would become so unbearable that the stifling audience would cry out: "Burn the Juniper! Burn the Juniper!" The juniper is an evergreen shrub which emits a strong and pleasing odor when burning, as does our cedar, and it was kept on hand in the theatres to camouflage the amalgamated stinks, that filled the Augean stables they called theatres in those days.

Filth was considered both holy and healthful. Terrestrial life was regarded as utterly worthless. Man was a "lowly worm of the dust." Poverty, squalor, ignorance and filth were everywhere. Europe was a rotting, stinking cess-pool. Fears and superstitions made life burdensome. The body was looked upon with contempt and regarded as the mortal enemy of the spirit. Life was worthless and treated as such. Filthiness and abuse of the body were encouraged because these aided spiritual development. Man tried to immortalize his spirit by mortifying his flesh.

Under such unspeakably insanitary and unhygienic conditions (and I have not told more than a fraction of the story), epidemics of all kinds raged. Bubonic plague or the "black death" typhus and typhoid fever, epidemic or asiastic cholera, smallpox, English sweat and other diseases abounded. And why not? These people were living in a vertible continental cess pool, filled with fears of robber knights, devils, hob-goblins, hell, purgatory and other imaginary beings and places. They worked long hours, and lived in poverty, drank heavily of wine and ate like hogs. No man would attempt to raise hogs under such filthy conditions to-day.

Finally a revival of common sense began. The long dark night of Medieval super-stition was broken. The yoke of fendalism was thrown off also. Gun powder battered down the walls and dried up the motes around the cities. Shade trees grew where the motes had been. Suburbs sprang up. The cities spread outward. Garden-cottages took the places of slum-dungeons. As Heinrich Heine puts it, "men proceeded to fumigate their wives and sweep their houses, as after a weathered pestilence."

Diet improved. Monastic beer-cellars became root-houses. Waste fields were planted with fruit trees. The rising power of the trade unions began to better the working man's conditions. People learned to bathe. Averhoes instituted a crusade against municipal abominations. Streets were made wider and paved. Unpaved streets were kept clean. Windows were put into homes. People learned to sleep in well ventilated bed-rooms. Garbage was carted to suburban ravines. Jailers were forced to remove their prisoners from subterranean cess-pools to ventilated cells. Irremediable rat-hatcheries were torn down to make room for wider and cleaner streets. Later sewage systems were installed. Man of to-day lives in a heaven of cleanliness in comparison to the hell of filth in the Middle Ages.

Epidemics began to abate. Diseases began to lose their virulence. The black death retreated to Asia. Typhus soon followed and then cholera. The English sweat disappeared entirely. Small-pox declined also.

The pathological demon of the middle ages had been tamed down to a hobgoblin, years before that Prince of Charlatans, Edward Jenner, grafted the milk maids creed onto the superstitious rite of the Georgians and promulgated his murderous method of exorcism.

In 1731 Frederick Wilhelm, father of Frederick the Great, declined to permit one of his generals to shift a manoeuvre (sham battle) camp on account of a smallpox out-break in a neighboring village. "Don't make such a fuss about trifles," he wrote in August of that year; "but all the same, it may do no harm to keep the boys in camp after dark." Vaccine advocates reveal their ignorance of the simplest facts of history in relation to epidemic diseases. In their ignorance they single out smallpox as the one and only exception to the fact that plagues retreat before the onward march of hygiene and sanitation. They doubtless assume that smallpox remained in Africa and Asia in ancient times and stayed out of Pagan Greece and Rome of its own accord. They surely know these nations had no vaccine to hold it back. Do they imagine that vaccination will prevent smallpox in the face of unhygienic and insanitary conditions? If so, they make the same childish mistake the medical department of our over-seas forces did during the war. They imagine vaccines and serums can make unclean living safe. The Public Health Report, Vol. 34, No. 13, for March 28, 1919, publishes under the title, "Typhoid Vaccination no Substitute for Sanitary precautions," a circular by the Chief Surgeon of the United States in which he charges that physicians with our overseas forces, having been lulled to sleep by their faith in the power of typhoid vaccine to protect from typhoid, had neglected sanitary precautions, with the result that typhoid broke out. It required a costly experience to show medical men that no form of pus or horse juice or dead bug squirts could make unclean living safe. Indeed most of them have not learned their lesson yet for they are still trying to substitute pus for clean living. They possess but little faith in the protective virtues of hygiene and sanitation. They have almost unlimited trust in the saving power of pus and filth.

The "*Report on Sanitary measures in India in 1879-80*" contains the following, (p. 142):

"The vaccination returns throughout India show the same fact, that the number of vaccinations does not necessarily bear a ratio to the smallpox deaths. Smallpox in India is related to season and to epidemic prevalence; it is not a disease, therefore, that can be controlled by vaccination, in the sense that vaccination is a specific against it. As an endemic and epidemic disease, it must be dealt with by sanitary measures, and if these are neglected, smallpox is certain to increase during epidemic times."

In the "*Memorandum of the Army, the Army Sanitarium Commission for the Punjab* (1879), the following is found:

"Vaccination in the Punjab, as elsewhere in India, has no power apparently over the course of an epidemic. It may modify and diminish the number of fatal cases (it really increases both of these. Shelton), but the whole Indian experience points in one direction, and this is that the severity of a smallpox epidemic is more closely connected with sanitary defects, which intensify the activity of other epidemic diseases than is usually imagined, and that to the general sanitary improvement of towns and villages must we look for the mitigation of smallpox as of cholera and fever."

Will those who advocate contamination of the human blood stream be capable of comprehending the meaning of the simple facts in these reports? I fear not. And it is just this inability to comprehend the simplest facts of life and their under-lying principles that causes such minds to declare that anti-vaccinationists think that smallpox just "died out," of its own accord. We insist that smallpox ceased when the unhygienic and unsanitary conditions that gave rise to it were removed and that vaccination had absolutely nothing to do with its decline.

There are a few facts about smallpox in the Middle Ages that we should get into our minds and keep there in any consideration of vaccination.

First: Smallpox made its appearance in Europe only after the collapse of Roman and Greek civilization and the hygienic and sanitary systems and methods employed by these. Throughout the long period of Greek and Roman Civilization, no small-pox ever entered Europe. But with the lapse of Europe into Barbarism and filth during the long medieval nights of superstition, smallpox was prevalent.

Second: At no time was smallpox ever half as prevalent or half as deadly as we are led to believe. Smallpox was a generic term applied to eruptive fevers. It was not until Sydenham, in the seventeenth century, differentiated measles from smallpox, that these were regarded as separate diseases. Prior to this time, every case of measles was considered a case of smallpox and every death from this disease was considered a death from smallpox. Compare the present prevalence of measles and the present death rate in this disease with the present prevalence of smallpox in unvaccinated districts and the present death rate in smallpox in these unvaccinated people and you get some idea of how much was done by Sydenham to decrease smallpox.

Third: Sydenham did more than this. In 1666, more than a century before Jenner, he published his famous "*Treatise on Fevers*," and demonstrated that the sweatbox tortures to which all fever patients were subjected, was deadly and that a cooling treatment was far less so. His biographers always state that he "discovered the efficacy of a cooling regimen in smallpox, by which discovery he saved many thousand lives." I shall say more of this medieval plan of treatment later.

Fourth: The pathological demon of the Middle Ages had been tamed down to a mere hobgoblin years before Jenner came on the scene. Smallpox, was already passing when Jenner arrived. Fear of it, which was never great, (people actually courting it for themselves and their children that they might have the disease and be done with it) was dying when Jenner stole the milk-maids' creed.

The death rate in smallpox and other fevers during the Middle Ages was largely due to the medical profession of that time. Patients were bled profusely and drugged hugely. Mercury and antimony were given in huge doses. The patient was smothered in blankets, allowed no water, no fresh air and stuffed with milk and brandy or wine. A fever patient would be clapped into a vapor-bath chamber on the theory that they could "sweat the impurities out of the system." If he cried for a drop of cold water, he was insulted with elder-blossom tea. If he gasped for a change of air they carried him into a dry-hot room for a while, and then carried him back into the steam trap. Many such patients must have died of heat stroke. Many more were bled to death.

Physicians of that day kept the smallpox patient "wrapped up warmly in bed, the room kept heated, the doors and windows carefully closed to the exclusion of every breath of air, and stimulating sudorifics (drugs to induce sweating), with wine and cordials, administered freely."

Caddiston, who lived in the fourteenth century, and who was the first court physician and one of the earliest English medical writers, recommended that the patient should be surrounded with "red curtains, red walls, red furniture of all kinds, so that everything he saw should be red, under the idea that there was something glowing or otherwise beneficial in that color."

Sennertus, who wrote at the beginning of the seventeenth century, advised:

"That while using these means, every attention is to be paid, especially in winter, to the exclusion of cold air. The patient, therefore, is to be tended in a warm chamber and carefully covered up, lest by closing the pores of the skin, the efforts of nature should be impeded, the humors driven on internal organs, and matter which ought to be expelled, retained within the body, to the imminent danger of the patient, and the certainty of increasing restlessness, fever, and other symptoms."

Diemerbrock, a contemporary of Sennertus, speaking on the same subject, says:

"Keep the patient in a chamber close shut. If it be winter let the air be corrected by large fires. Take care that no cold gets into the patient's bed. Cover him over with red blankets. Not that the color is material, but because all the best thickest and warmest blankets are dyed red. Never shift the patient's linen till after the fourteenth day, for fear of striking in the pock to the irrevocable ruin of the patient. Far better it is to let the patient bear with the stench, than to let him change his linen, and thus be the cause of his own death. Nevertheless, if a change be absolutely necessary, be sure that he puts on the foul linen that he put off before he fell sick and above all things, take care that this supply of semi-clean linen be well warmed. Sudorific expulsives are, in the meantime, to be given plentifully, such as treacle, pearls, and saffron."

Think of keeping a smallpox patient in bed for fourteen days without changing the linen—either the bed linen or the patient's linen—or if it must be changed, putting on him the dirty linen he discarded before becoming sick! That was medical science in the Middle Ages. Men who believed in such practices could easily believe that the introduction of pus into the body would prevent smallpox, but no intelligent man in these days of hygiene and sanitation can believe such non-sense.

A breath of cool air was dangerous. A drink of cool water was deadly. Fires in the closed room in winter consumed the oxygen and left the patient to gasp. The patient wallowed in putrescence. The wonder is that any of them ever lived—not that they frequently died. It is eloquent testimony to the inherent fighting powers of the body that the European races lived through such a long dark night of filth, superstition and murderous medical methods.

Mirabeau, before his death, was robbed by his physicians, of nearly a hundred ounces of blood in forty-eight hours. George Washington, in his last illness, was relieved in fifteen to twenty hours, of about ninety ounces of blood. A noted Scotch physician declared, when Washington died, that he was bled enough to kill any ordinary man and that he took enough calomel and antimony for either of these to have killed him. Ten grains of calomel were administered him at one dose. Yet this was a small dose of either calomel or antimony in those days. THE SICK DID NOT DIE, THEY WERE MURDERED. By far a large majority of those who die today are murdered, also.

Hygiene and sanitation prevent smallpox. Vaccination does not. Two historical examples will show this to be so.

In one little spot in Europe there remained a little sanitary Eden, a place where pork and alcohol were forbidden by religion, where everybody took a daily bath, where free public baths existed and every family occupied a home of its own. I refer to Moorish, Spain, a little country south of the Ebro Valley where the light of Pagan civilization had not been extinguished. Their towns were not crowded. They had the finest public parks in Europe and they maintained a regular system of street cleaning. Every well-to-do family maintained a tree-shaded court-yard with a cooling fountain, an *alguador*.

They had no vaccination but those cleanly Mussulmans enjoyed immunity from smallpox while it drove their northern neighbors to frenzy. Rabidly persisting in the insane idea that smallpox was due to insufficient abuse of their wretched bodies, some of the roving bands of self-torturers, north of the Ebro, flayed themselves with knotted thongs, tore their hair, mixed wormwood with their food and implored every passerby to kick them for pity's sake.

Their idea was that the way to prevent smallpox was to abuse the body. This is the same idea that forms the basis of the filthy practices of vaccination and inoculation. These modern practices are as disastrous as were those of the medieval fanatics.

Well-to-do Spaniards renounced their religious dogmas and sought refuge south of the Ebro. A King of Aragon sent his two sons to Cordova with royal presents to a Moorish physician who cared for and nursed them for a few weeks while the epidemic raged in Barcelona and the hamlets of the Pyrenees. Velez Malaga, the seaport town of Moorland, became crowded with refugees. Smallpox broke out among them. Instead of going into Board-of-Health convulsions the city fathers contented themselves with isolating the suffering refugees. No vaccination was used and no epidemic started.

Moorish doctors were persuaded to visit several of the cities of Christian Europe but these were unable to help stay the epidemic. Against the worse than pig-stye conditions their prescriptions were as ineffectual as a pad-lock on a night club.

Bigots of the Moorish faith ascribed the troubles of the Northland to their unbelief and when their physicians proved to be helpless in staying the disease they were, more than ever, confirmed in their belief that "the immunity of Moorland was due to talismans that lost their power in a country of the Cross."

Further south in Nubia and Abyssinia smallpox raged. During the hunting seasons, when the people were outdoors, it would die down, but would soon spring up again when these people returned to their beastly domestic habits.

Scholasticism, the classical revival in Italy, the Reformation in the North, the collapse of feudalism, with the rise of better and less crowded cities, improved diet, the rise of trade unions, Averhoos crusade against municipal abominations—these and other influences improved the living conditions of the people and revived common sense in the care of the body. Smallpox in Christian lands had to pass. Its passage began long before Jenner stole the dairy-maids creed and induced the British Parliament to pay him a huge sum for his "wonderful benefit" to the race.

The Franco-Prussian War supplied a memorable test of the efficacy of vaccination in preventing smallpox. Nearly all the German soldiers had been vaccinated in childhood. All of them, without a single exception, had been re-vaccinated at the recruiting depots. Thousands had been re-re-vaccinated. They were "protected."

But the camps were shifted so rapidly that it was not possible to enforce sanitary regulations. Whole regiments were forced to bivouac in rainstorms or among hillocks or poorly-buried carcasses. In some of the camps, galloping horses kicked up bits of putrefying flesh for the so-called graves were mere depressions covered over with a thin crust of earth.

In the smaller towns the barracks, churches and municipal halls did not begin to garrison the enormous numbers of cannon-fodder. Thousands were stationed in private residences or huddled together in barns and factories. The soldiers spent their leisure time picking vermin from their bodies. The sanitary condition of the camps became almost as bad as that of medieval European towns.

The result was that 53,288 able-bodied men, fully "protected" by Jenner's calf-pus had smallpox as virulent as any ever seen before. The death rate was high.

It is customary for vaccine apologists to say that such epidemics start among the "unprotected" and then become so virulent that nothing will protect against them. This is utterly false. It is a mere alibi. Keen eyed observers were on hand in 1870 who thought it worth recording that in Cologne, "the first unvaccinated person attacked by smallpox, was the 174th in order of time, in Bonn, the same year, the 42nd, and in Liegnitz, the 225th."

Prof. Adolph Vogt, an impartial observer and careful collector of statistics, stated that "the Bavarian contigent, which was revaccinated without exception, had five times the death rate from smallpox that the Bavarian civil population of the same ages had, although re-vaccination is not obligatory among the latter."

Vaccination failed to protect in this case when sanitary and hygienic conditions were ripe for an epidemic. It not only failed, but those who were most vaccinated suffered most. Vaccination as a protection against disease is like a burglar-proof-safe —alright until the burglar comes along.

Hygiene and sanitation immunized Spanish Moorland in the Middle Ages. Smallpox raged in the rotting, stinking pest-hole that was Northern Europe, but little Moorland remained safe. Personal and municipal cleanliness and sensible living did what vaccination can never do. Vaccination can never make unclean living safe and those who live cleanly are in no danger.

The British found by their experience in India that vaccination could not be substituted for hygiene and sanitation. They found that when these latter were neglected, smallpox and other endemic and epidemic diseases abounded and that smallpox could be eradicated only by those same hygienic and sanitary measures that prevented the other diseases that is by the same improvement in living conditions that wiped out cholera and typhus fever in this country. Only the Boards of Health(?) and Health(?) Commissioners are unable to learn this lesson. They talk as though they never heard of these things. They probably know nothing of the sanitary conditions of European towns in the Middle Ages and perhaps have not heard that the other epidemic diseases that ravaged Europe at that time have vanished without the aid of vaccine. Perhaps they have not heard that sanitation and hygiene and not a vaccine protected the foreign section of Shanghai, China, from cholera last year while the disease raged in the native section.

No serum or vaccine conquered the Black Death or Typhus fever. No pus punching banished Yellow Fever or Cholera. No form of blood pollution eradicated English Sweat. Did these diseases just "die out" of their own accord or did bath tubs, modern plumbing, better housing, better food, better working conditions, cleaner cities, sewage and sanitary systems, railways, refrigerators, and improved individual hygiene and the eradication of fear from religion have anything to do with their disappearance? When the bath tub was first introduced into this country the medical profession opposed its use, just as it has vigorously opposed every other advance in hygiene and saniatation. Just as they opposed Graham's dietary and hygienic reforms and continued to oppose dietary reform until ten years ago. They attempted to secure the passage of laws forbidding the use of bath tubs on the ground that they would cause disease.

We will probably be met with claim that these diseases are caused by germs that breed in filth. Let this be granted. We must still clean up the filth. We cannot control the germs except by controlling the filth. We cannot, by the use of serums and vaccines, make unclean living safe. Every epidemic proves this. They who are the worst livers, are the ones who suffer most. As Graham truly says:

"Disease is therefore not only induced by disturbing causes in the first place, but it is kept up by the continual action of such causes. It is true that when the action of disturbing causes has induced diseased structure in our organs, this, while it remains, will in the absence of all other morbific causes keep up diseased action to a greater or less extent in the system. But as a general law, in chronic complaints, where change of structure has not actually taken place and gone too far for vital redemption, diseased action will not long continue, after the entire removal of the disturbing causes; and hence, chronic disease is in almost every instance kept alive and cherished from day to day, from month to month, and from year to year, by the constant action of those disturbing causes which are mostly to be found in our dietetic and other voluntary habits. But whatever irritates our organs and disturbs their functions, not only tends to originate disease in the system, but always com-

445

mensurately diminishes the power of our bodies to resist the action of foreign morbific pestilential causes."

Those who have broken down their resistance are the ones who succumb, as a true physiology reveals. But where is a true physiology to be found? Not in the schools, as Trall said, but outside these, for it is still true, as he declared:

"When I intimate there is no physiology in the world, I mean, of course, the medical world. Out of the regular profession this science has been more prospered. Untrammeled by the theories of the schools, individuals, not of the order of medical men, have, as I shall hereafter show, demonstrated the true science of life, and laid the true foundation for a medical practice, whose most powerful remedies, so far from being the most potent poisons, known on the surface or dug from the bowels of the earth, are the very agencies by which the whole vegetable and animal creations are developed and sustained."—*Hydropathic Encyclopedia*. Vol. 1.

EARLY RECOGNITION OF SUPPRESSION
CHAPTER XXXIV

"**A** PATIENT has a sour stomach, and the doctor gives him soda; another is afflicted with worms, and the doctor administers something to poison them to death; another has gravelly concretions, and the doctor administers chemical solvents; another has acrid bile which corrodes his throat, and the doctor prescribes lubricating mucilages, and so on to the end of life. But who cannot perceive that all this practice as a part of the *healing* art, is absurd and ridiculous? Who is so stupidly blind as not to see that it is a mere patch-work, tinkering at effects without removing causes."—*Hydropathic Encyclopedia.* Vol. 2, pp. 11.

The above quotation from Dr. Trall draws a fairly accurate picture of medical practice of this day. The practice in general has not changed any since the dawn of history. It was always a system of suppression. It never concerned itself with causes, but always devoted its attention to the eradication or smothering of effects. Symptoms are such only and not causes but the medical profession never found this out, or, if they did, they never changed their practices to conform with their knowledge. All *schools of healing,* in all ages have been content to give "relief" from symptoms. If the symptom could be made to disappear, or to cease to annoy and distress, this was enough. It did not matter that this made the true condition of the patient worse. It was of no consequence that the patient's sufferings were prolonged, intensified and changed; that acute disease was converted into chronic disease and that a simple curative process was made the occasion for killing the patient.

How true are the following words of Jennings? *"Philosophy of Human Life."* pp. 214-15.

"Notwithstanding the medical profession have failed to define the general and special nature of disease—a true knowledge of which is essential to the establishment of a correct system of therapeutics—yet it is obvious from the general tenor of their instructions and practice, that they regard the difficulty as consisting essentially in a defect in Nature's balance-wheel, or self-controlling principle and power; a defect too that may be remedied to a greater or less extent by artificial force of various kinds and degrees, with various modes of application. Accordingly, in practical medicine, the object to be effected is to ascertain where nature fails to perform her accustomed duty and apply the necessary admonitory correctors. If there is too much action in any portion of the machinery, give her to understand, through the influence of some potent depletory, counter-irritant or revulsive process, that she must restrain or restrict her forces in that direction. If there is too little action, spur her up to greater vigilance and activity in the supply of efficient forces.

"Every Heteropathic system of medicine is underlaid with a deep conviction, that in an impaired or diseased state of the human system, its capabilities will not be realized to their fullest extent, without the intervention of some compulsory means of an impulsive or restraining character; and that the necessity of such interference is enhanced in proportion to the increase or exaggeration of the disease.

"The belief has been quite general if not universal, that in most diseases of any magnitude to which man's physical nature is liable, the cases would be more protracted and severe, and much oftener fatal, if left to the unaided and unrestrained powers of life, with the best possible regimen, than they would be under the direction and influence of even ordinary medical skill and means. The quantity of artificial remedial force supposed to be requisite to secure the speediest and best cures, have varied much under different systems of medicine, and different states of society. But there probably never was a period in the world's history since medicine began to be practiced as a science and an art, when the quantity of *medicine,* or compulsory interference with the natural vital operations in disease, which the public sentiment, medical and non-medical, would fix upon as that which was best calculated to secure the happiest results, was less than it is at the present time. Yet many schools, teachers and practitioners of medicine still inculcate, theoretically and practically, the importance of taking disease by storm, when practicable, and giving it no quarter till it is exterminated; and the most moderate of them think it best to 'give nature a little jog.'

"Just here is the broad line of demarcation between Heteropathy and Orthopathy. Orthopathists discard this doctrine of armed intervention as opposed to the law of the animal economy and unphilosophical; AND THEY REJECT IT AS MUCH IN ITS MINIMUM AS IN ITS MAXIMUM."

It was Dr. Jenning's conviction that the vital energies never have to be reminded of their duties; but, on the contrary, that they must of necessity, at all times and under all conditions, act according to law and always for the best advantage of the body. As well to think that gravitation requires to be reminded of its "duty" in bringing the stone that has been thrown upward back to earth again as to think that the forces of the vital economy do not constantly and ceaselessly obey the *laws* that control them. Every move of the forces of life, in health or disease is lawful and orderly and, in the very nature of things, cannot be otherwise. For this reason, if a given evil has occasioned a certain course of action in the body, an equal or greater evil will be required to suppress that course of action, although, a lesser evil may modify it. Well did Jennings say: *Philosophy of Human Life.* pp. 164 and 165:

"The symbols of distress will not exceed the reality, that is the real danger or difficulty that existed in this case in a latent form, back of all the symptoms, was fully commensurate with the aggregate of phenomena that will be manifested in the whole progress of development: for it would require at least as much attractive force to change the current of vital action, as it would to continue it in its natural or usual channel. The symptoms then, or the deviations from the natural condition in function and structure, are the spontaneous and necessary result of an embarrassed state of the vital funds, and the latter can only be improved, and the former restored by the regular administration of the vital economy, with but little aid directly from the hand of art. * * * * and it would be unwise, if it were practicable, to compel a return of that sooner or faster than it will return by due course of law, after the object for which it was withdrawn is accomplished; for it is now doing more good where it is, than it could do if it were immediately remanded back to its old position. * * * * Large bleedings, a free use of cold water and other powerful perturbating or annoying means might probably bring decided and temporary relief to this woman; not by 'helping nature' in any wise, but by compelling her to desist from her present purpose, and send home detached forces against the ruthless hand of art."

Is not this principle of diverting the energies of life from one "field of battle" to another field, to defend the body against another foe, the principle upon which medicine always worked. Indeed, did not Galen's "*law of antipathies.*" (*contraria contrariis curantur*), and Hahnemann's "law of similiars" (*similia, similibus, curantur*), or the cure of one disease by producing *another—opposite* or *similiar,—disease*, really recognize this fact that they subdued one disease by producing another. This idea that one disease can be made to antagonize, neutralize or supercede another was called a "law of the animal economy." Trall declared, *Hydropathic Encyclopedia,* Vol. 2, pp12-13, that it is really no law at all, but:

"It is the *resistance* that the vital powers make to morbific agents, which pathologists have misnamed a law of the animal economy. Two diseased actions, or diseases in two different parts of the body, are obstructing or offending materials in two or more parts or organs, will manifest different phenomena from what are observed when one part or organ only is affected, because vital resistance is then distributed to several points instead of being concentrated at one.

"If a person is laboring under a fever, that commotion of the organism which we denominate the *febrile paroxysm* is the manifestation of the vital struggle to defend the organic domain against some morbific cause, or to expel some injurious matter. If the vital powers are making the principal effort to the surface, the introduction of a cathartic dose of epsom salts would divert some part of the vital effort to the bowels to meet, defend against, and expel the new enemy which is committing its ravages there, and thus purgation would result, while the depurating or remedial effort to the skin would be materially diminished. The seat of war would be changed or the battle-field divided, but so far from being a 'friend in need' the saline purgation, by drawing off and wasting a portion of the vital power would only prove a 'foe in deed'."

The above fully explains and makes clear what Dr. Jennings meant when he declared that "curative" measures, if they are to draw off all the vital powers from a local seat of disease, must at least be equal in "attractive force" (that is, equally as injurious as the cause of the primary disease) as the cause of the struggle. Drugs or other measures, by dividing the body's forces, by calling for a supply of blood and energy to be sent to other parts of the body, easily and quickly diminish the symptoms of the disease, yet they do so, not by any influence they exert upon the cause of the original defense, but because, by their own injuriousness, they call for part of the body's army of defense to be sent against them. This both prolongs the disease, weakens the patient and, perhaps, results in death.

Dr. Felix L. Oswald, in *Nature's Household Remedies*, pp. 14-15, (1890), says, upon this same point:

"Drugs can rarely do more than change the form of the disease, or postpone its crisis. Mercurial salve, which conscientious physicians have almost ceased to regard as a lesser evil of an alterative, was once a favorite prescription for all kinds of cutaneous diseases; it cleansed the skin by driving the ulcers from the surface to the interior of the body. A drastic purge counteracts constipation—for a day or two—by inducing a still less desirable state of dysentery. Combined with venesection the same 'remedy' will suppress the symptoms of various inflammatory affections by compelling the exhausted system to postpone the crisis of the disease; in other words, by interrupting a curative process."

He continues this thought in *Physical Education*, pp. 188-199, (1901):

"opiates stop a flux only by paralyzing the bowels—i, e., turning their morbid activity into a morbid inactivity; the symptoms of pneumonia can be suppressed by bleeding the patient till the exhausted system has to postpone the crisis of the disease. This process, the 'breaking up of a sickness,' in the language of the old-school allopathists, is therefore in reality only an interrupting of it, a temporary interruption of the symptoms. We might as well try to cure the sleepiness of a weary child by pinching its eyelids, or the hunger of a whining dog by compressing his throat. * * * * It is not only the safer but also the shorter way to avoid drugs, reform our habits, and, for the rest, let Nature have her course; for, properly speaking, disease itself is a reconstructive process, the expulsive effort, whose interruption compels Nature to do double work; to resume her operations against the ailment after expelling a worse enemy—the drug. If a drugged patient recovers the true explanation is that his constitution was strong enough to overcome both the disease and the druggist."

Sylvester Graham explained, suppression in the following words, *Science of Human Life*, p. 424:

"It is true, however, as we have seen, that by the continued application of such remedies, the original symptoms for which they were applied may, upon the principle of counter irritation, be removed and other symptoms be established, which will disappear when the remedies are abandoned; and thus, in some instances, health may be restored; in other instances, the old symptoms will return after a short time, and probably in a more aggravated form, and in other instances, new symptoms, and perhaps of a much more serious character, may be permanently established, while the patient himself, and very often his physician also, will never suspect that the new symptoms have been produced by the very remedies by which the old symptoms were removed."

At this point I desire to quote extensively from Dr. Trall:

"Pain denotes the presence of some morbific agent, or some abnormal condition—The practice of 'curing' pain by means of opiates, narcotics, bleeding, etc., is founded on an erroneous theory of the nature of disease. Opium is more extensively employed in medicine than any other drug because it is the most convenient agent to allay pain. But it does this by silencing the outcries of Nature. The vital instincts of Nature proclaim that there is an enemy within the vital domain, and in the language of pain they call for help—for such materials and influences as they can use in expelling the morbific cause and in repairing the damages. The doctor poisons them with the drug, which is resisted with such intensity in another direction as to suppress the original effort—and this he calls a cure! The whole process is resolved into curing the disease by killing the patient. Hygienic agencies relieve pain by supplying the conditions which Nature required to expel its cause."—*Hygienic Hand Book*.

" * * * Should this struggle, this self-defensive action, this remedial effort, this purifying process, this attempt at reparation, this war for the integrity of the living domain, this contest against the enemies of the organic constitution, be repressed by bleeding, or suppressed with drugs, intensified with stimulants and tonics, subdued with narcotics and antiphlogistics, confused with blisters and caustics, aggravated with alterativaes, complicated and misdirected, changed, subverted, and perverted with drugs and poisons generally? * * * "

"To give drugs is adding to the causes of disease; for drugs always produce disease. Indeed, they cure one disease, when they cure at all, by producing others. Can causes cure causes? Can poinsons expel poinsons? Can impurities deterge impurities? Can Nature throw off two or more burdens more easily than one? No. Poisoning a person because he is impure, is like casting out devils through Beelzebub, the prince of devils. It is neither scriptural nor philosophical.

"The effect of drug-curing or drug-killing, as the case may be—I mean drug medication—is to lock up, as it were, the causes of the disease within the system, and to induce chronic and worse diseases. The causes should be expelled, not retained. The remedial struggle—the disease—should be aided, regulated, directed, so that it may successfully accomplish its work of purification, not subdued nor thwarted with poisons which create new remedial efforts (drug diseases), and thus embarrass and complicate the vital struggle."—True Healing Art.

Again:

"In Peoria, Illinois, I examined and prescribed for several similiar cases before an audience of nearly a thousand persons. Among them was a Mr. Gorsuch. He was twenty-eight years of age—of originally excellent constitution. Five years ago he had the ague, for which he took quinine in huge doses. This treatment so paralyzed the functions of the liver that it became greatly congested and enlarged; for which mercury was prescribed. The mercury induced chronic inflammation of the duodenum—mercurial duodenitis—for which antimony and opium were administered. These drugs extended the inflammation to the kidneys, prostrated the external circulation, and torpified the action of the skin; for which more mercury, in the shape of blue-pill, with narcotics was given. These remedies so exhausted the vital energies, that the next phase of the disease was termed 'nervous debility,' and then strychnine was prescribed. After the nervous debility had been sufficiently cured with strychnine, the doctors diagnosticated 'spinal disease,' and proceeded to blister and cauterize the back. Lastly, neuralgia 'set in,' and the doctors resorted to henbane.

"The condition of the patient, as I explained it to the people, in the presence of several drug doctors, was this: An enlarged liver, ague-cake of the spleen, and semi-paralysis of the abdominal and dorsal muscles, catarrh, laryngitis, duodenitis or 'canker in the stomach,' albuminuria or degeneration of the kidneys, constant heat and tenderness throughout the abdomen, inability to lie in the horizontal position, coldness and torpor of the extremities, and a thoroughly ruined constitution.

"The doctors worked at this young man for four long years, continually killing him with their curings, every one of his maladies, except the original ague, being nothing more nor less than the disease occasioned by the drugs administered for the preceding disease. Had the patient been let alone, as I stated to the audience, and had there been no doctors in the world, he would have been well and sound in a month; or had he been put into the hands of a competent Hygienic physician he might have been well in a week, in either case avoiding the expense of a five years' course of drug palliation, and the inconvenience of a ruined constitution, and the horrors of carrying about a shattered and frail organism for the remainder of his days."—True Healing Art.

"Do you know how many drug medicines, or poisons, you are liable to take into your system, for example, during an ordinary course of fever? Two or three kinds of medicines are usually administered several times a day, each probably compounded of several ingredients, so that a dozen drugs, on the average, may be swallowed daily. These are changed for new ones, to a greater or less extent, nearly every day, and in a month's sickness fifty to one hundred poisons—rebels, if you please—are sent into the domain of organic life.

"No wonder there are nowadays all sorts of 'complications,' and 'collapses,' and 'relapses,' and 'sinking spells,' and 'running down,' and 'changing into typhoid,' etc. No wonder that new diseases seem to hover around the patient and infest the very atmosphere, like a brood of malignant imps or voracious goblins, ready to 'set in,' or 'supervine,' or 'attack,' whenever the medication has brought the patient to the vulnerable point, or within range of their influence. Under Hygienic treatment these occurrences are wholly unknown. * * * *

"Commodore Perry died very suddenly and unexpectedly in New York, two years ago. The colchium relieved the gout, but the paitent died.

"How strange, that no sooner had the doctor subdued the rheumatism, than the typhoid 'set in,' and carried off the patient! Queries.—Where was the typhoid while the patient was being doctored for the rheumatism? How did it exist before Senator Douglas had it, or before it had him? Where did it come from? and where did it go? and what is it? I answer, it was the prostration of the patient caused by the treatment. Maltreat any form of febrile inflammatory disease; reduce the patient sufficiently by bleeding, blistering, or drugging, and the typhoid will be sure to make its appearance."—*True Healing Art.*

Well did Dr. Chas. E. Page, *The Natural Cure*, pp. 154 (1883), give the term "rear guard" to the professional subterfuge: "I shall bring him out of this alright if no new complication arises." For, as Dr. Page remarks: "he (the physician) prescribes a drug or a compound of drugs, which tend to provoke the complication."

Complications arise as a result of the suppressive and obstructive methods in vogue—methods which Page declared are "aimed at the removal of symptoms and not at the removal of their causes." If decomposing food in the intestine calls for a diarrhea to clean it out, how are the "over-active" bowels to be whipped back into a semblance of normal movement except by methods that paralyze their action? Their action will become normal again as soon as they have completed the house cleaning, but this is not the theory upon which the Heteropaths work. To them the diarrhea is "wrong action" and must be suppressed. But the suppression of the diarrhea holds the decomposing food up in the intestine and colon and adds the poisonous drug or drugs employed to the toxins which result from the decomposition. These facts shall be more fully explained in the next chapter.

SUPPRESSION OF DISEASE AND ITS RESULT

CHAPTER XXXV

IN the previous chapers the nature and purpose of disease have been made sufficiently apparent. Many references have been made to the evils wrought by the suppression of acute disease—that is, by the efforts to subdue and *cure* disease. It is deemed advisable to give the reader a more detailed explanation of this evil that he may better understand how to avoid suppressive methods.

If a sick man presents such "symptoms" as fever, diarrhea, skin erruption, a cold, coughing, sneezing, loss of appetite and "prostration" and everyone of these represent purifying and conservative measures, he surely has an excellent chance of getting well. It would at least seem so. Yet, many do die, apparently from acute disease. Why? Throughout this book the why has been made tantalizingly apparent. The reason is this—*the efforts to "cure" are all opposed to the curative process.* Symptoms are such only and are not cause and every effort to cure (suppress) them has been an obstacle to recovery. As an illuminating example, a medical author says of complications in measles:

"While the average case of measles runs a favorable course, the danger of the disease lies almost entirely in its complications. These are to be expected when the rash suddenly fades and the disease 'goes into the system,' to use a popular expression. A fading of the rash is often coincident with the development of a complication. Persistant fever after the disappearance of the rash is also highly suspicious."

Dr. Robert Walter declared (Exact Science of Health. pp. 188-9):

"The prevailing cry of all classes is, We must assist nature; and not knowing how nature works, nor what disease is, men proceed to obstruct and thwart her operations, not to aid her. If she vomits they proceed by force to stop her vomiting; if she purges the same truth applies; if we are weak we proceed to a forced strength; if we are sleepless we compel sleep without removing the occasions of the insomnia. Not knowing what nature is trying to do, we proceed to thwart her processes by any means at hand. As long as disease continues to be regarded as our enemy so long will medical practice continue the work of destroying life in the vain endeavor to destroy disease."

It is evident that the suppression of the effort at elimination through the skin (the measles rash) resulted in the use of "complications" or efforts to eliminate the causes of the disease through other channels. The most common seat of these "complications" is the respiratory tract. Inflammation in the bronchial tubes (bronchitis) and of the lungs (pneumonia) and of the pleura (pleurisy) result. The pleurisy is often accompanied with fever and night sweats. Other mucous surfaces, as the nose, eyes, eustachain tubes, ears, and the glands as well may become involved in this latter effort at elimination. All these "complications" and sequelae are the direct result of suppression and never develop in untreated cases.

The right of the body to control its own affairs in *disease* has been denied by the members of all schools of healing in all the ages and every effort has been made to force the body to act as the physician thought best. In this respect the sick body has been regarded as an ill-mannered child that must be whipped or forced into good manners or good health. And this is what we mean by suppressing disease.

If the temperature is above normal, antipyretics forcibly reduce it; if it is below normal it is forced up. If there is pain this is deadened with morphine or other anodyne. Coughing is checked with cough "remedies," tonics are given to stimulate an appetite, when this is lacking, and food is forced upon the body. Night sweats and foot sweats are suppressed; a "feeble" heart is *sustained* with stimulants until it is exhausted. Vomiting and diarrhea are checked. Constipation is broken up. Glands are stimulated or inhibited as the physician thinks should be done. Skin eruptions are suppressed . Stimulants force increased action in those organs presenting reduced action, thus preventing energy conservation. Depressants check the activities of accelerated organs, thus defeating the efforts at cure. Thus we might go on indefinitely with our recital and we would find the physicians of all schools busily engaged in trying to produce a forced state resembling that of *health.* In short, accelerated functions are depressed and decreased functions are accelerated. This is simply an effort to force the body to act normally in spite of the presence of causes that require a different course of action. If the reader is laboring under the prevalent delusion that this work of suppressing disease is done only by drugs and serums he should know that it can be done by heat, cold, electricity, kneading, pressure, manipulations, mechanical means and various other methods that are in vogue. In fact, anything that will alter these curative and conservative efforts without removing their occasion or cause is truly suppressive.

In the chapter on inflammation it was shown that inflammation is a process of defense and repair from first to last and that it follows a definite, well ordered and lawful course. The essential part of inflammation is a great excess of blood in the part, this being controlled by the neuro-vascular systems. It is possible, by various means to suppress this process. Any measure which forces the blood out of the inflamed area, or which draws the blood away from this area to another region of the body will impede and suppress the inflammatory process.

Bleeding, dry cupping, leeching, lead water and laudanum, and amonium are among the local measures that are employed to suppress inflammation. Cold compresses and ice bags are favorite "remedies" for inflammation. The cold acts by depressing the vitality of the tissues, contracting the blood vessels and reducing the circulation in the part. It also prevents absorption of the exudates.

Counter-irritants are employed to draw blood out of an organ. If there is inflammation in the lungs, for instance, a blister placed over the back or chest causes the blood to be sent to the surface. One drugless school teaches that if the inflammation is on the surface of the body or in the extremeties, increase it; but if it is in the internal organs, decrease it. Hydrotherapy, neuropathy, heat, electricity and other methods are employed for this purpose. Drugless men are as much afflicted with sympto-phobia as are medical men (all schools are Heteropathic in theory and practice) and spend their energies in "combatting disease."

Before we turn to a detailed discussion of suppressive measures let us explain that in general, the effects of suppression are:

(1) To lengthen the course and severity of the disease and build complications.

(2) To lock up the poisons in the system and these, with the drug poisons added, produce chronic "incurable" diseases.

(3) To kill the patient.

Suppression is a devastating practice regardless of the methods by which it is accomplished.

Medical men regard each disease as separate and distinct from every other. Diseases are said to be specific, having a specific cause and requiring specific treatment. Thus pneumonia is separate and distinct from typhoid, their causes are different and thus they must be treated differently.

But medical men do not have specific treatments for these so-called specific diseases. Quinine for malaria, mercury for syphilis and antitoxin for diphtheria are about the only claimed specifics and there does not exist unanimity of opinion about these. While, even in treating these diseases with their supposed specifics, other measures are employed with which to attack symptoms. In few words, medical measures are always symptomatic treatment and never specific.

Let me first explain this last statement and then give an example or two. About the first thing a physician does when called to see a patient is to give a physic. If fever is present, quinine or anti-pyrin or some other coal-tar drug is given to reduce the temperature. If the patient is in a state of "collapse" or "semi-collapse," heart stimulants—strychnine, digitalis, aromatic spirits of ammonia, caffeine, nitroglycerine, strophanthus, camphor, etc.,—are administered. When the heart fails to respond to one of these, another is substituted. If there is severe pain opium or its derivatives—heroin, morphine, codea,—or some of the coal-tar products is given. If he is sleepless an opiate, a bromid or chloral is administered. The opiates and bromids are used to stupify and paralyze the brain and nerves.

A partial list of the classifications of drugs and therapeutic measures will show that medical methods are all aimed at symptoms.

DRUGS THAT INCREASE ACTION

Tonics; stimulants—"Drugs increasing the functional activity of the body or any of its organs."

Diaphoretics, sudorifics; "Drugs inducing perspiration."

Cathartics, purgatives; "Drugs which cause a vigorous and copious bowel evacuation."

Laxatives; "Drugs producing a mild cathartic action."

Diuretics; "Drugs which excite the urinary flow."

Ecbolics, Oxytocics: "Drugs inducing uterine contractions."

Emmenagogues: "Drugs inducing or increasing menstrual flow."

Emetics: "Drugs which induce vomiting."

Expectorants: "Drugs increasing bronchial secretion."

Galactogogues: "Drugs increasing the secretion of milk."

Counterirritants, vesicants: "Drugs which redden or blister the skin when applied locally."

Rubifacients: "Mild counterirritants, intended to be applied with friction."

Cerebral Stimulants: "Drugs which stimulate the higher brain centers."

Astringents: "Drugs which cause tissues to contract."

Myotics: "Drugs producing contraction of the pupil of the eye."

Vasoconstrictors: "Drugs causing a constriction of the blood vessels of the body."

Cardiac Stimulants and Tonics: "Drugs causing increase of force or rapidity of the heart beat."

Aphrodisiacs: "Drugs stimulating the sexual centers."

DRUGS THAT DECREASE ACTION

Anodynes, Analgesics: "Drugs which diminish pain."

Anaesthetics: "Drugs abolishing sensation."

Narcotics: "Drugs causing extreme depression of the activity of the brain shown by stupor."

Antispasmodics: "Drugs depressing the spinal cord."

Anaphrodisiacs: "Drugs depressing the sexual centers."

Anti-emetics: "Drugs preventing vomiting."

Antigalactogogues: "Drugs decreasing milk secretion."

Antihydrotics: "Drugs diminshing the excretion of sweat."

Antiphlogistics: "Applications which reduce inflammation."

Antipyretics: "Remedies that reduce fever."

Antisialagogues: "Drugs decreasing salivary secretion."

Cardiac Sedatives: "Drugs which diminsh the work done by the heart," either by depressing the heart or its nerve centers or by depressing the vasoconstrictor nerves.

Demulcents: "Drugs which have a sedative action on the mucuous membrane of the alimentary tract."

Mydriatics: "Drugs producing dilitation of the pupil of the eye."

Refrigerants: "Saline drugs usually used to combat fever."

Respiratory Depressants: "Drugs depressing the respiratory center in the medulla."

Somnificients: "Drugs which produce sleep."

Vasodilators: "Drugs causing a dilitation of the blood-vessels of the body."

Other than these there are caustics or Escharotics which are used in local applications to destroy tissue; Germicides, Disinfectants, Antiseptics which destroy germs and drugs to kill worms, parasites, etc.

The reader will note that in the above two lists of drugs, named acording to their action, none of them are aimed at the removal and correction of causes. These drugs produce their effects upon the body and act in the same way as do the causes of disease. Indeed they are causes of disease. There are numerous drugs that have these effects and most of them are used to produce more than one of these effects. The effects of a drug are often different when given in doses of different sizes—or, perhaps it were better to say that the body reacts to it differently when given in doses of varying in size.

This list is sufficient to reveal to the reader that the practice of medicine is one of suppressing sypmtoms. Look at its folly for a minute before we go on. If there is high fever there must be a cause; a need for it. If the cause is corrected the temperature will again become normal. Does the physician bother with its cause? He does not. He administers an anti-pyretic which reduces the temperature by reducing heart action and paralyzing vital functions. Fever is treated as though it is its own cause or as though the functions of the body have rebelled against vital law and have become anarchistic. This is often continued until the heart is greatly weakened and then the physician resorts to heart stimulants which are often employed until they completely exhaust the heart and produce death. If there is restlessness and mental distress there is a cause for these and they will cease as soon as cause is removed. But the physician does not attempt to find and correct cause. He administers a bromid or other nerve and brain paralizing drug and thus clubs the brain and nerves into insensibility and stupor. The restlessness and distress are temporarily suppressed but appear again as soon as the body has eliminated the drug. Another dose is then given and this process is kept up until permanent damage is done to the nervous system. The same is true of pain. The nerves of sensation are sandbagged into insensibility by an opiate or a coal-tar product. The cause of the pain, the condition that gives rise to it still exists—all the drug does is to paralize the nerves, and weaken the functions of the body thus effectually interfering with every curative process that is going on.

Observe that in reducing temperature, "relieving" pain, allaying restlessness and delirium, etc., the drugs used all accomplish their effects by reducing the functions of the body—that is by paralizing the nerves. In doing this, they impair every function in the body. Take opium—it produces constipation (impaired bowel function), reduces secretion and execretion (impaired glandular function), etc. More of this later.

Drugs can be divided into two classes—namely, stimulants and depressants. These are subdivided into many classes as shown above. But all come under two general heads. The one increases action by irritating the system, the other decreases action by paralizing or depressing the brain and nerve centers. Neither process is any way reparatory or curative. Neither process gives any aid to the body in its work of cure, or exercises any influence upon the cause of the trouble. They are one and all poisonous and foreign to the body. They have no business ever being introduced into the body. They spend their whole force against the powers of life.

No stimulant can add any power to the body. Stimulants of all kinds only force the body to expend the power it already possesses. To stimulate a sick body is like applying a long shank spur to a tired horse. It causes increased activity and hastens exhaustion. Every period of stimulation is followed by a period of depression, the depression being equal to the former period of stimuation. Nothing is accomplished by this except the exhaustion of the patient.

The above facts relating to methods of increasing and decreasing physiological activities are true regardless of the means employed to bring these about. Drugs are not the only things that will accelerate and inhibit function and thus suppress symptoms and exhaust the body.

BY SUPPRESSING THE HEALING EFFORTS OF NATURE, MEDICINE BUILDS COMPLICATIONS AND SEQUELEA, AND KILLS THE SICK. Practically all medical methods are aimed at suppressing symptoms. These are regarded as evil and the chief duty of the physician is to club them out of existence. But symptoms are such only and not cause and should receive no attention. The fool who directs his attention to the suppression of symptoms and ignores cause cripples and kills his patient.

A standard work on materia medica says:

"Disease is a departure from the normal, and the aim of the physician in giving a medicine is to change an abnormal function into a normal one." "A symptom is an abnormal manifestation of some function or other. Symptomatic treatment is the giving of a drug which will produce an effect just opposite to the effect produced by the disease."

This definition of disease is that it is abnormal action while this definition of symptomatic treatment implies the assumption that by disease is meant the thing that causes the abnormal action. Ignoring the evident lack of clearness in the definitions let us put these two definitions together and see what can be made of them.

455

Diarrhea is an "abnormal action." It follows a more or less prolonged period of constipation or some unusual dietetic indiscretion. Its purpose is to empty the digestive tract of a mass of fermenting, putrefying food. It is a protective or defensive measure. Now, symptomatic treatment would be the giving of a drug that produces "an effect just opposite to the effect produced by the disease." That is to cure diarrhea a drug would be given that produces constipation. They do, indeed, "cure" one disease by producing "another."

But what is the effect of checking the bowels? The decomposing food is retained in the body to poison and kill its cells. By suppressing the purifying effort of nature the physician has laid the foundation for serious trouble.

Suppose the patient is constipated—he is given a drug that produces diarrhea. Purgatives, laxatives, etc., are used for this purpose. How do they produce their effects? By irritating the digestive tract and causing it to increase its peristaltic action. They also cause it to pour out much liquid and mucous in washing away the irritating drug. No power has been added to the body. None of the causes of constipation have been corrected or removed. What has really occurred? The bowels and, with them the whole digestive system, have been further weakened and the disease made worse. The whole system is weakened by the loss of fluid.

A standard medical author declares:

"While these toxins of germs may be called the 'cause' of the elevation of temperature, yet the word 'reason' is better. Fever seems to be one of the protective measures of the body, a means to an end, and that end is a fight against the germ. The body seems to fight the germ better at a higher than at normal temperature, and so the fever is really rather a part of the defense than a direct result of the toxin in the sense in which the headache is such a result. We emphasize this point because so many persons think the fever is an evil and try to lower it by drugs. They can do this easily, but with no benefit—perhaps always with injury—to the patient. We like to see the temperature fall, as after a cold bath, but only when we are sure the reason for the fall is victory over the toxin, or that the total result of the bath is beneficial."

He agrees with ORTHOPATHY about the beneficial nature of fever and deplores its reduction by drugs as never beneficial and perhaps always injurious, but does not object to its suppression by means of the cold bath. He does not seem to realize that when victory over the toxins has occurred the temperature will fall as naturally and spontaneously as it rose.

The average physician is not averse to reducing fever with drugs. He looks upon it as an evil to be suppressed. It is a "departure from the normal" and a drug must be given that has an "effect just opposite to the effect produced by the disease." He administers a drug that reduces vital action throughout the system and down comes the temperature. Part of Nature's defense is thus broken and all her curative operations are reduced. The foundation is laid for much worse trouble. Complications develop. Sequalea follow. Perhaps the patient is killed.

Parker's *Materia Medica and Therapeutics*, a text book for nurses, says (pp. 214);

"Fever is now recognized merely as a symptom and in infectious diseases as a protective condition in which antibodies are formed to counteract toxins. Unless, therefore, the temperature is very high no attempts are made to lower it except for the purpose of making the patient more comfortable."

It should be known that it makes no difference in the results whether the temperature is reduced to "cure" disease or merely to make the patient more "comfortable." It cannot be forcibly lowered by any metohd or for any purpose, without defeating the end served by the fever nor without greatly interfering with the vital curative activities. For instance, Parker says:

"The drugs which have some use as antipyretics are the COAL-TAR ANALGESICS, QUININE, and ACONITE. The coal-tar analgesics act by depressing the heat center. The heat center is now considered rather a coordinated mechanism and the exact method by which this mechanism controls body temperature is not known, but it is probable that when it is depressed *heat production* is decreased. THE DIFFICULTY, HOWEVER, IN USING DRUGS TO DEPRESS THIS MECHANISM IS THAT THEY ALSO AFFECT THE VITAL CENTRES AND

CAUSE A GENERAL DEPRESSION. PHENACETIVE, ANTIPYRINE, AND ACETANILID ARE ESPECIALLY DEPRESSING TO THE HEART if given continuously in long fevers, but they are used to some extent. They relieve the nervousness (by depressing the nerves. Author) which accompanies a high fever and are resorted to in cases in which baths cannot be given. QUININE is commonly employed as an antipyretic in the early stages of coryza. From two to four grains**** every four hours will break up a cold. ACONITE is safe only in short acute fevers and is being used less and less even in such cases, BECAUSE OF ITS TOXIC AC-TION ON THE HEART." (Capitals mine.)

The above are some of the results of measures that lower temperature by lessening *heat production.* There are other measures, such as fan baths, baths in tepid water, alcohol with much friction, hot drinks, Dover's powder, ammonium acetate and spirit of nitrous ether, which bring the blood to the surface, away from the scene of battle where it is needed. and thus increase the loss of heat. The salicylates also lower temperature by occasioning a marked dilatation of the cutaneous blood vessels and a consequent loss of heat. Vomiting, loss of appetite, a peculiar delirium, ringing in the ears and great kidney irritation are some of the results of the use of this class of drugs.

This is symptomatic treatment. This is supressive treatment. It cripples and kills the patient. The work on Materia Medica previously quoted says:

The three most important purposes for which drugs and medicine are given in disease are: (1) to avert collapse or death; (2) to eradicate, if possible, the cause of the disease; (3) to relive pain or other symptoms of disease.

"Most drugs and remedies belong to the first and third classes. Very few drugs, of themselves, can eradicate the *cause* of disease. Remedies that act as curative agents on the *cause* of the disease are said to be SPECIFIC remedies. Example, quinine cures malaria by killing the malaria parasite in the blood. Remedies that simply *modify* symptoms, and most drugs are of this class, are called SYMPTOMATIC remedies. Example, morphine causes insensibility to pain, but does not cure the cause of the pain."

Taking these three "uses" of drugs in the order named we have:

(1) *Drugs that avert collapse or death.* These are tonics and stimulants. They are the very causes of collapse and always hasten death. No drug can prevent death although any of them may cause it. This so-called use of drugs is based on the fallacy that life can be sustained on poisons—that the foes of life can be made to preserve it. For many years alcohol was the sheet anchor in "sustaining" the vital powers. It was regarded as a stimulant. It is now known to be a depressant from first to last and depresses every function in the body. It killed millions of the sick.

(2) *Drugs to eradicate the cause of disease.* This idea is based on the assumption that the cause of disease is some external thing or entity that attacks the body from without. It is a survival of the ancient belief in demons and evil spirits and is incarnated in the germ theory. Quinine is given as an example of this "class" of drugs. It is claimed to kill the blood parasite that is claimed to cause malaria. It probably kills all the parasites it comes in contact with, for it is a protoplasmic poison. It kills men and animals as well as parasites and will kill the patient long before it could possibly kill all the parasites that are claimed to be in the man's blood causing the malaria. H. C. Woods, Jr., London, says: (Pharmacology and Therapeutics):

Quinine is a protoplasmic poison and in sufficient doses is capable of destroying the vitality of nearly all forms of unicellular life." (P. 334)

Again:

"It is evident from a study of its germicidal properties that it is impossible to introduce enough of the drug into the blood to directly affect the growth of the micro-organisms without endangering the life of the patient." (P. 338).

Quinine does not cure malaria. This I know for a positive fact as I have seen it fail too often, both as a preventive and as a cure. We agree fully with Dr. A. S. Bleyer, of Washington University Medical School, St. Louis, Mo., when he said in a lecture before the mothers at the Community School, as reported in the St. Louis Globe-Democrat, March 19, 1920:

"SANITATION, NOT QUININE, ERADICATED MALARIA."

Quinine depresses all the functions of the body and is frequently the cause of serious nervous and mental troubles, blindness and even death. It is employed as an

457

antipyretic (a drug that reduces fever) because it depresses vital activity throughout the system and thus reduces heat production. In reducing vital activity and heat production it impairs every effort and process of the body that is engaged in the work of cure.

(3) *Drugs that relieve or modify symptoms.* Morphia is given as an example. It produces insensibility to pain by its paralyzing effect upon the nervous system, but does not affect the cause of the pain. Morphia is the principal narcotic alkaloid of opium. The same authority who offered morphia as an example of this third class of drugs says of the effects of this drug:

"Small quantities of opium produce a condition of mental abstraction; large doses result in a drowsy condition . . . but, if still larger doses are given, sleep comes, sleep which is deep, merging into torpor as the poisonous dose is reached."

"Morphine abolishes pain by depressing the areas of the cerebrum which govern sensation and thought . . . On the medulla it has the effect of depressing the respiratory centre and the vasoconstrictor centre."

"Morphine and opium cause a contraction of the portion of the stomach which is joined to the intestine. After hypodermic injection, morphine is soon found in the stomach and intestine, passing into these organs through the mucous membrane. A marked action in impairing the secretion and movements of the intestine follows the use of morphine and opium in man."

I shall not deal with the symptoms of poisoning by morphine. These are simply greater degrees of the above and a few other effects. Indeed the above effects are symptoms of poisoning. Morphine (1) Depresses the higher centers of the brain, producing drowsiness and torpor; (2) impairs or suspends thought; (3) paralizes sensibility; (4) depresses the respiratory centre thus interfering with breathing; (5) causes a constriction of the arteries thus interfering with circulation; (6) causes a contraction of the pyloric end of the stomach; (7) impairs the secretion of the stomach and intestine and colon—produces indigestion and favors decomposition; (8) impairs the movements of the stomach, intestine and colon—constipates.

These are but the most apparent of its effects. It depresses function throughout the body generally, directly by depressing the brain centres and indirectly by interfering with breathing and circulation. It relaxes all of Nature's defenses. It is used in *coughs* to "dull the sensibility of the respiratory centre, so that the impulse to cough is not felt so frequently." It is employed in "*diarrhea, peritonitis, typhoid hemorrhage,* and in similar conditions . . . to check the intestinal movements and secretions." Its use is always to suppress some symptom and in doing so it impairs every function in the body and by this very action lessens one's chances of recovery. People pay dearly for a brief respite from pain or other symptom. What is true of morphine is true of all drugs, or other means of suppression. It is true, as well, of all drugless means of suppression. The fact that morphine is soon found in the stomach and intestines following its injection into the blood is proof that the body uses these organs as organs of elimination.

Every disease, and every symptom of disease is beneficial in its action and represents vital effort in self-defense. Every method of treatment that is aimed at the removal or suppression of symptoms and not at the correction and removal of cause is evil and destructive. It is a combat against the body and the powers of life. *It does not cure, but kills.*

Dr. Walter is, so far as I have been able to find, the first man to emphasize the fact that the prevailing types of disease in any period are determined largely by the medical theories and practices of that time. He says (Exact Science of Health, P. 180):

"Opium, arsenic, digitalis all produce the very diseases they seem to remove. And history well proves that any class of diseases thrives and multiplies in close ratio to the practice that cures them. When bleeding and purging were the accepted methods of cure, blood-and-bowel diseases became correspondingly frequent and alarming, but when the theory of cure changed, and physicians began the practice of sustaining the patient's strength by nervines, tonics, stimulants, etc., nervous diseases, and especially nervous weaknesses, correspondingly increased. So, wherever a medicine produces sleep it does so by taking away the power of sleep. What cures a headache will invariably make a headache, of which coffee is a fine example."

Again:

"But they (drugs) destroy and kill by appearing to save and cure.*****All the while drugs are giving the appearance of strength they are exhausting the patient. They arouse vital resistance and expend vital power, all the while they seem to give the power. They also change the symptoms of the disease and so relieve the patient's fears, all the while new, and perhaps worse symptoms, are being produced. The patient thus feels stronger while he is being made weaker. Old symptoms are relieved but worse are taking their places. But as they have not yet attracted attention the patient is still deluded into the belief of improvement. By and by, when the new symptoms become established, and reported to the doctor, a new disease or complication is diagnosed, and new remedies prescribed. How long it takes to reach the end under such circumstances depends chiefly upon the constitutional capacities of the subject who is being tampered with. No greater paradox, therefore, exists in our day than that the treatment which seems to be curing is the treatment which is killing; the more faithful the physician the greater the danger to the patient; the more nearly correct the diagnosis the worse the result."

To prove that the medical method of treating disease is merely one of treating symptoms let us look into the treatment employed in typhoid fever. A standard medical author says: "The treatment is largely supportive and prophylactic." He then says: "Fever should be controlled by sponging, by the wet pack, and by the full bath *****the medicinal treatment includes the use of antipyretics, intestinal antiseptics, and antityphoid serum.

"Abdominal pain, tympanitis, and tenderness are best treated with fomentations and terpentine stupes, while meteorism may be relieved by the internal administration of turpentine and by the use of the rectal tube or injections of milk of asafetida***** Diarrhea, when it exceeds 4 or 5 stools daily, will require the withholding of all food except milk, and the administration of opium, bismuth, codein, naphthalin, etc. C n-stipation should be relieved every two days by enemas containing soap suds.

"When hemorrhage occurs, the foot of the bed should be elevated, and ice-bag or iced cloths should be applied to the abdomen, morphine should be given hypoder-mically, and opium should be administered by the mouth every three hours***** Alcohol, ammonia, strychnin, digitalis, etc., should be used if heart failure supervenes. Nervous symptoms are greatly lessened by hydrotherapy, but nerve-sedatives may be necessary."

With secretion suspended and digestion impossible in this disease, and with opium and other drugs frequently administered, which further impair secretion, this author says:

"The diet should be liquid, largely milk, and should be administered every 3 hours. The modern tendency is toward a more liberal diet, and the high calorie diet***** adds to the comfort of the patient, shortens the convalescence and lowers the death rate."

Comment upon this would be superfluous. Here is the treatment as given:

(1) Heat and drugs to relieve pain.
(2) Drugs to check the bowels.
(3) Enemas to empty the bowels.
(4) Ice-bags (cold) and drugs to stop hemorrhage.
(5) Heat or cold and drugs to allay nervousness.
(6) Antipyretics and baths to reduce fever.
(7) Intestinal antiseptics to kill germs, etc.

Is there any wonder complications and sequelea develop and the death rate is so high? Such barbarous treatment would kill a well man or an ox. Not one thing in the whole treatment is done to remove cause. It is symptomatic treatment from first to last.

For pneumonia, we find:

"Milk diet and the administration of fractional doses of calomel, followed by a saline in the early stage. The nervous symptoms and temperature may be controlled by applying ice-bags or compresses wrung out in cold water******to the chest or by the use of warm or cold wet pack. The heart and pulse should be sustained by the administration of alcohol, strychnin*****atropin, caffein, strophanthus, and nitro-glycerine. · Digitalis may also be employed*****In young, vigorous, and plethoric adults, with hyperpyrexia (very high fever) and a high tension pulse, bleeding may be beneficial in the first 48 hours. Convalescence should be guarded, and tonics, stimulants, etc. will be found very useful in this period of the disease."

Medical men frankly admit they have no cure for pneumonia. Their whole treatment for this disease is symptomatic. The control of symptoms is what they seek and this is what kills the patients.

In the treatment of acute rheumatism we are told: "fractional doses of calomel (gr. ¼ every hour for 6 hours) should be administered followed by a saline purgative. Salicylic acid or its derivatives may be given in full doses, and diuretics are especially indicated. Hyperpyrexia may be controlled by phenacetin*****. During convalescence; tonics are of decided advantage. Locally, lead-water and laudanum or belladonna liniment may be used."

These examples must suffice. The treatment of other diseases is the same. It is all symptomatic, and very much the same drugs are used in all of them. In the whole field of present day medicine there is little evidence of intelligence. Symptophobia has eclipsed all intelligence and *education* has destroyed all power to reason. Knowledge is hid away so that the professions and the public alike are in dense, dark ignorance, which they appear to enjoy.

We will now give an example or two of how drugs suppress symptoms. In doing so we use for the basis of our remarks standard works on Materia-Medica. Quinine, which is used to suppress fever, will do to begin with.

Quinine is a powerful protoplasmic poison which is rapidly diffused through the body and slowly eliminated. It acts upon the nervous centers, causing mental confusion, color blindness, noises in the ears, deafness, headache, giddiness, vomiting, and often prostration, due to its effect upon the spinal cord and circulation. A standard work on Materia-Medica says:

"Quinine appears to reduce the amount of nitrogenous excretions, of urea and uric acid, and probably also carbonic acid, as determined both in healthy and fevered animals, and in man.

"These two sets of effects, taken together, point to a powerful action of quinine in reducing the metabolism of the body, of which heat and excretions are the two most measurable products*****. We may, therefore, conclude that the effect of quinine in the body is to check metabolism by interfering with the oxygenation of protoplasm generally, with oxygenation, and with the associated action of ferments. Thus the fall of temperature produced by quinine is due to the diminished production of heat in the body, not to increased loss of heat." (Diminished heat production from diminished vital activities. All the body's activities are diminished and the work of cure retarded. Author.)

Another standard author says:

"CIRCULATION: In small doses the cardiac action is increased; large doses, by acting on the cardiac motor ganglia, depresses the heart, sometimes causing it to intermit (miss beats), and finally arresting it in diastole; the blood pressure is lowered.

"THE TEMPERATURE: In health is very slightly influenced, if at all; in fevers a rapid decline takes place, due to the depressive action on the blood and circulation.

"NERVOUS SYSTEM: Small doses stimulate the cerebral functions, large doses cause cinchonism, i.e., a constricted feeling in the forehead, giddiness and tiniitus aurium (ringing in the ears), with impairment of hearing and sometimes of vision. After toxic doses these symptoms are aggravated and delirium, weak pulse, coma, sometimes convulsions, and in rare cases death, supervene. It probably reduces the reflex excitibility of the spinal cord."

He also says the drug "interferes with the oxygen-carrying function of the red corpuscles, and diminishes their number." It evidently destroys these corpuscles, or else it prevents their production. Perhaps it does both. Looking back over the matter, we find that quinine:

1. Impairs elimination thus locking up in the system the poisons that are causing the trouble.

2. It interferes with the normal tissue changes of the body (called metabolism) thus preventing the repair of tissue and elimination of waste.

3. It decreases the oxygen-carrying power of the blood and decreases the number

of red blood cells. The latter effect produces anemia, the former causes the physician to wheel in the oxygen tank to save life.

4. It depresses the heart and in some cases produces death by heart failure—arrests it in diastole.

5. It paralizes the nerve and brain centers, thus reducing the activities of the whole body and producing nervous and mental troubles.

6. It reduces body temperature, and thus reduces molecular activity, by paralizing heat production.

In malaria it is supposed to kill the germs that are supposed to be the cause of the disease. It is stated by good authority that a dose sufficiently large to kill the germs would also kill the patient. However, this is nothing new. Killing their patients to cure them has always been the practice of physicians. In a popular treatise on "Infectious Diseases of Children" a medical author declares of whooping cough:

"The main reliance is to be placed on the internal administration of quinine. This is a most effective remedy and seems to exert a direct destructive influence on the causative germs."

Its real affect is that of depressing the centers in the medulla and cord. It checks the cough by depressing the nerve center.

If quinine suppresses nature's curative processes and builds chronic disease, the bromides are even worse. A standard work on Materia Medica says:

"The great vital centers of the medulla are depressed by the bromides; respiration becomes weaker and slower, whence, possibly, part of the value of the drug in whooping cough. The heart is also slowed and weakened in its action.***** The spinal centers, nerves and muscles are all depressed by bromides, the latter so much so that the convulsions of strychnin poisoning cannot be induced."

Let us separate these effects. The drug:

1. Depresses the vital centers in the brain.
2. Impairs respiration.
3. Impairs heart action.
4. Depresses the spinal centers and the nerves and muscles.

What does all this do? It does not have the slightest influence upon cause. The whole force of the drug is spent against the body and the forces of life. The depression of the brain and nerve centers impairs organic action in the whole system. Elimination is checked and recovery prevented. The impairment of respiration and heart action checks elimination, impairs the circulation, deprives the body of oxygen and checks recovery, if indeed, it does not prevent recovery altogether. Brain and nerve diseases follow. The symptoms of bromism, which means bromide poisoning, are: Brom-acne (seen in drug treated epileptics), a yellowish discoloration of the skin with formation of blisters, salivation, (revealing its effects upon the glands), catarrh, headaches, dizziness, and general depression, melancholia, impotence (more impaired glands), diminished reflexes, nervous and muscular weakness especially in the lower limbs, difficult breathing, loss of identity often, loss of self-consciousness, premature old age and paralysis.

The chlorine treatment for colds, catarrh, "influenza," etc., presents a striking example of the law of dual effect. When the victim enters the chlorine chamber and the chlorine gas is turned on he is immediately siezed with violent coughing which raises from the throat and lungs mucous in large quantities. There is smarting and running of the nose, smarting and watering of the eyes which lasts, sometimes for two days. Pains are felt throughout the body, but especially in the throat and bronchial tubes. Mucous is poured from the mucous surfaces of the nose and throat in excessive quantities in an effort to wash away the source of irritation. These tissues are left weak and exhausted as a result.

In one case which came under my observation the coughing was so violent that the mucous was tinged with blood. During the second treatment the doctor in charge took the man from the chamber and gave him a glass of milk to allay the irritation and stop the severity of the cough. His eyelids became inflamed and remained so for several days. His nose was sore and dry and for two days the nose felt stiff and breathing was painful. The flanks of the nostrils were puffed up and swollen. The amount of mucous that was discharged from his nose and throat on the following day was much less than previous to the treatment, but on the second day thereafter, the catarrh was as bad as ever. Three treatments are considered enough in most cases but three treatments in this case only made the man much worse.

A process of this kind, if continued long enough, and three treatments are enough in many cases, will result in paralysis of the mucous surfaces of the nose, eyes and throat and perhaps also of the nerve endings in these membrances. The first effect of the chlorine treatment is an exaltation of function, its secondary effect is a dimunition and even abolition of function. When the function of the mucous membranes of the nose and throat is paralyzed no more mucous will be excreted and the cold or catarrh, or "influenza", etc., will be pronounced cured. But the blood and flesh condition back of it will not have been changed for better in this way. On the contrary, it will have been made worse.

A man seffering with catarrh goes to a chlorine "clinic" and is given treatment. He is told to "EAT PLENTY OF GOOD NOURISHING FOOD," which means that he must overeat on bread, potatoes, cereals, eggs, meat, milk, etc. This will invariably make the systemic condition that produced the catarrh worse. Such treatment is a crime. It is to be regretted that the truth about the matter cannot be told where the truth hurts advertising. Thousands are being deceived and misled and hurled into an untimely grave because the great god, ADVERTISING, will not permit real health truth to be told. But, then, who cares how many die so long as profits are made and dividends are paid.

A patient of the writers who had suffered with catarrh of the bladder for years stated that during all this time he had not had the slightest catarrh of the nose and throat until the doctors treated his bladder with injections of silver nitrate. He immediately developed a marked catarrh of the nose and throat. He did not understand why this was so. The explanation is, that silver nitrate, by converting the mucous lining of the bladder into a semi-living leather, had practically suppressed the catarrh and the body had to develop another outlet for the matter that was being eliminated through the mucosa of the bladder. The suppression of catarrh in one part of the body must be followed by the development of catarrh in another part of the body or else by more serious troubles.

A man once consulted me. He had been sick for years and, as is usual in those who seek my advice, had spent all his money with medical men in a vain effort to recover health. Instead of regaining health he had grown worse. He had lived the conventional life of the bachelor, good fellow, big eater, late hours, etc., considerable drink and all the garnishings. His diet had been the usual denatured, pie-cake-white bread-meat-coffee bill of fare. He weighed about 300 pounds, had indigestion, catarrh, hyperacidity of the stomach, constipation, a suppurating jaw bone, catarrh of the nose and throat and had been until a few days before consulting me, unable to breathe through his nose.

In one of New York's largest hospitals, he had been prescribed for dietetically as follows:

Breakfast: Toast (white bread) and tea.

Lunch: Meat, bread (white), butter and tea.

Dinner: Some starch food (potatoes, macaroni, etc.), bread (white), butter and tea. In addition to this he was permitted to have alcohol in "moderation."

This diet was worse than the diet he had lived on the most of his life. To cure the effects of such eating they performed twenty-eight operations on his nose and mouth and pulled sixteen sound teeth. They frequently scraped the suppurating mandible. Of course such treatment failed. It did not remove cause. To overcome the fermentation and acidity of the stomach, inevitable on such a diet, particularly in the profoundly enervated, and to relieve him of distress from the gas that must form, he was advised to take rhubarb and soda.

Finally, the gentleman tried chlorine gas and this "cured" him. Cured him without removing the cause. He was still eating the above diet. He still had the hyperacidity of the stomach. He was still constipated. He was still using tobacco and alcohol. He was taking no exercise. He was unable to walk. His jaw was still suppurating. The slime and filth resulting from such living and such conditions, and that was being leaked out through the mucous membranes of the nose and throat,

462

would either have to be sent out elsewhere or it would kill him in a short time. *On a diet and regimen of this kind a man needs a chronic catarrh to get rid of the blood condition that must result.* The catarrh acts as a safety valve and saves his life. If this safety valve is closed the man must either develop another elsewhere or die shortly. If Nature selects another outlet, he will have "another" disease, thanks to the paralysis of the function of the safety valves of the nose and throat. Of course, no one but an ORTHOPATH would ever connect the "new" disease with the forcible suppression of the "old" one.

This man knew more about diet, fasting, exercise, etc., than I, so I let him go. He knew that his trouble was in his mouth, not in his blood and his manner of living had nothing to do with his condition. The chlorine gas had stopped the discharge of mucous from the nose, and throat and enabled him to breathe well. Now if he could only find a remedy that would work the same wonderful cure for his other troubles.

It was plainly evident that this "cure" was merely *suppression*. A fool could have seen that cause had not been removed, or corrected. How did the Chlorine act? I do not know, but I am confident that it paralyzed the execretory functions of the mucous membranes of the nose and throat. It is the theory of those medical men who employ this form of poisoning the sick, that the chlorine gas destroys the germs which they say causes colds. They do not know which germ causes colds and therefore do not know that any germ causes colds. This aside, however, there is little doubt that the gas kills germs. But if it kills germs, what does it do to the cells of the body—those with which it comes into contact. The results of its use in the war answers this question. IT DESTROYS THEM.

A standard work on Materia Medica says:

"Chlorine is a yellow gas, very irritating to the respiratory passages, and was employed in the European war as an asphyxiating agent for that reason. It is extremely toxic to bacteria and the lower forms of animal and vegetable life, ranking next only to bichloride of mercury in effectiveness."

It will be objected, of course, that they do not employ enough gas, in their treatment of colds, influenza, tonsilitis, etc., to injure the body. True, they do not employ sufficient quantities of it to produce as much injury as was produced by it during the war, but the fact remains that *if they use enough gas to kill the germs in the respiratory passages, they employ enough to injure the cells lining these passages.*

Perhaps these cells are not killed outright. Perhaps they are only paralyzed, as I suggested at first. No matter, they are injured and Nature's safety valve is rendered inoperative. *The filth and excess nutriment that nature was leaking out through the mucous membranes of the nose and throat is now pent up in the blood.* The supposed cure is only suppression and the patient is worse than ever. It is inevitable that suppression, by whatever means accomplished, shall make one's condition worse.

I have seen the claim by one company that is exploiting the chlorine gas treatment of colds, bronchitis, influenza, etc., that it forms a metallic layer or coating over the lining membranes of the nose and throat and throughout the lungs and thus protects these from germs. If this were true, the metallic coating would prevent the free exchange of oxygen and carbon dioxide in the lungs and the poor victim would die of asphyxiation—oxygen starvation and carbon dioxide poisoning or suffocation.

The taking of drugs in repeated small doses is like the repeated use of coffee, tea, tobacco, alcohol, opium, etc. That is, their effects are cumulative. They are slowly, and with difficulty, eliminated from the system and are a most fruitful cause of chronic disease. In fact, chronic diseases increase in direct ratio to the increase of suppressive drugs and serums. The more efficient physicians become in suppressing acute disease, the faster chronic disease multiplies. Suppressive methods build the very troubles they appear to *cure.*

Thus far I have talked only of medical methods of suppressing disease. There are many other methods of suppressing disease than by the use of drugs and serums. The drugless men have developed numerous methods of suppression. These will require some attention at this point.

"Elimination, is the key to success"; we hear this from all sides and we are offered thousands of ways of promoting elimination. The idea seems to prevail that elimination can be forced.

Elimination of toxins is absolutely essential to recovery but if this is all we eliminate we have not accomplished half the cure. The organism is equipped with organs of elimination and these organs are normally able to keep the blood stream pure. However, enervation lowers their functional vigor so that they do not perform their function as efficiently as they should. Thus, if the enervation is not overcome, we must again become toxemic soon after any temporary house cleaning we may undergo, if we allow that such house cleanings can be forced.

The body as an association of organs and parts works as a unit. The labors of each of its parts are essential to its normal well being and, if at any time any of these fails, wholly or in part, in the performance of its function, the work must be taken up by some of the other organs. The normal organ is capable of doing much more work than it is ordinarily called upon to do. Were this not so there would be no provision for emergencies—the heart and lungs, for instance, would fail if suddenly we were called upon to have a little foot-race with a bear. It is this ability to do extra work that enables one organ to compensate for deficiencies in other organs or parts. Thus the stronger organs of our body are constantly compensating for the failure of the weaker ones, so that disease appears only after the stronger organs are no longer able to perform the work of compensation.

Enervation, not only lowers functional efficiency in the weaker organs, but lowers the functional powers of the stronger organs as well. When this point is reached disease puts in an appearance and usually it shows up first in the weaker organs, although the symptoms may be so slight as not to be noticable until it has affected some of the stronger organs or parts.

When this condition is reached we may succeed, by stimulating methods, in whipping up the activities of the stronger organs so that temporarily they again compensate for the failures of the weaker ones and we produce a temporary semblance of health. We have produced a wonderful (?) "cure" for which the patient is very grateful. So grateful, indeed, that he or she sits down and writes a testimonial in which is told in glowing terms the great benefits derived from the treatment. However the true test of any system or method of "healing" is the condition of the patient six months or a year later. Those who write glowing testimonials often find their old troubles return.

These men fail to take into consideration in their treatment of patients that there is fatigue of the nervous system—enervation. They get hold of a patient and start stimulating his vital activities with little or no consideration for what the after effects of such stimulation will be. It is, however, like whipping a tired and overloaded horse up hill. He may pull much harder and reach the top much quicker but exhaustion is the result.

Such methods are positively injurious. They not only exhaust the patient but there is always present the tendency of both physician and patient to become obscured by his method and he is led to neglect cause. He falls into the common error of trying to "cure" the disease. He has a water cure, a diet cure, a spondylotherapy, a neurotherapy, zonetherapy, chromotherapy, electrotherapy or some other cure or therapy.

Attempts to force elimination through the skin, kidneys, and bowels by having the patient drink large quantities of water, are popular. An increase in the amount of water eliminated is sure to follow but very little if any increase of solids or waste is induced. Elimination is a physiological process, not a mere mechanical one. We can easily wash out a sewer pipe by flooding it with water, but the kidneys, skin and bowels don't work that way.

The change in the urine following the drinking of large volumes of water can be seen with the unaided eye. Whereas before the urine may have been highly colored and may have given off a very offensive odor, after large quantities of water have been taken, the urine is clear and the odor almost absent. Such a change cannot denote increased elimination of waste matter, but it does denote that the kidneys are being called upon to handle so much water that they are not permitted to give much attention to the elimination of waste. This same is true of elimination through the skin. Chemical analysis of both urine and sweat show this to be so. There is an absolute and not merely a relative decrease in the amount of solids in these excretions.

There is often an increase in bowel action following such a practice, but such is not always the case. Besides this increased bowel action does not continue but soon begins to decrease with the result that the constipation that may have existed previously is made worse. Such a practice has little justification and we feel that over-drinking like over-eating is a foolish practice.

The artificial induction of sweating is often used as a means of promoting elimination through the skin. The idea is that since sweating is, among other things, an eliminative process, any increase in the amount of sweat poured out must always mean an increase in the elimination of waste, of toxins, etc. This is just as false as the idea that increase of urine, due to increased intake of water, means an increased elimination of toxins and waste.

Sweating is a physiological process. The sweat glands, like all other glands of the body, possess the poyer of selective action. Among other things sweating does, is to regulate the temperature of the surface of the body. Artificially induced sweating is an effort to regulate the surface temperature. The attention of the glands is directed to this end. The elimination of waste must lag. The confounding of heat regulation with elimination has led to many ludicrous practices which are not always without their harmful effects. For instance the subjection of a patient to prolonged intense heat in a cabinet or in a steam room to induce sweating weakens the patient. It is no uncommon thing for weak patients to faint under such treatment. We know of one death which occurred during the third cabinet bath and of one lady who became temporarily insane after about seven such treatments.

The following words from Dr. Moras' "Autology", are of interest in this connection:

"If you are eating or drinking or behaving so bad that you need Turkish or steam baths, or anything else than the old-fashioned soap and water—why not resort to blood-letting or starved leeches? You'd get a heap more good out of one such treatment than you can ever derive from a legion of 'sweat baths.'

"If you really want a good 'sweating out,' one that won't merely sweat the water out of the skin or fat, but that will stir up and burn and remove impurities from your very flesh and marrow—take a brisk five mile walk. Then lie down and sleep it off, if you want too. Artificial or 'passive' sweating is a delusion."

Again he says:

"In the first place, anyone at all familiar with the chemistry of sweat and the chemistry of 'impurities' knows that in four gallons of sweat there isn't two ounces of solid matter—and that these two ounces are nearly three-fourths table salt with a little fatty matter. Think of having to sweat four gallons to get rid of about one-fourth to one ounce of urea—when the mere eating of a few bites less would accomplish the same result, without imposing any work on skin or internal organs. Don't imagine for an instant that sweating a gallon doesn't perturb internal organs—which must hustle to head off the vacuum produced."*****"Bathing or washing cleans the skin, but I never knew that it scoured the internal organs, although it does 'hold them up' on the water supply."

The experiments of Dr. H. Lahmann, confirm our views in this matter. From some of his patients he gathered the perspiration produced by ordinary exercise in the sunshine. He evaporated this and analyzed it and found that it contained small amounts of powerful toxins. These were powerful enough to kill rabbits. He then produced profuse sweating by artificial means in his patients and analyzed the sweat thus induced. He found that it contained practically no toxins.

Thus, did Dr. Lahmann's experiments prove that mere sweating, because of external heat, and the elimination of waste are different things. They prove that artificially induced sweating is not an eliminating process and that as we have already claimed, the organism cannot be forced by stimulants, irritants and by artificial measures to eliminate toxins and wastes but that it does its elimniation in its own way and knows better how to do it than the doctor. The foolish attempt of many to make the body behave as they think it should is thus apparent. They are only abortive efforts at cure or elimination.

At this place we desire to say a few words concerning another very popular past time that passes for rational treatment of the sick—spinal treatment. Since it was learned that so much could be done towards stimulating or inhibiting the activities of an organ through the spine, a number of methods of doing this have been developed. Chiropractic, Neuropathy, Spondylotherapy, Naprapathy, etc., are methods of tampering with the spine. Since spine tickling became so popular the Osteopath, the Mechanotherapist, the Masseur, the Electrotherapist, the Hydrotherapist, etc., are all giving more and more attention to the spine. It is a sort of fiddle upon which they play any old tune they desire.

I need hardly devote any space to a discussion of electrotherapy as a means of suppression. I believe it is generally conceded to be such, even by its most enthusiastic advocates. It is chiefly used for purposes of "stimulation," and "inhibition," to produce chemical changes and to destroy tissues. It is not claimed to remove or correct causes. It is not selective in its action. It destroys healthy as well as the unhealthy tissue and produces chemical changes that are not wanted as well as those that are supposed to be desired.

Of vibration but a few words. Chas. S. Neiswanger, M. D., says *Electro-therapeutical Practice*, (1922):

"The author does not wish to convey the idea that vibratory stimulation is not an excellent adjunct in the hands of the physician, because we have an accumulation of evidence to the contrary. The statement, however, that vibratory stimulation, such as is obtained by the use of the various mechanical devices on the market, can restore a normal vibration to nerves that have lost their normal vibratory tone, we believe to be erroneous.

"Vibratory stimulation, like massage, is irritating. It increases the activity of the skin and acts as an irritant to muscles, producing contractions which cause an increased blood supply; greater temperature and increased nutrition." (Page 323).

Again:

"Mechanical vibratory stimulation to motor points of the body is very similar in its action to that of rapidly alternating induced currents—faradism—first, by irritation of the nerve, and second, by sedation or loss of function by prolonged application." (Page 325.)

Vibration and electricity as well as most other methods of stimulating (exciting) and inhibiting nervous activity secure their effect by irritation. Prolonged irritation reduces or suspends function. Short applications of any irritation excites action—in defense.

Such methods, while they do "control" to some extent the activities of our internal economy, and further weaken and exhaust the nervous system, do not give any attention to the cause or occasion for the trouble. Such methods may increase the action of the kidneys or of the liver, but they do not remove the thing that is occasioning the sluggish action of these organs. They may inhibit the action of these organs but they do not destroy the reason for their excessive action. These methods are truly suppressive. They lead both patient and physician astray.

Then, there are mthods of stimulating physiological activity through the periphreal nerves. These methods further enervate the patient and give no more attention to the cause or occasion for the trouble, than the methods mentioned above. Men who use such methods simply ignore all previous study and observation of how the organism is intended to act and spend all their time and efforts in an attempt to force it to act the way they think it should.

They have learned how to force contracted tissues to relax or relaxed tissues to contract, by the application of heat, cold, vibration, electrical currents, etc., and they content themselves with such procedures. The fact that a few minutes after they cease their application, the tissues are again contracted or relaxed, as the case may be, does not enter into their consideration.

They seem prone to forget that normal tissues are not contracted or relaxed and that when such conditions exist there is a reason for them. Some irritating or disturbing element, some weakness is interfering with their function. These tissues must remain in such condition until the irrigating or disturbing element is removed. After it is removed the tissues will, of their own accord, by virtue of their inherent tendency toward health, return to normal, provided, of course, no irreparable damage has been done to them. They may force, by their methods, a temporary contraction or relaxation but it can be only temporary as long as the hindering element is present. They may keep up such methods until the degeneration of the tissues has reached the point where regeneration is impossible. Or Nature may succeed, in spite of their meddlesome interference, in removing the obstructing, irritating or hindering element and a return to normal be accomplished. In this case the practitioner and his method will receive full credit for the "cure."

It was found that by tickling the seventh cervical vertebra the action of the heart can be controlled to a certain extent. A patient comes into the office gasping for breath, a sense of fear gripping him, he feels that he is going to pass out. The physician examines his heart and finds it dilated. He gets out his little hammers or perhaps he uses his closed fist and starts beating on the seventh cervical. Presto! In a few seconds the heart has returned to its normal size and the disagreeable symptoms have vanished as if by magic. Wonderful! So the patient thinks. So the doctor thinks.

But why was the heart dilated? What has been done to correct the condition that produced the dilatation? What is to prevent the heart from becoming dilated again in a few minutes? Would it not return naturally and easily to a normal condition if the condition that produced it be corrected? Are not such methods, as the one above described, suppressive methods?

The following statement of Dr. J. H. Tilden expresses a great truth the acceptance of which will revolutionize the healing art. He wrote:

"The idea that disease can be cured is absurd. It is as reasonable to believe that a remedy can be given to overcome the effects of a knockdown blow over the head. It is as reasonable to believe that a remedy can be given to cure the tire following work or exercise or to cure the effects of inebriety while drinking is continued, or that a serum can be used to restore potency to those practicing sensuality."

Heat or cold applied to the body have varying effects depending upon the amount of heat or cold applied, the length of time they are applied, and the condition of the patient. Every action these occasion is vital action and is accomplished by vital power.

Short applications of cold water increases the heart action, the circulation, respiration and nerve activity. In short, short applications of cold water are stimulating. The one who is accustomed to taking cold baths knows this. The cold bathing habit fastens itself upon its victim in such a manner that if he misses his daily cold splash he feels miserable the whole day through. Such a practice indulged in regularly is truely enervating.

Like all methods of stimulation the cold bath is followed by a reaction. In a few minutes or a few hours—two to four—the stimulating effect ceases. The feeling of exhilaration gives way to a dull listless feeling.

Prolonged applications of cold water produce another effect. The temporary exhilaration of function is soon subdued by the cold so that the heart action is reduced, circulation slowed down, nervous activity decreased, respiration depressed. The feeling of warmth that came with the reaction from the first shock gives way to a feeling of cold. The patient is chilled and weakened.

Prolonged application of cold to the chief trunk of any nerve will greatly diminish or entirely abolish its activity. A short application of cold produces the opposite effect because of the resistance offered.

Short applications of cold increase muscular activity while a prolonged application decreases its activity even to the point of stopping such activity altogether if the cold is great enough and applied long enough.

The stimulating or inhibiting effects of cold have been shown to affect the whole organism, and not merely the superficial structures. This general effect comes through its stimulating or inhibiting influence upon the nervous and circulatory systems. Cold applications to the surface of the body are claimed to increase the absorptive powers of the lining membrances of the intestinal canal. This is claimed to aid in the process of nutritive assimilation. These same cold applications are said to increase the secretions and excretions of the body and to further tissue changes in the body. These are some of its stimulating effects. Its inhibiting effects are the exact opposite.

It will be noticed from the above that the effects of such applications do not differ materially from those secured by other methods of stimulating or inhibiting physiological function. The use of this method for such purposes amounts to nothing more nor less than an attempt to force the organism to work normally when its internal condition is such as to prevent normal functioning. Such treatment gives no attention to the reason for the abnormal function but simply ignores it.

Heat is applied to the body by means of water as well as by other means. For this purpose, hot water, hot packs, hot fomentation, steam, etc., are used. The effects of applications of heat depends upon the temperature of the application, the duration of the application and the condition of the subject.

For instance, water at about 99 to 101 degrees Fahrenheit causes the surface blood vessels to relax, while 104 degrees and higher causes them to contract.

The general effect of hot water at moderate temperature is to produce dilatation to the arteries, capillaries, small veins and lymph vessels. This temporarily increases skin activity. If this be prolonged or repeated often, the result is a weakening of the skin and a lessening of its reactive power. Debility or exhaustion always follows prolonged or repeated stimulation.

A prolonged hot bath increases the rate of the heart beat, diminishes respiration, diminishes muscular activity and capacity for work, increases nervous activity, yet if long continued nervous exhaustion may be produced. Hot applications are claimed, also, to stimulate or increase the activity of the stomach, liver and other digestive organs. They will also relieve pain.

The inhibiting effects of hot applications are the direct opposite of its stimulating effects. The practice of "hydrotherapy," or, more properly, of "thermotherapy," does not differ in its essentials from other methods of tampering with the vital machinery. The following from Trall in comparing water treatment to drug treatment shows that this fact was early recognized.

"All the impressions made on the living body can only affect its functions as they produce or arrest action or motion, which action or motion is muscular contraction. Cold water and ice are assuredly the most powerful constringing agents that can be applied to the living structures without destruction or injury; and hot water, or steam is the most efficient relaxant that can be safely employed. For producing moderate contraction or relaxation, we have all degrees of temperature between the freezing and the boiling points."—*Hydropathic Encyclopedia*, Vol. 2, P. 10.

A writer says:

"Hydrotherapy is chiefly relied upon as a means of stimulating the vital activities necessary for the curative process. When cold applications are suitably applied every bodily function will be stimulated. By hot applications properly applied excessive action may be controlled, pains relieved, and blood diverted from congested parts. By various other applications most powerful sedative, alterative and restorative effects may be produced. Scientific hydrotherapy affords the most direct and most rapid means of influencing the great function of life, the circulation of the blood, the processes of the liver, kidneys, stomach, and bowels. There is no means by which various bodily functions may be so perfectly and so quickly controlled as by the hydriatic measures applied with intelligence and skill."

We have no doubt that water applications "afford the most direct and most rapid means of influencing the great functions of life" and of "stimulating the vital activities" another method of forcing the body to act the way we think it should.

In full harmony with what has gone before, the colder or hotter the application— that is, the more the application exceeds or falls below the temperature of the body— the more rapid and marked is the reaction providing only that the power of reaction is present.

Again he says:

"Cold applications, suitably managed, are essential to the production of strong and lasting tonic effects*****but the general cold applications must be progressively increased in intensity as a means of increasing vital resistance, and raising the general tone of the system."

But, for the life of us, we can see no logical reason for such "influence" or "stimulation." It only weakens the organism, and interferes with the vital activities in their efforts at cure.

After all has been said upon this subject it becomes apparent that hydrotherapy is only another method of "controlling" vital activity and that it bears no relation to removing the condition or occasion that is producing the trouble if we except drugs.

Commenting upon the statement, "Cold applications must be progressively increased in intensity as the means of increasing vital resistance and raising the general tone of the system," Dr. Walter said: "Why should there be vital resistance to treatment that is beneficial to the system? Are the vital organs fools?"

Dr. Walter further says:

"But we can help Nature, we are told. How does treatment which arouses 'vital resistance' help Nature? Why should Nature resist her friends? She resists violence and injury, and these are what cold baths are, just as certain as is whiskey, and no two things are more alike in their effects upon the vital organism than are whiskey and the cold bath. Nature resists them because they are exhaustive and destructive and, in the resistance, it gives a feeling of strength—the strength of excitement—the same which the burning building arouses when discovered."—*Life's Great Law*, page 262.

Such treatment as hot or cold applications or alternate hot and cold applications are but refined methods of torturing and exhausting the sick.

Elsewhere we discussed the use of artificial means of producing sweating and do not intend to deal with it to any great length here. However, we want to say a few words in regard to the use of the pack for this purpose. There prevails a wide-spread view that while sweating induced by the steam bath, electric cabinet, etc., may not produce the elimination desired, the pack works differently. This idea seems to have been born of the fact that when the pack is removed it usually smells and also that occasionally it is colored. However, no one has ever made any efforts to determine whether or not the odor was not already on the patient before the pack was applied, or whether the coloring found on the pack was not already outside the body. When we think of the small amount of perfume needed to fill a room with its odor and the small amount of coloring matter on the sheets when removed we can easily see that such is a possibility. The author is convinced that this is the case.

Of the elimination supposed to be secured by the pack, Dr. Trall wrote:

"If anyone doubts the purifying efficacy of this process, he can have a 'demonstration strong' by the following experiment. Take any man in apparently fair health, who is not accustomed to daily bathing, who lives at a 'first-class hotel,' where they fatten their own pigs and chickens on the refuse matter of the kitchens, takes a bottle of wine at dinner, a glass of brandy and water occasionally, and smokes from three to six cigars per day. Put him in the 'pack' and let him 'soak' one hour or two; on taking him out, the intolerable stench will convince all persons who may be present that his blood and secretions were exceedingly befouled, and that a process of depuration is going on rapidly."—*Hydropathic Encyclopedia*, Vol. 2, P. 23.

I accept as true, every word in this description and the conclusions that the blood and tissues are foul and that a rapid depurating process is in progress and, yet, I deny that the pack did any more than hold that stench so that it did not pass off in the air as usual. This process of elimination through the skin is constant. The pack only collects and holds what is ordinarily carried away by the atmosphere. The extra blood brought to the surface may incerase elimination to a slight extent but at great expense to the body and with reduced elimination in the reaction.

Packs are said to have a drawing power, by which they are supposed to draw toxins out of the system. The absurdity of this becomes apparent when we consider that these can come out only as a result of the function of the glands of the skin. Any drawing power a pack may have is the patient's powers of resistance. If the patient's resistance is so low that he does not "react" there is no "drawing" done, yet if the pack did the drawing it should follow the application of a pack whether there was a reaction or not.

Hydrotherapy is a much abused method. It has been used for every abnormal condition which the human organism is subject to and heralded as almost a "cure-all." It is not a cure at all. Water, we are told, has been used from time immemorial in the treatment of disease, it is even mentioned a number of times in the Bible. "Let him wash himself," "go bathe," etc., are frequent expressions and it reminds us of instructions to keep clean, not instructions to produce sweating or to stimulate or inhibit vital activities.

The use of epsom salts, sulphur, and other chemical substances in the bath are to be condemned. They have no healing or curing power and can only serve to irritate the nerve endings in the skin. They are absorbed in small quantities and act as drugs. This same is true of the sulphur vapor bath, pine needle bath, etc.

Dr. Robert Walter says: *Exact Science of Health.* (P. 258-9-60):

"The great typical sanatory appliances are baths and bathing. The craze for these began more than fifty years ago when Priessnitz, a German peasant, discovered that he could produce with water, variously applied, the same results that physicians were accomplishing with drugs. He was able to offer to the invalid world stimulant baths, tonic baths, sedative baths, derivative baths, alterative baths, etc. He used, indeed, the phraseology of the schools to commend his system. And why not? Were his methods not sufficiently violent to produce 'vital resistance' and vital activity? The physicians gave poisons, sometimes in well-nigh deadly doses, but how much less violent were the baths of Priessnitz? To get out of a warm bed on a cold morning and stand under a stream of cold water, falling directly upon one's spinal column and nerves, under heavy pressure from a considerable height, need only be tried in order to prove its exciting character.*****Or be wrapped in cold wet sheets and kept in them for hours at a time. Can anyone doubt the tonic, stimulating, sedative, narcotic properties of such treatment as this? Will even the most powerful drugs arouse vital activity with greater certainty than this treatment will?

"But the fanaticism of cold bathing having practically worn away, Turkish and Russian baths soon began to attract attention. These are constituted of air, heated to a very high temperature, to be followed by cold plunges or shower-baths. The leading object is extremes of temperature. The cold applications are made all the colder from the preceding heat, and the effects of the heat are greatly enhanced by the succeeding cold. If, therefore, the heat is stmiulating, and the cold is equally so, it follows that the hot, followed by the cold bath, is the perfection of stimulating treatment. No whiskey ever drunk can exceed in quality of stimulation the alternate hot and cold applications. And this is especially true when the cold is applied in the form of a shower-bath or douche. By these means every nerve of sensation in the body is powerfully excited, and the sensations thus aroused induce extreme vital activity, which is but another name for stimulation.

"*****We have already clearly shown that such treatment prevents recovery rather than aids it. Quickening vital activity exhausts vital power—the power of cure. Its effects are the exact opposite of those of rest and sleep; they are analogous to the effects of whiskey, fright, excitement, labor; they are exhaustive rather than recuperative processes."

Someone once defined medicine as "the art of entertaining the patient while Nature restores him to health." Hydrotherapy is an excellent method of entertainment. There are hundreds of novel ways of applying it, all of which appeal to the patient. Like the little violet streak that jumps through the electrode of the high frequency applicator these many forms of water application appeal to the imagination of the patient. He thinks something is being done *for* him. In reality something is being done *to* him.

Hydrotherapists are not agreed on what are the best methods of application. Some will use only cold water, thinking it a crime to weaken the patient with warm or hot. Others use only the warm or hot, thinking it equally a crime to shock and stimulate the patient with cold water. Still others use any temperature from as hot as can be borne to as cold as can be withstood but professing to adapt the temperature to the condition of the patient. These latter are wise, indeed, since they know in advance just what temperature to use. There are those who attribute almost miraculous powers to the sitz bath. They fall out and argue among themselves with all the dogmatism that characterizes a theological controversy.

Each one is sure he is right and points to his experience to prove it. This is only another evidence of the folly of attempting to build a practice on experience. Experience has proven all methods to be good until, of course, it was later discovered that they were bad.

The curing is accomplished from the inside by the inherent powers and functions of the organism. The outside "treatments," although they may have been harmful, destructive, or at least worthless, get the credit.

Therapeutics is the art of meddling with the functions and operations of an organism, that is struggling to throw off a disease influence, on the absurd idea that the meddler (doctor) knows more about how the organism should act under the condition than the inherent power of the organism itself. Such meddlesome operations are not always the harmless or helpful things they are thought to be.

Repair of tissues and elimination of toxins is a specialty of vital power working through the organs and functions of a living body. Given an opportunity the vital forces do their work well. They often succeed in spite of destructive or obstructive treatment. But we cannot force desirable results.

While I was still in the curing business, a lady was once under my care who suffered, at times, with considerable pain and congestion in the lumbar region. By means of radiant heat and massage, I easily managed, in a very few minutes, to relieve all pain and to break up the congestion and restore normal movement. But, and here is the crux of the whole matter, in two or three hours her back was as bad as ever. I temporarily broke up the local trouble, but as I did not correct its cause, it returned.

Perhaps it will be said that adjustments would have corrected the condition permanently. Well, these had been tried, under the care of another, for some weeks, as had also traction, but to no avail. What is more, I could find nothing in the spine to adjust, and I never did believe that an adjustment could be made where there was nothing out of adjustment.

Another case, that of a man who came to me with a cold and with severe pain and congestion in the neck and shoulder, extending down to about a level with the fifth dorsal vertebra. The glands of the neck were enlarged, endurated and painful. By the use of massage, radiant heat and mechanical or manual means I "cured" all this except the clod in the head in about twenty minutes. The next day the man developed "rheumatism" in the left knee and ankle. I had temporarily broken up the local condition, thrown the toxins back into the general circulation and they produced congestion elsewhere. I had not corrected the cause.

In the first case the toxins continued to be returned to the same location, day after day. In the second case they were sent elsewhere. In this case the body had handed the work of detoxification and subsequent elimination of the toxins over to the glands and mucous membranes of the neck, nose and throat. I had succeeded in draining the glands, throwing the toxins back into the general circulation, and had thus effectually suppressed Nature's purifying effort. This led to trouble elsewhere. I dare say every naturopath and drugless man of experience has had many such experiences in his own practice. But how many of them ever connect the subsequent trouble with the suppression of the antecedent one? Not many, I fear. Yet they do reason just this way when medical men suppress a disease with drugs. Are they afraid to apply their own reasoning to themselves?

By massage or heat or vibration, we succeed in breaking up a deposit in some part of the body. The local trouble disappears, the patient is "cured," and we are satisfied with the "results that count." What have we done? Simply thrown back into the general circulation a mass of morbid matter that Nature had deposited out of it. Did we get it out of the body? We did not. Not by such methods. It is simply thrown into the circulation to be redeposited, either at the same or some other place.

You may say that Nature eliminates it after you break it up. My experience does not confirm this. Let us consider a minute why it was ever deposited. So long as the organs of elimination are capable of keeping the body clean there is nothing to deposit. It is only after they are so weakened that they are no longer able to meet the demands regularly made upon them that pathoferic matter accumulates in the body to produce trouble. When this occurs nature either eliminates it by means of acute disease or deposits it out of the general circulation and at the fartherest remove from the vital organs. If we break up the deposit, thus throwing the pathoferic matter back into the circulation, the over-taxed organs of elimination will not be able to throw it out. Perhaps the body will develop a crisis and eliminate it in that way, but it seldom does this except under natural living. The body usually redeposits it at the original or at some other point, then the patient has "another" disease. The "cure" is only a change.

A few years ago a well known naturopath developed a "cold" which was accompanied with sharp pains in his chest, coughing, headache, slight fever, malaise and loss of appetite. He suspected pneumonia.

Retiring to his office, he lay face down upon his table, while his assistant played a powerful Alpine lamp over his lumbar and gluteal regions for over an hour. This relieved him greatly. The next day, or the second day following, the process was repeated.

He explained that he had, by this means, "drawn" the blood away from the lungs and thereby avoided pneumonia. At that time I seriously doubted that this could be done, but I am now convinced that it can be.

What were the results? He avoided, or thought so anyway, pneumonia. But he never felt better after that, and in the course of four or five weeks he developed tuberculosis of the lungs. If by vaso-motor dilatation in another part of the body he had succeeded in draining the lungs sufficiently to suppress the work of purification nature was beginning there, he paid a big price for his relief. He has had a long, hard struggle in an effort to gain health.

Dr. Isaac Jennings wrote, Tree of Life:

"A man came to me with his left hand badly inflamed and swollen, apparently on the border of suppuration. I prescribed a warm, soft poultice. Two or three days subsequently he called again with his right hand inflamed and swollen, and told me that the swelling had gone from the left hand into the right hand. The left hand had recovered its natural condition, and the right hand was less fortunate, it passed through a tedious suppurative process to its former state."

Dr. Tilden records a case of rheumatic fever, treated by him early in his practice, in which the sufferer and her husband demanded that she be given relief from pain. This he refused to give, and they discharged him. Unfortunately, the next physician gave her "what she wanted", and in twenty-four hours there was a sudden death. He adds:

"That early in my professional career I had it demonstrated to me that it was very dangerous to use local applications, rub inflamed joints, or tamper with palliatives of any kind; and from that day to this I have never treated rheumatic fever patients in that way."

Rheumatism has a habit of wandering around in the body from place to place, and when forced out of one location by massage or hot and cold applications or electrotherapy, or other palliatives is just as likely to wander into the myocardium or the dura mater as elsewhere. And what is true of the poison of rheumatism is just as true of the toxins causing other diseases. Palliation and suppression by drugless methods lack the poison of the drug, but otherwise they are the same and productive of the same harm as drug suppression.

Is is hardly necessary to multiply cases of this kind. The cases given are sufficient to make my meaning clear, while any naturopath or any drugless physician of experience can think of a number of such cases that have come under his care and observation.

No doubt the drugless physician will reply: "It is here that our methods of promoting elimination are effective, and if these are employed in connection with the methods that break up the deposit, or congestion, or that drain the glands, the toxin will be eliminated and a real cure is accomplished."

How often is this the case? How often is one of your "cured" cases actually free of "disease"? How many of them are not sick or ailing again in a short time after you have "cured" them? How many of them fail to come back to you or go to someone else for more treatment in a short while after they are "cured"? How many who are financially able do not develop the "sanitarium habit" and make regular and frequent trips to the sanitariums for repeated "cures"? I think the man of experience and the man who has spent some time in each of several sanitariums will bear me out when I say that such cures are seldom, if ever, permanent.

Why is this so? In "Fundamentals of Nature Cure," I long ago pointed out that these efforts to increase elimination are all methods of stimulating physiological activity. I pointed out, also, that stimulation is a wasteful process—it is a forced expenditure of power, and this in an organism that hasn't a bit of power to waste. Its first and temporary effect is acceleration of funcion; its secondary and lasting effect is lessened function and exhaustion. This is all in accord with the law of dual effect. In this I have the support of Jennings, Graham, Trall, Dewey, Walter, Carrington and Tilden. The late Dr. Lindlahr recognized this principle to a limited extent, even going so far as to declare that elimination can not be forced. With this last Dr. Tilden agrees.

The more we stimulate a patient the more exhausted he becomes. The body of the patient was filled with toxins, when he came to you, because his excretory functions due to enervation (nerve fatigue) were unable to keep up with the work they were daily called upon to do. If you apply the whip or spur to these functions and force a temporarily increased output of toxins and succeed in producing a semblance of health you only weaken and enervate them that much more, so that the subsequent reaccumulation of toxins is more rapid than before. It is like whipping a tired horse up hill. He pulls harder and reaches the top quicker, but falls from exhaustion when he reaches the top. The condition of our patient is much worse than before.

The intelligent teamster, in driving that horse, would permit him to rest a bit instead of applying the whip and spurs. Thus with renewed energy, he would reach the top in good shape. This is the method originated by Jennings, Dewey and Walter. This is the method followed by Dr. Tilden.

But we can do more than just let out horse rest; we can lighten the load. In the case of our excretory horse, we lighten the load by stopping the manufacture and intake of toxins as much as possible. I have often compared, the effort to purify the body by stimulating the organs of elimination, without cutting off the supply of pathoferic matter, to the effort to dip a fountain dry with a bucket without cutting off the water supply. We may dip and dip until our backs ache and find that there is as much water in the fountain as when we commenced.

Medical men used to say: "Disease may be said to consist in the totality of its symptoms." Again: "The symptoms constitute the disease, or all we know of it." It is the orthopathic doctrine that symptoms are such only and not the cause. It is our idea that, back of the symptoms, there lies an efficient cause. We hold, also, that disease is a summing up or consummation of a long series of physiological abuses and not a sudden development. If we are correct, and I am fully convinced that we are, then the causes in each of the cases above described existed in the bodies of these patients before any symptoms appeared—cause must precede effect. Before the symptoms appeared the patient was called healthy. *Was he healthy?* After the symptoms are suppressed he is again called healthy. *Is he healthy?*

Popularly and professionally, if a man appears well and feels well, this is enough; no matter if he is on the verge of collapse, the most vital organs so impaired and deficient in vital power that as soon as they begin to falter the whole system is broken up and the spark of life goes out. If a person is sick, the anxious desire of all is to get rid of the symptoms, and at these the whole artillery of medical "science" (drug and drugless) is directed. When the symptoms are made to disappear, no one thinks to inquire whether the cause of the symptoms is removed or not. It is enough that a temporary simulation of health has been established

THE DELUSION OF CURE

Chapter XXXVI

"From time immemorial, man has looked for a savior; and, when not looking for a savior, he is looking for a cure. He believes in paternalism. He is looking to get something for nothing, not knowing that the highest price we ever pay for anything is to have it given to us.

"Instead of accepting salvation, it is better to deserve it. Instead of buying, begging or stealing a cure, it is better to stop building disease. Disease is of man's own building, and one worse thing than the stupidity of buying a cure is to remain so ignorant as to believe in cures.

"The false theories of salvation and cures have built man into a mental mendicant, when he should be arbiter of his own salvation, and certainly his own doctor, instead of being a slave to a profession that has neither worked out its own salvation from disease nor discovered a single cure in all the age-long period of man's existence on earth."—J. H. Tilden, M.D., in "Toxemia Explained."

IN this chapter I propose to show that Dr. Tilden's words quoted above are correct and that the delusion of cure is the chief obstacle in the way of a rational and successful solution of human health problems and, incidentally, that this idea in its religious, social, political and economic bearings also stands in the way of the solution of practically all the problems of these spheres of human activities. I shall show that the whole idea of cure is basically wrong—that is, that in the attempts to cure evils and diseases we are attempting the impossible and wasting our energy by directing our efforts at effects.

Medicine is the offspring of ancient priestcraft and its old and fundamental dogmas are mere superstitions derived from the ancient priesthoods. For this reason the fundamental ideas of CURE and IMMUNITY are identical with certain ancient fallacies in what passes for religion. This I shall show. The definitions which follow are all taken from Funk and Wagnalls PRACTICAL STANDARD DICTIONARY and are chosen because of their clearness and conciseness:

ATONE; To make expiation or amends for. To propitiate, appease; reconcile; To make an expiation for sin or a sinner.

ATONEMENT; Satisfaction, reparation, or expiation made for wrong or injury; something suffered, done, or given by way of satisfaction.

ABSOLVE; To set free; as from obligation or liability. To free from sin or its penalties; forgive; pardon; acquit.

ABSOLUTION; An absolving or being absolved; forgiveness. The act of a priest pronouncing sin, its eternal punishment, or the canonical penalties attached to it, remitted by authority of the priestly office. The act of releasing from censure without the sacrament of penance.

CONFESSION; The contrite acknowledgment to a priest of any mortal sins committed; a part of the sacrament of penance and a condition of absolution.

INDULGENCE; An act of compliance, grace or favor. Remission by those authorized, of the temporal or temporary punishment still due to sin after sacramental absolution, either in this world or in purgatory. The granting of liberties by the Declaration of Indulgence.

PENANCE; To inflict a penance on. Sorrow for sin of fault evinced by outward act; suffering, detriment, or punishment to which one voluntarily submits as an expression of penitence. The performance of some specific act of mortification voluntarily undertaken, as an expression of sorrow for and atonement of sin. The discipline or act of reparation or austerity imposed by the priest after sacramental confession and forming an integral part of the sacrament of penance. The sacrament of penance consists of contrition, confession, and satisfaction or penance on the part of the penitent, and of absolution on the part of the confessor.

TO DO PENANCE: To perform an act or acts of penance.

The above five doctrines form the basis for the false morality that exists in the world and are directly and indirectly responsible for much positive evil. These doctrines actually encourage sin and wrong doing. They belong to religion. But life is religion. Even atheists have their religion. If they do not worship Jehovah or the Unknown God or Spencer's Unknown Unknowable, or Matter, Motion and Force, or the atom, they worship humanity or the concept of progress or else. Whatever becomes the object of their worship forms the hub around which they build up their religious dogmas. And few, if any of them, have ever escaped the above doctrines.

Whatever is contained in a Man's religion becomes a part of his "science," his politics, his philosophy, his life. The above doctrines permeate present day medicine, law and politics. The high priests of medicine may repudiate these doctrines, as superstitions, in religion, but they exalt them, as scientific principles, in medicine. The theory of vicarious atonement is considered a religious dogma. Men who pose as rational profess to scoff at it. Scientists pretend to ridicule it. But these only scoff at and ridicule the idea in its *religious* bearings. Those who scoff loudest at its *religious* significance are the ones who are surest that vicarious atonement can be accomplished in medicine. A physician who rejects the doctrine of vicarious atonement in religion can still believe, though not logically, in artificial immunity. They may scoff at the practice of the ancient priesthoods in atoning for the sins of their peoples by sacrificing bulls and goats; but they assure us with grave dignity that immunity can be secured by the suffering and death of animals. Where, in heaven's name, is the difference!

This dogma of so-called religion and pretended science holds that a third thing can come between man and his violations of the laws of life and suffer the penalty for him, or turn the penalty aside so that he will not suffer. Conventional *religion* and *medicine* alike hold that man is the victim of agencies and forces which attack him from without. *Religion* thinks this enemy is the devil and his imps; *medicine* thinks it is germs. They both hold that a third power must come between man and his foes, else he will suffer disease and death. They attempt to save man from the penalties of violated law—they do not attempt to show him how to save himself by obeying the law.

For many hundreds of years humanity has believed and preached this false system of ethics. They have held that a fault may be atoned for by suffering that has no direct and inevitable connection with and does not arise out of the fault. Either one may atone for his fault by *penance,* or by the purchase of *indulgences,* or some one else may suffer for him. It is equivalent to the belief that one may put his hand in the fire and another be burned for him. The old idea of Christ's sacrifice was that I sin and Christ suffers for me—I put my hand in the fire and he gets his fingers burned. The old doctrine of hell was that I sin *now* and suffer in the *hereafter.* There was no necessary connection between my present sinning and my future suffering. The sin did not produce the suffering, and I would escape suffering for my sins altogether, but for the agency of a third thing that inflicts the punishment upon me. I was to be punished *for* my sins not by them.

But the opposite of this is the truth—no fault can be atoned for. No one can escape the results of his actions by any means. No doctor can dose, drug or treat away the effects of your evil actions. No one can immunize you against the natural consequences of your violations of the laws of life. If this could be done, it would enable you to go heedlessly on in your evil doing, and escape the penalties that are part and parcel of the transgression.

The many practices that have been in vogue in times past, or, which are yet in vogue to appease and propitiate the anger of the irascible deities cannot be listed here. Most of them consist in some form of sacrifice and are called "atonements." Anciently men sacrificed the most valueless and useless property which they possessed. Gradually, man learned to believe that the angry gods demanded their best in sacrifice. But it did not end here. Human sacrifices, followed animal sacrifices. And, as a climax to this bloody practice, they dragged the God of Heaven off his throne and sacrificed Him. The idea became current that the amount of favor bestowed by the gods was proportionate to the value of the sacrifice.

There was another widespread method of escaping the consequences of one's acts by means of a "scape-animal." By means of a formal hocus pocus process a man or woman was placed on the horns, head or back of some animal. The animal was then driven in to the wilderness or into some remote region where it could not find its way back to the people with its load of sins. The actual sinners were not placed upon the back of the animal. Instead, a cloth or fabric, dipped in blood, or of red or scarlet color in semblance of blood, was tied to the animal. Exposed to sun, wind and rain, the fabric would ultimately fade and become white. This is the significance of Isaiah's declaration: "Though your sins be as scarlet (red), they shall become as wool (white)." Not all people used the same animal to carry off the load of their sins. The ancient Mexicans had their "scape-lamb" and "scape-mouse"; the Tamalese their "scape-hen"; the Jews their "scape-goat"; the Hindoos their "scape-horse"; the Egyptians their "scape-ox"; the Chaldeans their "scape-ram", and the Britons their "scape-bull."

Later, when animal sacrifices led up to the sacrifice of God himself every nation had its "scape-god." The ancient Birmese believed that while the sacrifice of common property in burnt-offerings, (they were burned so that the smoke and incense might ascend up to heaven), would procure the temporary favor of the gods, the sacrifice of human beings would secure their good will for a thousand years. The Hindoos, holding this idea, carried the principle a step further, and in 1200 B.C., crucified their sin-atoning savior, Krishna, and thus gained the perpetual good pleasure of the gods. Thus ended animal and human sacrifices, in India. Anterior to Krishna, the Brahmans, or Priests, sacrificed as many as a thousand head of cattle in a single day. The sacrifice of the cows took the place of good behavior.

The "scape-goat" or the "scape-god" took away the sins of the nations. The sins were put upon the animal, or they were put upon the god. These were mere expedients by which guilty men and nations attempted to evade the effects of their conduct and tried to shift their retributive consequences to the innocent.

"Without the shedding of blood (of the innocent) there is no remission of sin." This was the ancient doctrine throughout Europe, Asia, Africa, the Americas and the far off Islands. It was a religion of butchery and blood-shed. It punished the innocent that the guilty might escape. *It went so far as to murder the gods that man might sin without suffering.* It was an immoral underworld punishing the moral over-world, that the underworld might prosper. It is strange, indeed, that such doctrines still persist throughout the world and that millions still believe them—BOTH IN RELIGION AND IN MEDICINE.

A belief in the propitiation of God by bloody sacrifices, dominated the whole Jewish and pagan world from the remotest antiquity. Religion consisted in the placation of the gods by gifts and sacrifices; *"holiness was a ceremonial cleanliness without moral quality."* If the gods were hostile *they could be bribed; if they were angry presents would appease them.*

Today, in India the religious "purity" of water is of far more importance than its chemical purity. The orthodox Hindu prefers to drink water from the muddy Ganges, which he believes will purify his soul, than to accept clear water from a person of lower caste. The lower caste person, he believes, taints the water which will then defile his soul should he accept it of him.

Usually these sacrifices were of animals or grains and fruits; sometimes they were human sacrifices. The belief in a man-god who would die and thus save the world was common to all pagan religions except that of Judaism. Bel-Merodach of Assyria and Babylon was the son of Hea (God) and was revered as the Prince of Light, the Conqueror of the Dragon, the Redeemer of mankind and Giver of life. The Babylonians used to address him in their prayers: "Merciful one among the gods, Generator who brought back the death to life." He was supposed to have descended into the underworld, broke the gates thereof, subdue death and returned to the living domain, having released the dead from captivity. He was a savior-god who died and conquered death. His resurrection occurred three days after his death and in both Babylon and Phoenicia a kind of Good Friday and an Easter was observed in his honor.

Osiris, of the Egyptians, died and arose to new life. Mithras in the Mithriac (sun worshippers) religion was the mediator between God and man, the viceregent of God on earth, the judge on the day of resurrection, was born of a virgin and was called the "Righteous Incarnate." He was the saviour of mankind and was to lead the good in their battle against the hosts of Ahriman, the evil one or devil. The Mithriasts dedicated the first day of the week, Sun-day, to the worship of the sun.

Numerous other examples of god-man saviours might be cited in pagan religions all over Europe, Asia, Africa and North and South America. Only the Jews rejected this idea. They were satisfied to be saved by the sacrifice of bulls and goats. But all had their victims bound upon an altar and slain to appease a wrathful God.

Propitiation of God by blood sacrifices, and the transfer of righteousness from the innocent to the guilty were the central ideas of these pagan doctrines. The only way by which mankind could escape their inevitable doom was through the rites and mysteries. The Savior-god had paid the full price, all guilt was upon him, man could secure an interest in the price the god had paid to propitiate the wrath of God. The guilty, if afraid, could put the slain man-god in his place and slip away.

Saint Paul gathered all these doctrines together and joining them with certain of the Jewish doctrines manufactured what later became known as Christianity after the Greek Christ. Out of the gigantic labors of this man and his successors came the Church—or the Churches. The Jews would not accept Paul's fusion of Jewish and Pagan doctrines. They would have nothing to do with his Greek Christ. They continued to look for the Jewish Messiah who would liberate them and enable them to place their heels on the necks of the gentiles. To this day the Jew continues to believe he is God's chosen people.

Paul reasoned with them in a strange manner. He believed their laws to be ordained of God, but argued with them that they were of but temporary value. Having been once fulfilled he declared, they were no longer binding. His Christ had fulfilled them perfectly, they were now null and void. What matchless logic! If a law is once perfectly obeyed, it may thenceforth be set aside. Atonement is obedience by proxy. This idea still prevails.

The Roman Church says:

"It was a sacrifice most acceptable to God, offered by his Son on the altar of the cross, which entirely appeased the wrath and indignation of the Father."

The Greek Church says:

"He has done and suffered all that is necessary for the remission of our sins."

The Presbyterian Confession of Faith declares:

"The Lord Jesus by the sacrifice of himself hath fully satisfied the justice of the Father, and hath purchased reconciliation for all whom his love hath given him."

The Protestant sects sing:

"Jesus paid it all."

These ideas are survivals of the old pagan ideas that an angry God can be appeased by pain and that a victim can be substituted for the offender—an innocent being can take the place of the guilty one and pay his penalty for him. When put thus baldly men do not accept these dogmas. They know that for justice to accept the innocent as a sacrifice for the guilty, that the guilty might go free, would be to violate the very constitution of the universe.

Before the time that Jesus is claimed to have lived, the Pagans had almost wholly abandoned their bloody sacrifices. They had substituted the "Mysteries", "Baptism", the "Eucharist", etc. The Jews clung tenaciously to their altars of blood. In vain did the Prophet declare unto them:

"Thus saith the Lord, what purpose is the multitude of your sacrifices to me? I am surfeited with burnt offerings of rams and of the fat of beasts and I delight not in the blood of bullocks or he goats."

In vain did Samuel admonish them:

"Hath the Lord as great delight in burnt offerings and sacrifices as in obeying the voice of the Lord? Behold to obey is better than sacrifice, and to hearken than the fat of rams."

God pleaded through the prophet Hosea that their cities were polluted with iniquity and blood, and their priests commit lewdness and adultery and waited for a man like troops of robbers while He;

"desired mercy, and not sacrifice; and the knowledge of God more than burnt offerings."

Jesus approved of the answer of the Sadducees that there is but one God and: "to love Him with all the heart, (emotions) and with all the understanding (intellect) and with all the soul, (being), and with all the strength, and to love his neighbor as himself, is MORE THAN ALL THE BURNT OFFERINGS AND SACRIFICES."

Theirs was a "religion of the shamble, and the medicine-men", and Jesus, who never brought even so much as a dove to the altar, advised them to bury it out of sight.

Among the Pagans Varro protested against sacrifices because the gods did not require them while the false gods made of copper and stone, could not care for them. Menander, the comedian, taught on the stage that it was vain to try to propitiate God by sacrifices of bulls and kids, by garments of gold or purple, or by images of ivory or emerald, instead of refraining from adultery, theft, murder, or covetousness; and declared that God delighted in righteous works.

Tibullus, in a Panegyric on Marcella, said: "A little cake, a little morsel of bread, appeased the divinities." This reveals the true nature of the "Lord's Supper" or the "Eucharist" or "Sacrament," practiced alike by the Essenes, Persians, Pythagoreans, Gnostics, Brahmins and ancient Mexicans. Like animal sacrifices, it was an effort to appease the wrath of the angry gods.

An English Archbishop says: "this reversion to the worst ideas of pagan sacrifice, savoring of the heathen temples and reeking with blood," is woven into the very fabric of the sacrifice of the mass, confessions, liturgies, articles, etc. And I declare that medicine in all its bearings is a survival of these same bloody sacrifices and superstitions of ancient paganism. Vaccination or inoculation was originally practiced among the Circassians to propitiate the gods. Lady Montague introduced it into England from there in the year 1721 since which time the sacrifice of animals, that man may live uncleanly, has stained the altars of pseudo-science every second of the day and night.

The idea that faults can be atoned for or blotted out and their consequences avoided by sufferings, penances, and sacrifices not directly connected with the act, or by the suffering and sacrifices of another, or that indulgences can be secured which will remit all or part of the penalty or that absolution can be had, and which encourages people to let the sacrifices of another wipe out their daily debits in the score of morality, is an actual demoralizing influence. In the middle ages the doctrine took on many strange forms and some of those we now refer to as saints earned their fame by the abuses and indignities they heaped upon their bodies. Flagellation which became so widespread in the 13th and 15th centuries was employed as a means of penance or atonement. People whipped themselves or had themselves whipped as a means of atonement and as a means of mortifying the flesh. It was regarded as a means of emancipating the soul from sensuality. The church was finally forced to oppose it because it served to increase sensuality.

As soon as people learn that punishment is a consequence drawn upon themselves, they learn to avoid the cause of punishments. So long as they believe that they can flirt with the causes and sidestep the penalties they will attempt to do so. For this reason, all pretended systems of cure that hold out to man the hope of immunity from, or cure of the effects of violation of the laws of life, while he continues to violate them, are evil and debasing. "Men are punished by their sins, not for their sins."

We are not punished for using alcohol. The use of alcohol itself punishes us We are not punished for overeating. Overeating administers its own penalties. We are not punished for excesses and dissipations. We are weakened by the excesses and dissipations.

Man has created God "in his own image;" and as man-made laws are subject to the State's enforcement officers, so, in his mind he has made the operation of the Creator's laws subject to the Creator's enforcement officers.

Nature's laws need no extraneous power to enforce them. The law enforces itself. Every abuse of mind and body administers its own penalties. Every good use of mind and body brings its own reward. The penalty or reward is concurrent with the act—is inherent in the act.

For this reason we can no more escape the penalty of bodily abuses than we can lift ourselves by pulling at our boot straps.

Each man is judged and punished according to his work—not hereafter, BUT NOW! We see the judgment falling daily, but we are blind and perceive not.

If we put our fingers in the fire we are burned. We are not burned for putting our fingers in the fire. We are burned by putting our fingers in the fire.

Our fathers and grandfathers had an idea that disease is a punishment sent upon man by God because of sin. This principle is not altogether wrong. Disease is a punishment—a disciplinary measure. But we bring it upon ourselves. We transgress the Laws of Life, that is, we sin, and the sin produces its own penalty.

Our fathers thought that when God punished them with disease, the punishment was just and merited. They felt, with one of Job's counselors, that God metes out no punishment where it is not deserved, and that He administrers no more punishment than is due.

This principle is fundamentally correct. The fact that we are punished by, and not for, our sins, makes it impossible for this to be other than true. It is the practice in applying the principle that is wrong.

Our fathers made the grave mistake of thinking that, while the punishment was deserved and just, it was possible to evade it by drugging and dosing it away. They believed that they could cheat God out of His "vengeance" by the magical power of the primitive medicine man and his poisonous concoctions.

This belief has come down to us from the past. We still believe that it is possible to dose or treat away the penalties of violated law. We vainly imagine that we can put our fingers in the fire and then dose away the burn. We imagine that we can find a drug, serum or vaccine that will enable us to put our fingers into the fire and not be burned.

We are forever looking for some magical power that will enable us to wallow in the mire without getting filthy. We do not want to give up wallowing, nor do we want to pay for keeping it up. We want to be clean but we also want to wallow. This desire keeps humanity chasing will-o'-the-wisps, over the bogs and swamps of magic and mystery, in our vain search for a philosopher's stone that will transmute unclean living into good health.

The Rev. Dr. Talmage used to say:

"We are constantly praying to Heaven for that which we could easily get for ourselves by correct diet."

It is fortunate for man that Heaven never does anything for him that he can do for himself. Heaven only does that which earth cannot. Heaven is pledged wholeheartedly and unalterably to the principle that no man shall have more than he deserves. There are those who appear to get more than they deserve. But these only appear to. Eternal Justice will not and cannot be denied.

Heaven will not encourage laziness. If man can do a thing for himself, Heaven will not give it to him. If man can acquire a thing by his own efforts Heaven will not give it to him free. There is no effortless achievement, despite what the mataphysicians say. Heaven is not an alms house. Man is not intended as a beggar. That which can be achieved by the sweat of the brow cannot be attained by prayer.

God is the giver of all good gifts, as the Bible declares. But He does not give that which can be secured by work. To do so would be to encourage idleness and laziness. The greatest gift of God, to man, is the power and ability to do for himself. He expects man to use this power and ability. Man is so constituted that the more one does for him the less he does for himself. To do for man what he can do for himself is to demoralize him. He would have remained in Eden leading an endless life of ease and idleness had he not been kicked out. He had to be forced to do for himself.

Neither God nor Heaven are in the curing business. They will not give us health in exchange for prayer; for, health we can attain and maintain for ourselves. If we are sick it is our own fault and Heaven cannot be induced to remit the penalty or any part of it. Heaven cannot be bribed or cajoled into remitting just penalties. Heaven will not be bargained with. And if Heaven will not remit penalties or make it possible to escape them, she has made it impossible that others may remit them.

479

No doctor can remit the penalties for your sins against your body. No drug, serum, or vaccine can immunize you against the natural penalties of your transgressions of the laws of being. There are no vaccinal indulgences. Nature does not absolve us of our sins—she demands obedience to her laws. No doctor can grant you absolution. No pill, powder, plaster, potion, knife or saw can grant you immunity.

Remedies do not exist. The full penalty for every infraction of natural law must be paid. There is no way to shorten the penalty. Penalties can be avoided by obedience. Nature will accept no substitutes for obedience. She will accept no sacrifices and sin offerings. Her decree is "Behave or take your punishment." Doctors who try to cure the punishment but reveal their lack of intelligence. The sick man can return to health if he but deserves health. Until he earns it, he must remain sick. Doctors and physicians of all schools have this fact to learn.

We must banish our faith in magic. We must throw off the spell that was cast over us by the fairy tales which we were taught as mere children in school, and which were ingrained still deeper in the university. We must free our minds of the "cure complex." We must learn that there is no such thing as a *cure for disease.*

If we want to keep clean, we must keep out of the mire. If we want to keep sober, we must keep booze out of our bodies. If we want good health we must live right—obey the law. Treatment will not keep a man clean while he wallows in the mire. Treatment will not keep a man sober while he continues to drink. Treatment will not keep a man well while he disobeys every law of his being.

There are no magical doses nor formulas that cure inebriety in a man who drinks. There are no magical pills, powders, nor potions that will or can restore health while you continue to disobey the laws of your being.

No pills can prevent fire from burning you. No potion can prevent excessive venery from weakening you. No powder can prevent fear from having its destructive effect upon your nervous system. If you want health, you must avoid fear, fire, excessive venery, etc.

If you want health you will have to reform your mode of life. When you cease to transgress the Laws of Life, the transgressions cease to punish you. Take your finger from the fire and the fire ceases to burn you. Cease the use of alcohol and alcohol ceases to consume you. Cease your excesses and excesses cease to enervate and degenerate you.

The punishment for violating the law is automatic and inevitable. The cessation of the punishment, when you cease the wrong doing, is automatic and inevitable, also.

When you stop injuring your body, it at once begins repairing its injuries, without treatment of any kind, and you are sooner or later restored to health, depending upon the severity of the injuries, sustained.

When you cease to burn your fingers, the burn soon heals. No treatment of any kind is necessary, and none can hasten or help the repairing process.

The power of repair is inherent in the body. It does not inhere in anything else. The living organism cures itself. Nothing else can cure.

The power of cure is the power of repair; the power of repair is the power of reproduction; and the power of reproduction is a function of the living body. There is and can be no cure outside of the powers of the body.

The body cures itself when the cause is corrected. There is, then, no cure other than *correction of causes.*

To correct causes, no magic, no mystery, no theurgy, no thaumaturgy, no drugs, no serums are needed, nor can they help. These things belong to the *curing professions and healing combines.* Nature can not use them, nor does she recognize them. She persistently and consistently refuses all plans of cure that do not have as their sole end and aim the *correction and removal of causes.*

Nature's decree ever and always is, *sin and you must suffer.* Her penalties are sure; her rewards are certain.

The child learns that fire will burn if he comes in contact with it. And if he continues to place himself in contact with the fire he soon learns that fire always burns. It does not burn him at one time, threaten him at another and bribe him at another. The burning is inevitable. The child soon learns that he can avoid the burning only by avoiding its cause. This is nature's strict and inflexible disciplinary measure. Violations of her laws are not punished at one time and overlooked the next.

If a mother slaps a child for touching the fire he can see no natural or necessary connection between his action and the slap. When mother is not looking he will touch it again. Slapping is not the natural and certain result of touching the fire, but burning is. The child will be burned every time he touches the fire but he soon learns that if he is clever enough, he can avoid the slaps. The slapping increases his tendency towards deception, but does not improve his morality nor strengthen his character. Rather it builds a false morality—one that suppresses faults under certain circumstances and allows them to break out when it is felt no punishment will follow.

This is the same kind of morality medicine engenders. It holds out, by implication rather than by direct assertion, that the laws of nature can be cheated if we are only clever enough. And the various schools of medicine all claim to be clever enough to outwit these laws. The doctrine of immunity, in particular, encourages people to believe that they can disobey the laws of old Mother Nature and escape her spankings.

Every effort that has ever been made to cure disease has been an effort to save man from the penalties of sin—violated law. They do not seek to prevent man from *sowing* to the flesh, but to save him from *reaping* the harvest of corruption. They seek to save him *in* his sins, not to show him how to save himself *from* them.

Every man must save himself. No one can obey the laws of life for another. No one can receive the penalties for the violations of the laws of life for another. "The righteousnes of the righteous shall be upon him and the wickedness of the wicked shall be upon him." "When the wicked man turneth away from his wickedness that he hath committed, and doeth that which is lawful and right, he shall save his soul (being) alive."

We do not have to wait for the hereafter for the rewards and punishments for our thoughts and deeds. We reap them here—NOW. The greater our perfidity the greater is our retribution. It comes before death. *You cannot fly in the face of the eternal laws of being and get away without paying for it.*

When the writer was a boy the preachers used to tell us much about the recording angel who kept the Book of Life wherein the credit and debit sheets of each of us were carefully filled in day by day to be presented to us in the final day of judgment. I always thought this particular angel had his hands full recording the good and evil thoughts and deeds of each of us. I now know that he has an easy job. We are our own bookkeepers. We are our own recording angels. Our thoughts and actions write themselves in our characters. Every wrong is followed by an immediate punishment. If it is but a small wrong our character is injured but little. If it is a great wrong the downward step is greater. We cannot hide ourselves from ourselves. We cannot escape the great law of cause and effect. We bring our own degradation upon ourselves. If there is to be a final Judgment Day, the Great Judge before whom the small and great shall stand, will but need to look upon our characters. The recording of the record is automatic—just as are rewards and punishments.

Life cannot be repudiated. Its laws cannot be cast aside. John Boyle O'Reilly has beatifully expressed the law of compensation in the following lines:

"There is no ill without its compensation,
And life and death are only light and shade;
There never beat a heart so base and sordid
But felt at times a sympathetic glow;
There never lived a virtue unrewarded
Nor died a vice without its meed of woe."

The ideas of the CONFESSION and the PENANCE are the religious equivalents of the medical idea of CURE; the ideas of ATONEMENT and INDULGENCE are the religious counterparts of the medical idea of IMMUNITY, the one is Theurgic, the other Thaumaturgic. At base medicine is a religion, having its origin in the ancient priesthood and deriving its cardinal doctrines from this same source. Note:

CURE; To resore to a healthy or sound condition. To eradicate, as disease or evil. That which restores health or abolishes an evil.

CUREALL; That which cures all disease or evils; a panacea.

IMMUNE; Exempt as from disease; especially protected by inoculation.

IMMUNITY; Freedom or exemption, as from a penalty, burden, duty, or evil. Exemption from contagion or infection or from liability to suffer from epidemic or endemic diseases (freedom or exemption from a penalty is license—the freedom to do as one pleases without suffering the consequences.. Author).

IMMUNIZE: To make immune; protect as from infection by inoculation.

We daily meet with the unconscious idea among the sick that if they have made themselves sick by a certain habit or mode of living they can do *something*, or *take something*, or some one else can do *something* to them that will CURE them. They think that after they have been *cured* they may return to the habit or mode of living that was responsible for their trouble. Indeed, most of them think they can be cured while still practicing the habits that are responsible for their ills. They look outside of themselves for a forcible savior, for something that will come to their aid and save them in spite of themselves. It is seldom possible to disabuse their minds of this old medically fostered idea. After they have been shown the causes of their troubles, and have made a temporary reform, and are improving, they are exceedingly impatient to get back to the old habits and former mode of life. The reform is looked upon as a necessary temporary evil. It is a *cure*, which, having done its works, is abandoned.

The idea of cure is strikingly like the old idea of the efficacy of deathbed repentances. These repentances were supposed to fit the most hardened criminal and the most disreputable character for heaven. They permitted one to live as he or she pleased. One could live a life of sin, debauchery, shame and crime, and then, a few minutes before dying or being hung, he or she could cry out "Lord, be merciful to me a sinner," and Saint Peter was supposed to welcome him or her to the heavenly realms. His or her whole character, a character that had required a lifetime to build, was instantly changed and made over. Repentance cancelled all his debts against morality and he or she became an angel. Purgatory was simply a place where men and women were purged of sin and prepared for heaven through sufferings that had no connections with the sin. It was believed in by those who did not believe in the sufficiency of death-bed repentances. Even, in Purgatory others could secure more or less absolution for you. The fact that each man must save himself is strange to these people.

This idea actually encouraged sin. Men found it easier to repent at the end of life than to live as they should through life. They were led by it to believe that the penalties of sin were of the next world and not of this. In the middle ages suffering and disease actually came to be looked upon as evidences of divine favor.

Gautama said:

"If a man speaks or acts with an evil thought, pain follows him as the wheels follow the foot of the ox that draws the carriage." Again: "Our good or evil deeds follow us continually like shadows. Since it is impossible to escape the result of our deeds, let us practice good works."

This doctrine that punishment is the natural and inevitable consequence of wrong conduct, that the effect is as inseparably connected with its cause as a shadow is connected with the object that casts it has no fascination for the mind of man. He is continually searching for a means of escape from the results of his deeds—rather than following the advice to "practice good works."

A few hours before Gerald Chapman, notorious bandit, was hung for a crime he probably did not commit, a priest went to him and pleaded with him, saying:

"My boy, if you have done this thing, confess to your God before it is too late, don't go into that execution chamber with the stains of murder on your soul. Confess, be contrite, and I will grant you forgiveness as a priest of your church— Our Church."

Who was this man that he could grant Chapman forgiveness? From whence comes such power? Do otherwise intelligent men really believe that a priest has power to grant forgiveness in the name of God, and do they think this forgiveness can obviate an iota of the penalties of transgressed law? The bandit, himself, expressed a clearer conception of law and order than those who believe in such theurgic powers, when he replied:

"If I've lived the wrong life—and perhaps I have, I've paid while I lived. When I'm dead tomorrow no power can make me keep on paying."

Why cannot mankind see this truth—*We pay now for our wrongs: we are rewarded now for our virtues.* "The wages of sin is death!" When the supreme penalty is paid what more is there to pay? Every violation of law administers its own penalties. No power sets aside those penalties. No priest can grant absolution, no serum can confer *immunity*, no drug or serum can *cure.* Law and order cannot be destroyed. Only a fool hath said in his heart there is no law and order.

We pay while we live.

Were this not so experience would be void of content. Life would teach us nothing.

Knowledge of *good* and *evil* is derived from the results of the two courses. We learn that an act is good or *evil,* *beneficial* or *harmful* by its effects. If evil doings were not paid for while we live—if they produced no evil effects now—we could not know them to be evil or harmful. If a life of good were not rewarded while we live—if it produced no beneficial effects—we could not know it to be good. If this life did not reward good and punish *evil* there would be no lessons taught by experience. Experience would be meaningless. The present would possess no educational value.

But the Creator has wisely seen to it that every evil brings a sure and swift penalty—every good a sure and swift reward. We do not have to await a future life to discover whether we have lived well or ill.

Today is the judgment day. You are judged and rewarded and punished by your acts. You cannot be pardoned, forgiven, absolved or atoned for.

Forgiveness can do nothing toward changing the nature of the act forgiven, or toward cancelling the effects of the act upon the individual or upon society. Every wrong act has its consequent penalty attached to it and no act of forgiveness can set aside that penalty. The confessing and forgiving of sin supplies a license to commit sin. So long as the effects of sins can be so easily evaded they will be committed. The doctrine that sins can be forgiven is a demoralizing doctrine.

The cure idea does not differ from this idea of forgiveness and atonement. Men are led to believe that they can live as they please and then, when their repeated abuses of their bodies have produced disease, they can implore a doctor, who by the thaumaturgic power of pill, powder, plaster, potion or by the use of a knife and saw, can cancel their debts against the laws of life and free them from suffering. The idea actually encourages men and women in their violations of the laws of life. It holds out to them the hope of a complete or partial remittance of the penalties for their wrong doing and tells them to "go to it." They are encouraged to believe that effects (suffering) are not essential parts of causes (sin).

The very foundation of the serum and vaccine therapy is the idea that your misdeeds against your body may be vicariously atoned for. Through the sufferings of an animal immunity may be built for you. You may do as you please and the poor animal, victim of the fiendish tortures of the vivisectionist, can take all your sufferings upon itself and give you a clean bill of health. We have our "scape-vaccines," "scape-serum," "scape-antitoxins," etc. This is the basis of the whole idea of cure, whether by drugs, serums, vaccines, surgery, electricity, hydrotherapy, Osteopathy, Chiropractic, Naprapathy, Physiotherapy, Psychotherapy, Christian Science, New Thought, suggestion, or other pretended system of cure. If this idea were correct, morality would perish from the earth.

If the Abrams contraption or its imitations, or Paresco's so-called "Biological Blood-Washing Bath" could do the things claimed for them, then one could live in any manner that he desires, and by frequent resort to these "cures" or "immunizers," could escape the natural penalties of his misbehavior. When men learn that they cannot escape these natural penalties by any means whatsoever, they will cease the attempt to evade them. Then will the cures and immunizers be relegated to the limbo of forgotten things.

The following story is credited to C. H. Spurgeon.

"Once when I was in the vestry an Irishman came to see me. Pat began by making a low bow and saying, 'Now, your Riverence, I have come to ask you a question.'

" 'Oh!' said I, 'Pat, I am not a Riverence, but what is your question and how is it you have not been to your priest about it?'

" 'I have been to him,' he replied, 'but I am not satisfied with his answer.'

" 'Well, what is your question?'

" 'Just this: God is just, and if He be just He must punish sins. I deserve to be punished. If He is a just God He ought to punish me; yet you say God is merciful and will forgive sins. I cannot see how that is right; He has no right to do that. He ought to be just and punish those who deserve it. Tell me how you make out that God can be just and yet be merciful.'

" 'That is through the Blood of Christ.'

" 'Yes, that is exactly what my priest said; you are both in agreement there. But he said a good deal beside, that I did not understand, and that short answer does not satisfy me. I want to know how it is that the Blood of Jesus Christ enables God to be righteous and just and yet be merciful.'

"Then I saw what he wanted to know and explained the plan of salvation thus:

" 'Now, Pat, suppose you had been killing a man and the judge said, 'That Irishman must be hanged!'

"He said quickly, 'And I should have richly deserved to be hanged!'

" 'But, Pat, suppose I was very fond of you. Can you see any way by which I could save you from being hanged?'

" 'No, sir, I cannot!'

" 'Then, suppose I went to the very highest judicial authorities of the land and said, 'Please, sire, I am very fond of this Irishman. I think the judge was quite right in saying that he must be hanged, but let me be hanged instead and you will then carry out the law.' Now they could not agree to my proposal; but suppose they could—and God can, for He has power greater than all kings and queens—and suppose they should have me hanged instead of you. Do you think the policemen would take you up afterwards?'

"He at once said, 'No, I should think not; they would not meddle with me. But if they did, I should say, 'What are you doing? Did not that gintleman condescind to be hung for me? Let me alone; shure, you don't want to hang two people for the same thing, do ye?'

" 'Ah, that, my friend,' said I, 'you have it exactly; this is the way whereby we are saved! God must punish sin. Christ said, 'My Father, punish Me instead of the sinner.' And His Father did. God laid on His beloved Son, Jesus Christ, the whole burden of our sins, and all their punishment and chastisement, and now that Christ is punished instead of us, God would not be just if He were to punish any sinner who believes in the Lord Jesus Christ. If thou believest in Jesus Christ, the well-beloved and only begotten Son of God, thou art saved, and thou mayest go on thy way rejoicing and full of hope.'

" 'Faith,' said the man, clapping his hands, 'That's the Gospel.'

"Pat is safe now; with all his sins about him he'll trust in the Man who died for him, and so shall be saved by His sacrifice."

"*Pat is safe with all his sins about him.*" This is the great desire of all nations. It is the almost universal desire of the human race—the desire to be saved in sin. Man does not want to give up sinning. He desires some way that will enable him to sin without paying the penalties. He desires some one else to take his place, some one else to pay his penalties for him. The religious profess to believe that God could accept such a sacrifice and still be just—that God's justice is of a lower order than that of our courts.

This is seen not only in religion, but in medicine, as well. The most clear-cut case of this is the effort to establish immunity to disease by the products of the suffering and disease of animal—the desire to be saved by the animals' sacrifice.

To paraphrase Spurgeon—

"Faith," said the fool, defiantly shaking his empty head, "that's immunity." The fool is now safe with all his sins about him. He'll trust in the animal that died for him, and so shall be saved by its sacrifice.

The idea that man can be immunized against disease by the use of serums and vaccines grants him indulgences to do as he pleases. "Your child's life or the rabbit's," ask the high-priests of medicine, and the ignorant mob answers back, "Sacrifice the rabbit."

Why do they never stop to consider that to sacrifice the rabbit, while it gives them a false sense of security, and insures the wreck of the child, does not save the child? Because they have been brought up to believe in vicarious atonement and atonement sacrifices. In this they are no more advanced than the ancient Jews who prostrated themselves before the tabernacle while the high priest sacrificed the bull. The bull atoned for their sins, and they went back to their sinning. What more natural than that they should do so? When penalties are so easily cast aside, will not man ignore them? Dr. Claunch rightly declares: "The sacrifice of the rabbit is a sure guarantee that your child will be sacrificed."

If by theurgic and thaumaturgic powers a man can be cured of the sufferings inflicted by violated law or immunized against the natural consequences and effects of these violations, why should he not violate the laws of life? Why shall not one do as he jolly well pleases when the results, if they are not desirable, can be so easily brushed aside by the magical powers of a serum or potion? Not until man learns that he reaps what he sows and that he cannot lessen his sufferings by so much as one short second of time, or by so much as one slight twinge of pain, will we have a morality that is worthy of the name. He must learn that no "indulgence" will enable him to sin without paying the full penalty; no form of vicarious atonement will enable a man or woman to transgress the laws of life and escape the full penalty. No discounts can be obtained. *Nature cannot be bribed.* He must learn that no one else and nothing else can pay his debts for him—no one can take his place. Any other plan leads to physiological hygienic and moral lawlessness.

Our religious instructors teach us that we are fallen beings, incapable of attaining perfection, however much we may try. And yet, these same instructors teach us that our only hope of life and happiness in the world to come depends on our attainment of holiness or wholeness. Our imperfections are excused because we are fallen, and to lift up to our former high plane, atonements, penances, indulgences, death-bed repentances, etc., are substituted for holiness. Flaws in character are rounded out by these things.

At the 29th Annual Convention of the American Naturopathic Association, held in the Hotel Commodore, New York City, 1925, a Catholic priest, in a lecture, likened the doctor who gives a drug to relieve suffering, without requiring a reform in the mode of living that was responsible for the suffering, to a priest who would repeatedly absolve a man or a woman of a certain sin without making an effort to correct the sin—an effort to secure reform. He asserted that such a priest would be a monster and that such a practice would encourage sin. If the man or woman was granted absolution each time he or she entered the confessional, without having to give up the sin, there would be no reason for reform.

I fully endorse this principle and extend it to cover not only medical methods but the methods employed by all the various drugless and semi-drugless schools. I do not believe that any man has the power or authority to absolve the sins of another. I care not whether he tries it in the confessional or in the treatment room. The efforts to treat away the effects of an unphysiological mode of life without correcting the mode of life is like trying to treat away the effects of contact with fire while in contact with the fire. It amounts to an effort to erase effects while cause is operative.

All violations of natural law brings suffering. Were this not so, we could violate the law with impunity, this would encourage us in its violation. This would encourage vice, crime, immorality, wrong-doing. Progress would cease. The race would deteriorate. Moral and intellectual bankruptcy and physical degeneration would abound.

Our secientific instructors teach us that we are unfinished beings in the process of becoming. We are headed for perfection and may reach there a few million years hence. Whether one is a biologist, physiologist or psychologist, sin is simply the expression of the brute nature that remains in us. The fact that in a thousand ways we are worse than any brute is hardly explained this way.

Whether we are sub-angels or super-apes seems to make no difference. Either way we can find plenty of excuses or extenuating circumstances to justify our wrong doing. Often it seems that what is called psychology is nothing more than a search for metaphysical reasons (*indulgences*) for wrong doing.

What is more natural, when the doctrine of moral irresponsibility underlies all our system of "thought," than that man should seek to find ways and means of evading the effects of his wrong doing? When, theoretically, he has established his irresponsibility then the next step is to attempt to practically abolish the consequences of his acts. Logically, it could not be otherwise, although, man is seldom logical. He is led unconsciously to follow the bent of such ideas.

The ancient Jews who declared that man should give an account for every idle word had a cleaner insight into life than those who pretend to follow them.

When Jesus prescribed, for those who sought his aid, a simple "go and sin no more," he must have had no idea that so-called "imputed righteousness" has any merit. How vastly have his simple teachings been corrupted and perverted!

Imputed righteousness means that the excess righteousness of one can be transferred to another who lacks enough. During the middle ages the excess(?) righteousness of some of the saints was transferred, as *indulgences*, on certain conditions, to poor sinners who lacked the determination to be righteous themselves. This gave immunity

Virtue is its own reward. Evil is its own punishment. Nature is forever unassailable in her justice. She metes out rewards or punishments, as we deserve, with the same lavish hand. Effort, striving, development of power—these are their own reward. Rewards are bound up in *good;* punishments are part and parcel of *bad.* When we learn this fact, then will we develop a higher and truer morality than that which we now see about us.

A lady once wrote me that she had been to fifty physicians since suffering a "nervous break-down" fifteen years previous, and that not one of them had been able to tell her what her trouble was or what caused it.

"EFFECTS—everything.

"CAUSES—nothing. This is my trouble with the doctors," she wrote.

But effects cannot be *everything* and causes *nothing.* Back of every effect there lies an adequate cause. *Something cannot come out of nothing.* This lady's physicians had not sought for causes. They had sought for physical changes in the organs of her body. They had resorted to all the arts of refined and advanced diagnosis, in an endeavor to locate some organic change in her body, onto which they could saddle the blame for her symptoms. Failing to find any physical signs they probably put her trouble down as hysteria. It has gotten so now that when a doctor finds no physical sign responsible for your trouble, you are suffering with hysteria. But these organic changes that they search for, are themselves effects. They are end results of causes lying back of them. They are consequences of antecedent causes—causes the doctors do not look for—causes that they do not even recognize in practice. If they find a physical sign, they treat it. They ignore causes. Their whole practice is built upon the ancient fallacy that some drug or other agent can be employed to *cure* disease or *atone* for the sins of the patient. If this idea were correct, law and order would cease to exist, and chaos would reign supreme.

A lady read in one of my books that there is no such thing as a cure for disease— no cure for any disease. She decided from this that she could do as she pleased; that she would take no advice from any one. Strange reasoning, this!

The fact that there is no cure for disease is exactly the reason why one should behave. If disease could be *cured,* then one could do as he pleased. There would be no reason for behaving in such a manner as to avoid disease, no reason for reforming one's mode of living, and thus enable the body to overcome its injuries and incapacities, if disease could be cured. One could simply go and have himself *cured* every time his wrong living caused difficulty and could live as he pleased and disregard natural law.

If the effects of inebriety could be cured, alcohol could be consumed at will without injury. But just because there is no cure for the effects of alcohol, the addict must cease the use of alcohol before his body can evolve out of its decadent condition back into normal helath. If the fatigue following work or exercise could be *cured,* rest and sleep would be unnecessary. One could continue working day and night a whole lifetime, and as rapidly as he became tired he could have himself cured. But there is no *cure* for fatigue so we have to cease work or exercise and permit the body to restore its energies and substances during rest and sleep.

There is but one guarantee of good health, and this is an unceasing conformity to the laws of life. If you are not conforming to these, you are gradually undermining your powers of life, and laying the foundation for serious trouble. It is a common error to assume that because your state of health is fair now, is is an indication that your mode of living is correct. This is a pernicious fallacy. That you have what passes for good health now, is no proof that your mode of living is correct. It requires time for even the worst mode of living imaginable to enervate and weaken the body sufficiently to produce recognizable disease. Disease does not develop suddenly. Back of every physical sign there are months and years of the gradual accumulation of the effects of your constant, habitual transgressions of the laws of life.

It is the height of folly to think that the effects of these daily transgressions against the laws of being, can be set aside by some method of treatment and thus *cure* the patient. To imagine that some one can come along with some magical remedy and, in a short time or instantaneously, undo the work of months and years, as the miracle mongers claim to be able to do, is to display the mind of a child. Cure is an evolutionary process in reverse.

Methods and theories of cure and immunity may change, but they all circle around the ancient fallacy that sins can be vicariously atoned for. The great Hindu national leader, Mahatma Gandhi, has sensed this fact and very harshly, but very justly, criticizes Western Medical Science (?), for its efforts at vicarious atonement and its sale of vaccine and serum indulgences. His biographer, Romain Rolland, says of Gandhi's views:

"As for the medical profession, Gandhi admits he was attracted to it at first, but he soon realized it was not honorable. For Western medical science is concerned with giving relief to suffering bodies only. It does not strive to do away with the cause of suffering and disease, which, as a rule, is nothing but vice. In fact, Western medical science may almost be said to encourage vice by making it possible for a man to satisfy his passions and appetites at the least possible risk. It contributes, therefore, to demoralize people; it weakens their will-power by helping them to cure themselves with "black magic" prescriptions instead of forcing them to strengthen their character by disciplinary rules for body and soul. In opposition to the false medical science in the West, which Gandhi has often criticized unfairly, he places preventive medical science. He was written a little pamphlet on the subject entitled 'A Guide to Health,' which is the fruit of twenty years' experience. It is a moral as well as a therapeutic treatise, for according to Gandhi, 'disease is the result of our thoughts as much as of our acts.' He considers it a relatively simple matter to establish certain rules that will prevent disease. For all disease springs from the same origin, i.e., from neglect of the natural laws of health. The body is God's dwelling place. It must be kept pure. There is truth in Gandhi's point of view, but he refuses a little obstinately to recognize the efficacy of remedies that have really proved to be useful. His moral precepts are also extremely rigid."

Gandhi has a clearer conception of the truths stated in the above quotation than does Rolland, as will be seen from two of Rolland's statements. Rolland seems to still believe that there are remedies that really prove useful. Roland is not entirely free from the taint of ancient magic. Nor, if Rolland has correctly presented Gandhi's view, is Gandhi fully free of this ancient belief in the magic powers of remedies. He does not criticize Western medicine because it CANNOT help them to cure themselves by "black-magic" prescriptions, and CANNOT make it possible for men and women to disobey the laws of life at the least possible risk, but because they DO do these things. He plainly sees that to do these things is to demoralize the race. But he does not see that they cannot be done. *The race is demoralized by the BELIEF that these things can be done.* It will not learn self-control; it will not strengthen its character; it will not heed the simple laws of life, so long as it has this faith in the powers of remedies and immunizers.

Let me repeat, we must teach the race that every act administers its own consequence, and that no treatment ever devised, or that ever can be devised, will or can prevent or mitigate that consequence. Every cause will have its effect. Causes and effects are indissolubly bound up together.

Science—medical science—today, also, transfers the immunity of animals to man and grants him *indulgences*. Fundamentally the two ideas are identical and, historically, they antedate written memorials. The cardinal principles of that collossal system of humbug that boasts of the wonderful progress it has made during the past fifty years are superstitions received from prehistoric man. Medicine's boasted progress is all based on these fallacies and cannot long endure.

We must learn that things are to be avoided because they are in and of themselves evil or wrong and, therefore, essentially harmful; that we are to aim at good, not to escape hell and get to heaven, but because good is infinitely better and higher than evil and is essentially and intrinsically beneficial. We must not excuse our faults and failures because of a pretended incapacity for good. Such an idea is morally and ethically weakening and debasing. A man is only as strong as his faith in himself and his faith in the eternal good of things.

The docrine of total depravity must be eradicated from all our fields of thought. And, it must be remembered that, practically, there is little or no difference between this old dogma and the "scientific" dogma of man's inherent brutality.

A young lady once remarked to me: "Why should one have to live right all his or her life? Why must one always eat this way or that when one can take a pill if feeling bad and get over it in a few days? Why can't one enjoy life?" She followed this by saying she gets a thrill out of doing what is wrong. As soon as she learns that a thing should not be done, she does that thing.

Her idea about curing the effects of wrong living or wrong eating by taking a pill is the popular idea. It is the outgrowth of the old fallacy that we can transgress the laws of life and sidestep the penalties.

Her very remarks reveal the menace to health and life that inheres in this idea. Can you not see that her idea is that she can do as she pleases and by taking a pill, right all the wrongs? If this thing were possible, if it could be done, then would morality perish.

This lady was not of the low, sensual type. She was an average American girl, living a conventional life and holding down a responsible position. Her views are those that are gaining in favor among our so-called flaming youth.

This idea is perhaps best expressed by Warner Fite in his "Moral Philosophy," where, according to his reviewer, he contends: that: "No objective standards of conduct exist, there is no act which is in itself either right or wrong; and thus with one admission are destroyed all those systems which would make morality consist in any duty to do or to refrain from doing either this or that."

He says all the Christian philosophies "which in their modern form stem from Kant" and all the Non-christian ones "which are based upon utilitarianism" rest upon "the conception of an imperative, whether that imperative get its sanction from the will of God, the dictates of reason, or the duty of securing the greatest happiness to the greatest number."

He then claims that the idea of duty has no solid foundation, the existence of God who has definitely legislated and the right of the majority to command are both hypothetical. What then? "But if man has been cut off from all possibility of guidance from without there remains within the possibility of making a choice, and to live morally is merely to exercise in full consciousness the possibility of that choice."

Is he moral regardless of his *choice*? This is the growing conception. Can we have no *imperatives* based on natural law? Away with imperatives! We want to have our fling! To Hell with your natural laws! A pill will settle with them! Or a serum or vaccine will guard us from their operations.

What Charles Brandt calls the Vital imperatives which are based on what he calls the *law of the conservation of life,* (The Vital Problem, 1924) are not fictions, and the prophets and apostles of moral and hygienic nihilism and anarchy would do well to consider these things.

There still remain lines over which we cannot step with safety. Despite the cant of the moral nihilists the law of gravitation still operates and the laws of life are equally as inexorable and eternal. Virtue is still higher than vice, cleanliness than nastiness. Love and fidelity are still higher than lust and adultery. Purity and modesty are graces of the soul that no false philosophy can turn into shame. Men and women may mock at these, as indeed they do, but when impurity and brazenness take their place, and they are rapidly doing this, we will not escape the scorching fires of retribution. Theft cannot become honorable and honest and murder cannot be exalted into a virtue. Even the murder of war, and by the state, does great violence to the state and nation—violating its maternal instincts, hardening its character and debauching its youth. The times may change, but the pillars of the universe remain as adamant.

> "In vain we call old notions fudge,
> And bend our conscience to our dealing;
> The Ten Commandments will not budge,
> And stealing still continues stealing."

Man can choose as he always has—but he will have to pay if he chooses wrongly. Were this no so the power of choice would be meaningless. "I have set before thee, *life and death, blessings and curses—choose life that ye may live.*"

Along with this *delusion of cure* and, indeed, forming a part of it, is the *delusion of relief.* This idea is that the conscious and recognized suffering and discomfort that accompanies the results of body abuses can be palliated and suppressed, so that the sufferer is not aware of his suffering, until the work of cure is complete. The greater part of the practices of all schools of "healing" are efforts to give the sufferer relief. This has been so since long before I-em Hetep, the earliest known physician, came on the scene. So intelligent a physician as James J. Walsh, M.D., Ph.D., Sc.D., says: "International Clinics," Vol. 8, Series 33:

"It has been pointed out that nature herself seems to have indicated one very successful and enduring remedy for pain from the earliest days, for the poppy grew amidst the wheat almost by preference, and the staff of life and the solace for pain were thus placed together."

Of course, Dr. Walsh does not believe that all the weeds, flowers and grasses that grow in the wheat fields of the world are indicated by nature, as solaces for the relief of pain or as cures for disease. His machinery of logic only slipped a cog when he penned those lines in dealing with the "Therapeutics of Pain." If he had reminded his colleagues of the disciplinary office of pain, of the fact that it does not exist without cause, and ceases following correction of cause, he might, then, have pleaded with them to cease making drug addicts. Instead of this, he says:

"Probably nothing brings a doctor more reputation, ceratinly nothing gives him a place of importance sooner in the regard of patients than the ability to relieve pain. At the same time there is nothing that affords the physician himself more satisfaction than to be able to lift a burden of discomfort that perhaps has made his patient miserable for a prolonged period and secure him such grateful relief as makes life worth living again. It is by the relief of pain, particularly, that physicians have commended themselves to the consideration of mankind all down the ages and in any review of the therapeutics of pain it must not be forgotten that from very early times men have succeeded in finding various remedies for pain and many of them have been very effective and are part of the precious heritage of knowledge from centuries or even milleniums ago."

If only this "precious heritage of knowledge" of "very effective" "various remedies for pain" could be let slip gently over the precipice into oblivion and permitted to remain there with I-em-Hetep and Aesculapius, the human race would be a thousand fold more healthy. What matters the doctors' "reputation" or "satisfaction" or "importance" or the "regard of patients," or whether he can "commend" himself to his patients? These things, as Solomon would have said, are vanity. "Vanity and vexation of spirit!" Yet human life has been, all down the ages, and yet is being, sacrificed to them.

Relief of pain! How? *By methods that do everything else than correct cause! But methods which often produce worse pains than those they relieve, or that are the cause of the very pains they relieve.* Who does not know that the poppy that grows with the wheat produces worse pains than those it is given to relieve? Who does not know that it relieves the pains it produces only to make these worse? Who does not know that coffee will relieve the headache it has caused? Or, that tobacco will steady the nerves it has unsteadied? And by steadying them makes them more unsteady than ever. And yet, all one requires to be permanently rid of the pains of opium or coffee or the uneasiness of tobacco is to refrain from the use of these long enough for the body to repair the damages they have created.

"There is something like charm," wrote Dr. Trall," in the idea of sending down the sick person's throat a dose which silences his pains and quiets his distress with magical celerity. But the charm is at once dispelled when we look to ultimate consequences. The very pain which the potent and ill-advised dose of the doctor has subdued is generally (always) the warning voice of the organic instincts that something is wrong, or the effort of the organism to rid itself of an enemy. When the organic instincts proclaim to the whole domain of life, through the medium of the brain that an enemy is present, that proclamation is felt, not heard, and its language is pain. It is one thing to silence the outcry of nature for help, but it is quite another thing to relieve her by dislodging the enemy." *Hydrophtic Encyclopedia,* Vol. 3, p. 11.

Can it not be seen that the relief of pain by such methods does not correct or remove the causes or conditions that produce the pain? Can it not be seen that by the very action through which such methods relieve pain, they also interfere with the functions and processes of the body and impede its own curative work? Where is there an intelligent man who cannot understand that such methods not only retard recovery and do not afford any true relief, but that they stand in the sufferer's and the doctor's light, obscuring the sufferer's true condition and preventing the doctor from discovering what is causing the trouble?

A patient has a sour stomach due to overeating. The doctor gives him soda. This "relieves" him and enables him to eat again. Except for the "relief" he would be forced to fast or eat less and the trouble would be corrected.

A patient suffers with pain. Every time he eats the pain increases. The pain inhibits secretion and impairs digestion. The result of eating under such conditions is more cause of pain. The physician "relieves" the pain (sandbags the nerves), the patient takes a meal and is not conscious of his suffering. Both he and the physician are satisfied. This method of "relief" continues until there comes a "sudden" break. The physician is surprised. So is the patient, his relatives and friends. They all thought he was doing so splendidly. The truth is, he was being slowly and insiduously undermined, but due to the fact that he had destroyed all of Nature's warning signals, neither he nor the physician knew what was going on. His fancied relief enabled him to continue those very practices that were responsible for the pain.

If his pain had not been "relieved" Nature would soon have forced him to stop eating long enough for her to repair the condition. "Relief" prevented him from learning one of nature's great health truths. Our "precious heritage" of antiquated ignorance has prevented us from knowing the truth. But man was always a lover of antiques as well as a worshiper of ancestors.

A patient complains of anorexia (lack of appetite)—as plain an indication as nature could possibly give that he should stop his food intake until further notice. The doctor gives him a tonic, perhaps an "aid to digestion," and advises him to "eat plenty of good nourishing foods," meaning by this, meat, eggs, white bread, potatoes, etc. This is good therapeutics, but it is poor hygiene. It produces greater trouble.

A man finds that every time he indulges in extra dissipation he is constipated. He is given a cathartic or an enema or a rectal dilation and this "relieves" him. Thinking he can substitute a pill or a powder or an enema or a dilator for decent behavior, he continues his dissipations and indulgences and enervating practices. "Relief" again prevents a true cure, prevents nature from forcing the sensualist to turn from his evil ways.

Every symptom would soon paint its origin if not "relieved" or suppressed with some form of therapeutics. If it were not for the "cures" nature would force us into Natural Hygiene and teach us how to live. Real cure is accomplished by the organism itself after cause has been corrected and is accomplished easiest and best without the interference of treatments.

A sick man has pain, fever, a rapid heart, diarrhea, etc. The doctor "relieves" the pain, reduces the temperature, slows up the heart action and checks the diarrhea. How? With drugs that force these conditions. What is then the true condition of his patient? Who knows? His present state is a forced semblance of healthy function. But cause has not been corrected. This is a dear bought "relief." It is paid for with increased and prolonged suffering, invalidism and premature death.

Are these things true only of "relief" secured by means of drugs? They are not. Drugless Methods, although usually not so harmful as drugs, also produce much harm by giving so-called "relief" and they also obscure the condition of the patient. Any method of relief that does not correct cause is evil.

The late Dr. Henry Lindlahr used to say: "Suppressed pains are deferred pains." He had reference only to pains suppressed by drugs. The doctor had the unhappy faculty of being able to state a principle in simple, terse language, and then applying it to a very limited extent. He never freed himself of the belief in *cure*. In fact I doubt whether he really understood many of the things he said and wrote, or whether he fully appreciated many of the principles he subscribed to verbally.

"Suppressed pains are deferred pains"—no matter how they are suppressed.

A patient suffered with intense pains in the "small" of her back. Heat and massage were given. These brought complete relief in ten minutes. But the relief was short lived. The pain came back with greater intensity.

A man suffered with a severe frontal headache. It lasted four days. He resorted to zone therapy for relief. As long as pressure was applied the ache was practically abolished. The instant the pressure was removed the pains returned with renewed force.

Neuropathy was next tried. Results were the same. Spondylotherapy was employed. Same results. Then hot baths were used. Results were identical. All these methods gave temporary relief but when the pains returned they came with renewed intensity, no true relief was secured.

A girl lay suffering with encephalitis (inflammation of the brain) and inflammation of the optic nerve. Pains were intense. Efforts to relieve her were made. Hydrotherapy and neuropathy were both employed. Each brought temporary relief. But when the pains returned they were much worse than before the "relief" was secured. *The period of increased intensity of pain was, each time, equal to the period of "relief. The girl was not saved any actual suffering.*

That pains are increased after morphine wears off is known by every one. But this fact is usually thought to apply to drugs only. The evidence that it applies to drugless methods, as well, continues to pile up.

Suppression *per se* is the same by whatever means secured. Nature rejects all plans of vicarious salvation. *Every effort to prevent an action from having its full reaction meets with defeat. Penalties cannot be side stepped by any means. Acts have their consequences. These cannot be avoided.*

It may be urged that by the constant application of measures for "relief" pain can be kept *suppressed* until Nature has time to effect a cure, after which no pains return when measures for relief are abandoned.

Is this true? Can it be true? In a narrow sense it is true, but in a large sense it is as false as we would expect it, on general philosophic principles, to be. What actually happens under such conditions is the prolongation of the period of the disease, if indeed, the patient is not killed outright, and the other sufferings of the patient prolonged and intensified. Recovery is not only delayed, *it is not so complete,* the patient is greatly weakened and his ultimate restoration to normal health is long drawn out. He is usually left with some sequalae or chronic after effect, from which he recovers, if ever, only after a long time has elapsed.

Outraged Nature demands the full payment of every debt against her. The law of compensation is one of strict justice. It rewards and punishes with the same exactitude. To return to full health after health has been impaired by wrong living, the full price must be paid.

If you have a bad habit, you must give it up. When you do this, Nature begins immediately to bring about physiological readjustment. Readjustment requires time and is accompanied by pain, want, lassitude, depression.

For instance, you use coffee until you become nervous and suffer with head-aches when deprived of the drug. If coffee is now given up, readjustment begins immediately. But you suffer from headache for a few days, nervousness is increased, you are irritable, depressed and miss your accustomed coffee.

You suffer in the same way when deprived of tobacco, alcohol, opium or other drugs. And the more poisonous is the action of the drug, the greater are your sufferings. The longer you have used the drugs, the more of the drug you are in the habit of using, the more you suffer before readjustment is complete.

The pains and sufferings endured by the opium addict, when he is deprived of his drug, are equal to anything in the conventional hell or purgatory. He becomes temporarily insane, perhaps, and in order to relieve his sufferings, will commit murder, theft or any other crime that may enable him to secure the drug.

Coffee will "cure" the headache and nervousness is causes. But only to perpet-uate and make them worse. Tobacco will "cure"' the nervousness and irritableness it causes, but only to prolong and intensify these. Opium will "cure" the pains and sufferings it causes, but only to perpetuate and double these. These things bring "relief," but it is a dear bought "relief." Such "relief" is paid for at terrible price.

Food inebriates—those who habitually gorge themselves with rich, stimulating and highly seasoned foods, suffer pains, weakness, lassitude, nervousness, irritableness, etc., when placed upon a fast or sensible diet. A return to the old diet and the old manner of eating will give "relief." It is the same kind of "relief" the coffee or opium gives to the coffee or opium addict. It is a dear bought relief.

A patient cannot sleep. A drug is given to induce "sleep." The patient goes to "sleep" immediately. It is not sleep. It is stupor. Upon awakening in the morning, such a patient finds his "sleep" has not been refreshing. It has not re-newed and reinvigorated him. He has not been prepared, by it, for more activity. His "relief" from sleeplessness was paid for at a great price.

A person gives up one form of stimulation. The true condition of his system then becomes manifest. He finds he is enervated, depleted, weak. He is nervous, depressed, irritable. He does not desire to return to the old stimulant. He resorts to another and supposedly less harmful one. This has the desired effect. He gets "relief." But he forms a "new" stimulant habit and is no better off than before.

Or, perhaps he attempts to "taper off" on his stimulant habit. He gradually reduces the amount of the drug taken. This does not decrease the suffering he will have to undergo in overcoming the habit—it but prolongs it. Instead of suffering for a week, he suffers for a month, or longer, and then, probably fails in his effort to free himself from the grip of the poison.

Tapering off is like cutting off a dog's tail an inch at a time until it is the desired length—or desired shortness. Cut off the tail and wait for this to heal, then cut it again and so on until you have cut it all you desire. This is the way tapering off works. It is best to cut out the stimulant at once. Pay the price all at once and have it over with.

A man suffers with constipation. He takes enemas, pills, wheat bran, etc., and forces the bowels to move. But this only makes his constipation worse. To wait upon Nature and correct the causes give true and permanent relief.

If you are suffering in any manner, it is better for you to *tough it out* rather than to resort to means for "relief." Correct the causes and leave the rest to Nature. Bear in mind that you must pay the full price and that there are no thaumaturgic nor theurgic methods that will give you a discount. All such means, instead of giving real relief only add to your suffering.

When you once realize that you reap what you sow, AND ALL YOU SOW, you will then cease the effort to sow and avoid reaping.

You will bear your sufferings with the fortitude of an Indian, and with the full realization that the best is being done that can be done for you.

Your fear of pain will then force you to avoid its causes.

When once you realize that the Law of Compensation demands that every outrage against the body must be paid for with a price equal to the outrage, you will cease the stupid practice of trying to "cure" your discomforts—you will cheerfully pay the price and enjoy the resulting good health.

Let me end this chapter with the following words of Dr. George S. Weger: "We shed crocodile tears in profusion while we accept soothing ministrations. These are not tears of repentance. They are tears of self-pity—meaning nothing. Many, throughout their lives, thus deceive themselves into the false belief that they are putting something over on God—on the law. They little reckon that their sins are finding them out. There is no security in a cheaply-purchased immunity. Forgiveness, pardon and parole are effective only for those who 'go and sin no more'."

CRITICISM OF THE HYPOTHESIS OF THERAPEUTICS

Chapter XXXVII

PRIMITIVE man's reaction to disease was essentially one of intense fear and dread. He did not understand it. He did not know its causes nor its ends. He only knew that he was uncomfortable and that the suffered, even died. He quite naturally regarded disease as an enemy, an unseen enemy, bent upon torturing and destroying him. He early developed the idea that disease was an evil spirit or demon, an invisible, intangible enemy, that came out of the unknown and settled within his body to torture and destroy.

With this idea of disease as a premise primitive man built up his methods of combatting disease. He attempted to drive away the unseen and voracious monster that was eating at his vitals. If disease "settled" in his arm he mutilated the arm in an effort to destroy the disease. If the disease took up its abode in the interior of the trunk he filled himself with vile, bitter, nauseous and poisonous witch-broths and concoctions to drive the evil spirit out. His idea was that if by any weapon, poison, fire, violence, force, etc., he could make things unpleasant for the disease it would depart.

This was the origin of the belief in cure. All the ideas and theories of cure that have come into existence since, and all the therapeutic practices which have had or do now have their vogue have been and are built upon this strange misconception of the nature, cause and purpose of disease. Primitive man, unable to comprehend or explain the phenomena of disease, built up for the race an inheritance of fear and misunderstanding which has been the foundation of much suffering and evil. Not only has modern science failed to dispel this fear and misunderstanding, but much of what is now called science is actually based upon it. It is really difficult to overestimate the importance of this "fear reaction" and "cure complex" in our daily habits and in our intellectual life.

The idea that somewhere God had provided a remedy for every disease was developed early. Man's task was simply to find that remedy. As James J. Walsh, M.D., Ph.D., Sc.D., says in his CURES—The Story of the Cures that Fail:

"Men started out with the idea that while a beneficent Providence has permitted disease, he has created all around mankind the means of curing those diseases if only man would bestir himself and find out what they were. As a result of this impression every kind of material under the sun has been used for the cure of human ailments and practically all of them with reported good success, at least at the beginning. Every plant and herb and root has been treated in various ways to extract its healing qualities. Practically every animal product that we know, including the excretions and the very vermin that live on the animals, have been used as remedies. The mineral kingdom has been placed under similar contribution and always 'cures' have been reported from everything. Very often combinations of drugs were announced as proving so much more efficacious than the simple drug materials of which they were composed. Mankind has gone right on finding new remedies and working wonders with them and patients have announced themselves as *cured* by all sorts of materials, and then after a time further experience has shown that ninety-nine out of every hundred or more of these valued drugs have proved to be absolutely useless or even slightly harmful."

An old French physician once observed that the therapeutics of any generation are always absurd to the next. But why? Not because the next generation has cast off its belief in cure. Not because it has any better therapeutics. It may have worse. For, as Dr. Trall remarked:

"The ancient priests and monks placed their patients in airy, salubrious situations, enjoined strict abstemiousness or the simplest food, gave water for drink, and prescribed efficient washing or bathing for thorough cleanliness, and then performed their magical ceremonies. Their patients recovered; Nature worked the cure, and the doctor got the credit." (Also, the cash.) ..Hydropathic Encyclopedia, Vol. 1, PP. 52.

"The diligent student of medical history cannot fail to discover that the ancient and more ignorant practitioners were more successful in curing diseases than are the modern and wiser physicians. The remedial agents of the ancients were comparatively inert and comparatively harmless, and, while they inspired their patients with a due degree of confidence and hope by the charms and ceremonials of magic and mystery, they really relied on judicious hygienic regulations to 'aid and assist Nature' in effecting the cure. Modern intelligence repudiates the arts and incantations of a less civilized age; and in their stead has substituted the stronger potencies of modern invention, while the habits of living and thinking, with medical as with other men, have become so unnatural and artificial that, in managing diseases, voluntary habits and hygienic agencies are almost wholly overlooked."—*Hydropathic Encyclopedia,* Vol 1, PP. 34.

Fashions and fads in therapeutics change as rapidly as styles in women's clothes but the underlying basis of therapeutics, the misconceptions of disease and the belief in cure, remains always the same. Schools of healing have risen, flourished for a time and passed away. We usually speak of the so-called regular school as being three thousand years old. It is scarcely a hundred years old. The history of medicine has always been a history of rival schools which rose and fell on the ocean of time as the foam on the troubled waters of the Atlantic. Each school or cult drew from the other, each age nursed at the breasts of those that preceded, until finally, out of this mass of superstition, fallacy, error, and ignorance what is called "regular" medicine was born. It has evolved from chaos and, since it cannot rise higher than its source, is chaotic still.

The schools have been legion, but all of them have been the same fundamentally. They have all been Heteropathic and have all sought for cures for diseases. As Dr. Walsh so cleverly remarks:

"All down the centuries we have had all sorts of means for the cure of disease. They have come and gone. Nearly every substance on the earth or from under the earth or the heavens above has been used as a vaunted cure and has succeeded in a certain number of cases. Nearly every kind of persuasion, psychological, metaphysical, religious, superstitious, scientific, and, above all, pseudo-scientific, has been used efficaciously in the same way."

"Cures" were effected by all these things. Every cult and every method has been backed up by a record of thousands of marvelous cures which it has accomplished. Everything has appeared to cure, at least, so long as it was in vogue. But the principles laid down in this book clearly show why cured cases form a very slippery foundation upon which to build a system and a philosophy of therapeutics. Every school has cried, "RESULTS ARE WHAT COUNT, and here are our results." But RESULTS are not enough. We must show that the RESULTS were produced by our methods and not by the inherent forces of the organism working independently of art and perhaps being hindered by art. Every new method which appeared to cure led men to believe that some great new discovery had been made, some new principle uncovered, some new force set to work. Some great new curative agent had been placed into the hands of mankind. But disillusionment has followed disillusionment as time and investigation have shown that the vaunted "cure" not only did not produce cures, but could not do so.

It is manifestly impossible to reconcile the theories and practices of the antagonistic systems of medicine. If the large, heroic doses of poisons of Allopathy have any reason or truth on their side, then the highly attenuated and diluted doses of Homeopathy are worse than a fraud and delusion. If Homeopathy succeeds as well or better than Allopathy, this success would prove that the damaging and dangerous poisons of Allopathy are unnnecessary and should be abandoned. If the theory of health, disease and cure we are advocating in these pages is correct, there is no value in either of these systems and they are both attributing cures to their respective remedies that were accomplished by the unaided powers of the body. Both schools are deluded. If we are correct Homeopathy should be the most successful system because it is the least harmful. It does not *cure* more, it only kills less.

If the drugs of Allopathy and Homeopathy have any truth on their side all patients cared for by mental scientists and Christian Scientists should die. But if the success of the latter is as great or greater than that of the former, the drugs of neither are needed. If either of these systems are correct the Chiropractors are wrong, whereas if Chiropractic is correct all the others are wrong and are murdering their patients. Thus we might go through the whole list of modern and ancient medical cults and find the same thing.

The facts are that patients recover under all these systems and more recover under the less obstructive ones. The cure is accomplished by the inherent, ever-active powers of life and not by the "remedies" and mummery.

That people recover goes without saying. People have always recovered from disease. In all ages of the world, in all ranks of society, under all conditions of life and in the most serious diseases. By far a larger number of people have always recovered from disease than died. It does not matter with what they were treated, or that they were not treated at all, most cases of disease recover; even where the treatment was of the most crucifying kind they recovered.

One of the best attested facts of medical history is the fact that the human organism has demonstrated its ability to overcome morbid influences in spite of treatment and conditions that were positively obstructive; yes, even murderous! Imagine a patient suffering from typhoid fever being kept in an almost hermetically sealed room, smothered in blankets, allowed no water to drink, stuffed with milk and brandy, drugged with calomel, blue mass antimony and bled regularly. Was any treatment ever designed more destructive, more murderous? Yet within the lifetime of many now living this was the approved allopathic treatment of fever. Not a thing was done that could have been of any advantage to the patient in recovery; but, on the contrary, every single measure mentioned above was calculated to shorten the patient's life. In spite of it all a majority of such patients recovered. This but demonstrates the fighting powers possessed by the human organism.

There is an unfailing tendency on the part of the living organism towards health. The inherent effort of the system to preserve its structural and functional integrity and its never ceasing efforts to resist, overcome and throw off any and all morbid influences which may be brought to bear upon it assures us that a system that is properly organized and possessed of sound functions, will be able to promptly and completely, and unaided by any external influences whatsoever, oversome and throw off all morbid influences unless these are so virulent or in such overwhelming quantity that they destroy life at once. Health is maintained and the injurious action of disease producing influences overcome by the silent, unconscious but every active powers of defense and self-preservation of the body. Disease influences if these are sufficient to cause disease, are thrown off and normal health reestablished by the same silent forces, even in the face of crucifying treatment.

The following quotations from the works of Dr. Edward Hooker Dewey who was trained by the University of Michigan to believe that drugs cure disease and who served his internship in the U. S. Marine Hospital, at Detroit, Mich., then entered one of the Large Army Hospitals in Chattanooga, Tenn., at the beginning of Sherman's campaign in Georgia, will serve to show how patients recover in spite of obstructive and destructive treatment.

"As my experience enlarged so did my faith in Nature; and, since there was no similarity in the quality, sizes, and times of the doses for like diseases, my faith in mere remedies gradually declined."—The Fasting Cure.

"It had not escaped my notice, even before I began the study of medicine, that whether diseases were coaxed with doses too small for mathematical estimate, or whether blown out with solid shot or blown up with shells, the percentage of recoveries seemed to be about the same regardless of the form of treatment."—Fasting Cure.

"The features of my hospital service that impressed me most were the post-mortem revelations and the diverse treatments for the same disease. I soon found that, no matter what the disease, every surgeon was a law unto himself as to the quality, quantity, and times of his doses, with the mortality in the wards apparently about the same."—Fasting Cure.

"Most of the cases of disease that fall to the care of the physician are trivial, self-limited, and rapidly recover under even the most crucifying dosages; Nature really winning the victories, the physician carrying off the honors.

"This is so nearly true that it may be stated that, aside from the domain of surgery, professional success in the general sense depends upon the personal qualities and character of the physician rather than the achievements of the materia medica.

"People have a confidence in the power of medicine to cure disease scarcely less than the dusky warrior has in the Indian medicine-lodge of the Western wilderness, and a confidence about as void of reason.

"The physician goes into the rooms of the sick held to the severest accountability in the matter of dosage; and the larger his own faith in medicines the greater his task; and, if he is of my own, the so-called 'old school,' or Allopathic, the more dangerous he is to the curing efforts of nature."—*Fasting Cure.*

"I now see, as I did not then so clearly, that Nature's victories are often won against the desperate odds of treatments that are simply barbarious; and yet Nature is so powerful, so persistent in the attempts to right all her wrongs, that she wins the victory in the great majority of cases no matter how severely she may be taxed with means that hinder. The great majority of the severely sick of a hundred years ago recovered in spite of the bloody lancet and treatments that are the barbarism of today."—*Fasting Cure.*

"Cures" of all kinds have apparently won a remarkable success, in all parts of the world. However, they cured in about the same way the noise of the savage saves the sun in an eclipse. Here I am reminded of Cushman's remark about this latter cure. The Choctaws believed an eclipse was caused by a little black squirrel devouring the sun. They could save this heavenly body only by making a loud noise and thereby scaring the little gormandizer away. Cushman says he was more than once an eye witness to these performances and that he can testify from experience as to the virtue of the "music' then adds: "At least the sun came out all right."

The reader will get my meaning—the Indians "cured" an eclipse of the sun with a loud noise—their experience proved to them that the noise did the work. They mistook a mere coincidence for cause and erected their system of cure upon an apparent fact, just as systems for curing the sick human body have all been erected on appearances—coincidences. If a "remedy" is used coincident with recovery, the "remedy" receives credit for the cure. Those who understand the process and power of cure, know that the body cured itself and that the remedy had no more to do with the recovery than the Indians loud noise had to do with the sun's recovery. Verily, therapeutics is a heathen god.

In all ages recovery from disease under any form of treatment has been regarded as proof of the curative virtue of that form of treatment. Patients and physicians were deceived by appearances. Mere coincidences were mistaken for causes and effects. Cures that were accomplished in spite of "remedies" were attributed to the "remedies" because men did not know and did not understand the essential nature of disease and its essentially evanescent character. "An examination," says Dr. Emmet Densmore, *How Nature Cures,* P. 9, "of the methods of operation of orthodox old-school medicine shows that these physicians, although able, learned, earnest and scientific, have been utterly misled as to the nature of disease. They have considered disease an organized enemy and positive force, which has taken up a position within the body and is carrying on a warfare with the vital powers; and the legion of heroic remedies (so-called) which orthodox physicians have prescribed and are prescribing for suffering invalids are the shot and shell hurled at the invisible enemy, in the hope of dislodging and expelling it. Not understanding the law of cure—that there is always coincident with life a tendency toward health—these well-meaning physicians have accepted a recovery made in spite of their medicines as the result of their (so-called) remedies." Again, Pages 11 and 12; "And this failure, alike on the part of the physician and patient, to understand that all illness and pain is only an effort on the part of Nature to rid the system of disease, and that a tendency toward recovery and health is an inseparable part of life, explains why it is that for generations and for ages there has been a constant change in methods of doctoring, coincident with an undying faith in the efficacy of the doctor and his methods. A patient is taken ill, a doctor is called, and in a great majority of cases the patient recovers; superficially the sending for the doctor seems to have been wise. Upon reflection it will be seen that fetishism has the same justification for existence. Some wooden god is cringingly approached by the friends of a sick man, or the services of the 'medicine man' secured on his behalf, and as these methods are often merely ceremonial, and appeal rather to the imagination than to the stomach, and so give the system time for curative action, wonderful cures are of course the result. Only a few score of years ago bleeding was the orthodox fetish."

Is not the doctor a fetish? Are not his "remedies" mere fetishes? Does he not secure his cures in precisely the same manner that the Indians saved the sun when it was eclipsed? Trall quotes the medical historian, Bostock, as saying:

"In modern times and more remarkably in Great Britain, no one thinks of proposing a new mode of practice without supporting it by the results of practical experience. The disease exists, the remedy is prescribed, and the disease is removed; we have no reason to doubt the veracity or the ability of the narrator; his favorable report induces his contemporaries to pursue the same means of cure; the same favorable result is obtained and it appears impossible for any fact to be supported by more decisive testimony. Yet in the space of a few short years the boasted remedy has lost its virtue; the disease no longer yields to its power while its place is supplied by some new remedy, which, like its predecessor, runs through the same career of expectation, success, and disappointment."

A few months ago the *British Medical Journal* declared: "Remedies and modes of treatment, like systems of philosophy and fashions in dress, have their little day and cease to be. Back numbers (of the Journal) are the graveyard of dead theories."

President Jefferson once wrote a letter to Dr. Wistar in which he said: "I have lived to see the disciples of Hoffman, Borhaave, Cullen and Brown succeed one another like the shifting figures of a magic lantern; and their fancies like the dresses of the annual doll babies from Paris, becoming from their novelty, the vogue of the day, and yielding to the next novelty, their ephemeral favors. The patient treated on the fashionable theory sometimes recovers in spite of their medicine, the medicine, therefore, restores him, and the doctor receives new courage to proceed in his experiments on the lives of his fellow creatures."

Of similar import are the following words from Bichat:

"To what errors have not mankind been led in the employment and denomination of medicines! They created *deobstruents*, when the theory of *obstruction* was in fashion; and *incisives* when that of the *thickening* of humors prevailed. The expressions *diluents* and *attenuants* were common before this period. When it was necessary to blunt the acrid particles, they created *inviscants, incrassants*, etc. Those who saw in a disease only a *relaxation* or *tension* of fibers, as they called it, employed *astringents* and *relaxants*. *Refrigerants* and *heating* remedies were brought into use by those who had a special regard in disease to an *excess* or *deficiency* of *caloric*. The same *identical* remedies have been employed under *different names*, according to the *manner* in which they were supposed to act; *deobstruent in one case, relaxant* in another, *refrigerant* in another, the *same* medicine has been employed with all the opposite views.

"Hence the *vagueness* and *uncertainty* our science presents at this day. An incoherent assemblage of incoherent opinions, it is, perhaps, of all the physiological sciences, that which best shows the caprice of the human mind. What do I say? It is not a science for a methodical mind. It is a shapeless assemblage of inaccurate ideas, of observations often puerile; and of formula as fantastically conceived as they are tediously arranged."

Medicine has been a ceaseless round of changing theories and practices throughout the ages. But through it all, the sick have recovered. Thousands of different materials and means have been employed by physicians and many thousands of these are still listed in the official list of drugs. It is, however, generally admitted by medical authorities that there are only a handful of valuable drugs. It is a strange thing that the "useful" drugs are about the most deadly they possess—mercury, arsenic, quinine, opium and a few others.

Every generation has developed new drugs and discarded or "improved" old ones. All of them have been more or less harmful, many of them very much so, but they all appeared to cure in thousands of cases.

For thousands of years, bleeding was almost a panacea. The rivers of the world ran with blood spilled by the physicians. They spilled more blood than war and wild beast. It was an ingenuous practice. The practitioner had to know just where to bleed for each disease. He had to know on what days to bleed and not to bleed. The phases of the moon, position of the stars and many other elements of astrology had to be considered. The practice was much like the system of acupuncture which has "cured" millions in China during the past three to four thousand years. This is a system of sticking needles into the body to chase the demons of disease out. The acupuncturer must know at just what point on the body to insert his needle for each disease.

George Washington, in his last illness, was relieved in the short space of fifteen to twenty hours, of eighty to ninety ounces of blood. Blood-letting was the remedy for all your ills just as tonsilectomy, appendectomy, de-dention, endocrine therapy, pus squirting are now cures for every ill and just as ovarectomy was the cure for all of woman's ills a few years ago.

Shortly after Washington's death, a British author, Prof. Reid of Edinburgh, Scotland, publicly declared that he was trebly killed; that he was bled enough alone to have caused his death and that he took enough of antimony and calomel for either of these alone to have killed him outright, had no other medication been resorted to. Think of giving him ten grains of calomel at a single dose! But this is a small dose compared to some given in those days of heroic dosage. Salivation was the rule and, to quote Dr. Walsh, "a great many patients must have been seriously injured and their powers of resistance to disease greatly impaired or even their chances for recovery nullified by this purgation."

Well, I should say so too. But the fact remains that in the face of such crucifying treatment, a great majority of cases of all diseases recovered. If such results had not apparently followed this dosage and bleeding, the human race, the "civilized" portion, at least, would either have perished, or they would have crucified the doctors. The results, as they were, were bad enough that homeopathy, physiomedacilism and the water cure easily forced a reform in medical dosage, after which they each declined and bid fair soon to be remembered only as interesting bits of medical history.

Antimony, a drastic purgative, was, perhaps, as popular as calomel in these heroic days and was administered in equally large doses. Everybody was dosed with it; most of them recovered.

Returning now to bleeding, Dr. Walsh says:

"Washington is said to have died of diphtheria or cyanache as they called it then, but anyone who reads the account of his treatment will be inclined to think that the physician who bled him so freely had at least a hand in the death."

In describing the bleeding received by Mirabeau, who was robbed of nearly a hundred ounces of life's precious fluid in forty-eight hours, to cure his angina pectoris, Dr. Walsh says:

"Some from the left arm where the pain was, some from the right area because it was the opposite side of the body and might prove derivative, some from the foot on the left side, because that side seemed most affected, and then a little later some from the right foot because that was farthest from the heart where the pain was complained of and it was hoped that the pain might be attracted in that direction."

Was there ever seen such a grotesque and comical effort to cure as this indulged in by the educated members of Scientific Medicine? Well, gentle reader, this was the approved orthodox practice of the time and only quacks and cultists disapproved of it, and these were not licensed to practice.

One doctor in Louisiana wrote to a medical journal (a few years ago) that, "during an epidemic of yellow fever he drew enough blood to float the steamer General Jackson, and gave calomel enough to freight it."—Physio-medicalism, J. S. Thomas M. D., 1870.

Seventy and eighty years ago medical men were divided, as now, over the nature of inflammation. One portion of the profession held that it consists essentially in an increased action of the capillary vessels of that part which is the seat of it; the other portion holding that it consists in diminished actions of the same vessels. To most of us it would seem that these two theories were distinctive enough to call for different plans of treatment. But not so to the physicians of that time. Whichever theory the physicians accepted, the treatment was the same. If a patient suffered with some inflammatory disorder and this was accompanied with a full strong pulse, they said, "bleed, because it reduces the strength of the system, and abates the force of the arterial action." If another had inflammation of the same part with a weak, frequent, oppressed pulse, they said: "bleed, because it strengthens the vessels by taking off a part of the load which they have to carry." Whatever the condition of the patient he was bled. And most of them recovered. Every physician could point to a long list of "cured" patients and the population of the country continued to increase. More blood has been shed in America for the cure of disease than has been shed in all her wars and some of the old fellows who used to go regularly each spring to their physicians or to their barbers for a bleeding, are still alive to tell us about it.

But if opposite theories of the nature of inflammation both led to bleeding, so did they both lead to stimulation. Those on the side of increased action said, stimulate, "Because the action of the capillaries has been preternaturally augmented, and we must let the action down gradually, by applying stimulants of less intensity than the proximate causes of the diseased action," while those on the side of diminished action said, "Give stimulants, because the action of the capillaries has been preternaturally diminished, and thus excite them to greater action."

Neither on the depleting plan, nor the stimulating plan, did the theory and the practice have anything to do with each other. Whether they stimulated or depleted or both it was to correct "wrong action" and not to correct cause. It reminds us very much of the words of Trall in discussing the revival of the Hippocratean doctrines during the seventeenth century and the simultaneous advances made in the knowledge of human anatomy:

"Although the discoveries alluded to in anatomy had turned the attention of medical men more to vital actions, as affording a better explanation of the phenomena of disease, than chemical changes, and had generally restored the humoral pathology of Hippocrates, the practice of medicine did not undergo a corresponding change. The Anatomists were anxious of course to have their pharmacopœia include 'all modern improvements', hence they pursued a mixed or compound practice, by adding the mercury, antimony and opium of Paracelsus, and other drugs of more recent production to the bleeding, purging, sweating, etc., of the earlier physicians. In fact they incorporated nearly all that was known of a poisonous or destructive nature among their therapeutical agents, and omitted nearly all that was really worth preserving—attention to regimen, bathing, cleanliness, etc."—*Enc. or Hydrotherapy*, PP. 23-4.

Theirs was a spirit such as prevailed during the dominancy of the Arabian school during the 8th to 12th centuries as pictured by Trall: "The spirit of the age, then, among those eminent in the profession—not unlike the spirit of the present day—was that of emulation in writing the greatest number of books, and finding out new substances which could be taken into the stomach and applied externally, and called medicines."

There are, today, many who are anxious to include "all the modern improvements" in their armamentarium and who pursue a "mixed practice" and are continually searching for some new method or appliance that can be called a remedy. For some time, I have noticed that this spirit exists, even, among the non-allopathic schools. And they often remind me very much of the bleeding and stimulation practices in inflammation so much in vogue during the middle of the last century. The most contradictory conclusions are often deduced from the most opposite premises. Practice often bears no relation to theory. I will point to just one of these contradictions. Some hold that disease is due to subluxations in the spinal column and attempt to adjust these in order to cure. Others hold that disease is due to unnatural living. These also attempt to cure the trouble by attempted adjustments of the spinal segments. Just what relation spinal adjustment has to unnatural living is not clear.

Instead of making a study of the laws, conditions and requirements of life and complying with these the human race has for ages sought for some magic power, some occult and incomprehensible principle, some hitherto inoperative law or force, that will set aside the known laws of life and enable man to destroy law and order with impunity.

500

The ancient alchemist sought for a philosopher's stone which would enable them to transmute the baser metals into gold and an *elixir vitae* that would enable them to live perpetually. The modern scientist seeks for some sort of a philosopher's law that will enable him to transmute one species into another and for some gland extract or serum or vaccine or vibration that will enable him to eradicate disease and death.

The new hypotheses in physics regarding the nature and structure of matter have caused many to seek for cures in the field of what they term vibrations. Apparently, they think that the laws and forces governing the atoms and electrons are different to those governing the aggregate of atoms composing a stone or clod, and that if they can discover this law or force they can use it to smash all other laws and thus accomplish what the alchemist failed at. Of course, it is absurd to think that the laws of the infinitesimal differ from those of the great or that one law can be made to smash another.

When we have learned all that it is possible to learn about matter, motion and force and the laws that control these, we will find physiology doing her work at the same old stand, in the same old way, by the same old laws—the laws of life; its conditions and requirements will not have changed. It will still be necessary that we obey and fulfill these and if we do this, there will be no reason to seek for other means by which to restore or maintain health.

Dr. Flint once gave a golden rule whereby to judge of the relative, if not also the intrinsic merits of different therapeutic methods. He said: "The superiority of a method is shown by a *larger* number of recoveries, and by an average *duration* in a series of cases treated one way than in another series of cases treated otherwise." At first glance this rule looks good, and yet, Dr. Flint, himself, showed that the difficulties and fallacies besetting this rule are such, and so great, as for scientific purposes to render it valueless.

"No two series of cases," he said, "are in all particulars, exactly alike; and cases differ in the degree of severity and extent of diseases, in the constitutional condition of patients, in the existence or absence of complications, and in a great variety of circumstances pertaining to season, climate, age, habits, etc."

The lessons we derive from pure empirical *experience* in the treatment of disease must, in the very nature of things, be more or less uncertain and fallacious. Harvey (*First Lines of Therapeutics*), in discussing Cullen's objection to the *vis medicatrix*, says: "But what would Cullen have said, had he lived to see it done, in view of pneumonia being treated, and successfully treated, under three widely different and indeed opposite systems, so successfully as would have made it impossible even for him to determine which is the best? Would not the introduction of the *Vis Medicatrix* have tided him over this obscurity,—have helped him to explain the equality of results? For, on no other footing can we account for that equality. In the case of a broken bone, the agency of that power must needs be admitted. Why not in the case of pneumonia?"

Again, he says: "Too much is ignorantly claimed for art. And thus, while Nature is the real healer, two diametrically opposite remedies, or systems of treatment, may each of them have the most confident claims advanced in its behalf—and on the supposed sure ground of experience.

"What M. Gubler says is true. And God be thanked that it is so. Were it otherwise—were mankind directly beholden to our art for the cure of disease, sad were our lot; sad it would be for the earlier patients of the most distinguished of our young physicians and surgeons, and until experience had given them adequate skill. And the fact that his position is a sound one is a comforting consideration for one who feels strongly, as I do, the neglect of the study of natural therapeutics. The profession will continue to differ and to dispute about remedies and cures, and to appeal confidently to the criterion of experience. But Nature will continue to hold her ground, and (laughing in her sleeve) to cure even under the most opposite kinds of treatment,—and as regards many diseases with results that shall be inappreciably identical—statistically the same. In inflammatory disease, Dr. Ambercrombie bled freely. Dr. Todd spared the blood and poured in wine and brandy. Dr. Hughes Bennett gave his patients beef tea and neither bled nor brandied. Dr. Cullen says (as we have seen) that wherever the *vis medicatrix* is admitted, it throws obscurity on our system. In the case just now in view, does it not rather throw light upon it, and enable us to understand how under systems so opposite, the results should be so satisfactory? The essential factor here is surely the Vis Medicatrix—the organism 'qui se guerit lui-meme'."

"Take another case," says Harvey, "one of a kind of daily occurrences. We shall have Nature working her way towards the cure of a particular disease; and we shall have Art in the person of five or six different physicians, treat that same disease in as many different ways, some of diametrically opposite ways—one of the physicians however treating it with placebos alone or by regimen only—virtually doing nothing. Let the case supposed be the Acute Rheumatism, or Rheumatic Fever. The result, we shall assume, is the same, or it is inappreciably the same under each. Recovery follows in all the cases, and is alike satisfactory in all of them. And this experience (experiment) may be appealed to, and confidently appealed to, in behalf of each method of treatment. But what as to their respective merits—for they cannot all of them have been equally beneficial? And what as to the respective shares of Nature and Art in the cure? Here we have two large questions to solve if solve them we can. As to the first, the respective merit of the severals modes of treatment, how can it, in the circumstances, be determined? For in each and all of the Modes, Nature has been at work,—silently it is true. And what if Nature has secretly been counteracting wrong doing in one or more of the modes,—and putting this (seemingly) on a level with the right doing of others?"

Let our therapeutic advocates ponder these questions and make reply. The case now put before theem is being enacted every day in a hundred different forms. But don't, I beg you, say that when a broken bone heals without therapeutics, it was only an imaginary break or that it healed due to the influence of ineffectual treatment on the mind. For once, be honest, and admit that Nature heals.

Bostock declared that Cullen did more than any of his contemporaries to sweep away the rubbish of antiquity. Harvey says of the state of medicine immediately preceding and during Cullen's lifetime: "But as to large numbers of the people in this country (England) and over wide districts of it,—especially in Scotland they must to a great extent have been as destitute of medical men as of roads and many other of the conveniences of life,—and when sick left in a great measure to the unaided powers of Nature. It may be questioned whether in the '45, Prince Charles had a medical man attached to his army. He himself had, I believe, a body physician from this county of Aberdeen. But how as to his brave followers? And how, as to this, did the army of the Duke of Cumberland fare?" He then tells us that the great majority of the sick in those days were left in the hands of barbers, farriers, butchers (he is not speaking of surgeons), blacksmiths, mechanics, artificers, farmers, grooms, and "old women reputed sagacious and skilled." What were their remedies? "They comprised among other things familiarly known, such things as snails, the web of the spider, the powder of dead men's skulls, men's own urine, besides an infinity of herbs." Added to this practice, which he says "was largely futile and feeble" were drastic purgatives and copious bleedings.

Would those who contend that all apparent cures by ineffective means are cures of imaginary diseases, hysteria, have us believe that all who recovered under such a practice or under no practice, and under the most filthy and unhygienic conditions conceivable, as then prevailed, were only possessed of imaginary diseases? Can it be possible that none of the many thousands who recovered of diseases then presented any physical signs that could be seen? In other words, didn't people get sick in those days, or if they did, did all truly sick people die?

Commenting upon King David's statement in the 103rd Psalm: "It is God that healeth all diseases," Harvey says: "That is, as we should say, (speaking reverently) it is Nature, the ordinance of God, that healeth our diseases. Whatever may have been the precise idea in David's mind, we may fairly take it in a figurative sense, and regard the expression of it as of the same general import with the Hippocratic Vis, both expressions having their root in the fact obvious to all, and known to all, that diseases are often cured independently of Art. David, we read, 'died in a good old age.' We cannot but imagine that the circumstances of his reign, and the surroundings of his life, must often have required the services of his court-physicians, ordinary and extraordinary, if he had such. He was perhaps aware that their knoweldge of physic and their skill as physicians were by no means great; and he may have felt that he had in fact been beholden many times when sick to another agency than theirs. It must have been matter of familiar observation to him and his subjects that when they fell ill, they got well somehow without benefit of phy-sicians, or with small help from them. In as far, however, as they were destitute of them, they doubtless felt no want; and we may well believe that on the whole they did not fare badly, not worse probably than the refined Chinese and Japanese do in these our own days under a system which we deem crude in the extreme. They had, as these have, the mighty *vis medicatrix* on their side; and apart from their bloody wars with the Canaanites and others, they led simpler lives than we do who enjoy the *luxury* of the medical Art. In illustration of this I may adduce the fact that among the Hindoos at the present time, nothing is more remarkable than their recu-perative powers under capital operations performed on them by our countrymen in the East living among them. They recover from operations to an extent that is quite astonishing and altogether unknown in European hospitals. 'God tempers the wind to the shorn lamb.' And in view of what could not be but well known to him, well might David make the ascription he does in that psalm. It is of a piece with the Hippocratic maxim that 'our natures are the physicians of our diseases,' and it is because I regard it as such, and as the popular equivalent in those days of that maxim, and as exhibiting the popular *estimate* then formed on the relative powers of Nature and Art in the cure of disease, that I adduce it here. Widely different that estimate would seem to have been from the popular estimate of the days we live in."

Thus, while man has spent ages in seeking for cures for disease, the cure has always resided within his own body and has continued to restore him to health under all forms of treatment or under no treatment at all, and man has mistakenly attrib-uted cure to his art. The difficulty has been that man has had his eyes forever trained in the wrong direction. As Trall so appropriately remarked:

"A man who should look to the moon all his lifetime in search of the 'philos-opher's stone', might not discover it though lying at his feet. Medical philosophers, instead of rationally tracing the effects of riotous living and abused hygienic agencies, have expended oceans of midnight oil and centuries of brain labor in trying to think out some specific, strange, hidden, occult, mysterious, extra-natural thing, substance, element, or cause, whose existence should, in some magical manner, account for all the phenomena of fever. Of course, all their toil has been in vain. It has been rather worse than labor lost, for the writings and teachings of medical books and medical schools are so tinctured and mystified with the vagaries of medical professors, that the student of medicine is morally certain to get his mind more or less befogged, and his judgment to some extent warped by their influence."—*Hydropathic Encyclopedia,* Vol. 2, P. 75.

"We are told that Nature has provided a 'law of cure'. Here is another vexed question for us to settle, and I meet it by denying the fact. What is this law of cure? The Allopathists say it is 'contraria contraiis curantur'—contraries cure opposites. The Homeopathists proclaim 'similia similibus curantur'—likes cures similar. The Eclectics declare that the law exists in or consists in 'Sanative' medication, and the Physio-Medicals believe that the law is fulfilled in the employment of 'Physiological' remedies.

"They are all wrong; there is no law of cure in all the universe; Nature has provided nothing of the sort; Nature has provided penalties, not remedies. Think you, would Nature or Providence provide penalties or punishment as the consequences of transgression, and then provide remedies to do away with the penalties? Would Nature ordain suffering as the corrective discipline for disobedience to the laws of life, and then permit the doctor to drug and dose away the penalties? There is a condition of cure, and this is obedience.

"And now, if Nature has provided no law of cure, she has provided no remedies. What then becomes of the materia medica and its two thousand drugs? (Thousands more now. Also, Naturopaths and drugless practitioners, what becomes of your herbs and other drugs, and curative measures? Author's note.) And what becomes or should become of the hundreds of quack nostrums which are deluging the land, filling newspapers with lying advertisements, and robbing the sick and suffering of millions of their hard earnings annually? (Also, Naturopaths and drugless practitioners what should become of the hundreds of quack machines and apparatuses which are deluging the land filling the mis-called health journals with lying advertisements and robbing the sick and suffering of millions of their hard earnings annually; and preventing them by these same lies from seeking true aid? Author's note). The regular practice and the irregular trade are based on the same false dogmas; and when one goes to oblivion the other will soon follow."—*True Healing Art.*

"The minds—professional minds—of medical men of this day are as mystified and twistified, as superstitious and fantastical, as irrational and absurd, so far as medical logic is concerned, as were the minds of medical men in that by-gone age when charms, magic, incantations, and necromancy were among the remedial resources. And so their minds will remain until they have some fixed basis, some settled principle to reason from. A man may be in possession af any amount of book knowledge, he may know all the facts of all the sciences in existence, yet if he does not recognize the principles to which those facts relate, his writing and talking may be unintelligible jargon, and his practice a promiscuous medley of truth and error. A man may understand all the letters of the alphabet, and all the words of the dictionary, and yet make bad words and sentences unless he is also acquainted with the principles of the construction of language." *Hydropathic Enc.,* Vol 1, PP—

". . . The only acknowledged guide now is experience. But unfortunately the guide points all ways at the same time. . . .

"To ilustrate: Bleeding has been extensively employed in typhus fevers for three hundred years, yet physicians are divided in opinion whether it is good or bad practice. Opium has been in use over two thousand years, but medical men cannot agree whether it operates primarily as a sedative and secondarily as a stimulant, or exactly the contrary, primarily as a stimulant and secondarily as a sedative. Mercury has been employed more or less for about three hundred years and extensively during the last fifty years; and some doctors consider it a tonic, others a stimulant, others a deobstruent, or alterative, others a sedative, and yet others an antiphlogistic. Brandy has been freely administered in New York and elsewhere in the treatment of the cholera during two epidemics; the result of the experience is, about half of the physicians commend it highly, and the other half condemn it utterly. Within the last fifty years no less than four different methods of treating ordinary fevers have prevailed; the bark and wine practice, the cold affusion practice, the bleeding and saline practice, and the mercurial and opium practice. In about the same period, some scores of specifics for some of the most formidable diseases have been discovered, tried, proved, and then laid aside, to be followed by others which experienced a similar rise and fall of reputation. Digitalis, the effluvia of cow-stables, and a preparation of nitric acid and opium, have been among the vaunted cures for consumption. Twenty years ago iodine was found to be a specific for scrofula; but no one now thinks of it save as an auxiliary; and two years ago cod-liver oil was literally flooding the country under the auspices of the allopathic medical journals, and the right wing of the great medical army, the apothecaries, as a remedy, for consumption and scrofula; but its brief day is already drawing to a close.

"These facts are enough to show the utter fallacy of medical experience and the unsatisfactory nature of medical testimony, unless based upon some intelligible principle to which we can refer the phenomena they present."—*Hydropathic Enc.,* Vol. 1, P 35.

"Without some fixed and unalterable and demonstratable rule of judgment, all our reasoning may be in vain; facts may be misapplied; experience misinterpreted; observation deceptive; and logic perverted.

"Though an angel speak to us in the voices of the rolling thunders; though God send instrucion in the red lightings flash; yet without a principle of interpretation, without the recognition of some law by which to explain the phenomena, we only know that it thunders, and that the sky is ablaze. But with the knowledge of the law which determines the results, we may rightly apply all the data of science and misapply none; we may use all things, and abuse nothing."—*True Healing Art.*

"The person who is ignorant of the first principle of astronomy could affirm most conscientiously that the sun rises in the east and sets in the west, and passes around the earth once in every twenty-four hours. Does he not see it with his own eyes? But with a knowledge of the law of gravitation, he would know that this appearance was illusory, and that the earth revolved on its axis, while the sun stood still."—*True Healing Art.*

"I have asked many of the professors of the Drug Schools to explain to me how their remedies acted, and how their 'Law of Cure' operated—the why, the wherefore, the rationale? but not one of them could ever tell me; yet each referred to his own experience to prove that his method of drug prescribing was the best one. None of them ever thought of the primary question, Is any drug medical system right?

"Experience! What is experience? It is merely the record of what has happened. It only tells what has been done, not what should be. I would not give a green cucumber for all the experience of all the medical men of all the earth in all the ages, unless predicated on some recognized law of nature, and interpreted by some demonstratable rule in philosophy. Medical men have been curing (killing?) folks for three thousand years with drug medicines, and their experience has led them away from truth and nature continually. If a dozen persons are sick of a fever for one, two or three months, and the physician gives them half a dozen drugs half a dozen times a day while the fever lasts, and one half of them die and the other half recover, the question then arises, what the drugs had to do with the results? The drug doctor will of course assume that all who survive owed their lives to the medication, while all who die, die in spite of the medication. But one who reasons from another stand-point, who reasons from the law of vitality instead of the false dogmas of medical schools, will conclude that those who die are killed by the medicine, while those who recover, recover in spite of it. Such is medical experience."—*True Healing Art.*

Jennings quotes an excellent example of the opposite practices of medicine from an old work by one Dr. N. Smith on the *Treatment of Typhus Fever.* He wrote:

"The practitioners of medicine in New England have been divided on this subject and while one part have converts to the doctrine of blood-letting to a high degree in this affection, the other has condemned it toto; and, as though opposition had produced a kind of reaction on their part, they have had recourse to the most powerful stimulants both internally and externally, such as opium, wine, alcohol, and the most *acrid* stimulants, as cayenne pepper, arsenic, etc. Indeed, individuals of this latter class have carried their prejudices to such an extent as even to boast of having made their patients swallow three pints of strong brandy, accompanied with large doses of laudanum and cantharides. I have myself seen a prescription, in which opium, wine, alcohol, cantharides, and arsenic, were all to be taken several times in the course of twenty-four hours.

"It is remarkable, that though the practice of these two sects—for such they seem to be—is as opposite as possible, each considering the others mode of treatment as highly deleterious, yet all boast of success, and enumerate various cases which have fallen under their care, with scarcely the loss of a single patient.

"There are but two ways of accounting for the equal success of these two opposite modes of cure, for as far as I can judge, there is not much difference in the success which attends them. Either the disease is not so much under the control of blood-letting as they would have us believe, or these two extremes produce about an equal degree of mischief; for it is not conceded that if a patient does not require bleeding, he stands in need of opium, arsenic, cantharides, or alcohol."

Dr. Smith was right; these two opposite practices did produce about an equal amount of mischief. Neither method had the "disease" under control. A news item published a few years later reads: "A Typhoid Fever epidemic has been ravaging the North-western parts of South Carolina, which in numerous cases has proved fatal. It has been a fact noted in its progress, that the more powerful the remedies employed, the more fatal the disease. Those only have recovered that have taken no medicine." And why not?

Dr. Smith mentions a prescription he had seen, in which the unfortunate patient had been plied so bountifully with stimulants. This case occured near Middletown, Conn., about seventy-seven years since. It was called "sinking typhus." Dr. Smith was called to see a gentleman thought to be dangerously ill. He found the strictest medical surveillance, with the stimulants mentioned to "rally his vital forces" whenever they should manifest a disposition to go to sleep on the job. After a careful examination, the Doctor declared their alarmed apprehensions groundless and by a complete change in treatment, "which gave nature an opportunity to exhibit the true state of her affairs, the man was soon restored to his usual health."

In this connection Dr. Jennings relates an interesting story that serves well to illustrate the thought we are trying to convey to the reader. He says: "after this disease had been in progress awhile, and, had extended somewhat beyond its original bounds, I inquired of Dr. Joseph Foot, of Northhaven, whose field of labor lay between me and the infected district, whether there had been any cases of 'sinking typhus' in Northhaven. 'Not till quite recently,' replied the doctor. 'A sinking typhus physician moved into the place a few weeks ago, and since that I have heard that we were having some of the 'sinking typhus.'

"The thought was rather new to me at the time, that the type of disease was fashioned somewhat by the Doctors; but I became satisfied that there was some ground for such an opinion."

The cod-liver oil fad has bobbed up time and again since Trall's day, and just now, under cover of the vitamine hypothesis is staging a "come back." Whether it was given as a "respiratory food" or is given for its "vitamines," whatever these are, it always worked cures. So did the offal of animals, the bark and wine, the bleeding, purging and puking. Cures follow the use of all methods, good, bad or indifferent. Iodine cured scroffula, the profession swore by it and only the "quacks" rejected it. But its place was soon taken by some other cure, while today it both prevents and cures goitre. The iodine for goitre fad holds a place in present day medical practice equal to that held by the "foci of infection" fad.

In the face of thousands of years of such experiences man must still have his "cures," and the search for new ones is prosecuted with as much zeal as ever, while every now and then someone revives one of the old antiques and it enjoys another hey day of popularity; although, perhaps, under a different name, based on a new theory, and garbed in a new terminology and, perhaps, couched in a more profuse verbosity. With Bostock, I would say: "These circumstances are interesting, not merely as forming a part of the history of medicine, but as displaying a singular feature in the history of the human mind; demonstrating the difficulty which exists in eradicating from it errors and follies, even the most gross and palpable, when they have once become deeply rooted."

Have matters change since? Not much. While medical men disown all the theories that ruled their predecessors by turns, they endeavor to preserve and incorporate in their precsriptions, all the remedial measures these rejected theories have brought into favor. The size of the dose, only, has changed. If my Naturopathic friends will kindly pardon another wound from my pen, I will say that in this respect, the present day medical man resembles the Naturopath who rejects the theories of the Naprapath, Neuropath, Chiropractor, etc., and yet, adopts and employs, all the methods and measures that have grown out of these rejected theories. Today, in the entire medical world, whether one goes among the self-styled "scientific" dope dispensers, or enquires among the members of those who are called cults one finds a remarkable state of affairs: the most contradictory theories are supported by equal authority, and the most opposite practices recommended on equal testimony.

These facts are sufficient to demonstrate the utter fallacy of medical experience, and the unsatisfactory nature of medical testimony, unless based upon some intelligible principle to which we can refer the phenomena these present. At present the whole medical world is bent on establishing new systems, building new theories, the discovery of new remedies, and the concentration and "improvement" of the old ones, with little, if any, thought given to the discovery of the primary law or principle from which any truly natural healing system must work. "Cures" continue to follow the employment of all methods by all schools.

The words of Dr. Schrodt are so appropriate in this connection, that I cannot resist the temptation to set them down here. He wrote: "If we reflect upon the obstinate health of animals and savages, upon the rapidity of their recovery from

506

injuries that defy all the mixtures of Materia Medica; also upon the fact that the homeopaths cure their patients with milk-sugar and mummery, the prayer-Christians with mummery without milk-sugar, and my followers with milk-diet without sugar or mummery—the conclusion forces itself upon us that the entire system of therapeutics is founded upon an erroneous view of disease."

AN ERRONEOUS VIEW OF DISEASE! Exactly! That is just what I am here contending. Disease is considered an enemy that must be combatted and yet here are three methods that combat nothing and the sick recover. In his *"Medical Reform"* (p. 247) Dr. Jennings wrote:

"It is unnecessary for my present purpose to give a particular account of the results of homeopathy. What I now claim with respect to it is, that a wise and beneficent Providence is using it to expose and break up a deep delusion. In the results of Homeopathic practice, we have evidence in amount, and of a character sufficient, most incontestibly to establish the fact that disease is a restorative operation, or renovating process, and that medicine has deceived us. The evidence is full and complete. It does not consist merely of a few isolated cases, whose recovery might be attributed to fortutious circumstances, but it is a chain of testimony fortified by every possible circumstance. All kinds and grades of disease have passed under the ordeal, and all classes and characters of persons have been concerned in the experiment as patients or witnesses;****while the process of infinitesimally attenuating the drugs used was carried to such a ridiculous extent that no one will, on sober reflection, attribute any portion of the cure to the medicine. I claim, then, that homeopathy may be regarded as a providential sealing of the fate of old medical views and practices."

Facts may be likened to beads and first principles to the string upon which the beads are strung; to unify them, to cement them togehter, thus forming the necklace of science. The man who has the beads only can do no more than roll them about in an impirical manner, in a hit and miss fashion. He is the man who, surveying the whole field of medical history, decides there are curative powers or virtues in all things, even though, they may also possess destructive powers; or else he may decide that all cures are mental and that anything that affects the mind strongly enough and in the right manner, will accomplish a cure. This is the kind of an individual who, seeing cures occur under all methods of treatment, declares that there is good in all methods and that he believes in *selecting* the best from them all.

The rock on which the Nature Cure system was wrecked and converted into a spurious system called Naturopathy, was or is, eclecticism—or, small I say, collectivism. Such is the power of education to bias the mind that few seem able to comprehend how it is possible for a disease to be removed without a little medicine or a little treatment of some kind. "It may be little, infinitesimal, the thirtieth dilution, or a ten-millionth part of a drop of the tincture of a shadow, or the weakest decoction of catnip or canary seed; still it must be something unnatural, or nature cannot be assisted!" And if medicine or treatment of any kind or strength is employed as an auxilliary, notwithstanding, Nature is regarded as the true curative power, the little charming, mysterious influence of the drug or treatment will gradually increase its hold upon the imagination and, in the end, expel the natural part of the practice as surely as weeds will crowd out the flowers from an uncultivated field. "It is like mixing brandy and water to make a beverage. Every one will admit that in such a mixture the water is the only strictly necessary and useful part of the drink; yet by employing them in combination no man ever had his taste for water increase, and that for brandy decrease. The contrary is always the fact." The safety of the Nature Cure depends on keeping it free of all "entangling alliances" and out of all "foreign entanglements." The *eclectic*, or collectic policy is destructive to the truly natural system.

The ancient priests and monks seem to have had some knowledge of nature cure. They placed their patients in airy, salubrious situations, enforced strict abstemiousness or the simpliest of good, gave water for drink and prescribed sufficient water for cleanliness after and only after which, they performed their magical ceremonies. Their patients recovered, perhaps more of them than recover today, and certainly, there were fewer chronic sufferers then than now. Nature worked the cure, but the credit went to the doctor and his weird ceremonies.

How different it is with our more learned and scientific modern physicians.

These are supplied more abundantly with disease-killing missiles, and with more powerful agents with which to cure the disorder. They permit or recommend the grossest food, give drugged instead of pure water, pay scarcely any attention to hygienic regulations, pour down their powerful remedies, or squirt them into the blood-stream or into the tisues under the skin; and, when their patients die, nature gets the blame, and the doctor and his method are excused. For, surely, no one could have done more. Did he not do all that is known to science?

If patients, millions of them, could and did recover under the crucifying treatment accorded to patients in the past, who can say how many more would have recovered had such methods been treated as suggested by Holmes and the patients left to nature? Surely, every effort of the physician was directed, although, not intentionally, toward killing the patient, or, at least, hindering his recovery. It is, indeed, eloquent testimony to the self-curative powers of the living organism that so many recovered. And yet, there are millions of earth's intelligent beings who dare not trust this self-curative power, but must have some treatment of some kind, if sick. Yet, who will deny the truth of Trall's remark:

"It is with all schools of medicine as it is with each individual practitioner of the healing art—the less faith they have in medicine, the more they have in Hygiene; hence those who prescribe little or no medicine, are invariably and necessarily more attentive to Hygienic conditions—to good nursing—which always was and ever will be, all that there is really good, useful, or curative in medication. Such physicians are more careful to supply the vital organism with whatever of air, light, temperature, food, water, exercise or rest, etc., it needs in its struggle for health, and to remove all vitiating influences—all poisons, impurities, miasms, or disturbing influences of any kind. And this is Hygienic Medication; this is the True Healing Art. Nor God nor Nature has provided any other; nor can the Supreme Architect permit any other without reversing all the laws of the universe and annulling every one of his attributes."— *True Healing Art*.

During the reign of Galen's school, which lasted over nine hundred years, his disciples stoutly maintained the divine authority of his works, but with the discovery of his mistakes in anatomy came doubt as to his infallibilty, and for a short time the whole field of medical science was open to the genius of invention, and the stupidity and ambition of practitioners were stimulated to a high point to be the discoverers of some wonderful healing agent. But, for the most part, all the reforms and revolutions in the medical world, were only rearrangements of old material. They resembled the endless changes of the kaleidoscope; for by changing the position of the old materials it struck the beholder, at first sight, as being the desired thing, but when closely examined, it was found to be only a change in appearance, while the fundamental principles remained the same.

If space permitted it would be both interesting and instructive to thread back the maze of medicine for a few centuries and observe the changes in theories and practices which have been forced upon it by the system makers and fabricators of peculiar doctrines and notions. If it were possible for some motion picture producing company to present for our view, on the screen, a historically correct picture of the theories and practices that have ruled mankind by turns in all parts of the world, in all ages, among both "savage" and "civilized" peoples, not only would it be the most comical, but as well, the most mournful picture ever produced. Comical when we think of the many absurd and contradictory theories and fantastic and ludicrous practices that have been employed by the "medicine men," magicians, astrologers, priests, philosophers, and physicians upon their patients for the cure of disease, the exorcism of devils and the destruction of germs; pathetic, when we view the gross ignorance and stupidity in which the whole world was steeped and the murderous methods that were so frequently employed by ignorant doctors to cure diseases in their equally ignorant patients.

Such a picture would be, not only extremely interesting, but highly enlightening, as well. No one could view that picture, see the whole panaroma of medical history and the conditions under which human beings have lived, labored, fought, loved, and died, without coming away with a greatly enhanced faith in the marvelous curative and recuperative powers of the human body. Shakespear's admonition would be changed to: Cast *Therapeutics* to the dogs; although it would be well understood that the dog would reject the whole of the therapeutic bill-of-fare as surely as he would the physic.

In the Middle Ages a "precious jewel" taken from the head of the toad was supposed to make one immune to toothache, and was a sure antidote to poisons. Gregory, the XIV, was "kept alive" for days by the administration of gold and jewels. The horn of the fabled unicorn was supposed to have miraculous curative powers and doses from its supposed horns sold for fabulous prices. Bishop Berkeley cured himself and friends of all their ailments with tar water. Gregory of Tours obtained a powder, by scraping the tombstones on the graves of the "saints," of which he exclaimed:

"Oh, indescribable mixture, incomparable elixir, antidote beyond all praise- Celestial purgative (if I may be permitted to use that expression), which throws into the shade every medical prescription, which surpasses in fragrance every earthly aroma, and is more powerful than all essence; which purges the body as the juice of scammony, clears the lungs as hyssop, and the head like sneezewort; which not only cures the ailing limbs, but also, and this is much more valuable, washes off the stains from the conscience."

Snails, taken from their shells and soaked in white wine, were good for coughs and "tightness of the chest." Roasted mouse was good for nervousness. A compound made of adders, bats, angle worms, suckling whelps, ox bones, and greace was a sure cure for hypochondria. A mixture of calomel, sugar of lead and pulverized human bones cured gout. Red herbs cured inflammations and yellow ones cured jaundice.

Moss scraped from a dead man's skull, or mandrake gathered in a grave yard, in the dark of the moon, at midnight hour, when the ghosts walk, remedies compounded of the tissues of mummies, urine and dung of animals, various organs and parts of animals and poisonous drugs of all kinds were used and *produced results* for thousands of years. Not many decades since, one could still purchase "mummy" in the apothecary shops; but such mummy was usually ordinary meat soaked in preservatives. Nevertheless it freuently "cured" pains and headaches which had refused to yield to the skill and "remedies" of ordinary medical practitioners. Horse chestnuts carried in the pocket cured rheumatism. A belt, made of a piece of a rope with which someone had been hung, and worn about the waist both prevented and cured disease. Oliver Wendell Holmes was truly right when he said:

"The disgrace of medicine has been that colossal system of self-deception, in obedience to which mines have been emptied of their cankering minerals, the vegetable kingdom robbed of its noxious growths, the entrails of animals taxed for their impurities, the poison-bags of reptiles drained of their venom, and all the inconceivable abominations thus obtained thrust down the throats of human beings."

The ever-changing and uncertain character of Therapeutics is well expressed in Trousseau's famous remark: "Take this quickly, while it is still a cure." J. F. Baldwin, A.M., M.D., F.A.C.S., then president of the Ohio State Medical Association, said in his Presidential address to that body, in June, 1920: "An exceedingly weak point in our position is its possession of such an enormous array of useless drugs as presented in our pharmacopeia. No thinking observer can look over the pages of that book without being amazed at the credulity of a profession that tolerates such a farrago of nonsense—such a hodge-podge of trash." In this same lecture, Dr. Baldwin expressed it as his wish that every medical man might read MEDICAL REFORM, by Dr. Jennings.

A survey of medical history reveals that the human race has used practically everything imaginable, obtainable, and inventable in the effort to cure its diseases. And with a persistance that is appalling, a vast majority of all cases of disease have always recovered. The physician may have made a mistake in his diagnosis and treated the patient for the wrong disease, but he usually recovered. The Egyptian priest may have appealed to different deities to those appealed to by the Greecians or Babylonians, but the patients of all these usually recovered. The physicians of the 17th Century may have denounced the methods of the physicians of the 10th Century, but if the patients of those 10th Century physicians had not recovered, there would have been neither patients not physicians in the 17th Century.

If the patients who drank the teas made of sheep dung, or those who imbided the urine of bulls, or those who anointed their bodies with the dung of swines, had not recovered, 20th Century civilization would never have developed. If our grandfathers, who were given 20, 30 and even 40 grains of calomel, or blue mass or quinine, or antimony, when they were not defending their scalps from Indian hair dressers, had not recovered, we would not now be boasting of our assumed superiority over them.

There has been much change of theory and method all down the ages—theories especially have changed—but the one stupendous fact that most of the sick recover does not change. A new theory is calculated to develop some new methods and while this is generally the case, it is not always so. Often the new theory made little or no change at all in practice, often it only changed the mode of application of the old methods. Under the new theory it was found that, while the old method was good, it had not been properly used, although the patients did recover. The new theory found perhaps that the old method was good in one disease in which it had never been tried, but useless or even harmful, in another disease in which, under the old theory, it had been used with great success.

It was ever thus. Every new theory or revival of an old discarded theory, every new hypothesis, has adopted part or all of the old methods and it has always been claimed that the methods work better under the new theory than under the old. The "regulars" may scoff at the theories of the eunuch, Paracelsus, and denounce him as the Prince of Quacks, but they do not, for this reason, discard his remedies. They may smile an indulgent smile when reading the theories of Pythagoris and Hippocrites about the four humors of the body, but they do not, for this reason, reject the remedies that were developed under the humoral pathology to restore humoral balance. The various theories and practices developed by the Dogmatists, Empirics, Alexandrians, Heroics, Pneumatics, Eclectics, Galenists, Arabians, Monks, Alchemists, Chemicalists, Quacks, Anatomicalists, Metaphysical Physicians, Boerhaaveians, Hallerites, Semi-animists, Cullenists, Brounians, etc., may be laughed at, but their "curative agents" are still in very general use. There has been some change of methods, some remedies that "cured" their mililons in the past have been discarded, new ones have been discovered or invented, some of the old ones have been concentrated, modified, "improved" or renamed. Animal parts that were once used to restore humoral balance are now used to supply lacking harmones, and these are supposed to restore "balance," also. Iodine that was once a specific for scrofula is now a specific for goitre. Remedies that were once used to scare away the evil spirits are now employed to scare away malignant germs. The mystic rites and magic ceremonies of the ancient priests and magi, and their prayers to the reigning deities gave place in the Middle Ages to the magic and mystery of the monks and priests who called upon the various saints and the Virgin Mary. Polytheism became poly-saintism, sympathy healing became magnetic healing, magnetic healing passed into mesmerism, mesmerism became hypnotism and electrical psychology, and these, in turn, became suggestion. Suggestion broadened out into Christian Science, Divine Science, New Thought, Practical Metaphysics, Dowieism, the Emmanuel Movement, the New Psychology, Psycho-analysis, etc. Valentine Greatrix was followed by Schlatter, and he, in turn, was succeeded by Emil Coue.

Soloman, finding that his thousandth wife was just like the first one, declared there is nothing new under the sun. The student of Medical History, finding that the last "cures" are all like the first ones is also, inclined to say, there is nothing new on the earth. I believe it was Hegel who said the nationas never learn anything from history and I believe it can be said with equal truth that few individuals ever learn anything from history. History, being chiefly the handmaid of propaganda, is either distorted or its essential truths suppressed, so that there is some excuse for the vast majority. Indeed, not one individual in a thousand is even aware that there is a medical history.

Pharoah's daughter and her attendants were bathing in the Nile when she found the infant Moses. Hercules received his "refreshing" warm baths at the hands of Minerva and Vulcan. According to Althenaeus, it was the custom of antiquity for women and virgins to assist strangers in their ablutions. Hippocrates practiced hydrotherapy and the ancient Chinese and Romans practiced mechanotherapy. "Bone Setters" have flourished in nearly every nation in all ages and in modern times their practices have been systematized, fine spun theories have been invented to underlie them, and euphonious names have been appended thereto. The world moves on—in a circle.

510

The sick recover whether treated or not. They recover, no matter how or by whom treated. Many die under all systems and many more develop chronic diseases under all systems. Some chronics get well under all systems; many do not. We have the facts; what is the explanation? Is there good in all methods and systems? Is there healing virtue in everything? Will anything that affects the mind powerfully enough and favorably enough cure, regardless of what method it is, or, regardless of any other effects it may have? Does it make no difference what method is employed so long as the people get well when treated thereby? Many have seriously contended for these things and have endeavoured, by an appeal to the record of experience to establish these contentions. The record of experience gives results only, and not causes.

Are there conditions or methods of treatment that retard recovery? Are there conditions that enhance recovery? Does it make no difference which of these we employ in caring for the sick? If the method is harmful, beneficial or merely indifferent, does it make no material difference which is used, so long as it appears to answer to the pragmatic test of "does it work?" Is recovery under a given method alone enough to establish its curative virtues?

In previous chapters, I have shown unmistakably that the power of cure is inherent in the living organism. In these chapters, also, I have shown that the successful exercise of this power is dependent to a great extent upon the conditions or environment under which the organism lives and labors. There is ample historical evidence to show conclusively that the methods of treatment employed and the conditions surrounding the sick organism do make a big difference in the death rate and in the rate of recovery from disease. Besides this, there are ample physiological and pathological facts and principles to show the correctness of this deduction from the record of history.

Dr. Oswald wrote *Physical Education*: "For, rightly understood, the external symptoms of disease constitute a restorative process that cannot be brought to a satisfactory issue till the cause of the evil is removed." The popular methods of "breaking up a sickness," he said, is, "in reality, only an interruption of it, a temporary interruption of the symptoms." He declared of such *cures*, "we might as well cure the sleepiness of a weary child by pinching its eyelids, or the hunger of a whinning dog by compressing its throat." By silencing the whinning, the symptoms of hunger, we do not cure its cause, the need for food. Dr. Oswald further declared:

"In sickness stimulants cannot further the actual recovery by a single hour. There is a strong progressive tendency in our physical constitution; Nature needs no prompter; as soon as the remedial process is finished, the normal functions of the organism will resume their work as spontaneously as the current of a stream resumes its course after the removal of an obstruction."

I cannot too strongly impress upon the mind of the reader the importance of grasping the fact that disease is not something to be cured, but that IS IT THE PROCESS OF CURE. This fact is of fundamental importance in this discussion and must lie at the root of all further considerations of our subject. Keep in mind that in treating the visible parts of disease, the physician is treating the curative process and not touching the causes of the disease. The whole effort to cure is based upon the assumption that disease is something to be attacked, subdued, suppressed, driven out, or, in some other way, defeated by the treatment.

Truly did Jennings declare:

"Spontaneous or natural cures—and there are and can be none other—have to stand vouchers for all sorts and sizes of medical doctrines, whether they emanate from M.D.'s of loftiest standing, or are the spawn of charlatanical cogitation. Whatever notion is entertained respecting the nature of disease, whether it be that of wrong action, altered state of the vital properties, bad blood, or general depravation of the fluids, or anything of a heteropathic nature, the final appeal for vouchers to the correctness of their doctrines is to cures which have been performed by them respectively."—*Tree of Life*, P. 180.

He again declares in this same work (P. 170), "Providential Nature is not careful to distinguish in her cures between those attended by learned doctors and those prescribed by the vilest quacks."

Either "nature is always true to herself," as Jennings declared, "moving undeviatingly onward and onward in the prescribed path of eternal and immutable law, aiming always and steadily under all circumstances toward the acme of perfection," or, else, nature is capricious and unlawful.

In previous chapters a sufficient collation of verified and historical facts and principles have been presented to show that the orthopathic theory is the correct one, that is, that disease, as a modification of healthy action, is still subject to the laws of life that control all vital action, and, therefore, however much it may deviate from the usual standard of healthy action, it must always be RIGHT ACTION. We do not need to claim rationality for the unconscious powers of the organic world anymore than we need to claim the same for the forces that control the formation and repair of a crystal. Every force in man's body is governed by immutable law which disposes of them to the highest interests of life and which wisely adapts means to ends. Outside the voluntary powers of man, all matters and forces or agencies, are puncticiliously and eternally subject to law. These laws, uniform in all places and all times, shut up the involuntary actions of man's body to their designed ends. The economy of life cannot relax its grasp upon the working powers of man's body and permit these forces to take on wrong or subversive action and thus endanger life. The law of life, itself, cannot become recreat of its high trust and misdirect the forces of life, or any part of them, and by this treason, create discord in the body, disturbing its peace and threatening its destruction. So firmly and indellibly is the law of life impressed with the "instinctive" inclination, or tendency, or actual necessity to maintain life in its highest condition, that it must, at all tmes, and under all circumstances, employ the power it has—be this more or less—with a wise adaptation to the end in view—the preservation and prolongation of life.

The instruments of motion, action, function, are the same in disease as in health. The motive or vital power which animates, controls and operates the organism or machinery, in health, is not altered in either its nature or quality, in disease. The laws of life have undergone no change in disease. Indeed, they are not susceptible of change. They are always present to the last flickering of life—there in full force and are fully capable of controlling with perfect ease, any amount of forces that may be present. No organic power or property can possibly escape from under the control of the animal economy and become lawless or reckless in its course of action. It must operate in a lawful or correct manner and work, to the fullest extent of its ability, for the highest welfare of the organism. Life cannot repudiate itself. It is always upright and correct in its actions and processes.

Nature makes no mistakes and violates no laws. She is uniformly governed by fixed principles and all her actions harmonize with the laws that govern those actions. She always does the best she can under existing circumstances. Nothing could be more preposterous than the idea that the vital machinery is capable of wrong action. We might as well contend for wrong action in any other department of fixed law. It is like claiming that gravitation may become bewildered and inverted in its action, and cast stones upward and cause streams of water to run up hill. As well expect cohesive attraction to split rocks, or magnetism to arrange needles parallel to the equator.

The *Right Action* theory must be right. And if it is correct, what are the results that we should naturally expect to appear to flow from the practices of the different schools and cults of medicine and from the varying forms of domestic practice? If the tendency of all remaining vital activity is unfalteringly in the right direction—toward the restoration of normal health—if nature, with but one aim, moves majestically onward in her recuperative and reparative work, and accomplishes this work as rapidly and effectually as she can, under existing circumstances, should not the results be just what we find them to be? Dr. Jennings answers this question in the following words, *Tree of Life*, P. 208-9:

"In the cases where the perturbating treatment is the strongest, the natural order of the renovating process, is disturbed, irregular and protracted, and the event rendered proportionately doubtful. In cases where the hostile treatment is moderate, the general course of the recuperative work is not much disturbed in its progress or materially lengthened or hazarded in its issue. And where the treatment is truly hygienic, fulfilling the natural indications and conditions of impaired feeble life,

512

there is great regularity in the curative process, the period of duration the shortest, probability of final recovery the greatest, and recovered health the most firmly established. And what would most likely be the course and ending of diseases under the different kinds of treatment which they would get by regular and irregular practitioners, if disease was an antagonism to health, in its nature and tendency subversive of life, justly represented by a house being on fire, or a 'certain noxious something to be destroyed by medicine, as an acid by an alkali'? In this case the result would be, that physicians who had great depth of penetration and research, who had acquired extensive and accurate diagnostic knowledge and skill, had obtained a thorough and familiar acquaintance with means adapted to counteract disease, and an easy art of applying them, would make rapid and sure work of demolishing the enemy and restoring health.

"Under the treatment of physicians who possessed but indifferent qualifications for 'discerning, distinguishing, preventing and curing disease,' the chance of recovery would be small in most disorders. And if physicians were to make a mistake in the selection and use of remedies, administer coinciding instead of counteracting means; throw spirits of turpentine on the fire instead of water, disease would soon put an end to life, the building would burn down rapidly. And in cases where disease had got well established in the system and there was nothing done to check its progress, death would be inevitable. Now everybody knows that nothing like such results follow in the train of different kinds of practice. On the contrary, it would puzzle a lawyer to tell what practice was, apparently, attended with greatest success, if in a populous place he were to pass in review the multitudinous treatment of the sick. There is a difference, a great difference in the resulting effects between good and bad treatment of depressed feeble human life, manifest, too, to those who are competent to judge of such matters; but the populace do not discern it, and they are ready to accept and employ every description of pretenders to skill in curing diseases. And in a large majority of cases, Nature manages to restore her damaged machinery and revitalize it in spite of the most oppressive and cruel treatment. This state of things is only reconcilable with the idea of right action in disease. It can be rationally accounted for on no other principle. And the doctrine of right action can now be sustaned beyond doubt or cavil by incontestable evidence of both a negative and positive character."

The Heteropathic babel of medicine, including its theories and practices, is stamped with the seal of delusion. Such uniformity of results seemingly proceeding from such diversity of means and methods is only explicable on the orthopathic principle. If the Heteropathic doctrine were correct the human race would long ago have perished. The present universally choatic state of medicine, in connection with the irrationality and monstrous absurdity of its various theories of disease and the great, manifest incongruity of medical practice, its use of positively poisonous substances and damaging measures and violent disorganizing processes, used with a view to "help nature" all conspire to place a stamp of delusion upon therapeutics and corroborate the theory of Orthopathy.

This miscalled science has been fully organized and elaborately equipped for several centuries. It has absorbed such an enormous share of the total wealth of the world that no believable estimate can be made of this. It has been more lavishly encouraged by governments, communities and philanthropic individuals, than any and all other arts and sciences. A greater number of the bright minds of earth have devoted themselves to its problems, and more time has been given to the solution of these problems, than to all the other problems with which scientists and artists contend. And, with what results? Only this—they succeeded for a time in deluding themselves and the race and in estranging man from nature until the universal dupe seemed to consider himself helpless and utterly at the mercy of the arrogant, intolerant and all-grasping schools and confederations of schools. But they have not succeeded in finding one real cure for a single form of disease, and all of them have been forced to admit their failure. At present the fact is beginning to dawn upon the minds of a few that nature is not to be coerced or cajoled by the administration of poisons or by the application of drugless methods, but that she does her own repairing in her own way and has provided simply and adequately for this.

Some years ago a prominent attorney, in a trial of some prominence, asserted

513

that scientists or experts could be obtained who would furnish evidence of the truth of almost any theory along scientific lines, no matter how startling or absurd its nature. Nowhere has this been more true than in the field of medicine. It is indeed an incomprehensible paradox that the wildest and most baseless speculations relating to disease and curative methods have had no lack of extravagant encouragement from the educated and learned in all ages, if they were only artificial enough, or mysterious enough. Medicine is still what Bichat declared it to be, "an incoherent assemblage of incoherent ideas, and is, perhaps, of all the physiologic sciences, that which best shows the caprice of the human mind. It is a shapeless assemblage of inaccurate ideas, of observations often peurile and of formulas as fantastically conceived as they are tediously arranged." All of their great discoveries have been great mistakes; all their wonderful "cures" have either been indifferent or harmful and all the curing ever accomplished has been done by the living organism itself. Neither pompous titles, boasting self-sufficiency, fanciful theories, nor incongruous mixtures of any kind, have ever aided the body in any way in its processes of cure. The sick body has been forced to rely upon what little of the requirements of healthy action the learned ones were unable to shut out and wage a winning fight against the original cause of the disease plus the physicians remedies. All the poisons known to all the kingdoms of nature have been poured down the throats of the sick or injected directly into their veins and tissues by learned ignorance in an effort to cure disease. People living under the most unhygienic conditions imaginable, have been subjected, when sick, to the most murderous forms of treatment conceivable, and a majority of them recovered.

During the reign of Claudius and Nero there lived a physician named Andromachus, who compounded a cure containing sixty-one ingredients. It was a whole apothecary shop in itself, and was called the Theriaca. Its most essential ingredient, from which it also derived its name, was the dried flesh of vipers. This wonderful cure was retained in the pharmacopeas until the beginning of the nineteenth century and was prescribed by all regular physicians—the learned or "scientific" ones—for almost every disease of the nosology. Indeed, the fad for taking out the teeth and tonsils for every known disease which rages today, in the ranks of the "regular" or "scientific" pyhsicians, is not a greater hobby than was the viperous compound of Andromachus among the earlier physicians of the "scientific" school. Because of his skill in mixing together the most incongruous articles in the most non-sensical manner, Andromachus was honored by the Roman Emperor, who bestowed upon him the title of Archiator, or Principal Physician.

Medical practices of all kinds are still as ludicrous as those of Andromachus and correct medical principles are still lacking. No system can be a science unless predicated upon correct principles. Napoleon is credited with the statement: "Get your principles right and the rest is a matter of detail." When the principles of a science rest upon a firm basis, there can be no sects or parties among those who cultivate it. Occasional error may have crept into mathematical science, but there exist no sects among mathematicians. In medicine, on the other hand, doctrines have been unstable and fluctuating in every age; there have been as many sects as schools; and, at this moment, there are almost as many opinions as practitioners. I mean this literally and I include both the drug and drugless schools and sects in this indictment. What I say in this chapter I want it understood in its strictest application and broadest liberality as applying to the drugless professions as well as to the druging professions.

In few subjects have there ever existed greater fallacies and delusions, than in the estimates that have been formed of the efficacy of the drugs, vaccines, apparatuses, machines and methods which form the established routine of medical art. It would be a matter of little difficulty to trace to the fountain-head the source of these erroneous opinions, but for the present I shall content myself with the irrefragable proof of the fact.

This proof may be readily drawn from the ever-varying fashions which predominate in the administration of remedies. Lord Bacon observed: "Medicine is a science more professed than labored, and yet more labored than advanced; the labor having been, in my judgment, rather in circles than in progressions; for I find much iteration, but small addition." This remark is as well founded today as when he made it, is equally as applicable to the drugless schools as to the druging schools. Two years never elapse without the discovery of some new mode of treatment or the invention of some new machine for the manufacture of health and eradication of some intractable complaint. Great cures are published, great expectations raised, the new methods and machines are universally tried; hope is followed by disappointment; and in the course of a few years, they are abandoned and forgotten. In the drugless field we have had zone therapy, spondylotherapy, orificial therapy, Neuropathy, Duncan's Auto-therapy, Dinsha's spectro-chrome therapy, chiropractic, naparpathy, Neuropathy, rythmotherapy (mechanical vibration), the electronic reactions of Abrams, the Autopath, the Biological Blood Washing bath, Hosmer's Rythmometer treatment, Hosmer's Hydrovibrometer, his cosmopathy, Anston's pneumophore and respirotherapy, Immanuel's Theo-therapy, Leavitt's volotherapy, White's Bio-Dynamic Chromatic diagnosis and treatment, etc. It would be easy to enlarge this catalogue but it is hardly necessary as every drugless practitioner knows them as well as I.

This ceaseless change of methods and machines, this constant and eager search for new remedies, forms a pretty sure index to the present status of both the drugging and drugless professions. It is an acknowledgement that something more is needed in the care of the sick; it betrays a restlessness and uneasiness, a consciousness that much of the established practice is either useless or impotent, if indeed much of it is not actually harmful. It reveals that their instruments are not what they wish them to be, that they are not what they are taught in their schools to expect them to be. We find in this constant grasping after new methods and new machines a secret wish— a very laudable and benevolent wish—that more successful methods should be found or that the old methods should be improved.

It is quite evident from the history of medicine that it has, at no time, been established upon fixed and acknowledged principles; such as, being founded on just experiments, or a copious induction of ascertained facts and demonstrated principles, command the assent of all correct reasoners. This is the reason that medical doctrines have ever been a subject of contention and disputation.

So many strange and incomprehensible things have been done in the medical professions. Even as late as the days of James the First, of England, a knowledge of judicial astronomy was considered essential to the physician. Strange as it may seem, astrology is taught today in some of the drugless schools. Along with this goes the teachings of iridiagnosis and basic diagnosis. If they could only add palmistry and fortune telling with cards, their "science" would be perfect. A time arrived in the history of Rome when the Augurs could not look each other in the face without laughing. Both the drugging and drugless practices are rapidly approaching that stage today.

Medical practice today is so full of absurdities, contradictions and falsehoods that to harmonize the contrarieties of its doctrines is a task as impossible as was the attempt of Medieval mathematicians to figure out how many angels could stand on the point of a needle. Consulting the records of medicine we cannot help being disgusted with the multitude of theories and methods that have been thrust upon us at different times. Nowhere is the imagination displayed to a greater extent, and perhaps so ample an exhibition of human inventiveness might be pleasing to our vanity, were it not more than counterbalanced by the humiliating spectacle of so much absurdity, contradiction and falsehood.

The very principles upon which most of the theories that this conglomeration of methods and machines rest were never established. They are, and always were, false, and consequently, the superstructures that have been erected upon them are the baseless fabric of visions, transient in their existence, passing away upon the introduction of new doctrines and hypotheses, like the dew before the rising sun. Method after method has arisen, flourished, fallen and been forgotten in rapid and melancholy succession, until the whole field is strewn with the disjointed materials and one may search among the chaos of rubbish for ages without finding one well established fact.

Many have often felt impelled to apologize for the instabilitiy of the theories and practices of the physicians. Their practice has been very rich in theory but poor, very poor in the practical application. Indeed, the tinsel-glitter of fine-spun theory, and of favorite hypothesis which prevail in their ranks, so dazzles, flatters, and charms human vanity and folly, that, so far from contributing to the certain and speedy cure of disease, it has continuously proved a bane and a disgrace to man. In despair of making their practice a science, they have agreed to convert it into a trade.

Why have all these things been so? What has been the root of their errors? Why has all their progress been confined to their inventions and theory spinning? Why have they been kept so busy seeking new cures, new methods, new machines?

The answer to these questions is not far to seek. Their fundamental error has been that, they have considered disease an organized enemy, a thing to be combatted and driven out. Their drugs and serums, machines, baths, beautifully colored lights, magical metaphysical formulas, witch broths, brewed from some obscure weeds that grow in Africa or high up in the Andes, have all been the shot and shell which they have hurled at our invisible foe in an effort to dislodge him.

They have been trying to cure disease—trying to cure the cure. Their methods have been of apparent value so long as, by advertising, the interest and enthusiasm in them could be kept at such a high pitch that patients would continue to patronize them in large numbers. When a method becomes commonplace and enthusiasm can no longer be maintained, a new method is acquired. The following story from the annals of medical history will illustrate this point:

In 1796 Dr. Elisha Perkins of Norwich, Conn., who was described as a splendid American and a devoted hard-working physician, became convinced that he had observed beneficial results in his patients, when the diseased parts were touched with certain metals. This led him to fuse several metals into a pair of short tapering rods, with blunt points. They contained a little gold. The curative effects of these rods were astounding. "Tractorization," as the new practice was called, became the fad of the day. "Pains in the head, face, teeth, breast, side, stomach, back, rheumatism, and all joint and muscular pains," yielded to the tender mercies of the tractor according to Dr. Perkin's announcement. "The bent straightened up and walked erect. All maladies yielded to twenty minutes' downward stroking with the magic tractor."

This wonderful instrument was patented both in America and England. Clergymen were supplied with them free. Other professional men were supplied with them for five pounds, while less fortunate individuals had to pay ten pounds. Dr. Perkins became both famous and rich. He had proven himself a great benefactor to his fellow man. In London a magnificent hospital was erected and called the Perkins Institute. Lord Rivers was made president and Sir Wm. Barker became vice-president. Perkins' own son was in charge, and after three years, he published the details of 5,000 cases treated at the Institute. It was estimated that fully 1,500,000 persons had been cured by this marvelous tractor. England socialized the method, for it was considered wrong that so great a benefit to mankind should be confined to the well-to-do. In Denmark, where the rods were carried by Major Oxholm, who had been in this country on diplomatic service, the tractor became the rage. Rich women carried them to the homes of the poor and treated these. They could not be manufactured rapidly enough to supply the demand. Distinguished members of parliament and supreme court testified that they had been cured by the tractors. German and English physicians employed them. They proved equally as efficacious in Germany as in America, England and Denmark. In England, Dr. Walsh tells us: "There were no less than eight professors in four different universities, tweny-one regular physicians, and nineteen surgeons, and thirty clergymen, twelve of whom were Doctors of Divinity, among those bearing testimony to the efficacy of the new cure."

Finally some English doctors who held that the cures were the result of imagination, proceeded to test their theory. They made some "tractors" of wood and painted them to resemble the invention of Dr. Perkins. They obtained the same results with their little wooden sticks that had been obtained by Perkins' metal rods. When these results were published, the bottom fell out of the tractor market. No longer could interest and enthusiasm be kept up for it. But were the cures really due to imagination? Can man really be humbugged out of his diseases? The heads of the Perkins' Institute declared that they had performed multitudes of cures on infants, and even on animals. Horses were often "cured" by them. Dogs, too, recovered health while being treated in this manner. Surely there was no imagination in such cases. The infants and animals did not know that they were being treated or that they were supposed to get well by the aid of such things.

In our own day we have witnessed a similar rise of an influence-less method of treatment, which attained a world-wide popularity and produced (?) many remarkable "cures," and then waned. I refer to the Abrams' hoax. Many men of science and many medical men fell for its claims. This story can be paralleled by the history of hundreds of medical methods in all ages. The majority of patients get well, no matter how treated, and this enables physicians to report a wonderful success for any method of treatment. This enables them to loudly proclaim that experience has demonstrated the value of their methods. *As a matter of historical fact, experience has proven all methods to be good until they were later discovered to be bad.*

A few years ago, a critic of *therapeutic nihilism,* writing in *The Naturopath,* attempted to prove the curative value of certain drugless methods by an appeal to certain experiments. Briefly, some of these were:

1. Ink was injected into the joints of a rabbit's legs. One joint was massaged, the other was not. The rabbit was killed and the joins examined. The massaged joint was almost wholly free of ink. The unmassaged joint was full of ink. This proved the value of massage in breaking up and thus bringing about the elimination of toxic deposits.

2. Distilled water was injected into the abdominal cavities of two rabbits. The abdomen of one was massaged, that of the other not. The rabbits were killed and their abdomens examined. The abdomen of the massaged rabbit was practically free of water. That of the other rabbit was full of water. This proved the value of massage in dropsical and edematous conditions.

I shall take up these two *demonstrations* first. We do no doubt that the ink and OTHER MATTER was forced out of the joints, but we would like to know what were the results of forcing out the matter that normally belongs in the joints. Or, does massage have a selective action, and only force out what the operator wants forced out?

Suppose instead of a small quantity of ink injected into a normal, healthty, vigorous rabbit, we use one of those much talked of "deposits of morbid matter" found in the enervated, sick, weak human being—a patient. What are the differences? In the rabbit we have:

1. Good health.
2. Normal elimination.
3. Plenty of reserve force.
4. No bad habits to lower his supply of nervous energy and destroy his tissues.
5. The "foreign matter" (ink) injected in small amount once, into an otherwise pure blood-stream.

While in the man we have:

1. Enfeebled health.
2. Impaired elimination.
3. Little or no reserve nerve force.
4. Plenty of bad habits lowering his supply of nervous energy and destroying his tissues.
5. The "foreign matter" (deposit) habitually formed in or introduced into a blood-stream already saturated with toxins to such an extent that it is forced to deposit some of these in the tissues.

Obviously we are dealing with an entirely different set of conditions, resulting from an entirely different set of causes and calling for an entirely different method of correction. In the case of the rabbit and the ink; when the ink, by means of massage, is forced out of the tissues faster than the body normally carries it out, it goes into an otherwise pure blood-stream and is carried to eliminating organs which are more than equal to the task of eliminating it. The rabbit, being of good habits and having plenty of reserve force, if not killed, soon recuperates from the OTHER EFFECTS of the massage, and, as no more ink is injected and no more massage given, is not perceptibly injured.

In the case of the patient; when the deposit, by means of massage is forced out into the tissues, it is thrown into an already toxin laden blood-stream and is carried to eliminating organs which are already overburdened and are not equal to the task of eliminating it. The broken-up "deposit" is redeposited in the same or another place. If in another place the patient has *another* disease, mistakenly called a crisis. The patient being of bad habits and having little or no reserve force, does not readily recuperate from the OTHER EFFECTS of the massage, and, as more toxins are constantly accumulating in the blood and tissues and the massage is repeatedly given, the patient is perceptibly, perhaps permanenltly, injured. At the same time, the massage does nothing to correct the cause of the deposit, does not remedy its sources and does not increase the powers of elimination.

Deposits do not cause themselves. They are not self-evolving. A deposit is only one small part of a general systemic condition which has resulted from a syndrome of causes and effects extending backward over considerable time. This condition must continue to exist so long as these causes continue to operate. The body's own self-curing, self-renovating powers will accomplish a true cure in the shortest possible time when these causes are corrected. There is no true cure outside of correction of cause. Palliative methods are legion.

The same differences, only greater in degree, as listed above between the patient with the deposit and the rabbit with the ink injection, also exist between the dropsical patient and the rabbit with the distilled water in the abdomen. (While dropsy is usually worse than the deposits, the distilled water may not be as harmful as the ink). The same objections to forcing the dropsical fluid back into the circulation hold, that were offered against forcing the deposits into the circulation.

What does massage do to correct the condition that gives rise to the dropsy? If the dropsy is due to heart or kidney affections or to cirrhosis of the liver, what effect does forcing the lymph back into the circulation have on these organs? What does it do toward correcting the causes of the affections of these organs?

That the dropsical fluid can be forced back into the general circulation by massage, I freely admit. I have, myself, done this very thing in several cases. But, and here is the rub, it always forms again. It is just like what Dr. Richard C. Cabot says about surgical removal of the dropsical fluid: "WE PUT IN A HOLLOW NEEDLE, DRAW OFF THE FLUID, AND RELIEVE THE INDIVIDUAL, * * * THEN THE FLUID REACCUMULATES, AND SO ON. * * * UNTIL HE DIES."

It is not deemed necessary to carry this criticism of *therapeutics* further. It could easily be expanded into a book. But enough has been said to indicate to the student that all methods of therapeutics are evil and useless.

The truth should be self-evident that any method or system that destroys the independence and autonomy of the individual and makes him forever dependent upon another man or class of men is not natural. Any system that of itself creates a priveleged class who can, by law, or otherwise, lord it over their fellow men, destroys true freedom and personal autonomy. Any system that teaches the sick that they can get well only through the exercise of the skill of someone else, or through the operation of something else, and that they remain alive only through the tender mercies of the privileged class, has no place in Nature's scheme of things, and the sooner it is abolished, the better will mankind be. It was no more a part of the original scheme of things that man should be a supplicate at the feet of the healers than that lions or cod-fish should be. It cannot be that mankind will forever be dependent upon the tender mercies of the doctor and his bag of tricks. It matters not whether man is dependent on the doctor for his drugs, on the chiropractor to adjust his spinal column, the psycho-analyst for mental catharysis, or the miracle monger as a medium through which to receive the divine emanations, he is a slave to that class upon which he depends. Therapeutics makes slaves of men. This is an evil and cannot endure.

Printed in the United States
33679LVS00008B/20